Medical and Orthopedic Issues of Active and Athletic Women

Edited by

Rosemary Agostini, MD

WITH THE ASSISTANCE OF SID TITUS, MD

Sports Medicine and Family Practice
Virginia Mason Sports Medicine Center
Clinical Assistant Professor of Orthopedics
University of Washington School of Medicine
Team Physician, Cleveland High School
Seattle, Washington

HANLEY & BELFUS, INC./ Philadelphia
MOSBY/ St. Louis • Baltimore • Boston • Chicago • London
   Philadelphia •Sydney • Toronto

Publisher: HANLEY & BELFUS
             210 S. 13th Street
             Philadelphia, PA 19107
             (215) 546-7293
             FAX (215) 790-9330

North American and worldwide sales and distribution:

             MOSBY
             11830 Westline Industrial Drive
             St. Louis, MO 63146

In Canada: Times Mirror Professional Publishing, Ltd.
             130 Flaska Drive
             Markham, Ontario L6G 1B8
             Canada

V

A portion of the proceeds from this book will be donated to the American College of Sports Medicine
Task Force on Women's Issues in Sports Medicine.

Medical and Orthopedic Issues of Active and Athletic Women   ISBN 1-56053-019-7

Library of Congress Catalog Card Number 94-75825

Last digit is the print number: 9   8   7   6   5   4   3   2   1

DEDICATION

To my parents, Irene and William

CONTENTS

PART III: MEDICAL AND ORTHOPEDIC CONDITIONS

CONTRIBUTORS

SARA JOYCE AGASSIZ, BS, PT
Physical Therapist, Virginia Mason Sports Medicine Center, Seattle, Washington

ROSEMARY AGOSTINI, MD
Sports Medicine and Family Practice, Virginia Mason Sports Medicine Center, Seattle; Clinical Assistant Professor, Department of Orthopedics, University of Washington School of Medicine, Seattle; Team Physician, Cleveland High School, Seattle, Washington

ELIZABETH A. ARENDT, MD
Assistant Professor of Orthopaedic Surgery, University of Minnesota Medical School, Minneapolis, Minnesota

KELLI R. ARNTZEN, MD
Teaching Faculty, Virginia Mason Medical Center, Seattle; Clinical Instructor in Medicine (Dermatology), University of Washington School of Medicine, Seattle, Washington

NANCY P. BARNETT, MS
Department of Psychology, University of Washington, Seattle, Washington

GARY BEERMAN, ARNP/PA-C
Family Nurse Practitioner, Virginia Mason Medical Center, Seattle; Clinical Instructor, MEDEX Northwest Physician Assistant Program and Department of Nursing, Family Nurse Practitioner Program, University of Washington, Seattle, Washington

JENNIFER D. BOLEN, MD
Clinical Professor of Psychiatry, Section of Psychiatry and Psychology, Virginia Mason Medical Center, Seattle; Department of Psychiatry and Behavioral Sciences, University of Washington School of Medicine, Seattle, Washington

CHERYL D.P. CLAYPOOLE, PT
Sports Physical Therapist, Virginia Mason Sports Medicine Center, Seattle, Washington

JULIE WENTWORTH COLLITON, MD
Resident, Department of Physical Medicine and Rehabilitation, Tufts New England Medical Center, Boston, Massachusetts

M. ELAINE CRESS, PhD
Research Assistant Professor, Department of Medicine/Geriatrics, University of Washington School of Medicine, Seattle, Washington

CRAIG J. DAVIDSON, MD
Sports Medicine Fellow, Ball Memorial Hospital Sports Medicine Fellowship, Muncie, Indiana

LINDA A. DIMEFF, MS
Research Assistant, The Addictive Behaviors Research Center, Department of Psychology, University of Washington School of Medicine, Seattle, Washington

PAMELA S. DOUGLAS, MD
Associate Professor of Medicine, Harvard Medical School, Boston; Director, Noninvasive Cardiology, Beth Israel Hospital, Boston, Massachusetts

BARBARA DRINKWATER, PhD
Research Physiologist, Department of Medicine, Pacific Medical Center, Seattle, Washington

CATHERINE M. FIESELER, MD
Private Practice, Alexandria, Virginia

MAUREEN A. FINNEGAN, MD
Associate Professor, Department of Orthopedic Surgery, University of Texas Southwestern Medical School, Dallas, Texas

PAMELA J. FOYSTER, RN
University of Utah Medical Center, Salt Lake City, Utah

ELIZABETH M. GALLUP, MD, JD
Senior Vice President of Medical Affairs and Medical Director, Shawnee Mission Medical Center, Shawnee Mission, Kansas; Associate Clinical Professor, University of Missouri–Kansas City School of Medicine, Kansas City, Missouri

JAMES G. GARRICK, MD
Director, Center for Sports Medicine, Saint Francis Memorial Hospital, San Francisco, California

PATRICIA HELLMAN GIBBS, MD
Medical Supervisor, San Francisco Ballet; Preceptor and Guest Lecturer, University of California at San Francisco School of Medicine, San Francisco, California

MARILYN A. GUTHRIE, RD
Manager, Health Promotion/Patient Education, Virginia Mason Medical Center, Seattle, Washington

JO A. HANNAFIN, MD, PhD
Assistant Attending Orthopaedic Surgeon, Instructor in Surgery, and Associate Director of Laboratory for Soft Tissue Research, The Hospital for Special Surgery, New York Hospital–Cornell University Medical Center, New York, New York

SALLY S. HARRIS, MD, MPH
Department of Sports Medicine, Palo Alto Medical Clinic, Palo Alto, California; Volunteer Clinical Faculty, Department of Pediatrics, Stanford University School of Medicine, Stanford; Team Physician, Stanford University, Stanford, California

DENISE J. HARTY, ATC
Certified Athletic Trainer, Central Indiana Sports Medicine, Muncie, Indiana

PATRICIA A. HEBERT, MD
Physiatrist, Department of Rehabilitation Medicine, Shaughnessy-Kaplan Rehabilitation Hospital, and Department of Orthopaedics, Salem Hospital, Salem, Massachusetts

SUSAN R. HOPKINS, MD, PhD
Clinical Assistant Professor, Division of Sports Medicine, Allan McGavin Sports Medicine Center, University of British Columbia Faculty of Medicine, Vancouver, British Columbia, Canada

REBECCA JAFFE, MD, FAAFP, FACSM
Associate Professor, Department of Family Medicine, Jefferson Medical College, Philadelphia, Pennsylvania; Medical Director, Pike Creek Sports Medicine Center, Wilmington, Delaware

CATHERINE M. JANKOWSKI, MS
Assistant to the Director, Center for Research on Women's Health, Texas Woman's University, Denton, Texas

MIMI D. JOHNSON, MD
Clinical Assistant Professor, Department of Pediatrics, Division of Adolescent Medicine, University of Washington School of Medicine; Assistant Team Physician, University of Washington, Seattle, Washington

ELAINE C. JONG, MD
Clinical Professor of Medicine, Department of Medicine, and Director, David C. Hall Student Health Center, University of Washington School of Medicine, Seattle, Washington

ELIZABETH A. JOY, MD
Consulting Physician, Department of Family Practice, Hennepin County Medical Center, Minneapolis, Minnesota

KATHERINE A.F. KENAL, MD, MA
Sports Medicine Fellow, Department of Primary Care Sports Medicine, Hennepin County Medical Center, Minneapolis, Minnesota

LISA S. KRIVICKAS, MD
Clinical Instructor and Academic Chief Resident, Department of Physical Medicine and Rehabilitation, University of Medicine and Dentistry of New Jersey/New Jersey Medical School, Newark, New Jersey

PATTY KULPA, MD, FACOG, FACSM
Obstetrician and Sports Gynecologist, Pacific Sports Medicine Clinic, Tacoma, Washington

CONSTANCE MARIE LEBRUN, BSc, MDCM, MPE, FACSM
Clinical Assistant Professor, Department of Family Practice, Division of Sports Medicine, Allan McGavin Sports Medicine Center, University of British Columbia Faculty of Medicine, Vancouver, British Columbia, Canada

MARIE E. LEE, MD
Radiologist, Virginia Mason Hospital, Seattle; Clinical Assistant Professor, University of Washington School of Medicine, Seattle, Washington

DAWN P. LEMCKE, MD
Section Head, Center for Women's Health, Virginia Mason Clinic, Seattle, Washington

DONNA A. LOPIANO, BS, MA, PhD
Executive Director, Women's Sports Foundation, East Meadow, New York

JUDY MAHLE LUTTER, MA
President, Melpomene Institute for Women's Health Research, St. Paul, Minnesota

CAROL MACERA, PhD
Professor, Department of Epidemiology and Biostatistics, University of South Carolina School of Medicine, Columbia, South Carolina

BERT R. MANDELBAUM, MD
Orthopaedic Surgeon in Private Practice, Santa Monica Orthopedic and Sports Medicine Group, Santa Monica, California; Head Team Physician, Pepperdine University, Malibu, California; Team Physician, United States Soccer World Cup Team

G. ALAN MARLATT, PhD
Professor of Psychology, University of Washington, Seattle, Washington

LORNA A. MARSHALL, MD
Clinical Instructor, Department of Obstetrics & Gynecology, University of Washington School of Medicine, Seattle; Head, Reproductive Endocrinology, Virginia Mason Medical Center, Seattle, Washington

PHILIP MEASE, MD
Clinical Associate Professor, Department of Medicine, Division of Rheumatology, Minor & James Medical Clinic and University of Washington School of Medicine, Seattle, Washington

DAVID J. MUSNICK, MD, MPH
Staff Physician, Sports Medicine, Internal Medicine, The Sports Medicine Clinic, University of Washington Hall Health Center, Seattle, Washington

AURELIA NATTIV, MD
Assistant Clinical Professor, UCLA Division of Family Medicine, Los Angeles; Private Practitioner, Santa Monica Family Physicians, Santa Monica, California

CAROL L. OTIS, MD
Director, Specialty Clinics, UCLA Student Health Service; Assistant Team Physician, UCLA, Los Angeles, California; Chair, Task Force on Women's Issues, American College of Sports Medicine

JULIE PATTISON, MD
Center for Women's Health, Virginia Mason Medical Clinic, Seattle, Washington

MARGOT PUTUKIAN, MD
Team Physician, Pennsylvania State University, State College; Assistant Professor, Department of Orthopedics and Internal Medicine, Hershey Medical Center, Hershey, Pennsylvania

NORMAN ROSENTHAL, MD
Staff Physician, Virginia Mason Medical Center, Seattle; Clinical Assistant Professor of Medicine, University of Washington School of Medicine, Seattle, Washington

CHARLOTTE FEICHT SANBORN, PhD
Associate Professor, Department of Kinesiology, and Director, Center for Research on Women's Health, Texas Woman's University, Denton, Texas

MARIE D. SCHAFLE, MD, FACEP
Director, Sports and Performing Arts Clinic, Student Health Service, San Francisco State University, San Francisco, California

ROBERT B. SCHOENE, MD
Associate Professor of Medicine, Division of Pulmonary and Critical Care Medicine, University of Washington School of Medicine, Seattle, Washington

ANGELA D. SMITH, MD
Assistant Professor of Orthopaedics, Case Western Reserve University School of Medicine, Cleveland, Ohio

CHRISTINE SNOW-HARTER, PhD
Assistant Professor, Department of Exercise and Sport Science, Oregon State University, Corvallis, Oregon

BARRI KATZ STRYER, MD
Postdoctoral Fellow, Department of Child Psychiatry, University of California Los Angeles, Neuropsychiatric Institute, Los Angeles, California

ROBYN M. STUHR, MA
Exercise Physiologist, Virginia Mason Sports Medicine Clinic, Seattle, Washington; American College of Sports Medicine Health/Fitness Director and Exercise Text Technologist

KATRINA SULLIVAN, DPM, ATC, MS
Auxiliary Faculty, Department of Medicine, University of Washington School of Medicine, Seattle, Washington

SUZANNE M. TANNER, MD
Assistant Professor, Departments of Orthopedics and Pediatrics, University of Colorado School of Medicine, Denver, Colorado

LYNNE P. TAYLOR, MD
Clinical Assistant Professor of Medicine, University of Washington School of Medicine, Seattle; Neurologist/Neuro-oncologist, Virginia Mason Medical Center, Seattle, Washington

SIDNEY TITUS, MD
Virginia Mason Clinic, Seattle, Washington

KATHE WALLACE, PT
Private Practitioner, Seattle, Washington

PRISCILLA W. WRIGHT, PhD
Clinical Assistant Professor, Department of Psychiatry and Behavioral Sciences, University of Washington School of Medicine; Staff Psychologist, Veterans Administration Medical Center, Seattle, Washington

KIMBERLY K. YEAGER, MD, MPH
Assistant Director Public Health Practice, Graduate School of Public Health, San Diego State University, San Diego, California

PREFACE

My immigrant parents gave their children two gifts—the ability to dream and to work incredibly hard. As children when we fell while skiing, my father would not pick us up; he would sit down in the snow next to us and show us how to get up by ourselves.

At a national sports medicine conference in 1990, I was speaking with two friends, Chris McGrew, MD, and Wade Lilligard, MD, about the lack of women speakers and topics related to exercise and sports in women at all the sports medicine conferences. Their response: "Rosemary, you do it."

The first conference entitled **Medical and Orthopedic Issues of Active and Athletic Women** was held at the Virginia Mason Medical Center in Seattle, Washington in the spring of 1991. My three goals were:

1. To organize a conference on sports- and exercise-related issues for girls and women.
2. To facilitate and create opportunities for women physicians, health care providers, and scientists to speak. This would allow women to develop skills and experience so that more women presenters would be given such opportunities.
3. To create a syllabus that would become a book. The publishing of *Medical and Orthopedic Issues of Active and Athletic Women* fulfills this dream.

This book would not exist without the step-by-step guidance, kindness, encouragement, and tenacity of the editor, Michael Bokulich.

Sid Titus, MD, helped and guided, was continually encouraging, and provided the essential anchor when I would get overwhelmed.

I need to thank John Lombardo, MD, for giving me the opportunity to be the first primary care sports medicine fellow at the Cleveland Clinic, and John Bergfeld, MD, and Barbara Drinkwater, PhD, for being my most important mentors.

A "thank you" to Moe Mellion, MD, who gave me my first opportunity to write and guided me through 12 rewrites of my first chapter.

To all the women of the American College of Sports Medicine Ad Hoc Task Force on Women's Issues in Sports Medicine, especially Carol Otis, MD, Kim Yeager, MD, Mimi Johnson, MD, Connie Lebrun, MD, Aurelia Nattiv, MD, Suzanne Tanner, MD, Becky Jaffe, MD, and the ACSM Staff, for the support, love, and hard work, THANK YOU!

Thank you to the contributing authors who wrote the chapters found in this book.

And, finally, *thank you* to my parents, who taught me to dream, work hard, and know how to pick myself up when I fall down.

Rosemary Agostini, M.D.

My aim is not to be consistent with my previous statements on a given question, but to be consistent with the truth as it may present itself to me at a given moment.
The result is that I have grown from truth to truth.

—Gandhi

PART I
INTRODUCTION

Chapter 1: History of Women in Sports

REBECCA JAFFE, MD

Plato was wise enough to suggest that men and women be physically active together. However, it took hundreds of years before there was any acceptance and documentation of women in sports. This historical progression has not always been in a positive, forward direction. It was only in the late 1800s, coinciding with higher education for women and the advent of the bicycle, that female participation in sports was somewhat accepted. However, the medical profession stymied the regular participation with misconceptions about females' ability to withstand physical stress. Not until the 1960s and 1970s did women begin to fight for their own right to participate. In 1972, the U.S. Title IX legislation helped to lend support for women's participation in sport.

I. THE ANCIENT WORLD

A. **Ancient Egypt and Sparta**—before 1500 BC
   1. Tomb of Beni-Hassan. Frescos and statues illustrate women engaging in sports activities.
   2. Women participate in gymnastics, calisthenics, swimming, and competitive games according to writings and art works.
   3. Society allows women to participate in sports in the belief that it improves reproductive capabilities.

B. **Golden Age of Greece**
   1. 776 BC—Women are not allowed to participate in or watch any Olympic events. The punishment for any woman found in Olympia during the games is to be hurled off a cliff. The only exception is the priestess of Demeter, who presides over sacred rituals.
   2. 392 BC—Kyniska, the daughter of the King of Sparta, becomes the first female Olympic champion. As the owner of the horses that won the four-horse chariot race, she received the olive wreath, not the driver.
   3. The sisters Tryphosa, Hedia, and Dionysia are victorious in the Pythian and Isthmian games (ancient athletic festivals). They compete in and win one-lap races and chariot races in armor. (Evidence of their participation was uncovered in 1894, but not pieced together until 1909.)
   4. Womanly qualities of the time are beauty and the feminine arête: "chastity, modesty, obedience, and inconspicuous behavior."

II. HISTORICAL ROAD BLOCKS

A. **Moral issue:** The main argument against women's participation. It deals with coeducation, freedom of action, revealing attire, frequent absences from home, and loosening of parental control.
B. **Social approval:** Society's acceptance varies era to era, culture to culture, and location to location.
C. **Biological unknown:** The female should not impair her ability to have children. Much was written about this at the turn of the century; e.g., British medical literature stressed how exercise would compromise fertility.

1

D. **Religious view:** Religion often had a restricting influence. An example which continues through the 20th century is Islam, which regards women's clothing for sports participation as against their traditional religious beliefs.

E. **Historical influence:** The most notorious use of this rationalization in the last two centuries is by Baron Pierre de Coubertin in 1920, who excluded women from the modern Olympic games based on their lack of participation in the ancient games and his belief that they were not athletes. Male chauvinism is also evident in the lack of funding for women's sports and limited chances for international competition.

III. MODERN OLYMPICS

A. **History of women's participation:** (Table 1)

   1. 1896—First modern games held in Athens. The only woman participant is an unofficial runner of the marathon, Melpomene. She spent 3 weeks training in secret and ran the 40 km from Marathon to Athens in 4.5 hours, about 1.5 hours slower than the winner but ahead of other male contestants.

   2. 1900—Summer games in Paris (11 women)
      a. Women participate in golf and lawn tennis.
      b. Margaret Abbott becomes the first U.S. female gold medalist, in golf.

   3. 1904—St. Louis (6 women). Archery is the sole female sport; it is later dropped after the 1908 games.

   4. 1908—London (36 women)
      a. Archery, tennis, figure skating, and a gymnastics exhibition
      b. *The New York Times* reports that the U.S. Olympic Committee is "opposed to women taking part in any event in which they could not wear skirts."

   5. 1912—Summer games in Stockholm (>100 women from 10 countries). Competition includes swimming and diving but the U.S. does not send a team.

   6. 1916—Games are suspended due to World War I.

   7. 1920—Antwerp (64 women). Figure skating, tennis, swimming, and diving

   8. 1924—Games are separated into winter and summer sports.

   9. 1928—Amsterdam
      a. Five track and field events are added to the roster.
      b. At the end of the 800-m women's race, several runners collapse from heat exhaustion (not unlike what happened after the men's race in 1896). The press reports this situation poorly, and the International Olympic Committee (IOC) votes that women cannot compete in races longer than 200 m, leading to a 32-year ban on these races for women in the Olympics.

   10. 1932—Los Angeles. Mildred "Babe" Didrickson wins gold medals in javelin and 80-m hurdles, but wins silver in the high jump because of her "illegal" head-first dive.

   11. 1936—Berlin (Nazi Olympics). Women participate in only four sports: athletics, swimming, fencing, and gymnastics.

   12. 1940 and 1944—Games are suspended due to World War II.

   13. 1948—London (385 women)
      a. Women compete in 5 sports, compared to 18 for men, making up 12.7% of the total events.
      b. Fanny Blankers-Koen of Holland wins three gold medals as a 30-year-old mother of two children. (She was allowed to compete in only three events, although she held records in two others.)

   14. 1952—Helsinki (518 women from 41 countries)
      a. Women's individual gymnastics and equestrian events are added.
      b. Russian women dominate.

   15. 1956—Melbourne. Dawn Fraser wins the first of her three consecutive medals in swimming.

   16. 1960—Rome. Wilma Rudolf, who overcame partial paralysis of her left leg in youth, is dubbed the "black gazelle."

TABLE 1. History of Women's Participation in the Olympic Games, with Date and Place of First Olympic Competition

Summer games

Archery
Several events were held in 1904 and 1908, then discontinued. Individual. 1972, Munich Team. 1988, Seoul

Basketball
1976, Montreal

Canoeing
Kayak singles, 500 m.
1948, London
Kayak pairs, 500 m.
1960, Rome
Kayak fours, 500 m.
1984, Los Angeles

Cycling
1,000-m sprint. 1988, Seoul
Road race. 1984, Los Angeles

Equestrian
Events are not categorized by men's and women's competition.

Fencing
Foil, individual. 1924, Paris
Foil, team. 1960, Rome

Field hockey
1980, Moscow

Gymnastics
All-around. 1952, Helsinki
Side horse vault.
1952, Helsinki
Uneven bars. 1952, Helsinki
Balance beam.
1952, Helsinki
Team combined exercises.
1928, Amsterdam
Rhythmic all-around.
1984, Los Angeles

Team handball
1976, Montreal

Rowing
Single sculls. 1976, Montreal
Double skulls. 1976, Montreal

Rowing (cont.)
Quadruple sculls with coxswain. 1976, Montreal
Pair-oared shell with coxswain. 1976, Montreal
Four-oared shell with coxswain. 1976, Montreal
Eight-oared shell with coxswain. 1976, Montreal

Shooting
Sport pistol. 1984, Los Angeles
Air pistol. 1988, Seoul
Small-bore rifle, three positions. 1984, Los Angeles
Air rifle. 1984, Los Angeles
Mixed, trap shooting. 1900, Paris
Mixed, skeet shooting. 1968, Mexico City

Swimming
50-m freestyle. 1988, Seoul
100-m freestyle. 1912, Stockholm
200-m freestyle. 1968, Mexico City
400-m freestyle. 1920, Antwerp
800-m freestyle. 1968, Mexico City
100-m backstroke. 1924, Paris
200-m backstroke.
1968, Mexico City
100-m breaststroke.
1968, Mexico City
200-m breaststroke. 1924, Paris
100-m butterfly. 1956, Melbourne
200-m butterfly. 1968, Mexico City
200-m individual medley.
1968, Mexico City
400-m individual medley.
1964, Tokyo
4 × 100-m freestyle relay.
1912, Stockholm
4 × 100-m medley relay.
1960, Rome
Synchronized swimming, solo.
1984, Los Angeles
Synchronized swimming, duet.
1984, Los Angeles

Swimming (cont.)
Springboard diving.
1920, Antwerp
Platform diving.
1912, Stockholm

Table Tennis
Singles. 1968, Seoul
Doubles. 1988, Seoul

Tennis
Singles. 1900, Paris
Doubles. 1920, Antwerp

Track & Field
100 m. 1928, Amsterdam
200 m. 1948, London
400 m. 1964, Tokyo
800 m. 1928, Amsterdam
1500 m. 1972, Munich
3000 m. 1984, Los Angeles
10,000 m. 1988, Seoul
Marathon.
1984, Los Angeles
100-m hurdles.
1932, Los Angeles
400-m hurdles.
1984, Los Angeles
4 × 100-m relay.
1928, Amsterdam
4 × 400-m relay.
1972, Munich
High jump.
1928, Amsterdam
Long jump. 1948, London
Shot put. 1948, London
Discus throw.
1928, Amsterdam
Javelin throw.
1932, Los Angeles
Heptathlon/pentathlon.
1964, Tokyo

Volleyball
1964, Tokyo

Yachting
470. 1988, Seoul

Winter games

Luge
Single. 1984, Innsbruck

Figure Skating
Single. 1908, London
Pairs. 1908, London
Ice dance. 1976, Innsbruck

Speed Skating
500 m. 1960, Squaw Valley
1000 m. 1960, Squaw Valley

Speed Skating (cont.)
1500 m. 1960, Squaw Valley
3000 m. 1960, Squaw Valley
5000 m. 1988, Calgary

Alpine Skiing
Downhill. 1948, St. Moritz
Slalom. 1948, St. Moritz
Giant slalom. 1952, Oslo
Super giant slalom. 1988, Calgary

Alpine Skiing (cont.)
Alpine combined. 1936, Garmisch-Partenkirchen

Nordic Skiing
5 km. 1964, Innsbruck
10 km. 1952, Oslo
20 km. 1984, Sarajevo
4 × 5-km relay.
1966, Cortina

Compiled from Wallechinsky D: The Complete Book of the Olympics. New York, Penguin Books, 1988.

17. 1964—Tokyo
   a. Volleyball is added.
   b. U.S. women dominate in swimming.
   c. Ewa Klobukowska participates as a runner for Poland, but 3 years later she is the first woman to fail a sex-verification test.
18. 1968—Mexico City
   a. First woman to carry the U.S. flag in opening ceremonies
   b. Gender testing begins: "Competitors in sports restricted to women must comply with the prescribed tests for femininity"—buccal smear for Barr body. (This test is not 100% sensitive but is the only current test accepted, although the IOC is working on alternative methods to assess female status.)
19. 1972—Munich (1299 women, 15% of participants)
   a. Archery is added.
   b. Olga Korbut gains notoriety for female athletes through the media's coverage of her story and success.
20. 1976—Summer games in Montreal (1261 women, 20.6% of participants)
   a. Women compete in 13 sports with rowing, basketball, and team handball added.
   b. Nadia Comeneci of Romania earns the first "10" in gymnastics.
   c. Only 65% of nations send female competitors.
21. 1980—Moscow. Field hockey is added as the 14th women's sport, but the games are boycotted by the U.S., West Germany, and Japan.
22. 1984—Los Angeles
   a. The 3000-m and marathon are added in track for women. The last place finishers of both the men's and women's marathon have identical times of 2 hr, 52 min.
   b. Women's cycling, synchronized swimming, and rhythmic gymnastics are added.
23. 1988—Summer games in Seoul (2476 women). Added are 1000-m cycling sprints, 10,000-m track race, heptathlon, team archery, air pistol, 50-m freestyle swimming, singles and doubles table tennis, and a separate yachting event (470 class).
24. 1992—Barcelona (28.9% of participants are female); badminton and judo are added.

B. **Women's Olympics**
   1. Created out of the IOC's rejection of women's athletics at the 1920 games
   2. Federation Sportive Feminine Internationale (FSFI) created by Alice Milliat in 1921
   3. Four sets of games took place every 4 years from 1922 to 1934.
   4. The last year, in London, 19 countries sent teams.

IV. **WOMEN'S SPORTS IN THE UNITED STATES**

A. **19th century**
   1. Feminine characteristics are considered to be piety, purity, domesticity, and submissiveness
   2. Dress for women includes long, heavy skirts and pinched waists, which promote the inactive lifestyle.

B. **20th century**
   1. Early 1900s: "Sport for every girl and every girl in sport"
   2. 1971—The Association of Intercollegiate Athletics is created with 280 members; by 1979 there are 850 member institutions with 27 championships in 14 sports.
   3. 1972—Title IX legislation is passed, prohibiting discrimination on the basis of sex in educational institutions that receive federal funding. (This legislation forced some equality in sports for women athletes, but also had drawbacks. In coaching, for instance, with better pay more men have become coaches of female sports, creating an actual decline in the number of women coaching women's

sports. In 1972, 90% of all women's teams were coached by women, but in 1988 only 49% were. In 1972, 90% of women's programs were headed by female administrators, compared to only 16% in 1988.)

4. 1973—Golfer Terry Williams is the first woman to receive a full-tuition athletic scholarship (from the University of Miami).
5. 1974—The Women's Sports Foundation is established by Billie Jean King, Donna DeVarona, and other athletes.
6. 1977
   a. Release of the *Final Report of the President's Commission on Olympic Sports 1975-1977*, which recommends the establishment of programs to facilitate performance and eliminate discrimination.
   b. Janet Guthrie is the first woman to compete in the Indianapolis 500.
7. 1982
   a. Cheryl Miller scores 105 points in a single high school basketball game.
   b. Melpomene Institute for Women's Health Research is founded.
8. 1983—First all-woman's triathlon is held in California, with 950 participants.
9. 1984
   a. In a 24-hour run/jog race in Michigan, both the first and second place finishers are women.
   b. Victoria Roche, age 12 from Belgium, is the first female to play in the Little League World Series (she pinch hits in the 5th inning).
10. 1985
    a. Lynett Woodward is the first woman to play basketball for the Harlem Globetrotters.
    b. Libby Riddles is the first woman to win the 1100-mile Iditarod dogsled race in Alaska.
11. 1986
    a. Brooks is the first shoe company to open a women's division.
    b. A girl is given the right to play high school football.

V. MEDIA

Media attention is important to the continuing success of women's participation in sports. A study in 1988 found that less than 10% of women's sports events were covered by the written or televised media.

VI. SUMMARY

Women's participation in sports has come a long way in the last century, but there is much more to be done. Worldwide, there are not many women who have access, encouragement, or support for their participation in sports. With better understanding of the benefits of physical activity and participation for women, the barriers will hopefully come down and there will be an international cooperation to promote all people who wish to compete in the athletic arena.

RECOMMENDED READING

1. Guttnam A: Women's Sports: A History. New York, Columbia University Press, 1991.
2. Borms J, Hebbelinck M, Venerando A (eds): Women and Sport. Basel, Karger, 1981.
3. Borries E: The History and Functions of the National Section of Women's Athletics. Washington, DC, National Section of Women's Athletics and the American Association for Health, Physical Education, and Recreation, 1941.
4. Howell R (ed): Her Story in Sport: An Historical Anthology of Women in Sports. West Point, NY, Leisure Press, 1982.
5. Simri U: A Concise World History of Women's Sports. Netanya, Israel, Wingate Institute for Physical Education and Sports, 1983.

Chapter 2: Sociologic Considerations on Women and Sports

JUDY MAHLE LUTTER, MA

Finally, in the 1980s more girls and women began to participate in physical activity on a regular basis. This trend started in 1972 with the passage of Title IX, as young women by the tens of thousands took advantage of opportunities to participate in sports. Older women, encouraged by road races, masters' swimming events, and triathlons, were also trying competition. Many more women regularly attended aerobic dance classes or bought walking shoes. Yet, the acceptance of women and sports is not complete and has been marked by vacillating attitudes since the beginning of the century. A summary of that history helps put today's issues in perspective.

I. **THE VICTORIAN ERA**

In the mid to late 1800s, conflicting forces were at work. The image of woman dictated that she be seen as frail and delicate, but in reality, many women were working in the factories and fields. The fact that their lives were physically active was viewed as a disadvantage. The uterus and woman's reproductive organs were emphasized as central to her being, with women being encouraged to rest during their menstrual cycles and to avoid overstressing their physical or mental capabilities. Women's dress was designed to hide their bodies, which obviously limited participation in sports or physical activity, including work.

A. **Reality vs image**
  1. **Reality**
     a. Women working in factories
     b. Women forging the way West in America
     c. Black women working in the fields, often as slaves
  2. **Image**
     a. "True womanhood," the ideal, is characterized as passive, frail, delicate, ethereal, and soft.
     b. Women are placed on a pedestal.
     c. Her duty is to provide calm from the storm, the husband's safe refuge.
     d. Ideal is the unused, sheltered body:
        i. Society thinks that it is best to stay indoors.
        ii. Lack of muscles is seen as a virtue, meaning that the husband could afford to hire servants.
        iii. Attractiveness is a high virtue, and standards of dress and beauty develop (e.g., corsets to attain small waists, voluminous skirts).

B. **Importance of the uterus**
  1. **Reproductive organs central to a woman's being**
     a. All illness, headaches, heart conditions, etc., are believed to be related to the uterus.
     b. "Stressing the brain" (through education) is believed to harm the uterus.
     c. Menstruation is seen as a serious threat throughout life:
        i. Victorians believe women should greatly restrict physical and mental activity during menses.
        ii. Danger exists of "brain fever" if women study too much during cycle.

      d. Victorians believe women should consider themselves "indisposed" throughout pregnancy:

         i. Very moderate activity, i.e., walking, is approved by some.

         ii. Activity in the period after birth also is very restricted.

  2. **Women's natural state to be sick**

C. **Victorian dress and sport**

  1. The premise is that women should not show body parts.

  2. Regular clothes are heavy, long, and cumbersome.

  3. Sports were limited by the type of clothes:

      a. Activities that can be done in a long skirt and long-sleeved blouse are acceptable.

      b. Genteel sports of archery, croquet, and bowling are approved.

      c. Swimming is unacceptable at first; later, very cumbersome heavy wool costumes that conceal most of the body make real swimming impossible.

  4. Exercise during pregnancy is extremely limited, in part by modest attire.

D. **Class considerations**

  1. Factory workers, immigrants, and blacks are exempt from some restrictions because they have to work and cannot afford "genteel" clothing.

  2. College students receive a respite from restrictions until following graduation.

      a. They are exposed to easy play, though restricted during time of menses.

      b. Focus is on fresh air, cooperation and hygiene.

      c. The goal is to create a healthy lifestyle so they can produce healthy children

      d. Aesthetic appeal is key, as the most important thing is to look good.

  3. Upper and middle class women lead sheltered, physically inactive lives.

II. BREAKING THE BARRIERS 1900–1920

In the early 1900s, some major shifts occurred that paved the way for greater participation in sports. In the social and economic sphere, more women were working and the suffrage movement encouraged women to become more outspoken and active in politics. The introduction of the bicycle proved to be a turning point in providing greater accessibility to physical activity for women as well as changing some ways of thinking about dress for exercise.

A. **Factors influencing women's growing participation in sport 1900–1910**

  1. Suffrage movement

  2. More women entering the world of work

  3. Introduction of the bicycle

      a. Immediate acceptance by women

      b. Transportation as well as exercise

      c. A professional biking team formed

B. **Modifications in dress and sports costumes**

  1. Tennis attire, circa 1900, includes:

      a. Corset

      b. Starched petticoat

      c. Starched skirt

      d. Heavily trimmed blouse

      e. Starched shirtwaist dress, long sleeves, cuff links

      f. High collars with necktie

      g. Sneakers with large silk bows

  2. Biking: Bloomers, the first real breakthrough in women's clothing, featured split legs and elastic bottoms.

C. **World War I era**

  1. More women in factory jobs, with sports teams created for women in some factory settings

  2. First women athletes, despite continued restriction of some sports (e.g., baseball)

  3. Women get the right to vote.

D. **The 1920s**
   1. Relaxed standards of dress and activity
   2. Mobility
   3. New autonomy for women
   4. Single women in the labor force begin to live independently of family:
      a. Recreation is considered appropriate in leisure time.
      b. Company teams and facilities are available.
E. **Emergence of women as "professional" sports figures**
   1. 1922—Glenda Collett wins six amateur golf championships.
   2. 1926—Gertrude Ederle swims the English Channel, breaking the record by 2 hours.
   3. 1920s and 30s—Helen Wills dominates tennis with U.S. singles championships and 8 Wimbledon titles.

III. **PERSISTENT BARRIERS 1920–1940**

Despite progress, there were persistent barriers preceding World War II. These were seen at colleges and in the Olympics, which remained largely closed to women. The economic depression also led to a greater restriction of women's activities.
A. **Colleges discourage competition in favor of physical activity.**
   1. Walking is encouraged as training for wifely duties.
   2. Competition is seen as a negative.
      a. Leads to aggressiveness
      b. Encourages individual excellence
      c. Is counter to women's inborn sense of modesty and innocence
   3. "Play days" are introduced.
      a. Strict avoidance of competition
      b. Members of the same school do not "play together" at play day; there is no team spirit.
      c. Promotes a spirit of cooperation and friendship
   4. Minimal opposition to these attitudes is voiced by those encouraging competition.
B. **Resistance to women's competition at the Olympics**
C. **Economic depression in the 1930s**
   1. Discourages women's competition for "men's" jobs
   2. Pressures women to assume the role of wife and mother
   3. Promotes propaganda that sports participation will make women more masculine

IV. **WORLD WAR II AND CHANGED PERCEPTIONS OF WOMEN**

A. **Need for women workers**
   1. Four million women enter labor force in 1940–42.
   2. Fill a great variety of jobs, including those needing physical strength
B. **Changed perceptions and changed roles:** The press recruits women into the work force by depicting them as strong and capable.
C. **Women in sports:** An all-women's professional basefall league is formed. Although participants are required to attend charm school and wear ladylike costumes, they prove to be skillful athletes. The league is disbanded at the end of the war.

V. **POST-WAR ERA**

After the war ended, women were encouraged to leave their wartime jobs and return to the home, making way for the returning male soldiers. The 50s and 60s saw a swing backward for women in all arenas.

VI. **CURRENT TRENDS**

True equality between men and women's sports remains unrealized, as evidenced by the disparity in college budgets for athletic departments as well as coverage in the media. Despite the belief that girls in their school years have greater opportunities to participate in sports, and although talented girls are encouraged to play, various changes today in the educational system, family structure, and community are causing the great majority to have a smaller chance at introduction to sports and physical activity. The implications are obvious for the long-term goal of a healthy society of lifetime physical exercise.

A. **Equality is still a myth.**
   1. Women's athletic department budgets are significantly less than men's.
      a. University of Minnesota 1990 budget for women's sports was $3.4 million, vs $11.8 million for men.
      b. Vassar College, in its first coed year, had a men's budget twice that of women's (although women made up two-thirds of the student body).
   2. Since 1972, there has been a decline in the numbers of women coaches and athletic directors.
   3. Since 1972, there has been a decline in the number of separate women's athletic departments.
   4. The percentage of athletes who are women in college programs:
      Division I   31%
      Division II   32%
      Division III   35%
   5. Athletic scholarship grants are approximately $179 million per year greater for men than for women.
B. **Inequality in the media**
   1. Television
      a. In 1972–73, 366 hours of live men's sports were broadcast on national television, vs 1 hour of women's (Wimbledon).
      b. In May 1980, national television broadcast 200 hr, 39 min of men's sports, vs 5 min of women's (Olympic immortals).
   2. Newspapers and print media
      a. In the decade 1980–90, great increases were seen in newspaper coverage of girl's and women's sports events.
      b. A 1990 study of four major newspapers found that stories focusing exclusively on men's sports outnumbered those on women's sports by 23 to 1.
      c. Of front-page articles on sports, 3.2% covered women's sports, vs 95.3% for men's sports.
      d. Photographs of male athletes outnumber those of female athletes 13 to 1.
C. **Educational system**
   1. Fewer opportunities for both sexes in schools due to reduction in physical education hours
   2. Physical education required K–12 in only one state (Illinois)
   3. Fewer opportunities for less-talented, less-motivated individuals
   4. Lifelong sports is supposedly promoted, but reality is that teaching is spotty.
D. **Family and community concerns**
   1. Level of activity for girls depends on availability of community programs and the commitment of parents' time and money.
   2. In general, girls' participation in sports declines as the number of both-parents-working or single- parent households increases.
   3. Individual family structure, including its belief in the importance of exercise, has great impact on the child's activity level.
   4. In families with two working parents or single parents, the amount of time for unsupervised outdoor play is diminished.
E. **Girls and sports**
   1. Coed opportunities exist.
   2. Drop out begins at age 9.
      a. Deference to boys: "I'm not as good, I can't do it."

      b. Different expectations: girls are given permission to fail and are over-praised for athletic success.

      c. Changing body

      d. Skill level changes

      e. "It's not a cool thing to do."

      f. More support for boys' athletic efforts

      g. Good coaching is infrequent.

      h. Worried about physical changes, diet, menstrual cycle

  3. Role models, good teachers, and coaches are important.

  4. New resources/advocates organizations:

      Women's Sports Foundation

      Melpomene Institute

      Girls and Women in Sports

      YWCA

      Girl Scouts

F. **Elite vs competitive vs recreational activities:** Which ensures long-term lifetime physical activity?

  1. **Elite**

      a. Need to start training early (under age 10)

      b. Some sports where early entry is crucial: swimming, gymnastics, tennis, ice-skating

      c. Questions for child and parent:

         i. Who is making the commitment?

        ii. Who is making the choice?

        iii. What is the motivation?

      d. How does "training" for the sport fit into the child's overall development?

      e. What gains can be expected?

        i. Skill

        i. Maturity

        iii. Discipline

        iv. Rapport with adults

      f. What may be the negatives?

        i. Missing out on normal socialization process

        ii. Unrealistic attitudes and expectations

        iii. Burn-out

        iv. Injury

      g. Dedicated parent(s) is essential.

  2. **Competitive** (high school or college team member)

      a. High school boys participate at approximately twice the rate of girls.

      b. Most popular sports for girls in Minnesota (in rank order):

        i. Basketball

        ii. Track and field

        iii. Fast-pitch softball

        iv. Tennis

        v. Soccer

        vi. Cross-country

      c. Gains

        i. Skill

        ii. Maturity

        iii. Discipline

        iv. Fun

        v. Ability to work as part of a team

      d. Negatives

        i. Pressure and stress to achieve

        ii. Difficulty in balancing academic and sport life

        iii. Injury

   3. **Recreational**

     a. Most realistic for continued long-term activity

     b. Exposure through school classes, where instruction is provided

     c. A disadvantage is that it is hard to motivate a student once class is over; one-shot approach may not have staying power.

G. **Competition beyond school age**

   1. 1970s—Beginning of separate divisions for women in road races

     a. Still some inequality in number of women recognized

     b. If prize money was offered, there were still great inequities.

   2. 1980s—Encouragement to compete reflected in age divisions

     a. Team sports

        i. Volleyball

        ii. Basketball

     b. Individual sports (big earnings still far behind compared to men's competition)

        i. Tennis

        ii. Golf

        iii. Figure skating

VII. THE FUTURE?

A. More women will have a history of organized sport participation; at the same time, there will be fewer women with a history of informal unstructured play, regular outdoor exercise, or the need to use their bodies for transportation, thereby decreasing rates of physical activity.

B. Women most likely to remain physically active over their lifetimes will be well-educated and economically well-off.

   1. Demands of two-career, two-job families will make time for exercise a premium.

   2. Single working mothers and women at lower economic levels will be more likely not to participate.

   3. Society will need to create an atmosphere and opportunities for low-income women, women of color, women with disabilities, and larger women

C. There will be increased demand for equal prize representation in "citizen" athletic events.

D. Questions concerning health and physical activity will remain, including:

   1. Menstrual cycle change   5. Nutrition and diet

   2. Exercise and pregnancy   6. Body image

   3. Menopause   7. Injury

   4. Osteoporosis

RECOMMENDED READING

1. Acosta RV, Carpenter LJ: Women in intercollegiate sport: A longitudinal study—thirteen year update, 1977–1990. Brooklyn, NY, Brooklyn College, 1990.
2. Albohm MJ: Health Care for the Female Athlete. North Palm Beach, FL, The Athletic Institute, 1981.
3. Benoit J, Baker S: Running Tide. New York, Alfred A. Knopf, 1987.
4. Boutilier A, SanGiovanni L: The Sporting Woman. Champaign, IL, Human Kinetics, 1983.
5. Clarke MD, Edward H: Sex in Education, or a Fair Chance for the Girls. Boston, R. Osgood, 1873.
6. Drinkwater L (ed): Female Endurance Athletes. Champaign, IL, Human Kinetics, 1986.
7. Duncan ML, Messner M, Williams L: Coverage of Women's Sports in four Daily Newspapers. Los Angeles, Amateur Athletic Foundation of Los Angeles, 1992.
8. Dyer KF: Challenging the Men: Women in Sport. St. Lucia, Australia, University of Queensland Press, 1982.
9. Ehrenreich B, English D: For Her Own Good: 150 Years of the Experts' Advice to Women. New York, Doubleday, 1978.

10. Gerber EW, Felshin J, Berlin P, Wyrick W: The American Woman in Sport. Addison-Wesley, 1974.
11. Greendorfer SL, Yiannakis A: Sociology of Sport: Perspectives. West Point, NY, Leisure Press, 1981.
12. Howe W (ed): Sex and Education. Boston, Roberts Bros., 1974.
13. Howell R: Her Story in Sport: A Historical Anthology of Women in Sports. West Point, NY, Leisure Press, 1982.
14. Kaplan J: Women and Sports. New York, Avon Books, 1979.
15. Lindgren A: Is it feminine to be fit? Melpomene 8(3):2–5, 1989.
16. Lyons P, Burgard D: Great Shape: The first Exercise Guide for Large Women. New York, William Morrow and Co., 1988.
17. Melpomene Institute for Women's Health Research: The Bodywise Woman. New York, Prentice Hall Press, 1990.
18. Metheney E: Connotations of Movement in Sport and Dance. Dubuque, IA, Brown, 1965.
19. Miller Brewing Company: The Miller Lite Report in American Attitudes Towards Sports. Milwaukee, Miller Brewing Co., 1983.
20. Navratilova M: Martina. New York, Ballantine Books, 1985.
21. Oglesby CA: Women and Sport: From Myth to Reality. Philadelphia, Lea & Febiger, 1978.
22. Puhl JS, Brown CH, Voy RO: Sports Science Perspectives for Women. Champaign, IL, Human Kinetics Books, 1985.
23. Smith K: Title IX and Gender Equity. Minneapolis, MN, University of Minnesota, 1992.
24. Women's Sports Foundation: Gender equity in athletic educational fact sheet. New York, New York, 1993.

Chapter 3: Gender Equity in Sports

DONNA A. LOPIANO, PhD

The debate over gender equity in sport unfortunately has been portrayed to the public as a choice between a favorite college football team and adding more sports teams for girls who are not as interested in sports as boys. There is a myth that football will die if girls and women are given equal opportunities in sport. The myth claims that football is the proverbial "goose that lays the golden egg" and its revenues support all remaining men's and women's sports; if it dies, all others will also die. It is important to know that football will not die and football is not the golden goose.

I. **BENEFITS OF SPORTS FOR WOMEN**

Sports is simply too important to the physical, psychological, and sociologic well-being of our children to have it only benefit our sons. Sports participation for girls has significant health implications.

A. High school girls who play sports are less likely to be involved in an unwanted pregnancy, less likely to be involved with drugs, and more likely to graduate from high school.

B. As little as 2 hours of exercise a week may reduce a teenage girl's risk of breast cancer, a disease that will afflict 1 of every 8 American women.

C. Sports or weight-bearing exercises are necessary in laying down bone mass; our mothers and grandmothers were denied this opportunity, and 1 of every 2 women over age 60 is now suffering from osteoporosis.

D. Girls and women who play sports have higher levels of self-esteem and lower levels of depression.

E. Girls and women who play sports have a more positive body image and experience higher states of psychological well-being than girls and women who do not play sports.[7]

F. Sports traditionally teaches teamwork, goal-setting, the pursuit of excellence in performance, and other achievement-oriented behaviors—critical skills for success in the workplace. Daughters should not be less prepared for the highly competitive workplace than sons.

II. **TITLE IX OF THE 1972 EDUCATION AMENDMENTS ACT**

Title IX prohibits discrimination on the basis of gender in the provision of educational programs and activities in all secondary and postsecondary educational institutions that receive federal funds. For athletics programs, Title IX addresses three basic equal opportunity program requirements:

A. **Participation opportunities**

1. Schools are obligated to provide athletic opportunities for men and women in proportion to their enrollment in the general student body—e.g., if a college has 55% male and 45% female undergraduates, athletic participation should reflect this 55/45 mix.

2. Defenses for not providing these numbers of opportunities are that the institution has already fully met the interests and abilities of women athletes *or* shown a continuing expansion of opportunities for women over time (e.g., is on the way to providing equity).

3. This requirement does not refer to equal numbers of "teams." Rather, "participation opportunities" must be equitable. For example, if the undergraduate student body is 55/45 male/female and 400 athletic participation opportunities are provided, there should be 220 male athletes and 180 female athletes.

B. **Scholarship dollars**
1. Scholarship dollars must be provided to male and female athletes proportional to their athletic participation—e.g., if a school is spending $400,000/year on athletic scholarships and half of their athletic participants are women, then $200,000 should be funding athletic scholarships for women.

C. **Other athletic program benefits**
1. The institution must provide equal benefits for male and female athletes in the areas of athletic equipment, uniforms and supplies, provision of quality coaches, locker rooms, practice and competitive facilities, scheduling, travel, recruiting, and other athletic program areas.
2. An equal dollar benefit is not required. For example, if it costs $1,000 to outfit a football player, an institution is not required to spend $1,000 outfitting a woman basketball player. The institution simply must spend whatever is required to provide that woman basketball player with the same quality uniform and equipment provided to the football player.

III. **ARE EDUCATIONAL INSTITUTIONS COMPLYING WITH TITLE IX?**

A. **High schools and colleges have virtually ignored the requirements of federal law over the past 20 years. Various surveys reveal:**
1. Females comprised over 53% of college undergraduate students in 1990.[34] Of 282,512 student-athletes at NCAA institutions in 1991–92, only 96,467 (34%) were women.[26]
2. Men's sports participation has not suffered by providing participation opportunities for women. There were 16,242 more male athletes in 1991–92 than in 1981–82. For every 2 female participation slots created in this 10-year period, 1.5 male participation slots were added.
3. The NCAA Gender Equity Study revealed significant discrepancies in athletic opportunities at the institutional level:

Division	Males	Females
I	250 (69%)	112 (31%)
II	167 (68%)	79 (32%)
III	215 (67%)	116 (35%)

4. Female collegiate athletes receive <24% of the athletics' operating dollar and <18% of the athletics' recruiting dollar.
5. Female athletes receive <33% of the college athletic scholarship dollar. Average Division I and II athletic scholarship expenditures are as follows:

Division	Males	Females
I	$849, 130	$372,800
II	$319,543	$148,966

6. Male college athletes receive approximately $179 million more per year in athletic scholarship grants than their female counterparts.
7. In Division IA institutions, women's programs received only 18% of the total budget.[29]
8. The proportion of African-American athletes in women's sports programs is significantly less than in men's sports programs (primarily because of the large number of black athletes in football).

B. **Administrative positions are not open to women.**
1. In 1972, 90% of all collegiate athletics programs for women were governed by women administrators; today, that proportion is 16.8%.[2]
2. Among the 107 Division IA institutions in the NCAA in 1992–93 (institutions with the most competitive athletics programs and highest administrative salaries), only 2 women currently head a merged department of men's and women's

athletics. In Division IAA, 3 of 88 member institutions have women athletic directors. In Division IAAA (programs without football), 3 of 103 member institutions have women athletic directors.[1]

3. In 28% of athletics programs, there are no women athletics administrators (athletic directors, associate directors, or assistant directors), even though over 300 of those schools have at least 3 athletics administrator positions.[2]

4. There are more female presidents of NCAA institutions than athletic directors[2]:

Division	Female athletic director	Female president
I	11	15
II	23	27
III	65	69
Total	99	111

5. Only 9 women are included among the 105 athletics conference commissioners in the nation—4 of these women serve as head of women's-sports-only conferences. Five hold a commissioner's position in a conference governing both men's and women's sports, but none serve as head of a Division IA conference (2 are at IAA conferences and 3 are at Division III conferences).

6. The NCAA has failed to provide strong leadership for its member institutions with regard to Title IX compliance. Only 9% of the faculty representatives at the NCAA Convention are women.[24] Only 23.4% of all delegates to the 1992 NCAA Convention were women. Historically, the NCAA has argued against the inclusion of athletics in the Title IX regulations.

7. Less than a third of all committee positions in the NCAA are held by women, and that percentage drops to 20% among the NCAA's most powerful committees. These numbers reflect minimum representation limits established by the NCAA when they opened their doors to women sports in 1981. There has not been a significant increase since women were let in.[19]

8. Forty-eight percent of all women's teams are coached by women,[2] but <1% of all men's teams are coached by women.

9. About 5952 jobs existed in 1992 for head coaches of women's teams, and this number has increased by 812 in the last 10 years. Women, though, hold only 181 more coaching jobs than they held 10 years ago, while men hold 631 more as coaches of women's teams.[2]

10. African-American women coaches, administrators, officials, and athletics support personnel are virtually nonexistent.

11. Although high school financial data are unavailable, only 34% of all high school athletes are women, and there is reason to believe that the high school situation directly mirrors the college situations.

IV. **WHY HAVE INSTITUTIONS FAILED TO COMPLY?**

A. **Institutions argue that they have not had the financial resources to provide additional participation opportunities for female athletes.**
   1. Yet, there appears to have been no commitment to holding the participation of male athletes at their 1970 levels while gradually building new athletic participation opportunities for females.
   2. For every 2 new participation slots created for women college athletes in the last 10 years, 1.5 have been created for men.

B. **Institutions have been aware that the federal government is not enforcing the law.**
   1. Facing no threat of loss of federal funds (the penalty for noncompliance with the law), institutions are ignoring the law.
   2. As a result, increasing numbers of parents are suing in court for their daughters' rights and opportunities guaranteed by law, and they are batting 1.000.

C. **High schools and colleges have been unwilling to make the difficult decisions required to redistribute resources within athletics to provide equal opportunities for women.**

   1. The goal is to reduce expenditures on men's athletics without damaging the participation opportunities for male students and then to redistribute these funds to provide gender equity for female athletes.

   2. Institutions have been unwilling to reduce excessive expenditures on men's football and basketball, but rather are eliminating men's non-revenue-producing sports and blaming it on having to provide equal athletic opportunities for women.

V. **CAN INSTITUTIONS COMPLY WITH TITLE IX WITHOUT HURTING MEN'S ATHLETICS?**

Participation opportunities and direct educational benefits to student-athletes are the most important reasons for maintaining athletic programs in higher education. Other cost-saving and revenue-producing measures should be pursued prior to cutting teams or reducing squad sizes:

A. **Increase revenues of men's minor sports and women's sports at the institutional and conference level.**

   1. The women's sports market is virtually untapped and must be developed. According to Raiborn's study,[29] at least 13 Division IA institutions in 1989 had women's programs which generated $1.3 million or more and twice that number that generated $400,000 or more.

   2. There is evidence that the spectator and donor market for women's sports is a new market, different from that supporting men's athletics. Therefore, developing that new market will not put women's sports in a position of competing against an institution's men's program.

B. **Encourage college conference members and high school districts to adopt the same sports when expanding women's programs.** Doing so will realize the financial savings of competition within a reasonable geographic proximity.

C. **Establish conference-level presidential review requirements for the control of athletic administration staffing and the construction and renovation of athletics facilities.**

   1. At the college level, plush locker rooms and indoor practice facilities for football have become recruiting enticements. Controlling these expenditures is difficult at the institutional level where arguments include matching the commitments of traditional opponents.

D. **Create inducements for gender equity.**

   1. Prohibit the allocation of an automatic national championship berth to any institution that has not achieved gender equity or to any conference without a conference-level presidential review requirement for the control of athletics expenditures.

   2. At the high school level, prohibit advancement to postseason play for boys' teams if a school is not providing equal opportunity for girls.

E. **Reduce institutional expenditures that do not directly and positively affect the participation experience of student-athletes:**

   1. Downsize athletics administrative staffs.

   2. Eliminate "status-related" expenses, such as plush locker rooms and coaches' offices and conference rooms.

   3. Eliminate cellular phones for athletes and administrators.

   4. Place a moratorium on construction of new athletics-only facilities, including study or computer centers accessible only to student-athletes.

   5. Continue efforts to restrict off-campus recruiting activities.

   6. Eliminate housing athletics teams in hotels prior to *home* contests.

   7. Eliminate airplane travel over short distances.

   8. Restrict team travel distances during regular season play.

F. **Legislate within the NCAA reductions in the amount of non-need-based athletics aid that institutions may award in each sport.**
   1. The goals would include maintaining competitive distinctions between all divisions, maintaining the current number of student-athletes who may receive such aid, and not reducing the aid levels of athletes who qualify for aid based on need. Such reductions should be accompanied by changing all sports to "equivalency" rather than "head-count" sports, with limits placed on the total number of student-athletes who may receive any amount of aid.
   2. For example, football is currently permitted to have 85 grants awarded to no more than 85 student-athletes. This is commonly referred to as a "head-count" system where every athlete on aid counts as 1 grant whether they receive $1 or a full scholarship. Under an equivalency system, football might be limited to 70 full scholarships that could be split up and awarded as full or partial scholarships to no more than 85 players. In this example, a savings of 15 full scholarships (approximately $120,000) would fully fund the addition of another women's sport.

G. **Revise the NCAA revenue distribution formula to provide 1 unit for every men's sport over the minimum requirement and 1.5 units for every women's sport over the minimum requirement**—or similar more advantageous weighting for women's sports or more advantageous weighting for women's scholarships than men's scholarships.

H. **Increase NCAA scholarship limits for women's sports** in order to permit institutions to meet their compliance obligations for scholarships without adding excessive numbers of new women's sports.

VI. **WOULD THE IMPLEMENTATION OF TITLE IX REGULATIONS HURT FOOTBALL PROGRAMS?**

Compliance with Title IX will not affect the success of intercollegiate football programs. Football will always be popular on college campuses and of interest to television and other media. However, 43% of all the monies spent on athletics in some schools are spent on football and basketball, so the standard of living of many football programs will have to be reduced in order to redistribute funds for the cause of gender equity. Such reductions need not result in lowering participation opportunities for football players or scholarship support for athletes in financial need. Neither will such reductions result in the demise of football as many would ask us to believe.

A. **College football coaches and athletic directors are asking the public to choose between gender equity and football.**
   1. We should not be asked to choose between our sons and daughters.
   2. We are hearing the arguments of boys or men who think that sports is their protected domain and values like sharing and equal opportunity do not apply to them.

B. **In reducing the cost of men's sports, and men's football in particular, in order to support increased opportunities for women, such actions will be healthy for all athletic programs.**
   1. Athletics, especially Division I and II athletics programs, need to be downsized. They are spending beyond their means in a quest for television exposure and bowl bids.
   2. Contrary to popular myth, football is not offered as a sport or does not pay for itself at 91% of all NCAA institutions[29]:

Division	Institutions with Deficit Football Programs	Average Annual Deficit
I	45%	$638,000
IAA	94%	$580,718
II	97%	$247,000
III	99%	$69,000

3. While football generates significant revenues at many schools, few teams generate the net revenue to support the rest of the school's sport programs. The situation is no different for men's basketball.[29]

C. **On most college and high school campuses, athletics administrators offer significant resistance to cost-cutting requests.**

1. Sex-discriminatory practices may be entrenched and the majority of existing funds already committed to men's programs.

2. Efforts to cut fat in men's athletics may require the assignment of an objective member of an institution's central administration to analyze expenditures as they relate to competitive success.

3. Intercollegiate athletics budgets are complicated and most have not been developed by professional managers. Thus, cost/benefit analyses are extremely rare.

4. In an athletics budget, most expenditures on men's and women's athletics cannot be separated on the basis of sex, especially in the area of support services such as athletic training, training tables, sports information, marketing and promotion, etc.

5. Most perquisites given to coaches do not appear in athletics budgets (i.e., free cars, country club memberships, etc.).

D. **Athletic program management and accounting practices must be carefullly monitored.**

1. Administrators should demand a cost-benefit relationship for any proposed expense related to maintaining the competitive status of a program in relation to rival institutions.

2. Education must conservatively approach proposals to expand athletics facilities during the next 5–10 years. Commitments to large debt service in light of rising costs and continued athletics program deficits may be fiscally irresponsible.

3. While investments in the people who produce quality athletic programs (coaches) need to be maintained, the productivity of clerical and other support personnel involved in large ticket offices, concessions, game management, and other administrative operations should be carefully examined.

4. Transportation and travel arrangements should be evaluated for cost-effective practices. The number of days teams are spending on the road related to the number of days of competition should be examined and the entire travel package for all sports teams should be put out on bid to a travel agent.

VII. **ARE WOMEN LESS INTERESTED IN SPORT OPPORTUNITIES THAN MEN?**

The issue of interest of female athletes is a critical one. Opportunity drives interest and ability. Title IX's purpose includes redressing historic discrimination. There is no lack of interest and ability on the part of males or females to participate in the finite number of opportunities available at the collegiate level. Currently, over 3.9 million males and 1.9 million female athletes participate at the high school level, and there are many more girls participating in Olympic sports traditionally not offered in the high school athletic program. Currently, there are only 186,045 male and 96,467 female athletes on NCAA teams.

A. **It can be argued that institutions are "intentionally" discriminating against female athletes when they conduct sex-separate sports programs and fail to offer the same participation opportunities and support as they do male athletes.**

1. When an institution establishes a women's team, hires a coach, offers scholarship incentives, or allocates money to recruit incoming female student-athletes, the coach never comes back to the institution saying that he or she could not find any women with the interest or ability to play on the team.

B. **Institutions with football teams argue that they cannot offer enough women's teams to offset the high participation numbers of football and that they cannot identify enough sports in which women are interested.**

1. Washington State University, a Division IA program with football, under court order to have its athlete population reflect the gender mix in its student body

(45% female, 55% male), has already achieved a female athlete population of 44%. The success of its football program has improved during this period.

C. **The number of "walk-ons"** (non-recruited athletes who come from the general student body over and above the student-athletes acquired through recruiting and scholarship incentives) is higher for males than females (especially in football) and is used as an argument to show females' lack of interest in sports. Also, different rates of participation in men's and women's recreational sport programs on campus are claimed to reflect student interest (greater male participation numbers).

1. On examination, the sport and activity offerings of recreational sports programs have traditionally reflected male sports interests rather than female sports interests.

2. Institutions that offer recreational programs based on a survey of interests of their male and female students show roughly equal participation rates.

D. **At many institutions, the lack of female participants is due to a failure to offer a sufficient number of sports and a lack of institutional commitment to existing women's programs.**

1. Better paid or more competent coaches of men's teams find it easier to recruit participants than underpaid, part-time, or unqualified coaches of a women's team. Better pay for women's team coaches and better facilities for women's sports would attract more and better athletes, just as it has in men's sports.

2. Often, a men's team has a recruiting budget while the women's team in that same sport has none. Less than 18% of all recruiting dollars go to women's sports.

VIII. WHAT NEEDS TO BE DONE TO ACHIEVE TITLE IX COMPLIANCE?

A. **Better Public Education Efforts:** Education officials at the campus and community level, electronic and print media journalists, and the Office of Civil Rights must increase its efforts to educate the public on Title IX requirements in athletics.

1. Parents and daughters are receiving misinformation from athletic directors at high schools or colleges regarding Title IX requirements.

   a. They are told that women's sports are not receiving the same support as men's sports because women's sports do not make money.

   b. They are told that football is excluded from Title IX requirements.

   c. They are told that the institution does not have the money to increase the numbers of women's sports.

   d. Athletic directors are defending a sex discriminatory program and are not willing to give good information to parents and female athletes.

2. It would be helpful for school officials to mandate that a summary of Title IX requirements and common questions and answers be distributed to all male and female student-athletes, to club sport participants, and in response to any inquiry.

   a. This educational effort should be annually conducted by each institution's Title IX Compliance Coordinator (a position required by the regulations).

3. There should be a legislative initiative to include full disclosure of an institution's Title IX gender equity progress in the Student Right To Know Act. The Act should require disclosure of athletic participation rates by gender, the total athletic scholarship dollars by gender, and the proportion of operating and recruiting funds spent by gender.

B. **Better Education of Investigators:** The current Title IX regulations are sufficient, but the government simply needs to enforce the law.

1. Title IX enforcement should stay under the Department of Education. Congress needs to keep sending the clear message that educational sport and athletic programs are clearly a part of the educational process. If this is not the case, they should not be receiving the benefits of tax-exempt status.

   a. It has been suggested that enforcement of Title IX be moved to the Department of Justice. However, the Department of Justice is not set up to do the nonjudicial program review elements of Title IX that can be helpful to institutions.

    b. The Department of Education needs to do a better job of monitoring compliance agreements and should pass on to the Department of Justice those cases where institutions are not implementing those agreements or where institutions refuse to comply. The Justice Department now has the power to enforce Title IX, but the Department of Education has not referred any cases to them.

  2. Title IX need not be amended to codify damages.

    a. The Supreme Court has already ruled that damages are permissible. The courts can deal with the damages issue without further lawmaking.

    b. Parents who have filed lawsuits to date have not been interested in damages. They simply want their daughters to have an opportunity to play.

C. **Stricter Enforcement:** The public is not pursuing Title IX complaints in athletics because there is no trust that the Office of Civil Rights (OCR) is serious about enforcing the law.

  1. Parents and their daughters would rather turn to the courts than place their daughters' concerns in the hands of the OCR.

  2. The fact that parents and daughters are not well educated on the requirements of the law is contributing to the absence of complaints and lawsuits.

  3. OCR needs more financial support so that it has the time and manpower to do its job, and it needs to more effectively monitor compliance agreements. The federal government should assume the burden for enforcement of the law.

IX. ASSIGNMENT AND COMPENSATION OF COACHES

Equal opportunity in women's athletics programs involves the provision of quality coaches who are compensated in the same manner as their counterparts coaching men's sports. Generally, male and female coaches of women's teams are paid less than coaches of men's teams (who are predominantly male), and female coaches are paid less than male coaches who are coaching the same sport. These salary inequities exist even though research shows that female coaches are as qualified and experienced as their male counterparts.

A. **There are two different "pools" of coaching candidates in the marketplace:** an all-male coaches pool for revenue-producing men's sports, and a mixed pool of men and women for men's non-revenue-producing and women's sports.

  1. The marketplace value of coaches in the first pool is 2–5 times higher than the marketplace value of coaches in the latter pool.

  2. With the recent development of women's basketball as a significant revenue-producing sport, it will be difficult to justify not hiring coaches of women's teams from the revenue-producing sport pool or not paying female coaches of women's teams salaries equal to those of coaches in that pool.

B. **There has been a steady diminution in the number of women coaching men's and women's sports and the number of women in professional leadership positions.**

  1. Only 48.3% of the coaches of women's teams are female.[2] In 1972, >90% of women's teams were coached by females.[2]

  2. The percentages of women coaching women's sports in 1978 and 1990 are compared[2]:

	1978	1992
Basketball	79.4%	63.5%
Cross-country	35.2%	20.1%
Softball	83.5%	63.7%
Tennis	72.9%	48.0%
Track and field	52.0%	20.4%
Volleyball	86.6%	78.7%

C. **Employment discrimination in athletics has taken subtle forms.**
   1. When searching for coaches of women's teams, the administrator may only look at formal written applications and hire entry-level employees. When looking for coaches of a men's team, the athletic director will solicit applicants or hire good coaches away from other programs.
   2. It is not unusual, when checking on the credentials or references of female coaching candidates, to hear concerns that the applicant may have homosexual inclinations or references to her physical appearance as being more masculine than feminine. The reference checker seldom hears anything about the personal lives or appearance of male applicants.
   3. It is not unusual for female candidates to be asked if they are planning to have children, despite prohibitions against such queries.
   4. Descriptions of a candidate as a "feminist" are often used to imply that a job candidate is a "troublemaker."
D. Higher education officials must monitor carefully employment and program practices in intercollegiate athletics if women's sports are to grow into equal opportunity athletics programs, especially in merged administrative units.

BIBLIOGRAPHY AND RECOMMENDED READING

1. 1992-93 NCAA Directory. Overland Park, KS, National Collegiate Athletic Association, 1992.
2. Acosta RV, Carpenter LJ: Women in intercollegiate sport: A longitudinal study—fifteen year update, 1977-1992 [unpublished manuscript]. Brooklyn College, 1992.
3. Aiken v Lievallen, 39 Or. App. 779, 593 P.2d 1243, 1979.
4. Atwell RH, Grimes B, Lopiano D: The Money Game: Financing Collegiate Athletics. Washington, DC, American Council on Education, 1980.
5. Berry RC, Wong GM: Law and Business of the Sports Industry: Vol. II. Common Issues in Amateur and Professional Sports. Dover, MA, Auburn House, 1986.
6. Blair v Washington State University. 108 Wash. 2d. 558, 740 P. 2d 1379, 1987.
7. Chalip L, Villige J, Duignan P: Sex-role identity in a select sample of women field hockey players. Int J Sport Psychol 11:240-248, 1980.
8. Delano LC: Understanding barriers that women face in pursuing high school athletic administrative positions: A feminist perspective [doctoral dissertation]. Iowa City, University of Iowa, 1988.
9. Demo DH: Closing or widening the gender gap? Boys' and girls' interscholastic sports in Mississippi. Stud Soc Sci 24:33-40, 1985.
10. Education Amendments of 1972, P.L. 92-318, Title IX—Prohibitions of Sex Discrimination, July 1, 1972 (now codified as 20 U.S.C. § 1681(a)).
11. Fed Reg (11 December 1979). 44(239):71413-71423, 1979.
12. Gelb J, Palley ML: Women and Public Policies. Princeton, NJ, Princeton University Press, 1982.
13. Gender Equity Survey. Mission, KS, National Collegiate Athletic Association, 1992.
14. Isaac TA: Sports—The final frontier: Sex discrimination in sports leadership. Women Lawyers J 73(4):15-19, 1987.
15. Lopiano DA: A fact-finding model for conducting a Title IX self-evaluation study in athletic programs. J Phys Educ Recreat Dance 47(5):26-30, 1976.
16. Lopiano DA: Modern athletics: Directions and problems. Thresholds Educ 8(4):23-27, 1980.
17. Lopiano DA: A political analysis of the possibility of impact alternatives for the accomplishment of feminist objectives within American intercollegiate sport. In Lapchick RE (ed): Fractured Focus: Sport as a Reflection of Society. Lexington, MA, Lexington Books, 1986, pp 163-176.
18. Lopiano DA: A speech made at the NCAA President's Commission National Forum. Phys Educ 45(1):2-4, 1988.
19. Lovett DJ, Lowry C: Gender representations in the NCAA and NAIA. J Appl Res Coaching Athletics 4(1):1-16, 1989.
20. Mottinger SG, Gench BE: Comparison of salaries of female and male intercollegiate basketball coaches: An equal opportunity study. J Natl Asoc Women Deans Admin Couns 47(2):23-28, 1984.
21. Oglesby CA: Women and Sport: From Myth to Reality. Philadelphia, Lea & Febiger, 1978.
22. Orleans JH: Aggressive pursuit of a legislative exemption under Title IX for revenue-producing men's sports is not in the best interests of athletes or colleges. Educ Rec (Winter):41-44, 1982.
23. Otto LB, Alwin DF: Athletics, aspirations and attainments. Sociol Educ 42:101-113, 1977.
24. Parkhouse BL, Lapin J: Women Who Win: Exercising Your Rights in Sport. Englewood Cliffs, NJ, Prentice Hall, 1980.

25. Participation Study, 1981–82: Men's and Women's Sports. Mission, KS, National Collegiate Athletic Association, 1983.
26. Participation Study, 1991–92: Men's and Women's Sports. Overland Park, KS, National Collegiate Athletic Association, 1993.
27. Pogrebin LC: Growing Up Free: Raising Your Child in the 80's. Toronto, Bantam Books, 1980.
28. Raiborn MH: Revenues and Expenses of Intercollegiate Athletics Programs: Analysis of Financial Trends and Relationships 1981–85. Mission, KS, National Collegiate Athletic Association, 1986.
29. Raiborn MH: Revenues and Expenses of Intercollegiate Athletics Programs: Analysis of Financial Trends and Relationships 1985–89. Mission, KS, National Collegiate Athletic Association, 1990.
30. Schafer SP: Women in coaching: Problems, possibilities. Am Coach (Sep/Oct):4–6, 1987.
31. Survey of NCAA Member Institutions on the Elimination and Addition of Sports. Mission, KS, National Collegiate Athletic Association, 1988.
32. Uhlir GA: Athletics and the university: The post-woman's era. Academe 73(4):25–29, 1987.
33. Uhlir GA: For whom the dollars toll. J Natl Assoc Deans Admin Couns 47(2):13–22, 1984.
34. United States Department of Education: Digest of Educational Statistics. Washington, DC, National Center for Educational Statistics, 1990.
35. Wong GM, Ensor RJ: Sex discrimination in athletics: A review of two decades of accomplishments and defeats. Gonzaga Law Rev 21(2):345–393, 1985–86.
36. Yudof MG, Kirp DL, van Geel T, Levin B: Educational Policy and the Law. Berkeley, CA, McCutchan, 1982.

Chapter 4: Gender-specific Physiology

CHARLOTTE F. SANBORN, PhD
CATHERINE M. JANKOWSKI, MS

Swimming is an excellent example for comparing or contrasting female and male athletes. Prepubescent girls and boys have similar winning times for all strokes. In fact, at age 8 and under the times may be even faster for girls than boys. "Girls are further along their road to maturity than boys" at any given chronologic age.[16] Departure in swim times follows the changes that occur during adolescence in body size, body composition, energy metabolism, circulation, cardiorespiratory capacity, and endocrinology. This chapter addresses each of the above areas, highlighting the major gender-specific differences. Although the focus is on absolute differences between the genders, the relative changes and adaptations to training are basically similar for both athletes.

I. BODY SIZE

A. Height and weight

1. Height and weight follow a **double-sigmoid growth pattern** from birth to adulthood.[11]
   a. A rapid gain occurs in infancy and early childhood, followed by a slow steady gain during middle childhood.
   b. Another rapid phase begins during adolescence with a slow increase until cessation of growth around the second decade.
2. **Peak height velocity** for girls ranges from 10.5–13 years and for boys is 12.5–15 years.[16]
3. **Menarche** occurs approximately 1 year after peak height velocity.
4. **Adult stature** is reached by 17–19 years for girls and early 20s for boys.[9]
5. **Peak weight velocity** occurs about 6 months after the height peak.[16]
6. Women have a larger **surface area to mass**[13]
   a. A larger body surface area is advantageous in dry heat.
   b. A larger body surface area offers no advantage in humid heat.
   c. A larger surface area to mass could be a disadvantage in the cold, but the insulation resulting from a thicker layer of subcutaneous fat in women inhibits the heat loss.

B. Skeletal comparisons

1. **Skeletal maturity** is known as the age at which the closure (union) of the primary and secondary ossification centers occurs. Skeletal maturity is completed by age 18 for girls and 21–22 for boys.
2. The adult female has a wider and shallower **pelvis** than the male. A potential concern regarding the wide pelvis is the greater angle of the femur from the vertical (Q angle), which may result in knee problems.[13]
3. Women are four times more likely to develop **osteoporosis** than men. The reasons are women have thinner, lighter bones than men, experience a rapid loss of bone after menopause, and live longer than men.
4. **Amenorrheic athletes** have lower bone mineral density than regularly menstruating athletes.

II. BODY COMPOSITION

A. Body fat

1. Overall, adult women have 8–10% more body fat than men.

2. Body fat is classified as **storage fat** or **essential fat**. The absolute amount of storage fat is basically similar between men and women, but women have a higher relative amount of storage fat than men. Because of the inclusion of sex-specific fat, essential fat is higher in women (9–12%) than men (3%).

3. Most female athletes are lower in body fat than sedentary college-aged women (23–27%). Further, many female athletes, especially runners, gymnasts, and ballet dancers, have lower body fat (10–15%) than average college-aged men (15–18%).

4. **A major misuse of prescribing optimal body weight** is occurring among female athletes. Dangerously low percentages of body fat are being required or recommended for female athletes. An obsession to reduce body weight may result in disordered eating.

B. **Muscle tissue**

1. The **strengths** of girls and boys diverge markedly with the onset of puberty. On average, girls obtain the following percentage of boys' strength[7]:

11–12 years:	90%
13–14 years:	85%
15–16 years:	75%

2. **Muscle fiber and total muscle cross-sectional area** of women average 60–85% of men; the relative proportion of fast-twitch and slow-twitch fibers is similar.[5]

3. Generally, **strength differences** between the sexes are greater for upper body than lower body strength. The probable explanation is that girls and women tend to avoid upper body strengthening activities.

4. The differences in absolute strength between sexes can be virtually eliminated when strength is expressed relative to fat-free weight. Thus, the differences in muscle strength between trained women and men appears to be explained by muscle mass size.

5. **Weight training** in women and men elicits similar relative gains in strength and muscle hypertrophy.[5]

6. **Resistance training** should be a high priority when prescribing a fitness program for women. An increase in strength is beneficial not only for athletic performance, but maintaining or slowing the loss of muscle mass is also beneficial with the elderly and dieting women.[14]

C. **Body fat distribution (regional adiposity)**

1. Body fat distribution is described as gynoid or android.

   a. **Gynoid**—an accumulation of fat in the hips and thighs; typically associated with females.

   b. **Android**—fat accumulation in the abdominal region; typically seen in males, but women tend to develop an androidal fat pattern following menopause.

2. **Gynoid obesity** is characterized by an increased number of normal-sized adipocytes with low lipolytic activity and may be more resistant to reduction by exercise than androidal obesity.

3. The **ratio of waist circumference to hip circumference (WHR)** is an index of relative body fat distribution.

   a. Higher WHR correlates with a higher prevalence of heart disease.

   b. WHR risk categories for women are:

Low	<0.75
Medium	0.75–0.80
High	>0.80

III. **ENERGY METABOLISM**

A. **Resting metabolic rate (RMR)** is 5–10% lower in women than in men. The difference is not related to gender per se, but rather to the metabolic activity of specific tissues—muscle mass is metabolically more active than fat. When RMR is expressed relative to fat-free mass, the gender differences essentially disappear.

B. **The energy cost of an activity is directly related to body weight.** For the same duration and relative intensity of bicycle ergometry exercise, women expend 40% fewer calories than men. The difference could be even greater for weight-bearing activity.[17]

C. Trained women have an increased RMR compared with untrained women.

D. **Total energy expenditure needs to be considered when prescribing exercise for weight changes.** A higher percentage of fat fuel will be used with low-intensity exercise ("fat-burning exercise programs"); however, the total caloric expenditure will be less than in higher intensity programs for the same duration.[17]

E. **Many elite female athletes appear to be in negative caloric balance.** Women with low caloric intakes coupled with high energy expenditure should be evaluated for adequate nutrient intake and potential disordered eating.

IV. **CIRCULATION**

A. **Hemopoietic system**
1. Ten-year-old girls and boys have similar red blood cell counts (4.7 million/mm^3), hemoglobin (13g/dl), and hematocrit (38%).[15]
2. Adult women have approximately 6% fewer red blood cells and 10–15% lower hemoglobin concentration and hematocrit than men[15]:

	Average RBC ($\times 10^6$/mm^3)	Hb (g/dl)	Hct (%)
Female	4.8	14	42
Male	5.4	16	47

3. Women generally have a lower **oxygen-carrying capacity** than men because of the lower concentration of hemoglobin.

B. **Blood volume**: women have less blood volume than men: 4200 vs. 5500 ml, respectively.[9]

C. **Women have lower iron stores,** decreased dietary intake, increased absorption, and increased loss of iron compared with men (Table 1).

D. **Anemia**
1. Women are at greater risk of iron deficiency and anemia than men.
2. **Iron stores must be measured in order to diagnose iron deficiency anemia.** The following hemoglobin (g/dl) values are rough guidelines for true anemia[6]:

	Women	Men
Nonexercisers	12.0	14.0
Moderate exercisers	11.5	13.5
Elite athletes	11.0	13.0

TABLE 1. Iron Status in Women vs. Men

	Women	Men
Body iron (mg)		
Total	2450	3450
Hemoglobin	1750	2100
Tissue	300	350
Storage	400	1000
Serum ferritin	0.1	0.3
Dietary iron (mg/d)		
Recommended daily intake	15*	10
Intake	11	16
Absorption	1.3 (12%)	0.9 (6%)
Iron loss (mg/d)		
Urine, sweat	1	1
Menstruation	0.5	—
Pregnancy	2.5	—

* Pregnancy RDA = 30 mg/d.

3. For women athletes, the cause of iron deficiency anemia is typically low dietary intake of iron.
4. **Vegetarian female athletes** are at greater risk for developing low iron status than female athletes who eat red meat.[12]

V. CARDIORESPIRATORY CAPACITY

A. **Lung volume**
1. Women have a **smaller thoracic cage** than men, resulting in lower lung volumes.
2. Average adult **respiratory volumes**[4]:

	Women	Men
Total lung capacity (ml)	4200	6000
Vital capacity (ml)	3200	4800
Residual volume (ml)	1200	1000

B. **Heart size/stroke volume**
1. Women have a **smaller heart** (volume) than men, resulting in a lower stroke volume and thus a higher heart rate at the same VO_2 but a lower maximal cardiac output.
2. Women have a **smaller left ventricular mass** both in absolute terms and relative to lean body mass.

C. **Blood pressure**
1. Infants and children tend to increase systolic and diastolic pressures with age. Girls reach a plateau between 15–17 years and boys about 20 years.[9]
2. From 12–54 years, mean levels of blood pressure among females are less than in males, but from 55–74 years mean levels of women are higher.
3. Racial differences[10]:
   a. Black women have higher blood pressure than white women from age 25–74.
   b. The mean systolic pressure is lower in black females than in black males aged 12–44.
   c. Diastolic pressure increases to 50 years in blacks of both sexes, then declines or remains constant.
4. Low fitness scores in women are associated with a 1.52 relative risk for becoming hypertensive.[2]

D. **Aerobic power (VO_2 max)**
1. VO_2 max is similar in prepubescent girls and boys.
2. Absolute VO_2 max (L/min) peaks for both sexes between ages 16–20.
3. Differences in body composition and the oxygen transport system account for much, but not all, of the sex differences in VO_2 max.
4. The large 52% difference in VO_2 max (L/min) between men and women decreases to 20–30% when expressed as VO_2 ml/kg/min and then to approximately 15% as VO_2 ml/kg fat-free weight/min.
5. Moderately fit women (>9 METS [metabolic equivalents] or 31.5 ml/kg/min) have significantly less risk of mortality than sedentary women.[3]

E. **Heat tolerance**
1. Adaptations that occur with heat acclimatization include decreased heart rate, decreased rectal temperature, increased plasma volume, and increased sweat rate.
2. Heat tolerance depends more on cardiovascular fitness than gender.
3. Young girls tolerate exercise in hot climates less effectively than adult women because of the former's larger surface area to body mass ratio and slower onset of sweating and sweating rate.

VI. ENDOCRINOLOGY

A. **Menarche**
1. The median age at menarche in the U.S. is 12.8 years for white girls and 12.5 for black girls.

    2. Athletes tend to have a later menarcheal age than nonathletes. To date, the evidence suggesting that training delays maturation of girls is not convincing.

B. Menstrual cycle physiologic changes

    1. The most consistent variation is the rise in basal body temperature during luteal phase.

    2. Hormonal fluctuations do not influence exercise heat tolerance.

    3. No conclusive evidence that menstrual cycle phase affects physical performance.

C. Amenorrhea

    1. Athletes have a high prevalence of amenorrhrea.

    2. The etiology remains unknown.

    3. The extreme pressure to have a low body fat has resulted in a high prevalence of disordered eating among athletes. Is the amenorrhea related to exercise or is the amenorrhea a symptom of an eating disorder?

D. Pregnancy

    1. Some physiologic changes that occur during pregnancy are increases in oxygen demand, blood volume, cardiac output, vascular conductance, metabolic rate, minute ventilation, insulin resistance, and body weight.

    2. While the exercise prescription should always be individualized, the following recommendations were made by a recent meta-analysis of the literature[8]: a variety of exercise modes performed approximately 40 min/day, 3 times/week, at a heart rate of 144 bpm appeared safe for both mother and fetus.

REFERENCES

1. Artal RM, Wiswell RA, Drinkwater BL (eds): Exercise in Pregnancy, 2nd ed. Baltimore, Williams & Wilkins, 1991.
2. Blair SN, Goodyear NN, Gibbons LW, Cooper KH: Fitness and hypertension in men and women. JAMA 252:487–490, 1984.
3. Blair SN, Kohl HW, Parrenbarger RS, et al: Physical fitness and all-cause mortality. JAMA 262:2395–2401, 1989.
4. Comroe JH, Forster RE, DuBois AB, et al: The Lung: Clinical Physiology and Pulmonary Function Tests, 2nd ed. Chicago, Year Book Medical Publishers, 1962.
5. Cureton KJ, Collins MA, Hill DW, McElhannon FM: Muscle hypertrophy in men and women. Med Sci Sports Exerc 20:338–344, 1988.
6. Eichner ER: The anemias of athletes. Phys Sportsmed 14(9):122–130, 1986.
7. Komi PV (ed): Strength and Power in Sport. Oxford, Blackwell Scientific Publications, 1992.
8. Lokey EA, Tran ZV, Wells CL, et al: Effects of physical exercise on pregnancy outcomes: A meta-analytic review. Med Sci Sports Exerc 23:1234–1239, 1991.
9. Lowrey GH: Growth and Development of Children, 6th ed. Chicago, Year Book Medical Publishers, 1973.
10. Masaro E (ed): Handbook of Physiology in Aging. Boca Raton, FL, CRC Press, 1981.
11. Shangold MM, Mirkin G: Women and Exercise: Physiology and Sports Medicine. Philadelphia, F.A. Davis, 1988.
12. Snyder AC, Dvorak LL, Roepke JB: Influence of dietary iron source on measures of iron status among female runners. Med Sci Sports Exerc 21:7–10, 1989.
13. Wells CL: Women, Sport, and Performance, 2nd ed. Champaign, IL, Human Kinetics Books, 1991.
14. Williford HN, Scharff-Olson M, Blessing DL: Exercise prescription for women. Sports Med 15:299–311, 1993.
15. Wintrobe MM, Lee GR, Boggs DR, et al: Clinical Hematology, 6th ed. Philadelphia, Lea & Febiger, 1967.
16. Tanner JM: Growth at Adolescence, 2nd ed. Oxford, Blackwell Scientific Publications, 1962.
17. Tremblay A, Despres JP, Bouchard C: The effects of exercise-training on energy balance and adipose tissue morphology and metabolism. Sports Med 2:223–233, 1985.

PART II
GENERAL CONSIDERATIONS

Chapter 5: Women, Activity, and Health Profiles and Healthy People 2000

KIMBERLY K. YEAGER, MD, MPH
CAROL MACERA, PhD

I. HISTORICAL PERSPECTIVE

A. Societal myths

Women have not been the focus of health promotion efforts or epidemiologic studies in the area of physical activity for a number of reasons. This has to do in some part with societal bias against women being active, as evidenced by the following historical notes[10]:

1. Competition was not considered ladylike (better to look good than to win); women were encouraged to focus on the "joy" of the game, not on winning.
2. Women who participated in sports were thought to develop a masculine appearance.
3. When women first began to play competitive sports (i.e., basketball in 1896), only other women were allowed to watch.
4. Women were thought to be unable to withstand prolonged mental and physical strain; they had to overcome the stereotype of "needing protection."

Now that there is significant evidence to support the role of physical activity in the prevention of several chronic diseases and conditions, it is imperative that women are encouraged to be active and that the gender-specific benefits and risks of physical activity are studied.

B. Scientific literature

In 1953, Morris et al.[17] published the first article that linked occupational activity to risk of death from coronary heart disease (CHD). Before 1970, most studies examined occupational physical activity, but since then, most have examined leisure-time physical activity.[18] By definition, the early studies excluded women, although more recent studies have included them (Table 1).

II. PHYSICAL ACTIVITY: AN ISSUE ON THE HEALTH AGENDA FOR THE 1990s

A. Definitions

1. **Physical activity** is a complex and multidimensional behavior that involves bodily movement, results in energy expenditure, and is correlated with physical fitness.
2. **Sedentary behavior** is defined as no leisure-time physical activity.
3. **Irregular activity** is defined as leisure-time physical activity <3 times/week.
4. **Sedentary lifestyle** is defined as either no leisure-time physical activity or irregular (sporadic) physical activity (<3 sessions/week).
5. **Regular activity** is defined as leisure-time physical activity at least 3 times/week. This category can be subdivided into **low-intensity** or **high-intensity** activity depending on the age of the person.

TABLE 1.   Summary of Epidemiologic Studies of Physical Activity and
Coronary Heart Disease (CHD) in Women

Study Location	Outcome	Findings
Framingham, Mass. (Kannel et al.,[11] 1979)	CHD mortality	No relationship
Netherlands (Magnus et al.,[16] 1979)	CHD	Strong relationship
North Karelia, Finland (Salonen et al.,[21] 1982)	Myocardial infarction	Equivocal
Gothenburg, Sweden (Lapidus et al.,[13] 1986)	Myocardial infarction ECG changes	No relationship

B. **Costs of a sedentary lifestyle**
1. More than half of the women in the U.S. (approximately 60% in 1988[4]) are not physically active on a regular basis.
2. Sedentary individuals are twice as likely to develop coronary heart disease as people who engage in regular physical activity.[18]
3. Physical inactivity is the only modifiable risk factor for coronary heart disease that has increased in prevalence over the past decade.
4. Cardiovascular disease accounts for $136 billion annually in health care costs and lost productivity in the U.S. Women consume 58% of the almost $60 million spent directly on cardiovascular disease-related health care (1985 figure) and 61% of the health care dollars spent on the care of patients with cardiovascular disease over 65 years.[23]

C. **The health dividend**
1. Evidence of the multiple benefits of regular physical activity is extensive and mounting. Regular physical activity can aid in the **prevention and management** of:
    a. coronary heart disease[15,16,18,20]
    b. hypertension[1]
    c. non-insulin-dependent diabetes[9]
    d. osteoporosis[9]
    e. obesity[9]
    f. depression and anxiety[6]
    It has also been associated with lower rates of colon, breast, and certain reproductive cancers[7,12] and stroke,[21] and it may be linked to reduced rates of lower back injury.[3]
2. With the growing **elderly population,** the majority of whom are women, there is an increasing need to enhance the opportunities and capabilities for functional independence and to improve musculoskeletal integrity to prevent falls and the associated morbidity. Physical activity plays a crucial role in these areas for those over age 65.[2,5,14]

D. **Physical activity: The nation's call to action**
1. The Centers for Disease Control and Prevention (CDC) provides overall scientific leadership in promoting physical activity and applied epidemiology, specifically in the areas of behavior change and risk factor modification as they relate to health outcomes. Since 1983, the CDC has provided scientific leadership in defining the role of physical activity in health and in conducting surveillance of this important behavior.
2. The U.S. Preventive Services Task Force issued a report entitled *Guide to Clinical Preventive Medicine Services* in May 1989, recommending:
    a. "Clinicians should counsel all patients to engage in a program of regular physical activity, tailored to their health status and personal lifestyle."

      b. For women, special emphasis was placed on **weight-bearing activities** to prevent osteoporosis and **moderate activity** to enhance weight-control efforts and to prevent and/or treat depression and reduce anxiety.

      c. This report also emphasized the importance of regular physical activity for women in the prevention and management of coronary heart disease, non-insulin-dependent diabetes, and hypertension, even though most of the data in these areas have been collected on men.

3. Office of Disease Prevention and Health Promotion, in September 1990 released *Healthy People 2000*, which summarizes the health objectives for the nation for the year 2000. The priority area of "physical activity and fitness" plays a prominent role. The objectives include:

      a. Increase to at least 30% the proportion of people aged 6 and older who engage regularly, preferably daily, in **light to moderate physical activity** for at least 30 min/day. (*Baseline:* 22% of people aged 18 and older were active for at least 30 minutes 5 or more times/week and 12% were active 7 or more times/week in 1985.)

      b. Increase to at least 20% the proportion of people aged 18 and older and to at least 75% the proportion of children and adolescents aged 6–17 who engage in **vigorous physical activity** that promotes the development and maintenance of cardiorespiratory fitness 3 or more days/week for 20 or more minutes per occasion. (*Baseline:* 12% of people aged 18 and older were active at this level in 1985; 66% of youth aged 10–17 in 1984.)

      c. Reduce to no more than 15% the proportion of people aged 6 and older who engage in **no leisure-time physical activity.** (*Baseline:* 24% for people aged 18 and older in 1985.)

      d. Increase to at least 40% the proportion of people aged 6 and older who **regularly perform physical activities** that enhance and maintain muscular strength, muscular endurance, and flexibility. (*Baseline:* data not available.)

      e. Increase to at least 50% the proportion of overweight people aged 12 and older who have adopted **sound dietary practices combined with regular physical activity** to attain an appropriate body weight. (*Baseline:* 30% of overweight women and 25% of overweight men for people aged 18 and older in 1985.)

      f. Increase to at least 50% the proportion of children and adolescents in grades 1–12 who participate in **daily school physical education.** (*Baseline:* 36% in 1984–86.)

      g. Increase to at least 50% the proportion of **school physical education class time** that students spend being physically active, preferably engaged in lifetime physical activities. (*Baseline:* Students spent an estimated 27% of class time being physically active in 1984.)

      h. Increase the proportion of worksites offering **employer-sponsored physical activity** and fitness programs.

      i. Increase **community availability** and accessibility of physical activity and fitness facilities.

      j. Increase to at least 50% the proportion of **primary care providers** who routinely assess and counsel their patients regarding the frequency, duration, type, and intensity of physical activity practices. (*Baseline:* Physicians provided exercise counseling for about 30% of sedentary patients in 1988.)

III. WOMEN AND PHYSICAL ACTIVITY: CURRENT STATUS

A. Prevalence estimates

1. Prevalence estimates were obtained from the 1988 Behavioral Risk Factor Surveillance System (BRFSS), a cooperative project between the CDC and state health departments. Thirty-seven states participated in the 1988 survey (32,852

women). The methodology of data collection and developing national estimates is discussed elsewhere.[8]

2. Physical activity levels are grouped into three categories:
   a. Sedentary (no reported physical activity)
   b. Irregular (occasional physical activity)
   c. Regular (physical activity sessions at least 3 times/week
   Sedentary lifestyle is typically defined as a combination of the first two categories (*see* section IIA).

3. Overall, the prevalence of sedentary behavior among women in 1988 was 32% and the prevalence of sedentary lifestyle was 59%, but subgroup variation was apparent (*see below*).

B. **Demographic profiles**
   1. Table 2 presents physical activity status by demographic characteristics (including ethnicity, age, and marital status).

C. **Activities preferred by women**
   1. Based on 1988 BRFSS data, the top five activities reported by active women and their frequency are:
      a. Walking   41.1%
      b. Gardening   8.6%
      c. Aerobics   8.3%
      d. Bicycling   5.3%
      e. Running   4.0%

D. **Health status profiles**
   1. Table 3 summarizes, by physical activity level, some key health status indicators of women. These are self-reported health status parameters from the 1988 BRFSS.

IV. CONCLUSIONS

A. **Summary**
   1. The historical, societal and scientific emphasis on the behavior of physical activity in sport and health has focused primarily on men, with women gaining recognition only recently.

TABLE 2.   Prevalence Estimates of Physical Activity Levels in U.S. Women by Ethnicity, Age, and Marital Status*

	No.[†]	Sedentary (%)	Irregular (%)	Regular (%)
Total	32,852	31.7	27.0	41.3
Ethnicity				
White	27,339	29.5	27.1	43.3
Black	2,902	44.9	25.5	29.6
Hispanic	1,415	36.4	28.4	35.2
Other	1,178	36.0	25.9	38.1
Age				
18–34	11,128	25.9	28.9	43.2
35–50	8,578	28.1	27.7	44.2
51–64	5,954	35.6	26.0	30.4
65+	7,192	44.3	23.4	32.3
Marital status				
Single	4,644	24.3	28.5	41.2
Married	17,375	30.5	26.9	42.6
Separated/widowed Divorced	10,369	39.7	26.7	33.6

[†] Sample size for all female respondents. Column totals may not equal the total sample due to missing data.

* Estimates are based on 1988 BRFSS data.

TABLE 3.   Prevalence Estimates of Selected Health Status Indicators by Physical Activity Levels in U.S. Women

	Sedentary (%)	Regular* (%)
Hypertension	24.6	14.7
High cholesterol	22.0	20.1
Obesity	28.6	16.5
Smoking	26.4	22.0
Diabetes	8.2	4.1

* This category includes those women who are regularly active at a low intensity.

2. There is increasing emphasis on the promotion of physical activity within the public health arena as evidence continues to mount regarding the numerous health benefits of a regular physical activity program.
3. The majority of women (59%) responding to the 1988 BRFSS are not physically active on a regular basis.
4. Women were more likely to report a sedentary lifestyle at older ages, especially if they are not white.
5. Less than 10% of women in our sample report an activity level adequate to allow for the improvement and maintenance of cardiorespiratory fitness.
6. Women who are regularly active may have an improved health risk profile compared to those who perform little or no physical activity. Specifically, highly active women report less obesity and lower rates of smoking as compared to less active and nonactive women.

B. **Recommendations**
1. Evaluating potential barriers, for women, to becoming more physically active is necessary to facilitate the design of physical activity promotion strategies and interventions.
2. The Year 2000 objectives and the U.S. Preventive Services Task Force recommendations provide direction for increased clinical and public health efforts in the area of physical activity promotion.
3. The medical and public health communities should collectively seek greater resources for additional research to better clarify the health benefits and risks of physical activity for women.

REFERENCES

1. Blair SN, Goodyear NN, Gibbons LW, Cooper KH: Physical fitness and incidence of hypertension in healthy normotensive men and women. JAMA 252:487–490, 1984.
2. Bortz WM: Disuse and aging. JAMA 248:1203–1208, 1982.
3. Cady LD, Bischoff DP, O'Connell ER, et al: Strength and fitness and subsequent back injuries in firefighters. J Occup Med 21:269–272, 1979.
4. Centers for Disease Control: Coronary heart disease attributable to sedentary lifestyle—selected states, 1988. MMWR 39(32):541–544, 1990.
5. deVries HA: Physiology of exercise and aging. In Woodruff DS, Birren JE (eds): Aging: Scientific Perspectives and Social Issues. Monterey, CA, Brooks/Cole, 1983, pp 285–304.
6. Farmer ME, Locke BZ, Moscicki EM, et al: Physical activity and depressive symptoms: The NHANES I epidemiologic follow-up study. Am J Epidemiol 128:1340–1351, 1988.
7. Frisch RE, Wyshad G, Albright NL, et al: Lower lifetime occurrence of breast cancer and cancers of the reproductive system among former college athletes. Am J Clin Nutr 45:328–335, 1987.
8. Gentry EM, Kalsbeek WD, Hogelin GC, et al: The behavioral risk factor surveys: II. Design, methods, and estimates from combined state data. Am J Prev Med 1(6):9–14, 1985.
9. Harris SS, Caspersen CJ, DeFreise GH, Estes EH: Physical activity counseling for healthy adults as a primary preventive intervention in the clinical setting. JAMA 261:3590–3598, 1989.
10. Henderson KA, Bialeschki MD, Shaw SM, Freysinger VJ: A Leisure of One's Own: A Feminist Perspective on Women's Leisure. State College, PA, Venture Publishing, 1989, pp 34–43.

11. Kannel WB, Sorlie P: Some health benefits of physical activity—The Framingham study. Arch Intern Med 139:857-861, 1979.
12. Kohl HW, LaPorte RE, Blair SN: Physical activity and cancer: An epidemiological perspective. Sports Med 6:222-237, 1988.
13. Lapidus L, Bengtsson C: Socioeconomic factors and physical activity in relation to cardiovascular disease and death: A 12 year follow up of participants in a population study of women in Gothenburg, Sweden. Br Heart J 55:295-301, 1986.
14. Larson EB, Bruce RA: Health benefits of exercise in an aging society. Arch Intern Med 147:353-356, 1987.
15. Leon AS, Connett J, Jacobs DR, Rauramaa R: Leisure time physical activity levels and risk of coronary heart disease and death: The multiple risk factor intervention trial. JAMA 258:2388-2395, 1987.
16. Magnus K, Matroos A, Strackee J: Walking, cycling, or gardening, with or without seasonal interruption, in relation to acute coronary events. Am J Epidemiol 110:724-733, 1979.
17. Morris JN, Heady JA, Raffle PAB, et al: Coronary heart disease and physical activity of work. Lancet ii:1053-1057 and 1111-1120, 1953.
18. Powell KE, Thompson PD, Caspersen CJ, Kendrick JS: Physical activity and the incidence of coronary heart disease. Annu Rev Public Health 8:253-287, 1987.
19. Public Health Service: Healthy People 2000: National Health Promotion and Disease Prevention Objectives. Washington, DC, US Department of Health and Human Services, Public Health Service, 1990.
20. Sallis JF, Haskell WL, Fortmann SP, et al: Moderate-intensity physical activity and cardiovascular risk factors: The Stanford five-city project. Prev Med 15:561-568, 1986.
21. Salonen JT, Puska P, Tuomilehto J: Physical activity and risk of myocardial infarction, cerebral stroke and death: A longitudinal study in Eastern Finland. Am J Epidemiol 115:526-537, 1982.
22. United States Preventive Services Task Force: Guide to Clinical Preventive Medicine Services. Baltimore, Williams & Wilkins, 1989.
23. Yeager KK, Macera CA, Merritt RK: Socioeconomic influences on leisure-time sedentary behavior among women. Health Values 17:50-54, 1993.

Chapter 6: Preseason Sports Examination for Women

MIMI D. JOHNSON, MD

Female athletes of all ages may benefit from a preseason sports physical. The physician will typically see junior-high, high-school and college-level athletes for this examination, as it is often required for sports participation. This chapter discusses the preseason physical examination in women athletes in these age groups.

I. **GENERAL CONSIDERATIONS**
   A. **Purpose:** The goal of the preseason sports physical is to reduce the risk of sports-related injury or death by identifying predisposing physical conditions, recommending appropriate rehabilitation and treatment, and counseling the athlete about sports in which she may safely participate.
      1. **Specific objectives of the examination**
         a. Determine the general health of the athlete
         b. Assess maturity
         c. Disclose defects that may limit participation
         d. Detect conditions that might predispose the athlete to injury (untreated injuries or illness, lack of conditioning, or congenital/developmental problems)
         e. Institute treatment that will bring the athlete to the optimal level of performance before the season begins
         f. Provide opportunities for persons who have physiologic or pathologic conditions that restrict them from unlimited participation in all sports to compete in activities appropriate for them
         g. Provide an opportunity to counsel youths and answer personal and health questions
         h. Assess the athlete's motivation for sports participation
         i. Acquaint the athlete with the local sports medicine system and establish a doctor-patient relationship that may continue if the need arises
         j. Meet legal and insurance requirements
      2. **Physician attributes** helpful in determining fitness of athletes for specific sports:
         a. Knowledge of the athletic profile of a sport
            i. Strength requirements
            ii. Flexibility requirements
            iii. Aerobic/anaerobic power utilized
         b. Knowledge of potential factors contributing to injury
         c. Knowledge of injuries commonly occurring in specific sports
         d. Knowledge of classification of sports
   B. **Type of examination**
      1. **Station-type mass examination:** Involving specialized personnel in sports medicine, athletic training, physical therapy, nutrition, and exercise physiology
         a. Time efficient
         b. Cost efficient
      2. **Office examination:** Provides opportunity for preventive health care and counseling on personal and health issues

C. **Timing and frequency of examination**
1. The preseason physical should take place 4–6 weeks before the season starts to allow time to further evaluate abnormal findings and rehabilitate musculoskeletal deficiencies.
2. One full examination should be performed at each school-entry level (i.e., junior high, high school), with an annual history and limited physical examination (to evaluate any sequelae from illnesses or injuries that occurred in the previous year) during intervening years.

II. DEVELOPMENTAL ISSUES IN FEMALE ATHLETES

Anatomic and physiologic changes which occur during adolescence can influence the injuries sustained while participating in sports. It is helpful to understand the changes that take place during puberty, not only to understand the etiology of some injuries but also to counsel young athletes on future expectations and avoidance of specific injuries.

A. **Pubertal growth**
1. Accounts for 20–25% of final adult height. Average growth spurt lasts 24–36 months.
2. Peak height velocity occurs about 18–24 months earlier in females than in males.
3. Pubertal weight gain accounts for 50% of an individual's ideal adult body weight. Peak weight velocity occurs 6–9 months after peak height velocity.
4. Menarche occurs 3.3 years after the start of the growth spurt and 1.11 years after peak height velocity.
5. Growth after menarche is limited and averages 7.4 cm, ranging from 4.3 cm at the 10th percentile to 10.6 cm at the 90th percentile.

B. **Strength** is not a meaningful indicator of maturity in girls.
1. The apex of strength occurs most often after peak height velocity and precedes peak weight gain in more than 50% of all girls.
2. Early maturers are stronger than late maturers at the same chronologic age, until 16–17 years of age, when the differences resolve.

C. **Maturity staging** in adolescent females
1. Not helpful in "matching" girls for sports
2. Can be helpful in counseling an athlete on general weight, height, and developmental expectations (Fig. 1).

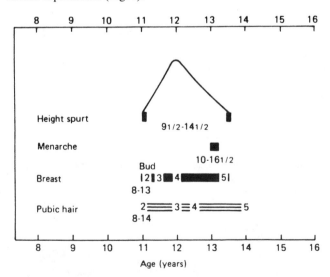

FIGURE 1. Biological maturity in girls. (From Tanner JM: Growth at Adolescence, 2nd ed. Oxford, Blackwell Scientific Publications, 1962; with permission.)

D. **Anatomic changes during puberty may predispose the athlete to injury.**
   1. Rapid growth, as in the growth spurt, leads to a decrease in flexibility, resulting in muscle-tendon imbalance and increased risk for injury.
   2. The growth cartilage at the epiphyseal plate, the joint surface, and the apophyseal insertions of the major muscle-tendon units are at increased risk for injury.
      a. Repetitive forces at the epiphyseal plate may cause damage, such as irregularity, widening, and premature closure of the distal radial physis in young gymnasts.
      b. Osteochondritis dissecans may be associated with repetitive forces at the joint surface.
      c. Tight muscle-tendon units may exacerbate traction apophysitis, most commonly seen at the tibial tubercle (Osgood-Schlatter disease) and at the calcaneus (Sever's disease).
   3. Many athletes are exposed to sport—and its associated repetitive stresses—for the first time during the growth spurt. The physician who is aware that the athlete is entering or going through a growth spurt can offer appropriate guidance toward increased flexibility.

III. SPORT-SPECIFIC INJURIES IN FEMALES

A. Most injuries in female athletes are sport-specific rather than sex-specific.
B. Specific musculoskeletal areas are more prone to injury in particular sports. These areas should be tested in the athlete during the musculoskeletal examination.
   1. Ballet: Feet, ankles, spine, knees, hips
   2. Basketball: Ankles, knees, feet, shoulders
   3. Gymnastics: Ankles, knees, spine, wrists, shoulders, elbows
   4. Ice skating: Ankles, spine, shins, feet
   5. Racquet sports: Shoulders, elbows, wrists, knees, ankles, feet
   6. Rowing: Spine, achilles, hands, wrists, shoulders, elbows, knees
   7. Soccer: Ankles, knees, feet, shins, hips, pelvis, neck, thighs
   8. Softball: Shoulders, elbows, ankles, knees
   9. Swimming: Shoulders
   10. Track/cross-country: Knees, ankles, feet, shins, hips, shoulders (javelin, shotput)
   11. Volleyball: ankles, knees, shoulders, hands

IV. COMMON INJURIES IN FEMALE ATHLETES

Because of anatomic variations, some injuries occur with a greater frequency in women than in men.
A. **Patellofemoral stress syndrome**
   1. Due to lateral patellar tracking, which can result from greater valgus angulation of the knee, femoral anteversion, and increased foot pronation.
   2. On knee examination, note patellar laxity and tracking during active and passive extension.
      a. If the patella tracks laterally, the athlete should strengthen the vastus medialis obliquus and stretch the lower extremity musculature.
      b. If foot pronation is present, orthotics may be beneficial.
B. **Rotator cuff injuries**
   1. Increased shoulder laxity and decreased strength of the rotator cuff muscles can lead to shoulder subluxation/dislocation or rotator cuff overuse injuries.
   2. Seen particularly in the throwing, hitting, or swimming athlete.
C. **Ankle injuries**
   1. Women have a higher risk of ankle sprains than men.
   2. Women involved in sports played on uneven ground (field hockey, soccer, softball) and sports that involve jumping (basketball, volleyball) should be encouraged to perform ankle strengthening and proprioceptive exercises, and Achilles tendon stretches.

D. **Overuse injuries of the lumbar spine**
   1. Women are often involved in sports that encourage increased lumbar lordosis (i.e., gymnastics, ballet, ice skating).
   2. As these can lead to overuse injuries of the lumbar spine, such as spondylolysis, abdominal and paravertebral muscle strengthening, along with hamstring and hip flexor stretching, should be encouraged.
E. **Foot pain**
   1. Women often have a predisposition for the development of bunions, corns and retrocalcaneal bursitis.
   2. To prevent development or worsening of these conditions, women should be counseled on appropriate footwear.

V. **MEDICAL HISTORY**

The medical history is the most important component of the preseason physical examination, identifying 63–74% of all problems. To increase accuracy, both parents and athlete should fill out the history form.

A. **General medical history**
   1. General health
   2. Past hospitalizations and surgeries
   3. Chronic disease
   4. Medication use
   5. Allergies
   6. Immunization status
   7. Missing organs
B. **Sport-specific history**
   1. **Respiratory:** To evaluate for exercise-induced bronchospasm, the athlete should be asked if she ever experiences wheezing or coughing during or after exercise.
   2. **Cardiac**
      a. History of sudden cardiac death or cardiac problems in family members <50 years of age might warrant further evaluation.
      b. Has she ever passed out during exercise or stopped exercising due to dizziness, chest pain, or palpitations?
      c. Has she ever been told she had a heart murmur, click, extra heart beat, high blood pressure, or heart abnormality?
   3. **Neurologic:** A positive history of concussion necessitates a thorough neurologic exam.
   4. **Heat-related illness:** It is unknown whether this is due to inability to dissipate heat or to poor aerobic conditioning. Questions about fluid replacement and fitness would be appropriate in an athlete with previous history of problems with heat.
   5. **Protective equipment:** The athlete should be questioned about eyewear and use of protective equipment.
   6. **Musculoskeletal**
      a. Focus on previous history of injuries and pain which limits exercise. Unrehabilitated previous injuries are strong predictors of subsequent injuries.
         i. Previous stress fractures should prompt questions about menstrual patterns.
         ii. History of scoliosis, which is more common in females, should be obtained. Scoliosis should be monitored until growth is complete.
         iii. History of recent growth spurt alerts the physician to look for growth-related injuries.
      b. Look also for training errors, poor alignment, muscular imbalance, or equipment misuse as possible causes of a prior injury.

C. **Female-specific history** (Fig. 2)
 1. **Menstrual and gynecologic history**
    a. **Age of menarche:** If the athlete is 14 years of age and prepubertal, or 16 years of age and premenarchal, she should be evaluated for primary amenorrhea.
    b. **Length and frequency of periods**
    c. **Date of last menstrual period:** If the athlete has not had a period in the previous 6 months or has missed 3 of her usual cycle intervals, she should be evaluated for secondary amenorrhea and encouraged to undergo treatment.
    d. **Amount of flow:** If heavy, could result in anemia.
    e. **Dysmenorrhea:** May interfere with sports participation and can often be treated adequately with antiprostaglandin therapy.

Name: _____ Age: _____

Directions: Please answer the following questions to the best of your ability.

 1. How old were you when you had your first menstrual period? _____
 2. How often do you have a period? _____
 3. How long do your periods last? _____
 4. How many periods have you had in the last year? _____
 5. When was your last period? _____
 6. Do you ever have trouble with heavy bleeding? _____
 7. Do you have questions about tampon use? _____
 8. Do you ever experience cramps during your period? _____
    If so, how do you treat them? _____
 9. Are you on birth control pills or hormones? _____
10. Do you have any unusual discharge from your vagina? _____
11. When was your last pelvic exam? _____
12. Have you ever had an abnormal Pap smear? _____
13. How many urinary tract infections (bladder or kidney) have you had? _____
14. Have you ever been treated for anemia? _____
15. How many meals do you eat each day? _____ How many snacks? _____
16. What have you eaten in the last 24 hours? _____
    _____
17. Are there certain food groups you refuse to eat (meats, breads, etc.)? _____
    _____
18. Have you ever been on a diet? _____
19. What is your present weight? _____
20. Are you happy with this weight? _____ If not, what would you like to weigh? _____
21. Have you ever tried to lose weight by vomiting? _____
    Using laxatives? _____ Diuretics? _____
    Diet pills? _____
22. Have you ever been diagnosed as having an eating disorder? _____
23. Do you have questions about healthy ways to control your weight? _____
24. How often do you drink alcohol? _____
25. How often do you use drugs? _____
    Smoke cigarettes? _____
26. Do you wear your seat belt when in a car? _____
27. Do you wear a helmet when you bike? _____
28. Do you have any questions about health or personal issues? _____
29. Do you own any guns? _____

FIGURE 2. Health history for the female athlete.

    f. **Oral contraceptive or hormonal therapy**

    g. **Date of last pelvic exam:** If the athlete is 18 years of age or older, or has been sexually active, she should be encouraged to undergo a pelvic examination.

    h. **Unusual vaginal discharge**

    i. **Abnormal Pap smears**

    j. **Urinary tract infections:** Some athletes tend to restrict fluids which could aggravate urinary tract infection.

    k. **Breast support:** Adequate support should be encouraged, especially in running and jumping athletes. A good sports bra is firm, made mostly of nonelastic material, and has good absorptive qualities (*see* Chapter 18).

    l. **Tampon use:** Young athletes may have questions about tampon use during sports activity. Their use in sports is appropriate as long as they are changed frequently.

2. **History of eating patterns**

    a. All female athletes, particularly those with menstrual irregularities, should be questioned about eating patterns. Up to 32% of college female athletes are involved in disordered eating patterns (*see* Chapter 20).

    b. Eating patterns

        i. Number of meals and snacks per day

        ii. 24-hour food recall

        iii. Avoidance of certain food groups

        iv. Satisfaction with present weight

        v. What does the athlete consider to be her ideal weight?

        vi. Use of dieting, vomiting, laxatives, diuretics, or diet pills to lose weight

    c. If disordered eating is suspected, it should be evaluated further and treatment begun by a nutritionist, physician, and therapist trained in the management of eating disorders.

    d. With appropriate questioning, it may be determined that the young athlete is having concerns about weight control. Detected early, this athlete can be counseled about healthy weight control, and dissuaded from disordered eating patterns.

D. **Health habits:** Other health concerns can be discussed during the office exam, with an opportunity for the patient to ask questions about these or other issues.

1. Drug and alcohol use
2. Cigarette use
3. Unprotected sexual activity
4. Seat belt and helmet use
5. Guns

VI. PHYSICAL EXAMINATION

A. **General assessment:** An assessment of body habitus will include:

1. Initial estimation of maturity
2. Nutritional status
3. Body fat
4. Presence of any syndromic features, such as those of Marfan syndrome

B. **Vital signs**

1. **Height and weight:** Used for evaluating overall growth and development, and nutritional status.

2. **Resting heart rate:** Suggests cardiovascular fitness and may be abnormal in anemia, cardiac disorders, drug use, and anorexia nervosa (heart rate <50 beats/min).

3. **Blood pressure:** Upper limits of normal for the athlete 11 years or younger is 130/75 mm Hg and for 12 years or older, 140/85. To confirm elevated blood pressure, three abnormal measurements should be found on different occasions.

TABLE 1. Classification of Sexual Maturity Staging in Girls*

Stage	Pubic Hair	Breasts
1	None	Prepubertal. No glandular tissue
2	Sparse, long, straight, lightly pigmented on labia majora	Breast bud. Small amount of glandular tissue
3	Darker, beginning to curl, extend laterally	Breast mound and areola enlarged, no contour separation
4	Coarse, curly, abundant, less than adult	Breast enlarged, areola and papilla form mound projecting from breast contour
5	Adult type and quantity, extending to medial thigh	Mature, areola part of breast contour

* Adapted from Tanner JM: Growth at Adolescence, 2nd ed. Oxford, Blackwell Scientific Publications, 1962, pp 28–39.

   C. **HEENT examination**
      1. Assessment of visual acuity and evaluation for anisocoria, especially in contact athletes
      2. Evaluation for otitis externa and tympanic membrane perforation (in swimmers and divers)
   D. **Respiratory examination**
      1. May be helpful in the athlete with symptoms of atopy and exercise-induced bronchospasm
   E. **Cardiovascular examination**
      1. Palpation of radial and femoral pulses
      2. Inspection, palpation, and auscultation of the heart
      3. Approximately one-third of all adolescents will have an audible murmur. If the murmur is considered functional or physiologic, no further evaluation is necessary. If the murmur is abnormal or greater than grade II/VI, a cardiologist should be consulted.
   F. **Abdominal examination**
      1. In athlete with recent history of Epstein-Barr infection, viral illness, or hematologic disorder, check for enlargement of liver and spleen.
   G. **Pubertal staging**
      1. Appropriate in pubescent athlete (Table 1)
      2. If the sports physical is part of the annual physical examination, a breast examination can be performed, with instructions on self-examination.
   H. **Skin examination**
      1. Check for infectious skin disease (herpes, scabies, impetigo, boils).
   I. **Neurologic examination**
      1. If there is a history of concussion, a thorough neurologic evaluation is required.
   J. **Musculoskeletal examination**
      1. Include a general assessment for all athletes (Table 2).
      2. Focus on areas most prone to injury:
         a. Areas of previous injury or pain: Check for residual swelling, laxity (if joint), pain, or weakness. Compare to opposite extremity.
         b. Areas of increased risk for the athlete's specific sport (*see* section III above): Test for general strength and flexibility
      3. Check joint stability and record for future comparison if injury occurs.

VII. **LABORATORY ASSESSMENT**

   Although most school physical forms require a hematocrit or urinalysis, neither has been found to identify an athlete who warrants disqualification. If an athlete complains of fatigue or increased menstrual flow or has a history of anemia, then hematocrit, hemoglobin, and serum ferritin should be measured.

TABLE 2.   The Two-minute Orthopedic Examination

Figure*	Instructions	Observations
3	Stand facing examiner	Acromioclavicular joints, general habitus
4	Look at ceiling, floor, over both shoulders; touch ears to shoulders	Cervical spine motion
5	Shrug shoulders (examiner resists)	Trapezius strength
6	Abduct shoulders 90° (examiner resists at 90°)	Deltoid strength
7	Full external rotation of arms	Shoulder motion
8	Flex and extend elbows	Elbow motion
9	Arms at sides, elbows 90° flexed; pronate and supinate wrists	Elbow and wrist motion
10	Spread fingers; make fist	Hand or finger motion and deformities
	Tighten (contract) quadriceps; relax quadriceps	Symmetry and knee effusion; ankle effusion
11	"Duck walk" four steps (away from examiner with buttocks on heels)	Hip, knee and ankle motion
12	Back to examiner	Shoulder symmetry, scoliosis
13	Knees straight, touch toes	Scoliosis, hip motion, hamstring tightness
14	Raise up on toes, raise heels	Calf symmetry, leg strength

* See figures 3–14 below and on following pages.
Reprinted with permission from Sports Medicine: Health Care for Young Athletes. Elk Grove, IL, American Academy of Pediatrics, 1991.

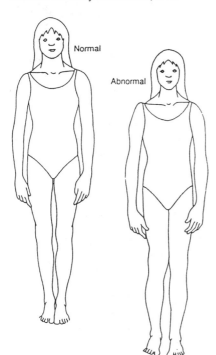

Stand straight with arms at sides.

Symmetry of upper and lower extremities and trunk.

Common abnormalities:
1. Enlarged acromioclavicular joint
2. Enlarged sternoclavicular joint
3. Asymmetrical waist (leg length difference or scoliosis)
4. Swollen knee
5. Swollen ankle

FIGURE 3

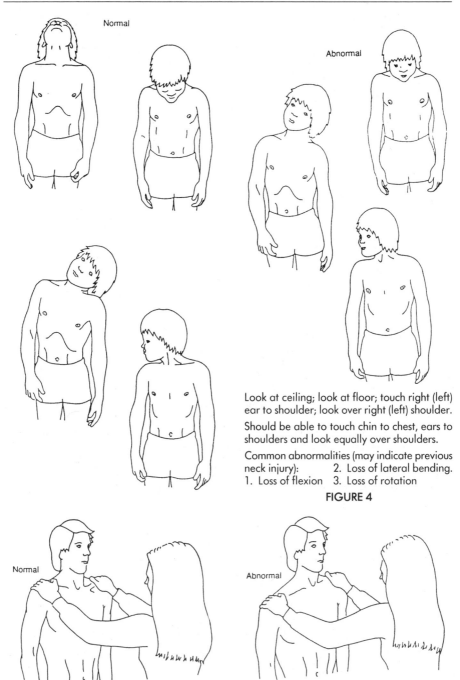

Look at ceiling; look at floor; touch right (left) ear to shoulder; look over right (left) shoulder.

Should be able to touch chin to chest, ears to shoulders and look equally over shoulders.

Common abnormalities (may indicate previous neck injury):   2. Loss of lateral bending.
1. Loss of flexion   3. Loss of rotation

FIGURE 4

Shrug shoulders while examiner holds them down.

Trapezius muscles appear equal; left and right sides equal strength.

Common abnormalities (may indicate neck or shoulder problem):
1. Loss of strength   2. Loss of muscle bulk

FIGURE 5

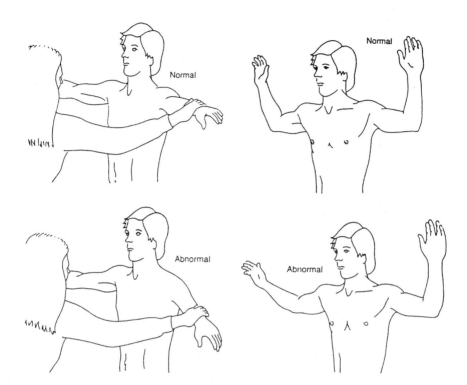

Hold arms out from sides horizontally and lift while examiner holds them down.

Strength should be equal and deltoid muscles should be equal in size.

Common abnormalities:
1. Loss of strength
2. Wasting of deltoid muscle

FIGURE 6

Hold arms out from sides with elbows bent (90°); raise hands back vertically as far as they will go.

Hands go back equally and at least to upright vertical position.

Common abnormalities (may indicate shoulder problem or old dislocation:
1. Loss of external rotation

FIGURE 7

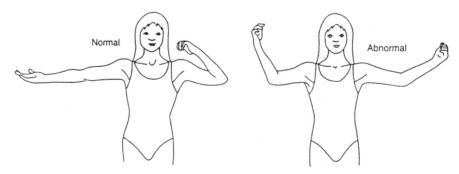

Hold arms out from sides, palms up; straighten elbows completely; bend completely.

Motion equal left and right.

Common abnormalities (may indicate old elbow injury, old dislocation, fracture, etc.):
1. Loss of extension   2. Loss of flexion

FIGURE 8

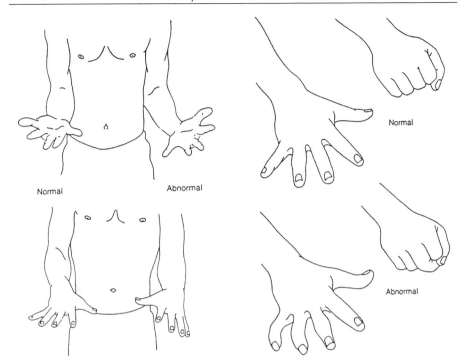

Hold arms down at sides with elbows bent (90°); supinate palms; pronate palms.

Palms should go from facing ceiling to facing floor.

Common abnormalities (may indicate old forearm, wrist, or elbow injury):
1. Lack of full supination
2. Lack of full pronation

FIGURE 9

Make a fist: open hand and spread fingers.

Fist should be tight and fingers straight when spread.

Common abnormalities (may indicate old finger fractures or sprains):
1. Protruding knuckle from fist
2. Swollen and/or crooked finger

FIGURE 10

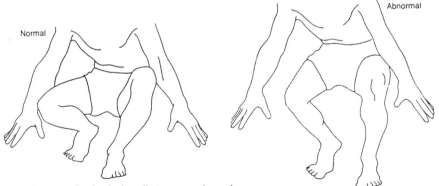

Squat on heels; duck walk 4 steps and stand up.

Maneuver is painless; heel to buttock distance equal left and right; knee flexion equal during walk; rises straight up.

Common abnormalities: 1. Inability to full flex one knee   2. Inability to stand up without twisting or bending to one side

FIGURE 11

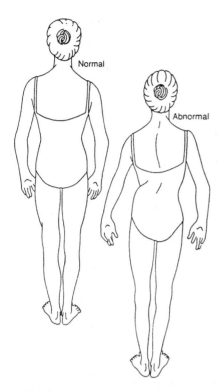

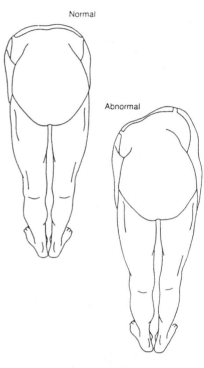

With back to examiner stand up straight.

Symmetry of shoulders, waist, thighs, and calves.

Common abnormalities:
1. High shoulder (scoliosis) or low shoulder (muscle loss)
2. Prominent rib cage (scoliosis)
3. High hip or asymmetrical waist (leg length difference or scoliosis)
4. Small calf or thigh (weakness from old injury)

FIGURE 12

Bend forward slowly as to touch toes.

Bend forward straightly and smoothly.

Common abnormalities:
1. Twists to side (low back pain)
2. Back asymmetrical (scoliosis)

FIGURE 13

VIII. **CLEARANCE TO PARTICIPATE**

    A. Based on the results of the preseason physical examination, the physician can make a disposition for the athlete's participation in sports. Options include:
        1. Clearance to participate in all sports
        2. Clearance deferred pending further evaluation, consultation, treatment, or rehabilitation
        3. Clearance for limited activities
        4. No clearance
    B. The American Academy of Pediatrics has issued guidelines for classification of sports as contact vs noncontact (Table 3) as well as recommendations for participation in sports for the athlete with limiting conditions (Table 4).

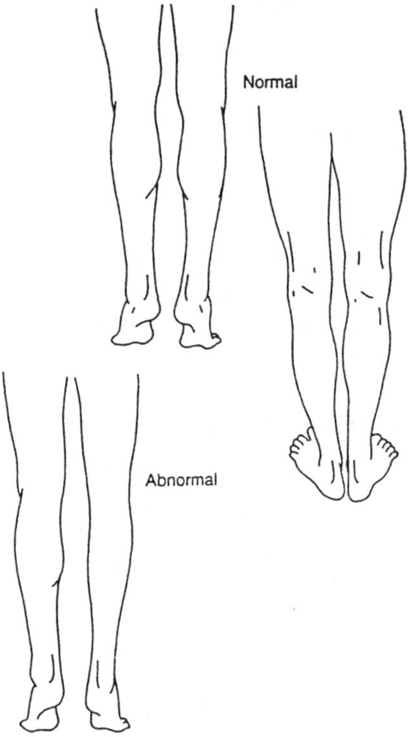

Stand on heels; stand on toes.

Equal elevation right and left; symmetry of calf muscles.

Common abnormalities:
1. Wasting of calf muscles (Achilles injury or old ankle injury)

FIGURE 14

Normal

Abnormal

TABLE 3. Classification of Sports as Contact vs Noncontact

Contact/Collision	Limited Contact/Impact	Noncontact		
		Strenuous	Moderately Strenuous	Nonstrenuous
Boxing	Baseball	Aerobic dancing	Badminton	Archery
Field hockey	Basketball	Crew	Curling	Golf
Football	Bicycling	Fencing	Table tennis	Riflery
Ice hockey	Diving	Field		
Lacrosse	Field	Discus		
Martial arts	High jump	Javelin		
Rodeo	Pole vault	Shot put		
Soccer	Gymnastics	Running		
Wrestling	Horseback riding	Swimming		
	Skating	Tennis		
	Ice	Track		
	Roller	Weight-lifting		
	Skiing			
	Cross-country			
	Downhill			
	Water			
	Softball			
	Squash, handball			
	Volleyball			

From American Academy of Pediatrics: Recommendations for participation in competitive sports. Pediatrics 81:738, 1988; with permission.

TABLE 4. Recommendations for Participation in Competitive Sports

			Noncontact		
	Contact/ Collision	Limited Contact/Impact	Strenuous	Moderately Strenuous	Non- strenuous
Atlantoaxial instability	No	No	Yes*	Yes	Yes
* Swimming: no butterfly, breast stroke, or diving starts					
Acute illnesses	*	*	*	*	*
* Needs individual assessment, eg, contagiousness to others, risk of worsening illness					
Cardiovascular					
Carditis	No	No	No	No	No
Hypertension					
Mild	Yes	Yes	Yes	Yes	Yes
Moderate	*	*	*	*	*
Severe	*	*	*	*	*
Congenital heart disease	†	†	†	†	†
* Needs individual assessment.					
† Patients with mild forms can be allowed a full range of physical activities: patients with moderate or severe forms, or who are postoperative, should be evaluated by a cardiologist before athletic participation.					
Eyes					
Absence or loss of function of one eye	*	*	*	*	*
Detached retina	†	†	†	†	†
* Availability of American Society for Testing Materials (ASTM)-approved eye guards may allow competitor to participate in most sports, but this must be judged on an individual basis.					
† Consult ophthalmologist					
Inguinal hernia	Yes	Yes	Yes	Yes	Yes
Kidney: Absence of one	No	Yes	Yes	Yes	Yes
Liver: Enlarged	No	No	Yes	Yes	Yes
Musculoskeletal disorders	*	*	*	*	*
* Needs individual assessment					
Neurologic					
History of serious head or spine trauma, repeated concussions, or craniotomy	*	*	Yes	Yes	Yes
Convulsive disorder					
Well controlled	Yes	Yes	Yes	Yes	Yes
Poorly controlled	No	No	Yes†	Yes	Yes‡
* Needs individual assessment					
† No swimming or weight lifting					
‡ No archery or riflery					
Ovary: Absence of one	Yes	Yes	Yes	Yes	Yes
Respiratory					
Pulmonary insufficiency	*	*	*	*	Yes
Asthma	Yes	Yes	Yes	Yes	Yes
* May be allowed to compete if oxygenation remains satisfactory during a graded stress test					
Sickle cell trait	Yes	Yes	Yes	Yes	Yes
Skin: Boils, herpes, impetigo, scabies	*	*	Yes	Yes	Yes
* No gymnastics with mats, martial arts, wrestling, or contact sports until not contagious					
Spleen: Enlarged	No	No	No	Yes	Yes

From American Academy of Pediatrics: Recommendations for participation in competitive sports. Pediatrics 81:738, 1988; with permission.

IX. REHABILITATION

The athlete with musculoskeletal conditions requiring rehabilitation can be instructed on the appropriate exercise program by the physician knowledgeable in sports medicine or by a physical therapist or athletic trainer. The athlete with medical conditions requiring treatment should be started on treatment or referred for further evaluation and/or treatment. A follow-up visit should be planned to assure appropriate rehabilitation or treatment was received, and to release for sports participation.

REFERENCES

1. Adams JE: Injury to the throwing arm: A study of traumatic changes in the elbow joints of boy baseball players. Calif Med 102:127–132, 1965.
2. Albanese SA, Palmer AK, Kerr DR, et al: Wrist pain and distal growth plate closure of the radius in gymnasts. J Pediatr Orthop 9:23–28, 1989.
3. Allman FL: Medical qualification for sports participation. In Ryan AJ, Allman FL (eds): Sports Medicine. New York, Academic Press Inc., 1974.
4. Allman FL, McKeag DB, Bodner LM: Prevention and emergency care of sports injuries. Fam Pract Rec 5:141–163, 1983.
5. Barnes HV: Physical growth and development during puberty. Med Clin North Am 59:1305–1317, 1975.
6. Committee on Sports Medicine, American Academy of Pediatrics: Recommendations for participation in competitive sports. Pediatrics 81:737–739, 1988.
7. Donahue P: Preparticipation exams: How to detect a teenage crisis. Phys Sportsmed 18:53–60, 1990.
8. Dyment PG: The sports physical. Adolesc Med State Art Rev 2:1–12, 1991.
9. Goldberg B, Boiardo R: Profiling children for sports participation. Clin Sports Med 3:153–169, 1984.
10. Goldberg B, Saranati A, Witman P, et al: Pre-participation sports assessment: An objective evaluation. Pediatrics 66:736–745, 1980.
11. Hunter LY: Women's athletics: The orthopedic surgeon's viewpoint. Clin Sports Med 3:809–827, 1984.
12. Hunter-Griffin LY: Orthopedic concerns. In Shangold M, Mirkin G (eds): Women and Exercise: Physiology and Sports Medicine. Philadelphia, F.A. Davis Co., 1988.
13. Jones R: The preparticipation, sport-specific athletic profile examination. Semin Adolesc Med 3:169–175, 1987.
14. Linder CW, DuRant RH, Selecki RM, et al: Preparticipation health screening of young athletes: Results of 1268 examinations. Am J Sports Med 9:187–193, 1981.
15. Lombardo JA: Pre-participation physical evaluation. Prim Care Clin 11:3–21, 1984.
16. Malina RM: Growth, performance, activity, and training during adolescence. In Shangold M, Mirkin G (eds): Women and Exercise: Physiology and Sports Medicine. Philadelphia, F.A. Davis Co., 1988.
17. McCaffrey FM, Braden DS, Strong WB: Sudden cardiac death in young athletes. Am J Dis Child 145:177–183, 1991.
18. McKeag DB: Preseason physical examination for the prevention of sports injuries. Sports Med 2:413–431, 1985.
19. McKeag DB: Preparticipation screening of the potential athlete. Clin Sports Med 8:373–397, 1989.
20. Micheli LJ: Overuse injuries in children's sports: The growth factor. Orthop Clin North Am 14:337–360, 1983.
21. Nelson MA: Medical exclusion from sport. Adolesc Med State Art Rev 2:13–25, 1991.
22. Ogden JA, Southwick WO: Osgood-Schlatter's disease and tibial tuberosity development. Clin Orthop, May (116):180–189, 1976.
23. O'Neill DB, Micheli LJ: Overuse injuries in the young athlete. Clin Sports Med 7:591–610, 1988.
24. Rosen LW, McKeag DB, Hough DO, et al: Pathogenic weight control behavior in female athletes. Phys Sportsmed 14:79–86, 1986.
25. Shaffer TE: The health examination for participation in sports. Pediatr Ann 7:666–675, 1978.
26. Shangold MM: How I manage exercise-related menstrual disturbances. Phys Sportsmed 14:113–120, 1986.
27. Whiteside PA: Men's and women's injuries in comparable sports. Phys Sportsmed 8:130–140, 1980.

Chapter 7: Nutritional Issues of Exercise and Performance

MARILYN GUTHRIE, RD

The belief that consuming special foods can enhance physical performance dates as far back in history as the early Olympic periods. In fact, many athletes today believe that consuming a high-protein diet helps in their physical endeavors, even though this particular theory was disproved nearly a century ago.

Good nutrition is essential to optimal physical performance. The well-nourished athlete has more energy and stamina than the under-nourished athlete and can therefore train harder. Women athletes may have additional nutritional concerns because of their unique nutrient needs as well as the demands of intense training and competition. For the most part, the same basic principles that promote good health for the general population will maximize performance for the athlete. However, a key point to remember in keeping the relationship between nutrition and performance in perspective is that nutrition is only one of many factors that affect physical performance.

I. **FACTORS INFLUENCING PERFORMANCE**
   A. **Training:** The type and amount of training and respective goals can vary.
      1. Intense training for elite competition
         Objective: any advantage in competition
      2. Physical training on a regular, but less competitive basis
         Objective: physical fitness
   B. **Genetic endowment:** The child's potential at birth to later become an athlete depends on inherited traits such as stature or body type or muscle type.
   C. **Physiologic status:** These are parameters of general physical fitness such as weight and body composition, flexibility, and muscular strength and endurance.
   D. **Nutritional status**
      1. Adequate long-term energy stores are determined by quality of training diet.
      2. Adequate short-term energy stores are determined by precompetition meal.
      3. Adequate nutrient stores are determined by quality of training diet.

II. **ENERGY EXPENDITURE AND FOOD INTAKE**
   A. **Caloric needs:** The calories necessary to support the energy expended in training as well as competition.
      1. Specific needs depend on body size, age, sex.
      2. Calories used vary according to sport (Table 1).
      3. Increased needs during weight training
   B. **Energy sources**
      1. **Protein:** Can be used as a source of energy; its more important function is in building and maintaining cells and tissues.
         a. Recommend to make up 15–18% of total caloric intake; typical American diet contains adequate protein to meet the needs of most athletes.
         b. Expensive as an energy source, as metabolism involves production of byproducts that need to be eliminated from the body; protein accentuates the potential for dehydration.
         c. Food sources of this energy source can be costly.
         d. Increased need for protein in weight training; 1.0–1.5 g/kg body weight/day.

50

TABLE 1. Energy Requirements for Various Sports*

Activity	Competition (cal/event)	Training (cal/hr)
Cycling	1000 (1 hr)	750
Football	100 (11 min)	250
Gymnastics	6.5 (1 min)	100
Racquetball	612 (1 hr)	612
Running		
2-mile race	215 (11 min)	852
4-mile race	384 (24 min)	852
6-mile race	540 (36 min)	852
Swimming	40 (4 min)	600
Wrestling	225 (9 min)	600

* Data from Costill DL: Carbohydrate for exercise: Dietary demands for optimal performance. Int J Sports Med 9:1–18, 1988.

    2. **Carbohydrate:** The primary energy source for physically active individuals.
       a. Recommend to make up 50–60% of total caloric intake; 5 g/kg body weight/day.
       b. Carbohydrates used during activity are released during anaerobic metabolism of glucose and the aerobic metabolism of glycogen.
       c. The preferred sources are complex carbohydrates and starches.
       d. Endurance athletes require additional carbohydrates (60–70% of total calories, 500–600 g).
    3. **Fat:** Can supplement carbohydrate as a stored energy source for physical activity.
       a. Energy released from aerobic metabolism and triglycerides.
       b. Fat is a less-efficient source of fuel; carbohydrate and protein needs should be calculated first.
       c. Recommend to make up 25–30% of total caloric intake.
    4. **Alcohol:** An empty source of calories. Recommend to make up ≤2% of total caloric intake.
  C. **Fuel mixture:** The proportion of protein, carbohydrate, and fat used during exercise.
    1. **Type of activity**
       a. Short-term, high-intensity activities require an immediate energy source generated by anaerobic metabolism, such as glucose or lactic acid; it is almost entirely from carbohydrate.
       b. Long-term, low-intensity activities require a sustained energy source generated by aerobic metabolism of stored glycogen and fats; it is from 50–60% carbohydrate and the balance from fats.
    2. **Duration of activity**
       a. Initial effort uses energy from anaerobic sources for a short period of time (2–4 minutes).
       b. There is a gradual increase in use of glycogen for fuel (4 minutes or longer).
       c. As the effort continues, proportionately more fat is used as a source of fuel (2 hours or longer).
  D. **Vitamins and minerals:** In exercise they function as coenzymes in the metabolism of fat, carbohydrates, and protein and in muscle function.
    1. No dramatic increases needed in athletes, except for a few (calcium, iron) that deserve special mention (*see below*).
    2. No advantage in taking excess amounts of vitamins and minerals; they can interfere with absorption and metabolism of other nutrients and produce potential toxicity.
  E. **Special considerations for women**
    1. **Calcium:** An important mineral in maintaining integrity of bone tissue and bone mass, muscle contraction, and nerve conduction.

      a. Often lacking in diets of most women; low levels increase the risk of osteoporosis.

      b. Accelerated bone loss may occur in some women who exercise at very intense levels—**"athletic amenorrhea"**—(a decrease in estrogen leads to decreased absorption of Ca^{2+} and deposition in bone).

      c. Recommend 1000–1200 mg/day for premenopausal women, 1500 mg/day for adolescents and postmenopausal women.

      d. Calcium intake at the recommended level is difficult to meet strictly from food sources (dairy foods, such as non-fat milk, yogurt, low-fat cheese contain approximately 300 mg/serving).

      e. **Consider supplemental form** such as calcium carbonate (Tums) or calcium citrate.

  2. **Iron:** Important in oxygen transport to the exercising muscle.

      a. Often lacking in diets of women.

      b. **"Sports anemia":** changes in blood characteristics of exercising women may compromise performance; possible causes may be dietary, mechanical (destruction of red blood cells), or metabolic (increase in blood volume).

      c. Screen for serum ferritin levels.

      d. **If iron deficiency is found,** provide nutritional guidance on iron-rich foods (heme iron in meats, fish, and poultry); consider supplemental form (ferrous salt).

F. **Fluids and electrolytes**

  1. **Water:** The most important nutrient affecting performance due to its role in thermal regulation.

      a. Available stores of water: 2–3% of body weight.

      b. At 5% or more of fluid loss, some compromise in performance begins.

      c. Replace fluids at same rate of loss: 1 pint for each pound lost during exercise.

      d. Gastric emptying time is a limiting factor.

      e. Fluids should be cool, taste good, and provide a carbohydrate source (6–8%) with a small amount of sodium to maximize absorption.

  2. **Sodium and other electrolytes:** Sodium losses are not as great as water loss and are easy to replace with foods.

      a. Salt tablets not appropriate; corrosive on stomach lining.

      b. Small amount of sodium in drink may enhance fluid replacement.

  3. **Fluid replacement drinks**

      a. Carbohydrate concentration of 6–8% is ideal for optimal fluid absorption.

      b. Some carbohydrates—either sucrose, glucose, or glucose polymers—enhance endurance; potential side effects of fructose are cramps.

      c. Consume 2 cups about 2 hours prior to event, followed by 2 cups approximately 15–20 minutes before endurance exercise.

      d. During exercise, consume frequent small servings (4–6 oz every 10–15 minutes) of plain cool water or other hydration beverage to prevent dehydration.

G. **Meal timing and composition**

  1. **Pre-event meal:** The primary objective of this meal is to stave off hunger.

      a. The composition should be easy to digest, primarily carbohydrate, low fat, light (500 kcal or less).

      b. This meal should be consumed 2–4 hours prior to activity.

      c. Choose foods that are familiar and comforting; avoid gas-forming (legumes, cabbage family) or laxative (high-fiber, fruits) foods.

      d. A liquid meal that provides a balance of fluids and nutrients may be better tolerated by athletes with precompetition jitters or gastric distress.

  2. **During competition:** The primary objective is to provide a steady source of available energy.

      a. In endurance activities of long duration (1–3 hours), carbohydrate source (fruit, juice, hydration beverage) may enhance performance by delaying fatigue.

      b. Fluids with carbohydrate (6–8% concentration) and some sodium can limit depletion of water and glycogen stores.

      c. Athletes should drink 4–6 oz every 10–15 minutes during activity, regardless of thirst.

   3. **Post-event meal:** The primary objective is to replace depleted stores of energy and fluid stores.

      a. Replace fluids with juices, fruits, etc. at the rate of 2 cups/lb of weight lost.

      b. Appetite may be suppressed; resume normal eating of high-carbohydrate diet when appetite returns.

      c. Consume carbohydrates (up to 600 g) within the first several hours to replace muscle glycogen stores.

III. WEIGHT AND FAT CONTROL

  A. **Body composition:** More appropriate standard than weight alone; preferred measure of an individual's health and fitness.

    1. **Typical levels of body fat for athletes:** 12–20% for well-trained women athletes. Levels vary between sports and between positions in a specific sport (Table 2).

    2. **Average levels of body fat for the general population:** 20–25% for women is considered acceptable.

    3. **Levels with potential health risk:** body fat levels >30% for women is considered a clinical indicator of obesity and a risk factor in the development of chronic disease. At the other end of the spectrum, low body fat levels are possible indicators of eating disorders (precise percentage is not known).

  B. **Type of activity:** Low intensity, longer duration better for fat utilization.

  C. **Recommendations for weight control:** Reduce body fat while maintaining lean body tissue.

    1. **Rate of weight loss:** Rapid weight loss promotes loss of lean body tissue and muscle, compromises nutrient intake, and increases likelihood of regain; it can also compromise endurance and impair both cardiac function and body temperature regulation.

    2. **Caloric needs:** Moderate reduction in caloric intake (not <1500 kcal) with <30% of energy from fat is more effective for achieving desired changes in body composition.

    3. **Ideal distribution of carbohydrates, fat, and protein** is similar to recommendations outlined in Dietary Guidelines for Americans and the Food Guide Pyramid (Fig. 1), with emphasis on complex carbohydrate foods (whole grains, cereals, breads, pastas, starchy vegetables, legumes, fruits).

    4. **Starvation or low-calorie diets** are not recommended; these can have an adverse effect on performance.

TABLE 2. Percent Body Fat for Athletes in Various Sports*

Sport	%	
	Males	Females
Basketball	7–12	18–27
Cross-country skiing	7–13	18–24
Gymnastics	3–6	8–18
Swimming	4–10	12–20
Track and field		
Running	4–12	8–18
Jumping/Hurdles	—	12–22
Discus	12–18	22–28
Shot put	14–20	23–30
Volleyball	—	20–23

* Data from Wilmore JH: The Wilmore Fitness Program. New York, Simon & Schuster, 1981.

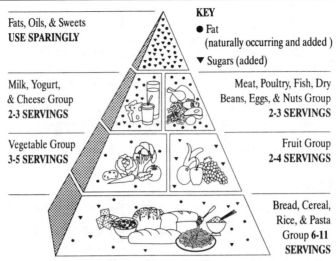

FIGURE 1.   The food guide pyramid.

D. **Recommendations for weight gain:** Increase caloric intake while weight-training to increase lean body mass, not fat tissue.
   1. Increase intake of high-calorie, high-carbohydrate, nutrient-dense foods (e.g., nuts, granola bars, milkshakes, juices, hearty soups, etc.).
   2. Increase frequency of eating; "mini-meals" or snacks 2–4 times/day are used to complement training schedules.
   3. Liquid meal supplements may be helpful in providing a high-carbohydrate meal in a ready-to-consume package.

IV. **FOOD AS AN ERGOGENIC AID**
   A. **Nutritional supplements**
      1. **Protein and amino acid supplements:** There is no evidence that excess protein improves performance or increases muscle mass.
         a. Use of amino acid and protein supplements is expensive.
         b. Amino acid oxidation can increase potential for dehydration because of the need to eliminate protein metabolic end-products via urine.
      2. **Vitamin and mineral supplements:** There is no evidence to support claims for ergogenic properties.
         a. Increased energy intake should provide the additional vitamins and minerals necessary.
         b. They may improve the nutritional status of individuals consuming marginal amounts of nutrients from food; if taken, recommend a multivitamin supplement that provides no more than 100% of RDA.
   B. **Nonnutritive supplements:** Scientific research does not substantiate claims for any ergogenic effect from substances such as bee pollen, brewer's yeast, caffeine, lecithin, etc.
      1. Some evidence suggests that caffeine increases the release of free fatty acids; they can increase urine production and potential for dehydration.
      2. These substances may provide certain psychological benefits rather than proven physiologic benefits.
      3. Use of these substances to replace sound nutrition practices may compromise health and performance.
   C. **Dietary regimens**
      1. **Carbohydrate loading:** A modification of diet and exercise regimens with concomitant changes in storage of glycogen. This practice is of value only in endurance activities beyond 90 minutes.

   a. Training phase: High carbohydrate diet (60–70% of total calories; 600–800 g/day) over 3–4 days; curtail training to limit utilization of muscle glycogen; can increase storage of glycogen 20–40% higher than initial level.
   b. Competition phase: Pre-competition meal.
2. **High protein diets:** For weight-training, athletes may require more protein than the RDA.
   a. The limiting factor for muscle protein deposition is energy intake, not protein.
   b. Athletes who wish to increase muscle mass should meet energy needs first, then ensure that protein intake is adequate (1.0–1.5 g protein/kg body weight).

V. SUMMARY

Both individual participants and professionals in the field of sports nutrition have long recognized the importance of diet and healthful food choices in optimizing health, fitness, and athletic performance levels. As new research findings emerge, there continues to be a need for sound interpretation and dissemination of this information. The registered dietitian or nutrition professional who has specialized in sports nutrition has the knowledge and counseling skills to act as an interpreter and provider of this nutrition information.

REFERENCES

1. American Dietetic Association: Nutrition for physical fitness and athletic performance for adults. J Am Dietetic Assoc 93(6):691–696, 1993.
2. Benardot D (ed): Sports Nutrition: A Guide for the Professional Working with Active People, 2nd ed. Chicago, IL, The American Dietetic Association, 1993.
3. Brotherhood JR: Nutrition and sports performance. Sports Med 1:350–389, 1984.
4. Coggan AR, Coyle EF: Reversal of fatigue during prolonged exercise by carbohydrate infusion or ingestion. J Appl Physiol 63:2388–2395, 1987.
5. Costill DL: Carbohydrate for exercise: Dietary demands for optimal performance. Int J Sports Med 9:1–18, 1988.
6. Hargreaves M, Costill DL, Coggan AR, et al: Effects of carbohydrate feedings on muscle glycogen utilization and exercise performance. Med Sci Sports Exerc 16:219–222, 1984.
7. Lloyd T, Buchanan JR, Bitzer S, et al: Interrelationships of diet, athletic activity, menstrual status, and bone density in collegiate women. Am J Clin Nutr 46:681–684, 1987.
8. Murray R: The effects of consuming carbohydrate-electrolyte beverages on gastric emptying and fluid absorption during and following exercise. Sports Med 4:322–351, 1987.
9. Murray R, Eddy DE, Murray T, et al: The effect of fluid and carbohydrate feedings during intermittent cycling exercise. Med Sci Sports Exerc 19:597–604, 1987.
10. Roberts KM, Noble EG, Hayden DB, Taylor AW: Simple and complex carbohydrate-rich diets and muscle glycogen content of marathon runners. Eur J Appl Physiol 57:70–74, 1988.
11. Wilmore JH, Freund BJ: Nutritional enhancement of athletic performance. Nutr Abstr Rev 54(1):1–16, 1984.

Chapter 8: Exercise Prescription for Women

ROBYN M. STUHR, MA

When prescribing exercise for women, it is not so much gender but individual physical status, needs, and goals that should determine program design. Certain challenges (low energy levels, fat loss) and obstacles (child care, recovery from pregnancy, juggling work and family responsibilities) may present themselves more frequently in the female population.

I. **INITIAL ASSESSMENT**

An initial assessment of patient goals, medical and activity history, fitness status, and exercise preferences can ensure a successful program. The assessment can be helpful not only to the practitioner but for the woman as a self-awareness, motivational, and personal planning tool. An initial assessment should include:

A. **Medical screening questionnaire** (Fig. 1)
   1. **Cardiac risk:** Age, family history, high blood pressure, high cholesterol/poor lipid profile, smoking history, diabetes, overweight, sedentary lifestyle, cardiac symptoms, and history.
   2. **Orthopedic status:** Previous and chronic injuries. Ask specifically about back, shoulder, and knee pain. Prior to initiation of a generalized program, it may be prudent to refer the woman to physical therapy for a program of strengthening and stretching to protect integrity of previously injured joints or muscles.
   3. **Personal history of physical activity:** Review any previous exercise programs— type, frequency, intensity, and length of participation. This can provide a reference point for activity recommendations. Is there a history of pain or urine leakage with exercise?
   4. **Other**
      a. **Medications:** Beta-blockers, calcium channel inhibitors, or other drugs which affect heart rate response to exercise should be considered.
      b. **Weight management history:** Assessment of previous attempts at fat loss through diet and exercise can be helpful in designing the current strategy and assessing patient knowledge of successful weight-loss techniques.
      c. **Child-bearing history:** Associated weight gain, morphologic changes.

B. **Assess patient's readiness for behavior change**
   1. **Pre-contemplation** (not interested): Advise of health risks related to sedentary lifestyle and exercise benefits.
   2. **Contemplation** (considering, maybe for years): Advise of health risks associated with a sedentary lifestyle and the benefits of regular physical activity. Emphasize the positive impact of a modest and reasonable amount of habitual exercise.
   3. **Preparation** (intends to take action, initial commitment to change): Reinforce pros of active lifestyle and provide exercise prescription guidelines.
   4. **Action** (begun an exercise program): Commend positive health behavior and review exercise prescription.
   5. **Maintenance** (currently in exercise program, yet risk of relapse): Provide encouragement, review exercise program, discuss obstacles and strategies.

C. **Individual goals**
   1. Assist woman in identifying personal goals related to physical activity: Why exercise now, at this time in her life?
   2. Identify specific personal goals; establish reasonable short- and long-term goals.

CONFIDENTIAL
HEALTH HISTORY

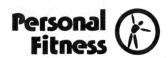

Name _____ Date _____

Address _____

City_____ State_____ Zip_____ Sex_____

Phone: Work _____ Birthdate _____

Home _____

Occupation _____ Employer _____

Nearest Relative_____

Personal Physician _____ Phone _____

FAMILY HISTORY

Please indicate which illnesses your blood relatives have had and fill in the approximate age of the first occurrence:

	HEART ATTACK		ANGINA		HIGH BLOOD PRESSURE		STROKE		DIABETES		AGE AT DEATH	CAUSE
	YES	AGE	YES	AGE	YES	AGE	YES	AGE	YES	AGE		
FATHER	☐	___	☐	___	☐	___	☐	___	☐	___	___	___
MOTHER	☐	___	☐	___	☐	___	☐	___	☐	___	___	___
BROTHER	☐	___	☐	___	☐	___	☐	___	☐	___	___	___
BROTHER	☐	___	☐	___	☐	___	☐	___	☐	___	___	___
SISTER	☐	___	☐	___	☐	___	☐	___	☐	___	___	___
SISTER	☐	___	☐	___	☐	___	☐	___	☐	___	___	___
GRANDFATHER	☐	___	☐	___	☐	___	☐	___	☐	___	___	___
GRANDMOTHER	☐	___	☐	___	☐	___	☐	___	☐	___	___	___

MEDICAL HISTORY

Please place an (X) in the blank(s) which apply to you:

YES NO
☐ ☐ High Blood Pressure
☐ ☐ Heart Disease
☐ ☐ Heart Attack
☐ ☐ Angina
☐ ☐ Heart surgery or coronary bypass surgery
☐ ☐ Stroke
☐ ☐ Chest pain or shortness of breath during exercise
☐ ☐ Heart murmurs
☐ ☐ Diabetes
☐ ☐ Chronic Bronchitis or emphysema
☐ ☐ Asthma
☐ ☐ Varicose veins

YES NO
☐ ☐ Epilepsy
☐ ☐ Allergies or hay fever
☐ ☐ Thyroid or other endocrine disorder (please specify) _____
☐ ☐ Kidney disease
☐ ☐ Recurring headaches, dizziness or blackouts
☐ ☐ Blurred vision
☐ ☐ Chronic nose bleeds
☐ ☐ Arthritis
☐ ☐ Have you ever been told you have high blood lipid levels (i.e. cholesterol or triglycerides)? If you remember what the value was, please list it here_____

FIGURE 1. Sample medical screening questionnaire. (Reprinted with permission from the National Center for Health Promotion.)

3. Example goal: Fat loss
    a. Long-term (1-year) goal—lose 24 lbs of fat. "Wouldn't you feel great if this time next year you were 24 lbs lighter?!"
    b. Short-term (monthly) goal—lose 2 lbs/month. (Calculate weekly energy expenditure level for desired caloric deficit.)
    c. Short-term (weekly) goal—walk 30–40 minutes 4–6 times/week. (Set minimum and maximum parameters so the woman can feel success on difficult days.)

If you are under the care of a physician, please describe the condition and its duration.

_____
_____
_____
_____
_____

Are you currently taking medication or other drugs?

_____

Type	Dosage	Age of Prescription

When did you have your last medical examination?

_____

Are you pregnant?   □ Yes   □ No

ORTHOPEDIC HISTORY

Indicate if you wear any type of brace, splint, orthopedic appliance.

_____
_____
_____
_____

Indicate area of injury, surgery or condition and explain (i.e. arthritis, low back pain, calcium deposits, nerve injury, fracture, tennis elbow, etc.)

	Description	Date injury occured
_____ Head		
_____ Neck		
_____ Shoulder, clavicle		
_____ Arm, elbow, wrist		
_____ Hand		
_____ Spine, back		
_____ Ribs		
_____ Hips and pelvis		
_____ Thigh		
_____ Knee, kneecap		
_____ Leg		
_____ Ankle		
_____ Foot		
_____ Other		

SMOKING

YES NO
□   □   Do you currently smoke? If yes, how much?
(Number of cigarettes, cigars, pipe) _____
_____

How long have you smoked? _____

If you do not smoke now, did you ever smoke?
How long? _____ When did you quit? _____

CURRENT PHYSICAL ACTIVITIES

Mark the appropriate description of your present physical activity level:

□ No physical activity.
□ Light to moderate exercise (golf, tennis, bowling, leisure cycling) less than 3 times each week.
□ Light to moderate exercise 3-5 times each week
□ Heavy aerobic exercise 3-4 times each week (jogging, stationary cycling, aerobic dancing, swimming).
□ Heavy aerobic exercise more than 4 times each week.

YES NO
□   □   Do you monitor your pulse rate during exercise?
If yes, what does it average? _____
How long have you been involved in these activities?
     □ Less than 6 months
     □ 6 months to one year
     □ More than one year

YES NO
□   □   Is your present exercise program consistent from month to month?

What other types of activities are included in your daily life? _____

DIET HISTORY

YES NO
□   □   Are you presently dieting? Please specify if you are on a prescribed diet (i.e. low sodium, low fat, diabetic, etc.)

_____
_____

YES NO
□   □   Do you drink alcoholic beverages, If yes, how many drinks do you consume each week (beer, cocktails, wine)? _____
What is your current weight? _____ Height _____
What was your body weight at age 21? _____

YES NO
□   □   Have you recently experienced a rapid weight gain or loss?
If yes, what amount? _____

OCCUPATION

How would you rate your daily occupation?

Sedentary		Moderately Strenuous			Strenuous			
1	2	3	4	5	6	7	8	9

(Please circle the number that represents your current job activity level.)

FIGURE 1 *(Cont.)* Sample medical screening questionnaire.

   D. **Exercise preferences and access**
      1. What fitness, recreational, and sport activity sounds appealing or has the woman successfully engaged in previously?
      2. What type of fitness equipment is available? Is an exercise club nearby and affordable? Exercise equipment in the home? Access to good walking or cycling area?
   E. **Fitness evaluation** (not mandatory, but helpful to enhance patient's awareness and motivation, provide a baseline for improvement, and set reasonable fitness goals)

1. **Blood pressure and pulse** (resting)
2. **Body composition**
   a. Possible measurement methods include hydrostatic weighing, bioelectrical impedance, skinfold calipers.
   b. An **ideal weight** can be established for an overfat woman using the formula:

$$\text{Ideal weight} = \frac{\text{Current lean mass}}{\text{Ideal \% lean mass}}$$

   The ideal lean mass can be selected using body fat tables and identifying realistic goals based on current level of overfatness or activity/sport requirements (Table 1).
   c. **Circumference measures** can provide a simple benchmark for body dimensions and changes over time. A woman can use this technique at home to assess progress.
3. Flexibility
   a. **Tests** can include sit and reach, trunk extension, and various range-of-motion tests involving different muscles, i.e., hamstrings, quadriceps, gastrocnemius, hip flexors and rotators, gross shoulder movement, and trunk rotation.
   b. **Tight muscles** can be identified, and specific stretches given to increase muscle flexibility.
   c. Discuss **proper stretching technique** and take woman through at least one stretch to make sure she understands and demonstrates the following concepts:
      i. Feel stretch or tension in the muscle, but avoid pain.
      ii. Apply constant hold; avoid ballistic movements in stretching.
      iii. Hold at least 20–30 seconds.
      iv. The best time for stretching to improve flexibility is *after* vigorous exercise, when muscle blood flow and temperature are highest.
4. **Cardiovascular endurance**
   a. While the high-risk individual may require a maximal stress test, submaximal evaluation is appropriate for most, using a bike ergometer, treadmill, or step bench.
      i. A high-risk person may be defined as one with two or more major coronary heart disease risk factors, symptoms suggestive of or known to have cardiac, pulmonary, or metabolic disease.
      ii. Major risk factors include cigarette smoking, hypertension ($\geq 160/90$), serum cholesterol ≥ 240 mg/dL, diabetes, or a family history of cardiac disease prior to age 65.
   b. Select testing protocol based on the woman's typical mode of activity, physical limitations, and equipment availability.
   c. Monitor heart rate and blood pressure, through various stages of the test to a submaximal endpoint and through recovery (75–85% maximum heart rate predicted).

TABLE 1. American College of Sports Medicine Body Fat Table for Women

Rating	Age (yrs)				
	20–29	30–39	40–49	50–59	60+
Excellent	<15	<16	<17	<18	<19
Good	16–19	17–20	18–21	19–22	20–23
Average	20–28	21–29	22–30	23–31	24–32
Fair	29–31	30–31	31–33	32–34	33–35
Poor	>32	>33	>34	>35	>36

From American College of Sports Medicine: Guidelines for Exercise Testing and Prescription. Philadelphia, Lea & Febiger, 1991, with permission.

        d. Workload, heart rate, and blood pressure response during exercise and recovery can provide good baseline for measurement of progress, apart from estimation of maximal aerobic capacity.

        e. Heart rate, perceived exertion ratings, and visual observation of the woman can validate standard target heart rate range for exercise training or suggest modification.

    5. **Muscular strength and endurance**

        a. Because strength is specific to the muscle involved and action performed, no one test is a sufficient indicator of overall strength.

        b. Standardized muscle endurance tests (abdominal curls, push-ups, flexed arm hang, bench and leg press) or one repetition max are common choices. An individual baseline can be established using the various pieces of strength training equipment that the woman will be using in her exercise regimen.

II. EXERCISE PROGRAM DESIGN

Practical considerations related to adherence and requirements for training pace and volume should be integrated. Table 2 gives a sample program design.

  A. **Match goals and needs with appropriate activity:** If a structured vigorous program does not seem feasible given the patient's physical status or level of motivation, encourage simple efforts to increase daily caloric expenditure—i.e., walking at every opportunity, taking stairs, active transportation options such as cycling or walking, fitness activities with children, pushing the lawnmower, dancing, etc.

  B. **Establish ideal recommended activity pattern:** Time, duration, intensity, and rate of progression. (*See* Table 2 for sample prescriptions.)

  C. **Identify obstacles** (i.e., time, access, child care, weather, fatigue) **and facilitate problem solving.** The woman may need to be reminded that she is skilled at problem-solving in other areas of her life (work, family) in which she has made a commitment. Is her physical, mental, and emotional well-being and her personal health no less a priority?

    1. **Identify support systems.** This can include exercise partner(s) or supportive family members and physically active friends and coworkers.

    2. **Institute a system of tracking exercise progress.** This may be as simple as giving the woman a box of stars to affix to her calendar on exercise days or an exercise diary recording specifics of the workout sessions.

    3. **Suggest an initial system of rewards** (until the intrinsic value of the exercise becomes the reward). Workout gear, massage, free-time activities, whatever is personally motivating to each woman can be identified for each successful week of compliance.

    4. **Behavioral contracts, discussion, or written exercises to clarify values, priorities, self-worth** in regard to personal health, self-affirmation, gentle self-love, and relapse prevention can facilitate a successful lifestyle change.

  D. **Identify equipment and athletic clothing needs** for function and safety: To prevent injury and avoid unnecessary discomfort during exercise, appropriate workout gear is critical, particularly athletic shoes and supportive bra.

III. SAMPLE EXERCISE PRESCRIPTIONS FOR SPECIFIC FITNESS COMPONENTS

  A. **Goal: Cardiovascular conditioning, increased energy and stamina.**

    1. **Mode:** Aerobic activities—Rhythmic, continuous, using large muscle mass, e.g., swimming, jogging, cycling, stair-stepping, rowing, aerobic classes, walking or hiking, dance.

    2. **Frequency:** 3–4 times/week

    3. **Duration:** 15–60 minutes/session. (Remember, this does not include 5–10 minutes of warm-up and cool-down, at a slow pace at the same activity.)

TABLE 2.   Sample Exercise Plan

Client: Female, 35 yr
  Married with 2 children, ages 3 and 6 yr
  Full-time job as bank teller
  No recent injuries, occasional low back pain
  No medications
  No cardiac risk

Fitness evaluation:
  64 inches, 150 lbs
  33% body fat—100.5 lbs lean mass, 49.5 lbs fat
  Resting heart rate 78 bpm
  Predicted maximal aerobic capacity 24 ml/kg/min (fair)
  Poor abdominal and upper body strength scores
  Hamstring tightness

Client's interest:
  Weight loss
  Improved energy level

Fitness interests: Walking, swimming, aerobics

Fitness goals:
  Long term: 25% body fat—102 lbs lean mass, 34 lbs fat
    136 lbs
    Predicted aerobic capacity 28–33 mL/kg/min (avg)
    Improved hamstring flexibility
    Decreased incidence of low back pain
  Short term: Focus on behavioral goals
    Walk at least 20–30 minutes at least 3–5 times/week (first week)
    1–3 lbs fat loss/month, decrease in circumference

Exercise plan:
  Mode: Walking
    * Incorporate stretching exercises for hamstrings, calves, back extensors and abdominal strength-
    ening at the end of home-based session
  Frequency: 3–7 days/week
  Duration: 10–45 minutes/session
  Intensity: 11–14 Borg Rating of Perceived Exertion
    Target heart rate 60–75%, predicted HRmax 111–139 bpm
    Karvonen formula target heart rate (60–75%) 142–158 bpm
  Lunch Walk: 10–15 minutes brisk, followed by hamstring/calf stretching
  Home Walk: 10–15 minutes brisk, followed by stretching and strengthening routine
    Add 2–4 minutes each week . . .
  Estimated calorie expenditure for 150-lb person, "normal-paced" walking on asphalt: 5.4 kcal/min
    30 min, 5 times/wk = 12 lbs lost/year
    60 min, 5 times/wk = 24 lbs lost/year
  Nutritional consultation with dietician is recommended for guidelines on decreasing dietary fat
  intake.
  After 3 months: Reassess
            Investigate convenient fitness facilities for lunch-hour aerobics/pool

Equipment:
  Good-quality, well-fitting walking shoes
  Acrylic/poly/cotton blend socks
  Outerwear jacket with hood for rainy days
  Watch with sweep hand or timer

Problem-solving:
  Child care: Exercise in the middle of workday.
        Ask husband to watch kids in evening.
        Check out child care in local fitness facilities.
        Home exercise equipment while kids are in bed?
  Fatigue: Just do it! I'll have more energy once I've started.
        Recruit a workout partner from work or neighborhood.
        Don't stay up late watching TV.

TABLE 3. Borg Perceived Exertion Scales

20-Point Scale		10-Point Scale	
6	No exertion at all	0	Nothing at all
7	Extremely light	0.5	Very, very weak (just noticeable)
8		1	Very weak
9	Very light	2	Weak (light)
10		3	Moderate
11	Light	4	Somewhat strong
12		5	Strong (heavy)
13	Somewhat hard	6	
14		7	Very strong
15	Hard-heavy	8	
16		9	
17	Very hard	10	Very, very strong (almost max.)
18			
19	Extremely hard		Maximal
20	Maximal exertion		

4. **Intensity:** 55–90% maximal heart rate
   a. Standard range choice of 70–85% should be modified upward or downward based on status of exerciser (novice/athlete, young/old), exercise goal, and ratings of perceived exertion.
   b. ± 15 beat variance should be taken into account in **maximum heart rate** if actual maximal heart rate data are not available.
   c. Individuals desiring a **reduction in body fat** should be encouraged to choose a lower intensity/longer duration balance in their new exercise regimen for greater success with fewer injuries.
   d. Perceived exertion ratings (Table 3) may be used, especially if the individual is taking beta-adrenergic blockade drugs or has difficulty finding her pulse:
      i. 12–16 (somewhat-hard to hard) on 20-point scale
      ii. 4–6 rating on 10-point scale
   e. Two methods of calculating **target heart rate:**
      i. First, estimate maximal heart rate (HRmax) using either:
         (a) 220 – age = predicted HRmax
         (b) 210 – ½ age = HRmax (a more liberal estimate)
      ii. Then, calculate a target heart rate (THR) range using desired percentages and either:
         (a) Standard formula
            HRmax × 0.70 = lower THR
            HRmax × 0.85 = higher THR
         (b) Karvonen formula
            [(HRmax – HR rest) × 0.70] + HR rest = lower THR
            [HRmax – HR rest) × 0.85] + HR rest = high THR
         Provide 10-second count by dividing by 6.
5. **Rate of progression in cardiovascular conditioning** (Table 4).
   a. Begin with shorter intervals and possibly frequent but shorter exercise bouts during the day.
   b. Increase to 20–30 minutes before increasing intensity.
   c. Increase time or distance by no more than 10% per week.
   d. Consider individual variations and past history of injuries.
   e. Allow 4–6 weeks for individual phase-in.
   f. For maintenance: variety should be encouraged to prevent overuse injuries, avoid boredom, provide for indoor/outdoor options, and expand range of familiar activities for lifetime choices.

TABLE 4. Sample Jogging Program Showing Increasing Exercise Times as Cardiovascular Conditioning Is Achieved

Week	Target Zone Exercising	Total Time in Minutes (warm-up + target zone exercising + cool-down)
1	Walk 10 min	20
2	Walk 5 min, jog 1 min, walk 5 min, jog 1 min	22
3	Walk 5 min, jog 3 min, walk 5 min, jog 3 min	26
4	Walk 4 min, jog 5 min, walk 4 min, jog 5 min	28
5	Walk 4 min, jog 5 min, walk 4 min, jog 5 min	28
6	Walk 4 min, jog 6 min, walk 4 min, jog 6 min	30
7	Walk 4 min, jog 7 min, walk 4 min, jog 7 min	32
8	Walk 4 min, jog 8 min, walk 4 min, jog 8 min	34
9	Walk 4 min, jog 9 min, walk 4 min, jog 9 min	36
10	Walk 4 min, jog 13 min	27
11	Walk 4 min, jog 15 min	29
12	Walk 4 min, jog 17 min	31
13	Walk 2 min, jog slowly 2 min, jog 17 min	31
14	Walk 1 min, jog slowly 3 min, jog 17 min	31
15	Jog slowly 3 min, jog 17 min	30
16 and after	Check your pulse periodically to see if you are exercising within your target zone. Remember that your goal is to continue getting the benefits you are seeking and enjoying your activity. Slowly continue to increase your jog time until you can jog at your target rate for 20–30 minutes without stopping.	

Reprinted with permission from Running for a Healthy Heart. Dallas, American Heart Association, 1989.

B. **Goal: Flexibility**
1. **Mode:** Static stretching
2. **Frequency:** Daily, before activity for injury prevention or after activity for improved flexibility.
3. **Duration:** Hold each stretch position 20–60 seconds.
4. **Intensity:** Slight discomfort or pulling sensation, but absolutely no pain.
5. **Stretches** should be chosen based on areas of tightness and muscle groups used in training activities. Recommended stretches for common activities are illustrated in Figure 2.
   a. Walking—exercises 1, 2, and 4
   b. Jogging—exercises 1, 2, 3, and 4 (hamstring, calf emphasis)
   c. Cycling and stair climbing—exercises 1, 2, 3, 4, and 5 (quadriceps, calf emphasis)
C. **Goal: Increase strength, muscular endurance, change body shape via muscle hypertrophy.**
1. **Mode:** Weight training, i.e., calisthenics, free weights, Nautilus/Universal/Eagle/Cybex machines, elastic bands
2. **Frequency:** 2–3 times/week or every other day
3. **Repetitions:** 8–12 reps, fewer reps and higher weight for hypertrophy and strength, higher reps and lower weight for endurance. 1–3 sets depending upon time, program goals, and utilization of different angles to maximize involvement of stabilizing and synergistic muscles.
4. **Intensity:** To momentary muscular fatigue. Note that it is important to allow a several-week phase-in before adopting a challenging weight-lifting regimen. Do not increase to higher weight until the same regimen is performed easily on two consecutive workouts.

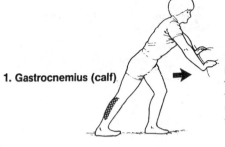

1. Gastrocnemius (calf)

Lean against a wall with your back leg straight and your front leg slightly bent. Keep your back heel on the floor and lean progressively closer to the wall until you can feel the stretch in your calf. Repeat with other leg.

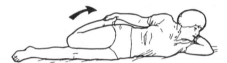

2. Soleus (calf)

Repeat #1 but keep back leg slightly bent.

3. Quadriceps (front of thigh)

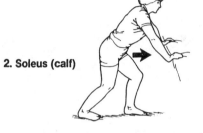

Lying on your side, reach back and grab your upper foot and pull it up toward your buttocks. Repeat with other leg while on your other side. Keep your knees together.

4. Hamstrings (back of thigh)

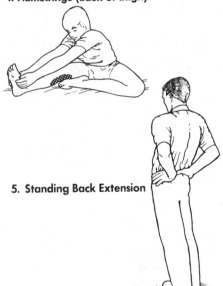

Sitting, bring the sole of your bent leg to the inner thigh of your straight leg. Lean forward and grasp the ankle of your straight leg with both hands. Keeping the leg straight, pull your upper body down towards your feet.

5. Standing Back Extension

Stand with feet comfortably apart, *knees straight*, and hands placed against the back of the pelvis. Arch backward as far as comfortably possible while pushing forward with the hands. Hold only 3 seconds. Repeat 5–10 times.

FIGURE 2. Common stretches: Each exercise should be held for 20 seconds, followed by a 5-second relaxation period. Each exercise should be done at least 3 times. Do this routine once a day or as specified.

5. **Technique tips**
   a. Work large muscle groups first; work from the center of the body out.
   b. Perform combination exercises (those which utilize numerous muscles) before isolation exercises (those which focus primarily on one muscle).
   c. Allow a 30–60-second rest period between sets or exercises.
   d. As a general rule, allow a day of recovery between training sessions involving the same muscle groups.
   e. Exhale during concentric work (muscle contraction) and inhale during eccentric work (controlled lengthening of the muscle).
   f. Always move in a controlled manner (particularly during eccentric work) to challenge the muscle most effectively.
D. **Goal: Reduction of body fat**
   1. **Mode:** Sustained cardiovascular/aerobic activity
   2. **Frequency:** 5 times/week (or more if a variety of activities, including low-impact options, are chosen)
   3. **Intensity:** 55–85% maximal heart rate
   4. **Duration:** 30–60 minutes
   5. **Considerations for weight loss**
      a. An increase in daily energy expenditure should be the focus of the program (300–500 kcal/session or 1,000–2,000 kcal/week).
      b. The intensity, frequency, and duration of variables should be manipulated to provide increased caloric expenditure within individual physical and lifestyle limitations.
      c. The beginning exerciser may see more success in achieving her energy expenditure goals through frequent, long-duration and low to moderate intensity exercise (i.e., brisk walking). This may improve adherence through providing a more pleasant exercise experience and alleviate the risk of injury with high-intensity, high-impact activity. The active individual who is dissatisfied with their rate of fat loss will want to increase training volume through additional exercise days, duration of sessions, or workout intensity and examine the diet for excess fat intake or other poor nutrition choices.
      d. Due to the risk of orthopedic injuries, particularly in the overweight individual, a combination of weight and non-weight-bearing activities should be suggested; i.e., cycling and walking, swimming and step aerobics, running and rowing.
      e. Supplementary resistance training may increase lean body mass, provide strength for endurance activities, and reduce injuries.
      f. A single bout of long-duration exercise may be more effective at utilizing free fatty acid oxidation than several short bouts involving the same amount of exercise.
      g. Regular aerobic exercise combined with a hypocaloric low-fat diet will elicit maximal fat loss results while preserving lean body mass.
      h. The individual should be encouraged to look at fat loss over months and years, rather than days and weeks. This will involve a gradual change in lifestyle related to nutritional choices and activity patterns.
      i. Many women still believe that performing leg lifts will remove fat from the thighs and that abdominal curls will remove fat from the stomach. It is important to address this myth and discuss the difference between muscle endurance training and aerobic training in relation to utilizing body fat stores and increasing metabolism during exercise.

IV. **CONSIDERATIONS DURING MENSTRUATION**
   A. No reason to alter exercise patterns (even swimming, as there is no risk of contamination).

B. Wearing supportive bras or two bras (one encapsulation model, one compression model) is helpful for tender breasts.

C. Use of tampons is helpful.

D. Testimonials relating exercise to control of PMS symptoms; no documented studies.

V. THE BOTTOM LINE

Epidemiologic studies show a strong, graded, and consistent inverse relationship between physical fitness/activity and coronary heart disease/mortality in both men and women, which is not confounded by age or other risk factors. The epidemiologists' definition of an active lifestyle includes blocks walked, stairs climbed, and calories expended through occupational, recreational, or fitness activities. This dose-response relationship between exercise and health status suggests that modest increases in physical activity elicit a positive health impact, which is particularly important for the lowest fit woman who may be discouraged or intimidated by standard vigorous exercise protocols.

It is beneficial, therefore, to encourage any efforts a woman can make to increase her average weekly caloric expenditure and establish the base for a more active lifestyle: riding a bike to the store or to the park with children, walking briskly and using stairs at every opportunity, going dancing or hiking, active gardening, as well as more traditional aerobics and fitness activities.

RECOMMENDED READING

1. American College of Sports Medicine: Guidelines for Exercise Testing and Prescription. Philadelphia, Lea & Febiger, 1991.
2. American College of Sports Medicine: Resource Manual for Guidelines for Exercise Testing and Prescription. Philadelphia, Lea & Febiger, 1988.
3. Berline JA: A meta-analysis of physical activity in the prevention of coronary heart disease. Am J Epidemiol 132:612–628, 1990.
4. Blair SN, et al: How much physical activity is good for health. Annu Rev Public Health 13:99–126, 1992.
5. Blair SN, et al: Physical Activity and Health: A Lifestyle Approach. Cambridge, MA, Blackwell Scientific Publications, 1992.
6. Borg G: An Introduction to Borg's RPE. Ithaca, NY, Movement Publications, 1985.
7. Brook GA: Exercise Physiology—Human Bioenergetics: Its Applications. New York, Wiley & Sons, 1984.
8. Butler RM, et al: Exercise and prevention of coronary heart disease. Prim Care 16:99–114, 1989.
9. Chandrashekar Y: Exercise as a coronary protective factor. Am Heart J 122:1723–1739, 1991.
10. Curfman G: The health benefits of exercise. N Engl J Med 325:574–576, 1993.
11. Fletcher GF, et al: AHA medical/scientific statement on exercise: Benefits and recommendations for physical activity programs for all Americans. Circulation 86:340–344, 1992.
12. Gordon NF, et al: The role of exercise in the primary and secondary prevention of coronary artery disease. Clin Sports Med 10:87–103, 1991.
13. Hagan RD, et al: Physical fitness is inversely related to heart disease risk: A factor analytic study. Am J Prev Med 7:237–243, 1991.
14. Haskell WL, et al: Cardiovascular benefits and assessment of physical activity and physical fitness in adults. Med Sci Sports Exerc 24:5201–5220, 1992.
15. Heyward V: Advanced Fitness Assessment and Exercise Prescription. Champaign, IL, Human Kinetics, 1991.
16. Howley ET, Franks BD: Health Fitness Instructor's Handbook. Champaign, IL, Human Kinetics, 1992.
17. Kendrick JS, et al: Re: A meta-analysis of physical activity in the prevention of coronary heart disease. Am J Epidemiol 134:232–234, 1991.
18. King AC, et al: Determinants of physical activity and interventions in adults. Med Sci Sports Exerc 24:5221–5234, 1992.
19. Manson JA, et al: Primary prevention of myocardial infarction. N Engl J Med 326:1406–1416, 1992.
20. Miller WC: Clinical symposium: Obesity, diet composition, energy expenditure and treatment of the obese patient. Med Sci Sports Exerc 23:273–297, 1991.

21. Paffenbarger R, et al: The associate of changes in physical activity level and other lifestyle characteristics with mortality among men. N Engl J Med 328:538–545, 1993.
22. Samitz G: Physical training programs and their effects on aerobic capacity and coronary risk profile in sedentary individuals. J Sports Med Phys Fitness 31(2):283–293, 1991.
23. Stefanick MD: Exercise and weight control. Exerc Sport Sci Rev 21:363–396, 1993.
24. Turock A: Getting Physical. New York, Doubleday, 1984.
25. Wells CL: Women, Sports and Performance. Champaign, IL, Human Kinetics, 1991.

Chapter 9: Exercise and Older Women

M. ELAINE CRESS, PhD

In projected estimates of the population by the year 2080, the Census Bureau places the number of people aged 85 and above at 18.7 million. Others set the figure much higher based on projections of increased lifespan. Although the majority of older adults (65+) recognize the importance of physical activity, less than 10% exercise on a regular basis. The need for scientific exercise programs is particularly great in retirement communities. The Healthy People 2000 goals (*see* Chapter 5) focus on the positive aspect of health and what people can do to influence their own health status. By maintaining a regular exercise program, we can substantially prevent or defer some of the physiologic changes associated with aging.

I. **PHYSIOLOGIC CHANGES WITH AGING**
   A. Aerobic fitness declines on the order of 1% per year.
   B. Lean muscle mass and strength decline in parallel, with a loss of about 30% between 30 to 70 years of age.
   C. The typical 80-year-old is below the threshold quadriceps strength necessary to stand from a chair.
   D. Bone mass declines are most rampant in the perimenopausal years but are exacerbated by a sedentary lifestyle.

II. **EXERCISE BENEFITS**

   Habitual exercise can help alter the physiologic changes of aging. The older adult responds to training in the same manner as a young adult.
   A. A 10–20% increase in cardiovascular fitness
   B. Strength gains of between 50 and 174%, depending on the extent of deconditioning
   C. Global effect of habitual exercise on aerobic fitness is equivalent to someone 20 years younger.
   D. Function is the bottom line justification for people in this age group to exercise. Staying active can mean the difference between independence and living a dependent lifestyle.
   E. In 1982, 20% of the total aged Medicare population was functionally impaired and living in the community.

III. **FUNCTIONAL STATUS**
   A. **Living status** (skilled nursing care, living in a retirement community either independently or assisted, or community dweller) is a reflection of functional ability, which in turn reflects physical capacity. The maximal ability to perform tasks necessary to maintain a house is higher than that required to live in a continuing care facility.
      1. **Instrumental activities of daily living**
         a. Light and heavy housework, laundry, preparing meals, grocery shopping, getting outside the house, going places out of walking distance, managing finances, telephone calls, medication management.
         b. Bathing. To get up from sitting out of bathtub requires calf strength, quadriceps strength, upper body strength, and balance and coordination.
         c. Bed making. To fling a comforter over the bed, one must have good grip strength and upper body strength in the arms and torso.
         d. When maximal ability declines to a level of minimal function, one finds these tasks exhausting or impossible.

2. Much of **functional performance** is hierarchical.
   a. If quadriceps strength is improved so that someone can rise out of a chair, then stair climbing is eventually made possible.
   b. With additional strength gains, new tasks are added to the program that reinforce the healthy behavior.
B. **Frailty** is a process of multiple-systems decline, and that person's ability is limited by the weakest link.
   1. If the respiratory system is compromised, then the heart and muscles decline to the level of use which is limited by the lungs. Exercising the weakest system to improve it can then achieve a general systems improvement.
   2. During a particular period of disuse (e.g., during a hospital stay or winter sedentary period), we lose fitness.
   3. For most, the loss of strength during winter does not compromise safety. However, elderly women (72 years old) in Madison, Wisconsin, lost 12% of their thigh strength over the 7 months of winter. A regular exercise program prevented this loss in an intervention group.
   4. A regular exercise program can prevent seasonal strength declines and help people stay aware of their capabilities.

IV. **EXERCISE PROGRAM GUIDELINES**
A. **Exercise modes:** Sessions should include the following:
   1. Strength
   2. Endurance
   3. Flexibility (under-taught)
   4. Coordination (under-taught)
B. **Duration:** Plan at least 1.5 hours for the program to allow time for each component.
C. **Exercise intensity:** The greatest strides in general health status are made by persons going from sedentary status to low or moderate activity. Use an intensity based on a heart rate (HR) of 40–60% to begin with, which can safely be increased to 75% of HR reserve. Over-intense exercise is a major cause of injuries.
   1. **Target heart rate:** HR reserve = HRmax – HRrest

   HR training = [HR reserve (0.60)] + HRrest
      a. Prescription by HR reserve is important in elderly because of their high resting HR. Percent HR max under-prescribes.
      b. Monitor HR in addition to using respiratory rate, perceived exertion, and pain scale to monitor intensity, since HR should stay below a 60–75% level.
      c. As other systems cease to be the limiting factor, switch to HR as a monitoring system.
   2. **Perceived exertion**
      a. The 20-point Borg scale correlates heart rate with perceived effort. 12 is "somewhat hard" and is a good intensity for people to feel as though they are working, to get a training effect without a negative experience.
      b. It is important to use this scale for persons on beta-blockers, with dyspnea, or otherwise limited by something other than the cardiovascular system.
   3. **Pain scale**
      a. 0 = no pain, 4 = severe pain.
      b. This has been used effectively in cardiac rehabilitation for ischemia and can be used by persons with musculoskeletal limitations such as rheumatoid arthritis or overuse injuries.
   4. **Respiratory rate**
      a. Usually persons who require a high respiratory rate will self-limit their exercise.
      b. Average maximal respiratory rate for elderly is 48 breaths/min.
      c. Persons with asthma or COPD should limit themselves to 9–10 breaths/15 seconds.

5. **Start low, go slow**
   a. Collagen in older people becomes less compliant as cross-linking increases with age, yet the muscle (be it heart or skeletal muscle) responds quickly to increased intensity. If muscle hypertrophies more rapidly than collagen adaptations, musculoskeletal injuries result.
   b. Increase duration before increasing intensity.
D. **Evaluation:** This can be a motivating tool with any group. The American Academy of Health, Physical Education, Recreation, and Dance (AAHPERD) has a low-tech method of evaluation for seniors, and norms are available. In lieu of a formal evaluation, elders will present anecdotal evidence of increases in function on a regular basis.
E. **Medical history and physical**
   1. Physician approval is required, and if cardiovascular disease is suspected, an exercise evaluation is required.
   2. AAHPERD has a physical form (Fig. 1) that is geared toward the older adult and is specific for exercise. These forms should be memorized in detail for medications and for chronic and acute conditions.

Name _____ Phone _____ Date _____
Street _____ City _____ State _____ Zip _____

PART I: TO BE FILLED OUT BY PARTICIPANT
A. ACTIVITY HISTORY
   1. How would you rate your physical activity level during the last year?
      ☐ LITTLE—Sitting, typing, driving, talking. NO exercise planned
      ☐ MILD—Standing, walking, bending, reaching
      ☐ MODERATE—Standing, walking, bending, reaching, exercise 1 day a week
      ☐ ACTIVE—Light physical work, climbing stairs, exercise 2–3 days a week
      ☐ VERY ACTIVE—Moderate physical work, regular exercise 4 or more days a week
   2. What exercise and recreational activities are you presently involved in and how ofen? _____
   _____

B. HEALTH HISTORY
   1. Weight _____ Height _____ Recent weight loss/gain _____
   2. Please list any recent illnesses: _____
   _____
   3. Please list hospitalizations and reasons during last 5 years: _____
   _____
   4. Please check the box if you *have* any of these conditions:

☐ Anemia	☐ Heart conditions _____
☐ Arthritis/bursitis	☐ Hernia
☐ Asthma	☐ Indigestion
☐ Blood pressure _____	☐ Joint pain in _____
☐ Bowel/bladder problems	☐ Leg pain on walking
☐ Chest pains	☐ Lung disease
☐ Chest discomfort while exercising	☐ Shortness of breath
☐ Diabetes	☐ Passing out spells
☐ Difficulty with hearing	☐ Osteoporosis _____
☐ Difficulty with visions	☐ Low back condition
☐ Dizziness or balance problems	☐ Other orthopedic conditions [List]

   _____
   5. Smoking: ☐ Never smoked   ☐ Smoke now [how much? _____]   ☐ Quit
   6. Alcohol consumption: ☐ None   ☐ Occasional   ☐ Often [how much? _____]
   7. List any existing health concerns _____
   _____
   8. Please list any medications and/or dietary supplements you take regularly _____
   _____

FIGURE 1.   Sample form for medical/exercise assessment in older adults *(cont. on next page).*

PART II: TO BE COMPLETED BY PHYSICIAN

A. PHYSICAL EXAMINATION—Please check if it applies to the patient.

☐ Resting heart rate _____   ☐ Resting blood pressure _____
☐ Chest auscultation abnormal   ☐ Thyroid abnormal
☐ Heart size abnormal   ☐ Any joints abnormal
☐ Peripheral pulses normal   ☐ Abnormal masses
☐ Abnormal heart sounds, gallops   ☐ Other _____

Present prescribed medication(s): _____
_____

B. CARDIOVASCULAR LABORATORY EXAMINATION [within 1 year of the present date if recommended by physician]   DATE: _____

1. *Resting EKG:*   Rate _____   Rhythm _____
                    Axis _____   Interpretation _____
2. *Stress test:*   Max HR _____   Max BP: _____   Total time _____
                    Max VO$_2$ _____   METS _____   Type of test _____
3. Recommendation for exercise. *Moderate* is defined as standing, walking, bending, reaching, and light exercise 3 days a week. Please *check* one:

_____ There is no contraindication to participation in *moderate* exercise program.

_____ Because of the above analysis, participation in a *moderate* exercise program may be advisable, but further examination or consultation is necessary: i.e., stress test, EKG, other _____

_____ Because of the above analysis, patient may participate only under direct supervision of a physician (cardiac rehabilitation program).

_____ Because of the above analysis, participation in a *moderate* exercise program is inadvisable.

C. SUMMARY IMPRESSION OF PHYSICIAN

1. Comments on any history of orthopedic and neuromuscular disorders that may affect participation in an exercise program, especially those checked: _____
_____

2. Message for the Exercise Program Director: _____
_____
_____

Physician: _____   Signature _____
          [Please type/print]
Address _____   Phone: _____/_____

PART III: PATIENT'S RELEASE AND CONSENT

_____ RELEASE: I hereby release the above information to the Exercise Program Director.
_____ CONSENT: I agree to see my private physician for medical care and agree to have an evaluation by him/her once a year, if necessary.

SIGNED: _____   DATE: _____

FIGURE 1 *(Cont.).*   Sample form for medical/exercise assessment in older adults.

F. **Precautions**
1. Elderly persons have reduced muscle mass and are particularly susceptible to heat.
2. By lowering intensity, one can assist in acclimation; also, provide plenty of water.
3. Diuretics (for hypertension) can exacerbate heat stress, as can coffee and tea consumption.

G. **15-beat rule** can distinguish between psychological and physiologic reasons for a person's not feeling like exercising:
1. Have elderly persons take their resting heart rate first thing in the morning (before coffee and activity). Do this once or twice a week on a regular basis.
2. When they question whether or not to attend exercise class, they should take their pulse. If it is 25% over the resting HR, they may be overtraining, dehydrated, or coming down with an infection and should skip class that day.

H. **Emergency procedures**
   1. The exercise leader must be CPR certified.
   2. Phone locations should be well known, and directions to the site marked above the phone.
   3. Designate one person to go for help, another to remove the class from the site of the emergency, cool down the class, and dismiss them.

V. **EXERCISE LEADERSHIP**

A. **Maturity**
   1. The leader must have a lot of interaction with the group to be successful.
   2. More than one leader may assist with the class to provide an alternate personality.
   3. Do not speak down to older adults in a patronizing fashion. Make compliments genuine.

B. **Knowledge**
   1. Know medications, what they do, and how they interact with exercise.
   2. Know exercise interactions with chronic conditions (*see* below).
   3. Know how to use blankets, pillows, straps, and chairs to modify exercise to different body types, tightness, injuries, etc.

C. **Confidence:** The art of confident exercise leadership is essential. We can be too timid because of our lack of knowledge.

D. **Enthusiasm:** Dare to be outrageous.

E. **Challenge:** Persons who lead the elderly in exercise should challenge themselves physically. This helps them to identify with the feelings of trying something new. It is also helpful if what they are learning in their challenge will broaden their knowledge base for senior exercise.

VI. **IMPLEMENTATION OF EXERCISE**

A. **Endurance**
   1. **Walking**
      a. It can be done anywhere, without lessons, with or without friends, and without much expense.
      b. It is good cardiovascularly and for lower extremity strength and bone density, as it is weight-bearing exercise.
      c. It is a good public health exercise recommendation.
   2. **Stationary cycle**
      a. Arms and legs (Schwinn) are nice, but standard Monarch style cycle is also fine.
      b. It is hard for older people to stay on the cycle for 30 min; work up gradually.
      c. Only one major muscle group (thigh) is exercised.
      d. The seat is often uncomfortable. Get large seats.
      e. Watch that there is not too much isometric contraction in the handgrip (which would be contraindicated in cardiac patients).

B. **Weightlifting:** Emphasis is on the legs, because legs lose strength faster than arms in aging and disuse and leg weakness cuts into independence dramatically. Upper body strength, however, is important for activities of daily living.
   1. Machine information
      a. ROM stops
      b. Low initial plate
      c. Small increments
      d. Not intimidating
      e. Variable cam
   2. Machines are generally safer than lifting with free weights
   3. **General principles for weightlifting:**
      a. First 2 weeks: 2 weeks range of weightlifting, no or lowest weight

       b. Setting intensity: 8 reps of low weight (after 2 weeks). Get to maximum in 2–3 weight increments. One maximal rep at weight where athlete does not lose integrity of lifting position. Work closely with the individual at first.

       c. Training intensity: 75% works fine in frail elderly without injury.

4. Leg extension
5. Leg curl
6. Leg press
7. Hip adduction
8. Hip abduction
9. Ankleciser
10. Upper body
11. Rotary torso
12. Abdominal
13. Upright row

C. **Flexibility**
1. Pool exercise for range of motion
2. Yoga is working actively where two muscles on either side of the joint are contracted and actively stretching the tissue over the joint. Combines flexibility with strengthening (upper and lower body) and balance.

D. **Integrated programs**
1. Tai chi: strength (lower body), flexibility, coordination, balance
2. Aerobic dance: coordination, aerobic exercise

VII. MEDICAL PRECAUTIONS

A. **Cardiovascular disease**
1. Ensure patient's cardiovascular status is well controlled and patient is on medication.
2. If in doubt, have the patient checked.

B. **Hypertension**
1. Extended **cool-down** period is important, as the peripheral vessels are vasodilated by medication and as the elderly, in general, have slowed autonomic reflexes causing blood to pool in their legs. Hot showers are contraindicated after exercise.
2. **Diuretics** cause reduced blood volume, higher heart rate, less sweat, and less thermal regulation.

C. **Chronic obstructive pulmonary disease (COPD)**
1. Persons with **asthma or COPD** may be on inhalants or oxygen. They should have their medications with them and be encouraged to stop upon dyspnea. Encourage long-term participation.
2. A training effect occurs so that the muscle is better able to extract O_2 as well as peripheral circulation being improved.
3. Exercise decreases the dependence on the lung for gas exchange.
4. Breathing deeply is important to maintain flexibility in the rib cage and healthy respiratory muscles. People over 80 have decreased breath excursion merely because of lung mechanics.

D. **Arthritis**
1. Range of motion and low-intensity exercise is the standard recommendation.
2. Recent evidence shows exercise improves functional ability in patients with arthritis.

E. **Diabetes**
1. The diabetes should be stable. Exercise perturbs this stability, so beware of symptoms of hypoglycemia.
2. To minimize this disruption, diabetics should eat, exercise, and take medications at the same time each day.

3. Beta-blockers attenuate the symptoms of hypoglycemia.
4. Because of decreased peripheral circulation, pay immediate attention to sores on feet.

VIII. SUMMARY

The exercise program for elderly individuals should be well rounded. We do not know how well exercise carries over into functional improvements, but we need to be aware of the importance of strength, endurance, coordination, and flexibility in the overall function of the older person.

Older adults respond to training in much the same way as younger adults, and we should not be timid about training them. The exercise environment is important and should be safe and comfortable. Health clubs could build up clientele at senior centers and invite them to visit the health club together, so that people do not have to develop the courage to come alone. Play appropriate music, and have club staff who are older and look it.

The elderly are a rewarding population to work with. However, you must win their confidence, so become a knowledgeable exercise leader skilled in the art of confident exercise leadership. Once committed, this group will stay with the exercise.

RESOURCES FOR SENIOR EXERCISE

1. American College of Sports Medicine: Guidelines for Exercise Testing and Prescription, 4th ed. Philadelphia, Lea & Febiger, 1991.
2. Corbin DE, Metal-Corbin J: Reach for It!: A Handbook of Health Exercise and Dance Activitites for Older Adults. Dubuque, IA, Eddie Bowers Publishing Co., 1990.
3. de Vries HA: Fit After 50. New York, Charles Scribners Sons, 1987.
4. Harris JA, Pittman AM, Waller MS: Dance a While: Handbook of Folk, Square, and Social Dancing, 5th ed. Minneapolis, Burgess Publishing Co., 1978.
5. Kisner C, Colby LA: Therapeutic Exercise: Foundations and Techniques. Philadelphia, F.A. Davis Co., 1990.
6. Lerman L: Teaching Dance to Senior Adults. Springfield, IL, Charles C Thomas, 1984.
7. Minton SC: Body and Self. Champaign, IL, Human Kinetics Publishers, 1989.
8. Rikkers R: Seniors on the Move. Champaign, IL, Human Kinetics Publishers, 1986.

VIDEOS

1. Harlow D, Yu P: The ROM Dance: A Range of Motion Exercise Relaxation Program. Madison, WI, WHA TV, 1993. (A version adapted for chair exercisers is available.)
2. The Complete Guide to Exercise Videos. Video Specialties, Inc., 1-800-433-6769.

Chapter 10: Breast Cancer Screening

MARIE E. LEE, MD

Breast cancer is not a problem unique to active and athletic women. The problem is pervasive, affecting 10–12% of all women and causing 46,000 deaths/year. Therefore, it is clear that all women should understand their risk and the importance of screening to prevent this disease.

I. **GENERAL PRINCIPLES**
   A. A screening procedure is performed in the absence of known or suspected disease.
   B. It divides the population into two groups:
      1. One group with low probability of disease
      2. One group with high probability of disease, in whom further evaluation is merited
   C. Mammography and physical examination are screening procedures for breast cancer detection.

II. **INCIDENCE OF BREAST CANCER**
   A. **Breast cancer affects 1 in 9 women.**
      1. 180,000 new cases are diagnosed each year.
      2. 46,000 deaths/year are caused by breast cancer.
   B. Breast cancer is most common in women over 50 years old ($\geq$75% of all cases).
   C. Its incidence in women under 50 is 22%.
      1. 35–50 years—19%
      2. 30–35 years—2%
      3. $\leq$30 years—1%
   D. **Detection and survival rates:** Breast cancer survival is determined by lesion size at the time of detection and lymph node status.
      1. The goal of screening is to detect the cancer at an earlier and more curable stage.
      2. Stages of breast cancer
         a. Premammographic period (5–7 years)
            i. Lesion size: First malignant cell to 2 mm
            ii. The cancer is undetectable during this period.
         b. Preclinical period (3 years)
            i. Lesion size: 2 mm–1 cm
            ii. The cancer is detectable by mammography during this period.
         c. Clinical period (2–3 years)
            i. Lesion size: 1–2 cm
            ii. The lesion is palpable during this period.
      3. In an optimal screening program, mammography is performed regularly so that cancer can be detected in the preclinical period.
      4. Breast self-examination in conjunction with regular mammography detects palpable lesions early.

III. **EFFECTIVENESS OF SCREENING**
   The need for effective screening is high since there is no known way to prevent breast cancer and its incidence is significant.
   A. **Despite public awareness about the benefits of mammography and breast self-examination, most breast cancers are detected by chance.**
      1. 75% of cancers are detected by the patient by chance.
      2. <25% of cancers are detected through breast self-examination.

    3. At detection, most tumors are 2–3 cm.

    4. At detection, axillary metatases are present in 40% of women and the average 5-year survival is 60–70%.

B. **The goal of screening is to detect breast cancers early and thereby reduce mortality.**

C. **Three major studies have assessed the effectiveness of mammography screening on survival rates and mortality.**

    1. **Breast Cancer Detection Demonstration Project (BCDD)**

        a. 5.54 cancers detected per 1000 women in the initial scan

        b. 2.65 cancers detected per 1000 women on second annual examination

        c. Proportion of nonpalpable cancers detected

            i. 47% if woman was <50 years old

            ii. 48% if woman was >50 years old

        d. 42% of all cancers were detected by mammography alone; 44% were noninfiltrating or <1 cm.

        e. 7% of cases were detected by physical examination alone.

        f. Findings emphasize the need for physical examination and breast self-examination and the correlation of physical and mammographic results.

    2. **Health Insurance Plan (HIP)**

        a. Screening mammography was shown to reduce mortality by 25% in all women and 40% in women >50.

    3. **Swedish Trials**

        a. 24% reduction of breast cancer mortality among women of all ages who received mammography

        b. For women aged 40–49, there was a 13% reduction.

D. **Screening mammography detects lesions earlier and at a smaller size.**

    1. 13–25% of breast cancers found by mammography alone are regionally or locally advanced.

    2. Mass detection lead time gained is 2.5–3.5 years.

    3. 25–40% of tumors detected by mammography are small (<5 mm) or wholly intraductal and are associated with a better prognosis and 20–25-year survival rate of 95%.

E. **Risk of radiation exposure during mammography is small compared with benefits of cancer detection.**

    1. Radiation is 0.1–0.2 rad, equal to the risk of 10 miles of car travel.

IV. **AMERICAN CANCER SOCIETY GUIDELINES FOR SCREENING**

A. **Screening recommendations by age groups**

    1. 20–35 years: Monthly breast self-examination

    2. 35–40 years

        a. Monthly breast self-examination

        b. Baseline mammogram

    3. 40–50 years

        a. Monthly breast self-examination

        b. Mammography every 1–2 years

        c. Clinical breast examination by a practitioner annually

    4. >50 years

        a. Monthly breast self-examination

        b. Yearly mammography

        c. Clinical breast examination by a practitioner annually

B. **Screening recommendations (controversy)**

    1. The Canadian National Breast Screening Study[4] has raised some question that mammography may not reduce mortality rates in women age 40–49. As a result, there currently is controversy surrounding the benefit of mammography for women in the 40–50 age range.

V. SUMMARY

Screening mammography in association with breast self-examination and regular physical examinations can detect breast cancer earlier and improve survival from breast cancer. With improvements in availability, acceptability, accuracy, and affordability, we can hope that screening with mammography and breast self-examination will lead to reductions in the mortality statistics for breast cancer.

REFERENCES

1. Balter S, Alcom F: AAPM tutorial to value of mammographic screening: Assessment of studies and opinions. Radiographics 10:1133–1139, 1990.
2. Feig S, et al: Diseases of the breast. In Theros E, Harris J, Siegel B (eds): ACR Syllabus. Reston, VA, American College of Radiology, 1988.
3. Nystrom L, Rutquist L, Wall S, et al: Breast cancer screening with mammography: Overview of Swedish studies. Lancet 241:973–978, 1993.
4. Miller A, Baines C, To T, Wall C: Canadian National Breast Screening Study: 1. Breast cancer detection and death rates among women aged 40–49 and 2. Breast cancer detection and death rates among women aged 50–59 years. Can Med Assoc 147:1459–1488, 1992.

Chapter 11: Effects of the Menstrual Cycle and Birth Control Pill on Athletic Performance

CONSTANCE M. LEBRUN, BSc, MDCM, MPE, FACSM

The female athlete is a unique species. From puberty through pregnancy and childbirth to menopause and beyond, she has to cope with a kaleidoscope of shifting hormonal patterns that undoubtedly affect her ability to train and compete successfully. The effects of exercise on the menstrual cycle, exercise during pregnancy, and exercise and bone health have been extensively investigated. Much less is known about how the various phases of the menstrual cycle and oral contraceptives might affect exercise performance.

I. PHYSIOLOGIC CONSIDERATIONS

It is commonly accepted that important biomechanical and physiologic differences exist between male and female athletes. Women also suffer from a higher incidence of problems such as iron deficiency anemia and stress fractures. There is also a very small risk of injuries to the breast tissue and/or reproductive organs.

A. **Biomechanical factors:** Distinct **skeletal system differences** may affect the way a woman carries out certain sporting activities (such as throwing a baseball) and may also cause an increased predisposition to specific injuries. For example, the "miserable malalignment syndrome" and excessive pronation can be factors in lower extremity stress fractures and patellofemoral problems. Some biomechanical factors in women are as follows:[59]
   1. Usually smaller and shorter stature
   2. Wider pelvis, larger Q angle, legs less bowed
   3. Shorter limbs (relative to body length)
   4. Narrower shoulders with more slope
   5. Greater "carrying angle" of elbows
   6. Greater percent body fat, less muscle mass

B. **Cardiovascular system differences**
   1. Smaller heart
   2. Faster heart rate
   3. Lower blood volume
   4. Fewer red blood cells (~6% less)
   5. Less hemoglobin (~15% less)
   6. Lower maximal oxygen-carrying capacity ($\dot{V}O_2max$) (up to 50% less), but when expressed in relative terms—i.e., per kg body weight—the difference shrinks to approximately 16%. When further corrected for percent body fat, the $\dot{V}O_2max$ per kg of lean body mass of an aerobically trained woman is only 9% less than that of a trained male.

C. **Response to training:** Many of the differences between males and females can be attributed to fundamental underlying endocrine differences and to the effects on the musculoskeletal system and other target tissues of the **gonadotropins**—luteinizing hormone (LH) and follicle-stimulating hormone (FSH)—as well as the **steroid sex hormones**—testosterone, estradiol, and progesterone. Females respond to training as do males, with:
   1. Increased $\dot{V}O_2max$
   2. Lowered blood pressure
   3. Lowered heart rate
   4. Reduced percent body fat

Therefore, participation in sports is a healthy and desirable outcome and *is to be encouraged* for women of all ages.

II. THE MENSTRUAL CYCLE

A. **Phases of the menstrual cycle:** The menstrual cycle is classically categorized into phases beginning with the first day of menstruation. Normal cycles range from 23–35 days in length, with an average of about 28 days.
   1. **The menses**—cycle days 1–5
   2. **Postmenstrual phase**—cycle days 6–13 or 14 (also termed the estrogenic, proliferative or **follicular phase**)
   3. **Ovulation**—cycle days 13–15. Here, the midcycle surge of estrogen triggers the LH and FSH bursts that subsequently cause ovulation. This phase is most susceptible to variability.
   4. **Postovulatory phase**—cycle days 15–28 (also called the progesterone, secretory, premenstrual, or **luteal phase**)
   The hormonal changes that take place over the course of a normal ovulatory menstrual cycle are shown in Figure 1.
B. **Molimina:** The cascade of hormonal events during a normal menstrual cycle causes various systemic effects, particularly in the postovulatory phase when progesterone levels increase, which are collectively described as **molimina**. In moderation, these symptoms can be interpreted to mean that the neuroendocrine system is working in a normal healthy fashion and that regular ovulation is occurring. These symptoms are hormone mediated.
   1. Appetite changes
   2. Breast tenderness (especially lateral breast tenderness)
   3. Fluid retention
   4. Mood changes
C. **Premenstrual syndrome:** In some women, these symptoms are exaggerated and become troublesome. These symptoms may potentially affect athletic performance, but it is frequently difficult to sort out the physiologic from cognitive components.
   1. Mood changes, including dysphoria and sometimes severe depression
   2. Breast tenderness and swelling
   3. Fluid retention, leading to edema, weight gain, sluggish feelings

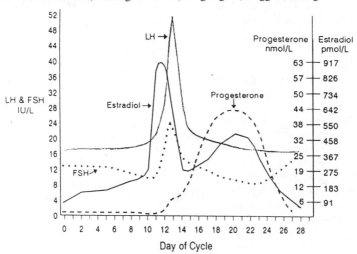

FIGURE 1. Hormonal changes during the menstrual cycle (courtesy of Dr. Jerilynn Prior). (Adapted by Dr. J. C. Prior from: Speroff L, Van de Wiele RL: Regulation of the human menstrual cycle. Am J Obstet Gynecol 109: 234–247, 1971, with permission.)

4. Abdominal bloating
5. Appetite changes, such as carbohydrate cravings
D. **Dysmenorrhea:** Some women experience significant discomfort or **dysmenorrhea**, associated with menstruation itself.
   1. Abdominal pain and low back pain associated with uterine contractions or ischemia during menstruation
   2. Due to prostaglandins released by the endometrium
   3. Antiprostaglandin nonsteroidal antiinflammatory drugs (NSAIDs) are often helpful.

III. **EFFECTS OF EXERCISE ON MENSTRUAL FUNCTION**
   A. **Vigorous regular exercise** has beneficial effects that may counteract the physical perturbations associated with the menstrual cycle phases, decreasing:[47]
      1. Menstrual pelvic pain
      2. Low back pain
      3. Headache
      4. Anxiety, depression
      5. Fatigue
      6. Use of analgesics
   B. **Athletic training** can have an adverse impact upon normal menstrual function and can lead to menstrual cycle variations:[52,59]
      1. **Delayed menarche or primary amenorrhea**—No menstruation by age 16, or the failure to develop secondary sexual characteristics (thelarche) by age 14
      2. **Secondary amenorrhea**—No menstrual cycles for at least 3 months, or less than two periods in 1 year, once regular menstruation has been established
      3. **Oligomenorrhea**—3–6 menstrual cycles/year, or cycles at intervals of >38 days
      4. **Short luteal phase**—<10 days in duration
      5. **Anovulation**—Regular menstrual bleeding may still occur, both in the absence of ovulation and in cycles with a short luteal phase.
   C. **"Exercise-related" or "athletic amenorrhea"** is a diagnosis of **exclusion.** Many other pathophysiologic processes that can cause disruption of the neuroendocrine axis must be ruled out before ascribing menstrual cycle variations to exercise.

IV. **EFFECTS OF THE MENSTRUAL CYCLE AND ORAL CONTRACEPTIVES ON PERFORMANCE**
   This is an extremely important topic for a number of reasons, including increasing participation of women in competitive sports, alteration of normal cycles by rigorous endurance training, common usage of oral contraceptive agents by athletes, and current concerns regarding prolonged amenorrhea in athletes and osteoporosis. Medical treatment may include replacement hormones, either as estrogen and/or progesterone, or oral contraceptives.
   A. **Components of athletic performance:** Many factors can contribute to athletic performance,[62] and there is a high degree of sport specificity:
      1. Sensory motor—simple reaction time
      2. Psychomotor—hand/eye coordination
      3. Sensory perceptual—pain threshold
      4. Cognitive—information processing
      5. Neuromuscular—strength
      6. Psychological
         a. Affective—mood
         b. Psychophysiologic—arousal
      7. Cardiovascular
         a. Heart rate
         b. Stroke volume

8. Metabolic
   a. Core body temperature
   b. Resting O_2 consumption
9. Aerobic capacity—$\dot{V}O_2$max

B. **Energy systems**
1. **Anaerobic systems:** The anaerobic systems function in the absence of oxygen and provide energy for short-duration, intense activity.
   a. **Phosphate system** uses creatine phosphate stores as a source of energy for activities up to 10 seconds in duration. Creatine phosphate splits to provide energy in the form of a phosphate molecule for resynthesis of adenosine triphosphate (ATP) from adenosine diphosphate (ADP).
   b. **Lactic acid system** provides energy for activities from 30 seconds to 2 minutes in duration. ATP is produced by the anaerobic metabolism of carbohydrate (i.e., glycogen). The major byproduct is lactic acid, which builds up in the exercising muscle and contributes to the onset of muscle fatigue. Once the activity stops, other enzyme systems come into play to reutilize the lactic acid for fuel and clear it from the muscle. The threshold for this lactic acid buildup can be increased through training, as the muscles will be able to clear the lactate more quickly.
   c. **Alactic system** uses other fuels for energy, but this system does not play a very important role in energy metabolism.
2. **Aerobic systems**
   a. Aerobic metabolism requires oxygen and provides energy for activities performed at a submaximal rate over a longer time (i.e., >2 minutes). Both glycogen and fat are metabolized in the presence of oxygen to ATP, H_2O, and CO_2. This type of glycolysis is very efficient and produces 38 ATP/glucose molecule, as opposed to 2 ATP molecules by the anaerobic metabolism of glucose. Fat is the body's most concentrated form of energy and yields 9 kcal of energy per gram, as compared to 4 kcal/g for carbohydrate or protein.
   b. The amount of aerobic metabolism that can take place, or the maximal aerobic capacity ($\dot{V}O_2$max) depends on:
      i. O_2-carrying capacity of blood (hemoglobin concentration)
      ii. Volume of oxygen-containing blood delivered to tissues:
         cardiac output = stroke volume × heart rate
         Even though trained athletes have a lower resting heart rate than untrained people, the output with each heartbeat is greater, and both the stroke volume and heart rate can increase in response to exercise to levels up to 5 times as high as the average sedentary adult.
      iii. Ability of the body to utilize O_2 at the cellular level. The enzyme systems in mitochondria can also be increased with proper training techniques.
   c. In reality, these various energy systems are not discrete, but rather they are recruited as a continuum depending on the type, intensity, and duration of exercise performed.
3. **Muscle strength and endurance**
   a. The type and number of muscle fibers are genetically determined to some extent but can also be modified by training. There are three types of muscle fibers:
      i. **Slow-twitch fibers** (slow oxidative) are the main type utilized for prolonged aerobic exercise.
      ii. **Fast-twitch** (fast glycolytic) are more useful for quick bursts of explosive power. They utilize muscle glycogen, do not require oxygen, but, because of this, are not capable of sustained effort.
      iii. An **intermediate subtype** (fast oxidative glycolytic) uses both muscle glycogen and oxygen.

    b. As the intensity of effort increases, the nervous system progressively recruits slow oxidative, then fast oxidative glycolytic, and finally fast glycolytic fiber types.

V. VARIABLES INFLUENCED BY HORMONAL LEVELS

A. The changing pattern of hormones during a regular ovulatory menstrual cycle may impact on both cardiovascular and metabolic variables:
1. Blood pressure
2. Blood volume
3. Heart rate
4. Vascular tone
5. Body temperature
6. Electrolyte and water exchange
7. Respiration/ventilation
8. Energy metabolism

B. **Each hormone has its own specific actions:**
1. **Estrogen**
   a. Causes **deposition of fat** (in breasts, buttocks, thighs)
   b. Decrease in total **cholesterol level**, increase in HDL cholesterol. This leads to a protective effect against atherosclerosis and is one beneficial aspect of female hormones.
   c. Increased strength of **capillary walls**
   d. Increased **glycogen storage in liver and muscle.** This effect has been shown in both animals and in humans and is important because it increases the amount of fuel available for exercise.[9]
   e. **Glycogen sparing during exercise**, shift to free fatty acids[9]
   f. Effects on **blood glucose and lactate**. The studies are somewhat contradictory on this aspect, and progesterone also plays a role.
   g. Facilitates **calcium uptake into bone** *(very important)*
2. **Progesterone**
   a. Increases **glandular elements in breasts** (in preparation for lactation)
   b. Increases **core body temperature**. The increased progesterone in the luteal phase of the cycle is responsible for the biphasic basal body temperature curve (increase of 0.3–0.5° C).
   c. Increase in **excretion of H_2O and sodium from kidney**
   d. Causes **hyperventilation in pregnancy** and during the luteal phase. This may cause some inhibition of maximal performance due to a subjective sensation of dyspnea (this is seen only in untrained individuals, not in trained athletic women).
   e. Possibly stimulates **ventilatory drives** during exercise
3. **Oral contraceptives**
   a. Most oral contraceptives contain both an **estrogen and a progestagen.** The specific effects are modulated by the balance of the two components, as many of the progestagens have antiestrogen effects. In addition, some newer contraceptives, such as Depo-Provera (medroxyprogesterone acetate), Norplant (a subdermal implant of levonorgestrel), and the progestin-only pill do not contain any estrogen.
   b. **Side effects** include:[46,50]
      i. Increased water retention
      ii. Weight gain
      iii. Breakthrough bleeding
      iv. Alteration of carbohydrate metabolism. This may show up as a potentiation of underlying diabetes, but may affect performance by altering the amount and composition of fuels available for energy.

       v. **Change in serum lipids**, potential effect on cardiovascular system
     vi. Alteration in **hemostatic mechanisms** such as clotting mechanisms and platelets. There may be a subtle physiologic effect of increased blood viscosity on oxygen delivery to the tissues.
   c. **Beneficial effects**, some of which may have implications for athletic performance, include:[46,50,52]
       i. Elimination or reduction of dysmenorrhea
      ii. Reduction in menstrually induced anemia
     iii. Reduced risk of endometrial and ovarian cancer
     iv. Reduced incidence of benign breast lesions, pelvic inflammatory disease, ovarian cysts, ectopic pregnancy, rheumatoid arthritis
      v. Reduced risk of endometrial hyperplasia
     vi. Prevention of premature osteoporosis in amenorrheic athletes. (This potential therapeutic effect is still being studied.)

C. **Problems with research to date:** Various methodologic and other problems with early studies on the effects of hormonal levels on athletic performance and various other factors in the later studies limit their generalizability:
  1. **Anecdotal or retrospective surveys.** Most of these studies are biased and, although interesting, are scientifically inaccurate.
  2. Marked discrepancies in **timing of testing**. This makes it difficult to compare different studies or to make generalizations about a specific phase of the cycle.
  3. Wide variety of **physiologic tests** used. Again, this makes it impossible to draw many general conclusions or to extrapolate to the clinical situation.[17]
  4. Inadequate documentation of **menstrual cycle phase**. Studies should at the least utilize basal body temperature monitoring to estimate the time of ovulation, preferably backed up by accurate hormonal determination. Improved laboratory measures, such as ability to accurately measure salivary progesterone or the newer urine testing kits that can pick up the luteinizing hormone surge, may also make it easier to do proper controlled studies.
  5. Difficulties with accurate **hormonal measurements.** The concentrations of both estradiol and progesterone rise with exercise,[27] and therefore blood for these hormones must be drawn before the subjects begin to warm up!
  6. Use of **untrained subjects**. Most studies have used subjects with relatively low fitness levels. The effects on performance may be more noticeable, as well as more critical, in high-performance athletes.
  7. **Small numbers of subjects** (<20 women in studies to date)
  8. Wide variation in estrogen and progesterone **composition of the oral contraceptive** used. Much of the earlier research used oral contraceptives with much higher dosages than those in today's formulations. No studies to date have looked at the effects of oral contraceptives containing either progesterone only (oral or injectable) or the newer progestins, such as gestodene, norgestimate or desogestrel.

D. **Physiologic variables over the menstrual cycle**
  1. Various **physiologic and psychological variables** have been studied over the course of the "normal" menstrual cycle:[22,53]
   a. Heart rate
   b. Blood pressure
   c. Cardiac output
   d. Hemoglobin
   e. Body temperature
   f. Sweating response
   g. Reaction time
   h. Perceived exertion

2. Results have been contradictory,[17,22,53] and it is difficult to draw any definite conclusions based on these studies unless there is proper documentation of menstrual cycle phase by ovarian hormone measurements.

VI. **EFFECTS OF CYCLE PHASE**

A. **Athletic performance**
   1. Early studies
      a. Most of the early studies are retrospective or anecdotal and have no documentation of cycle phase. The results are somewhat inconsistent, but they have generally reported:[2,16,64]
         i. "Best" performance during "intermenstrual" or "postmenstrual" phases
         ii. "Worst" performance during "premenstrual" phase or time of menses
      b. Postulated **mediators of cycle-related effects** include:[59]
         i. **Self-expectancies**
         ii. **Possible negative attitude toward menstruation**
         iii. **Cultural restrictions and myths** (e.g., it was previously thought that swimming during menstruation was harmful, but the advent of tampon usage during menses certainly had a positive effect.)
         iv. Coexistence of disturbing **premenstrual or menstrual symptoms.** The influence of these factors on performance is accentuated by the very nature of a retrospective survey.
      c. Records have been set and gold medals won during every phase of the menstrual cycle.
   2. **Studies without hormonal documentation:** These studies used either the calendar method or basal body temperature monitoring to establish the cycle phase and tested subjects at many different phases during the cycle. There was a wide range in fitness of the subjects, and testing included a variety of protocols. Results are presented in Table 1.
   3. **Studies with accurate hormonal documentation:** These researchers all documented the cycle phase by determination of ovarian hormones. Any differences in performance demonstrated between luteal and follicular phases were small and probably of borderline statistical significance. These studies are summarized in Table 2.

B. **Strength:** The small number of studies that exist have found:
   1. **Decreases in isometric handgrip strength and endurance of forearm contraction** during the "luteal" phase (perhaps secondary to the increase in core body temperature)[44]
   2. Best achievement in hip strength (flexion and extension) and standing broad jump during the "premenstrual" phase[58]
   3. No significant differences in:
      a. Grip strength or isokinetic knee extension[25]
      b. Leg press or bench press[48]
      c. Knee extension and flexion strength and endurance[13]
      d. Isokinetic strength of quadriceps and hamstrings (study done with accurate cycle phase documentation)[34]

C. **Body temperature:** Some studies have shown:
   1. **Variation in core temperature,**[24,55] but no differences in response to short-term heat exposure[60,61]
   2. Differences in the **thresholds for shivering and sweating** between the follicular and luteal phases[23]
   3. **No apparent effects of body temperature on performance.**[55] However, studies with hormonal documentation have found higher heart rates[24,45,51] and rating of perceived exertion[45] at the same level of exertion during the luteal phase. This may have implications for prolonged athletic activity at a high ambient temperature.

TABLE 1. Effects of Menstrual Cycle on Performance Tests: Studies Without Hormonal Documentation

Author	Subjects	Method	$\dot{V}O_2$max	Tests	Results
Doolittle and Engebretsen, 1972[15]	16	C[†]	—	$\dot{V}O_2$max (treadmill) 12-min run/walk 600-yd run/walk 1.5-mile run/walk	No significant differences
Wells and Horvath, 1974[61]	7	BBT	—	$\dot{V}O_2$max, $\dot{V}_E$, oxygen pulse: 40 min rest, 40 min work at 50% $\dot{V}O_2$max, 40 min rest	No significant differences
Gamberale et al., 1975[21]	12	C	2.18 L/min	O_2 uptake at 40% and 70% of $\dot{V}O_2$max (bicycle ergometer)	No significant differences At same HR, exercise perceived as more exerting in "menstrual" stage than in "pre-" or "postmenstrual" stages
Fox et al., 1977 (abstract)[19]	7 (UT) 8 (T)	C	—	Treadmill walk at 4.8 kph, 2% grade Maximal running at 10.4 kph with increasing grade	Untrained: no differences Trained: submaximal $\dot{V}O_2$ highest in "postmenstrual" phase
Allsen et al., 1977[1]	10 (T)	C	46.56–66.07 ml/kg/min	$\dot{V}O_2$max (treadmill)	No significant differences
Higgs and Robertson, 1981[25]	12	C		3 min run at 90% and 100% $\dot{V}O_2$max; knee extension, grip strength; all-out run at 7 mph, 7.5% grade	Perceived exertion at 100% $\dot{V}O_2$max higher premenstrually and day 1 compared to midcycle. Endurance run time decreased in premenstrual and day 1 phases
Stephenson et al., 1982[54,55]	6	C	2.6 L/min	$\dot{V}O_2$max (cycle ergometer) Submaximal $\dot{V}O_2$ Anaerobic threshold Time to exhaustion	No significant differences (Mean core temperature elevated on days 14 and 20, above days 2 and 8)
DeBruyn-Prevost et al., 1984[11]	7	C	2.4 L/min	Aerobic and anaerobic endurance (cycle ergometer)	No significant differences
Bale and Nelson, 1985[3]	20	C	—	50-m swim	Best on 8th day "postmensum" Worst at beginning of menses
Brooks-Gunn et al., 1986[8]	6	BBT[‡]	—	100-yd freestyle swim 100-yd best event	Both tests: fastest in "menstrual phase," slowest in "premenstruum"
Fomin et al., 1989[18]	164	C	—	5-km test race on standard track 12.5-km test on ski rollers	Best performance during "postovulatory" and "postmenstrual" phases
Quadango et al., 1991[48]	15	C	—	100 m and 200 m swim	No significant differences

This table is excerpted from Lebrun CM, reference 33.
C = calendar; BBT = basal body temperature; UT = untrained; T = trained; HR = heart rate.
[†] Blood taken for progesterone, postexercise; 1 subject did not ovulate, 2 others ovulated late or not at all.
[‡] 5 of 10 cycles biphasic, 2 monophasic, 3 biphasic with short luteal phase.

TABLE 2.   Effects of Menstrual Cycle on Performance Tests: Studies with Hormonal Documentation

Author	Subjects	$\dot{V}O_2max$	Tests	Results
Jurkowski et al., 1981[26]	9	41.8 ml/kg/min	Bicycle ergometer 20-min at 30–35% $\dot{V}O_2max$ 20 min at 60–66% $\dot{V}O_2max$ 85–90% $\dot{V}O_2max$ to exhaustion	Time to exhaustion longer in luteal phase (1.57 ± 0.32 vs 2.97 ± 0.63 min)
Schoene et al., 1981[51]	6 nonathletes 6 athletes (N) 6 athletes (A)	35.2 ml/kg/min 49.6 ml/kg/min 49.1 ml/kg/min	$\dot{V}O_2max$ (bicycle ergometer) Exercise time to exhaustion	Maximal exercise response better in follicular phase in nonathletes only
Robertson and Higgs, 1983 (abstract)[49]	14		12-min submaximal run at 90% $\dot{V}O_2max$; all-out run at 100% $\dot{V}O_2max$	Endurance performance decreased in early menses compared with midfollicular phase, and and increased in mid-luteal phase
Hessemer and Bruck, 1985[24]	10	2.81 L/min	Bicycle ergometer–15 min at temperature of 18°C, between 0300 and 0400	5.2% increase in mean $\dot{V}O_2$ during luteal phase, along with increase in metabolic rate of 5.6% and decrease in net efficiency of 5.3%
Dombovy et al., 1987[14]	8	34.4 ml/kg/min	$\dot{V}O_2max$ (bicycle ergometer), then constant load × 4 min above and below anaerobic threshold	No significant differences in $\dot{V}O_2max$, maximum duration of exercise, work efficiency, or maximum work load
Nicklas et al., 1989[42]	6	44.9 ml/kg/min	Bicycle ergometer–exercise to exhaustion, 90 min at 60% $\dot{V}O_2max$ followed by four 1-min sprints at 100% $\dot{V}O_2max$, 3 days rest, 60% carbohydrate diet; then exercise time to fatigue at 70% of $\dot{V}O_2max$; muscle biopsies for glycogen	Borderline increase in endurance time during luteal phase (p <0.07) (126 ± 17.5 vs 139 ± 14.9 min)
DeSouza et al., 1990[12]	8 athletes (N) 8 athletes (A)	53.4 ml/kg/min 55.4 ml/kg/min	$\dot{V}O_2max$ (treadmill) Submaximal test–40 min at 80% $\dot{V}O_2max$	No significant differences in $\dot{V}O_2max$ or in any submaximal tests in either group or between phases
Pivarnik et al., 1992[45]	9	43.2 ml/lg/min	Bicycle ergometer 60 min at 65% $\dot{V}O_2max$	No significant differences, but increase in cardiovascular strain and perceived exertion during luteal phase
Lebrun et al., 1993[34]	16	53.7 ml/kg/min	$\dot{V}O_2max$ (treadmill) Time to exhaustion at 90% of $\dot{V}O_2max$ Anaerobic endurance	Slight decrease in $\dot{V}O_2max$ in luteal phase (p = 0.04), no other significant differences

This table is excerpted from Lebrun CM, reference 33.
N = normal; A = amenorrheic.

D. **Cardiovascular and hemodynamic responses:** Studies have found:
   1. Conflicting results on hemoglobin and hematocrit with no phase difference,[33] luteal phase increases[26] and decreases.[14] Studies without hormonal measurement have shown no differences[21,61] or higher hemoglobin around day 13–14.[19,22,60] In general, any changes are small and likely do not affect exercise performance.

2. No changes in heart rate in the majority of studies, although several more recent studies[24,45,51] have documented a luteal phase increase in exercise heart rate.

3. No significant differences in vascular volume dynamics (study done without hormonal documentation).[20]

E. **Alterations in respiratory drives:** Some ventilatory changes take place during the menstrual cycle, largely due to the effects of progesterone:

1. **Decreased end-tidal PCO_2 and base excess** during the luteal phase. This is due to the hyperventilation caused by the higher level of progesterone and is also seen during pregnancy.

2. **Increase in hypoxic ventilatory response** (response to breathing air that is low in oxygen) and **increase in hypercapnic ventilatory response** (response to breathing air that is high in carbon dioxide) during the luteal phase.[14,51] Successful endurance athletes are known to have lower or blunted respiratory drives. This relative insensitivity to hypoxia and hypercarbia allows them to perform better during intense exercise. Therefore, anything that interferes with this mechanism may affect maximal performance. This study only demonstrated an effect on $\dot{V}O_2$max and maximum work time in the nonathletes.[51]

3. **Similar ventilatory changes in men** given medroxyprogesterone acetate, but no corresponding effect on performance.[5]

F. **Substrate utilization:** Studies have shown hormonal effects on substrate metabolisms: (These are reviewed in greater detail elsewhere.[33])

1. **Decrease in exercise-induced lactate** during the luteal phase[14,26,28,32] (associated with a doubling of endurance time[26,28]). This suggests a glycogen-sparing effect under the influence of the female hormones and a shift in metabolism toward the use of free fatty acids for fuel for the exercising muscle.

2. **No cycle phase influence on blood glucose,[6,29,42] lactate,[6,12,29,30] or free fatty acid metabolism.[12,39,32,42]** However, nutritional status also has an influence. One study[6] noted a lower luteal phase free fatty acid response in glucose-loaded vs fasting subjects. Another study[32] used a 24 h carbohydrate-poor diet to "unmask" a luteal phase decrease in blood glucose during exercise.

3. **Increase in muscle glycogen storage** during the luteal phase, as determined by muscle biopsy. Although this increase did not reach statistical significance, an associated trend was seen toward enhanced endurance performance during the luteal phase.[42]

4. Greater protein catabolism during exercise (shown by increased urea nitrogen excretion) during the midluteal phase.[31]

5. During prolonged submaximal exercise, females have greater fat utilization and less carbohydrate and protein metabolism than equally trained and nourished males.[56]

VII. EFFECTS OF ORAL CONTRACEPTIVES ON PERFORMANCE

The few studies that exist have utilized oral contraceptive agents (OCAs) with a large variety of estrogen and progestins. They have demonstrated the following:

A. **Cardiovascular system**

1. No difference in cardiac index, pulmonary artery distensibility, heart rate, or blood pressure between women on a combined pill, progesterone-only pill, or no pill at all. Higher cardiac output in women on estrogen-protestin pill.[37]

2. Higher cardiac output during exercise as well as increase in blood volume and stroke volume (monophasic OCA for 1–2 months)[36]

3. Increase in systolic blood pressure and cardiac output after 2–3 months of OCA, without any increase in heart rate[57]

4. No difference in maximal heart rate (low-dose triphasic OCA)[35]

5. Adverse effects on blood lipids and cholesterol

B. **Ventilatory system**
   1. Increase in O_2 consumption for standardized workloads on a cycle ergometer (monophasic OCA).[38] Hypothesized shift in substrate utilization towards fat.
   2. Increase in minute ventilation ($\dot{V}_E$ and $\dot{V}CO_2$), but no change in oxygen consumption ($\dot{V}O_2$) (2 monophasic OCAs)—effect greater at 3 than at 6 months[41]
C. **Substrate metabolism:** Effects of OCAs are determined by the balance of steroid hormones and modulated through counterregulatory hormones such as insulin and growth hormones. Progestins have contrainsulin effects and are responsible for the deterioration in carbohydrate metabolism seen in genetically susceptible women on OCAs. Growth hormone has a lipolytic and glucose-sparing effect that may be important for prolonged exercise. Growth hormone levels are increased by estrogen and decreased by progesterone. The implications for exercise responses are complex.[4a] Studies have shown:
   1. Increase in free fatty acid levels during mild exercise and lower blood glucose levels at rest and during exercise in OCA users compared to controls.[7]
   2. Lower blood glucose levels during prolonged exercise in OCA users (3 multiphasic and 5 monophasic OCAs) compared to controls, associated with a diminution of carbohydrate utilization.[4] A greater ability to spare carbohydrate may be advantageous for prolonged exercise, but lower blood glucose levels may potentially reflect decreased hepatic output.
D. **Aerobic capacity**
   1. Small but statistically significant decrease in $\dot{V}O_2$max after 2 months on an unspecified OCA, reversible 6 weeks after discontinuation of OCA. This was associated with a decrease in muscle mitochondrial citrate, suggesting a potential cellular mechanism for this change.[10]
   2. Small but statistically significant decrease in $\dot{V}O_2$max after 6 months on a low-dose monophasic OCA as compared to a control group on no medication, also reversible after discontinuation of OCA.[43]
   3. Smaller decreases in $\dot{V}O_2$max after 2 months of a low-dose triphasic preparation as compared to a control group on placebo, no follow-up after discontinuation of OCA.[35]
E. **Anaerobic endurance:** No effects of low-dose triphasic OCA compared to placebo.[35]
F. **Aerobic endurance**: No effects of low-dose triphasic OCA compared to placebo.[35]
G. **Muscle strength:** Extrapolation from the known anabolic effects of steroid hormones might lead one to expect an increase in strength on OCA, especially with the more androgenic formulations, but studies have shown:
   1. Decrease in forearm isometric endurance and muscle force output[63] (16 women on 8 different OCAs as compared to 10 normals)
   2. No differences in isokinetic strength of knee flexors and extensors after 2 months on a low-dose triphasic OCA, as compared to placebo[35]
H. **Other:** Fewer traumatic injuries in female soccer players on OCAs (perhaps due to a decrease in dysmenorrhea and its effects on coordination).[39,40]
I. These studies represent only a small number of women and OCAs. There is a wide variety of OCAs containing different combinations of hormones, and given the large number of athletic women who take OCAs at some time during their athletic careers and the large number of OCAs currently available in varying dosages and formulations, it can be seen that there is a significant gap in current knowledge in this important area.

VIII. **QUESTIONS FOR FUTURE RESEARCH**
   A. **What are the effects of different phases of the menstrual cycle (including midcycle or ovulation) on various aspects of performance?** If differences exist, are they due to estradiol, progesterone, or their combined effects?
   B. **What are the effects on performance of different OCAs**, including low-dose triphasic preparations and formulations containing the newer progestins or progesterone only?

   C. **Should there be standard phases of cycle for physiologic testing?** This would be important for researchers studying other aspects of performance, to eliminate any potentially confounding effects relative to cycle phase.

   D. **What are the implications for athletes with amenorrhea/oligomenorrhea,** especially if they are to be treated with either estrogen and progesterone or with OCAs?

   E. **What is the value/safety of artificially manipulating menstrual cycles with OCAs around major competitions?**

REFERENCES

1. Allsen PE, Parsons P, Bryce GR: Effect of the menstrual cycle on maximum oxygen uptake. Phys SportsMed 5(7):53–55, 1977.
2. Bale P, Davies J: Effect of menstruation and contraceptive pill on the performance of physical education students. Br J Sports Med 17(1):46–50, 1983.
3. Bale P, Nelson G: The effects of menstruation on performance of swimmers. Aust J Sci Med Sport (Mar):19–22, 1985.
4. Bemben DA, Boileau RA, Bahr JM, et al: Effects of oral contraceptives on hormonal and metabolic responses during exercise. Med Sci Sports Exerc 24:434–441, 1992.
4a. Bemben DA: Metabolic effects of oral contraceptives: Implications for exercise responses of pre-menopausal women. Sports Med 16(5):294–304, 1993.
5. Bonekat HW, Dombovy ML, Staats BA: Progesterone-induced changes in exercise performance and ventilatory response. Med Sci Sports Exerc 19:118–123, 1987.
6. Bonen A, Haynes FJ, Watson-Wright W, et al: Effects of menstrual cycle on metabolic responses to exercise. J Appl Physiol 55:1506–1513, 1983.
7. Bonen A, Haynes FW, Graham TE: Substrate and hormonal responses to exercise in women using oral contraceptives. J Appl Physiol 70:1917–1927, 1991.
8. Brooks-Gunn J, Gargiulo JM, Warren MP: The effect of cycle phase on the adolescent swimmers. Phys SportsMed 14(3):182–192, 1986.
9. Bunt JC: Metabolic actions of estradiol: Significance for acute and chronic exercise response. Med Sci Sport Exerc 22:286–290, 1990.
10. Daggett A, Davies B, Boobis L: Physiological and biochemical responses to exercise following oral contraceptive use [abstract]. Med Sci Sports Exerc 15(2):174, 1983
11. DeBruyn-Prevost P, Masset C, Sturbois X: Physiological response from 18–25 years women to aerobic and anaerobic physical fitness tests at different periods during the menstrual cycle. J Sports Med 24(2):144–148, 1984.
12. DeSouza MJ, Maguire MS, Rubin K, Maresh CM: Effects of menstrual phase and amenorrhea on exercise responses in runners. Med Sci Sports Exerc 22:575–580, 1990.
13. Dibrezzo R, Fort IL, Brown B: Relationships among strength, endurance, weight and body fat during three phases of the menstrual cycle. J Sports Med Phys Fitness 31:89–94, 1991.
14. Dombovy ML, Bonekat HW, Williams TJ, Staats BA: Exercise performance and ventilatory response in the menstrual cycle. Med Sci Sports Exerc 19:111–117, 1987.
15. Doolittle TL, Engebretsen J: Performance variations during the menstrual cycle. J Sports Med 12:54–58, 1972.
16. Erdelyi GJ: Gynecological survey of female athletes. J Sports Med Phys Fitness 2:174–179, 1962.
17. Eston RG: The regular menstrual cycle and athletic performance. Sports Med 1:431–445, 1984.
18. Fomin SK, Pivovarova VI, Voronova VI: Changes in the special working capacity and mental stability of well-trained women skiers at various phases of the biological cycle. Sports Training Med Rehabil 1:89–92, 1989.
19. Fox EL, Martin FL, Bartels RL: Metabolic and cardiorespiratory responses to exercise during the menstrual cycle in trained and untrained athletes [abstract]. Med Sci Sports Exerc 9:70, 1977.
20. Gaebelein CJ, Senay LC Jr: Vascular volume dynamics during ergometer exercise at different menstrual phases. Eur J Appl Physiol 50:1–11, 1982.
21. Gamberale F, Strindberg L, Wahlberg I: Female work capacity during the menstrual cycle: Physiological and psychological reactions. Scand J Work Environ Health 1:120–127, 1975.
22. Garlick MA, Bernauer EM: Exercise during the menstrual cycle: Variations in physiological baselines. Res Q Am Assoc Health Phys Educ 39:533–542, 1968.
23. Hessemer V, Bruck K: Influence of menstrual cycle on shivering, skin blood flow and sweating responses measured at night. J Appl Physiol 59:1902–1910, 1985.
24. Hessemer V, Bruck K: Influence of menstrual cycle on thermoregulatory, metabolic and heart rate responses to exercise at night. J Appl Physiol 59:1911–1917, 1985.
25. Higgs SL, Robertson LA: Cyclic variations in perceived exertion and physical work capacity in females. Can J Appl Sport Sci 6:191–196, 1981.

26. Jurkowski JEH, Jones NL, Toews CJ, Sutton JR: Effects of menstrual cycle on blood lactate, O_2 delivery and performance during exercise. J Appl Physiol 51:1493–1499, 1981.

27. Jurkowski JEH, Jones NL, Walker WE, et al: Ovarian hormonal responses to exercise. J Appl Physiol 44:109–114, 1978.

28. Jurkowski JE, Jones NL, Sutton JR, Toews CJ: Exercise performance and blood lactate levels in relation to the menstrual cycle [abstract]. Med Sci Sports Exerc 9:70, 1977.

29. Kanaley JA, Boileau RA, Bahr JA, et al: Substrate oxidation and GH responses to exercise are independent of menstrual phase and status. Med Sci Sports Exerc 24:873–880, 1992.

30. Lamont LS: Lack of influence of the menstrual cycle on blood lactate. Phys SportMed 14(11):159–163, 1986.

31. Lamont LS, Lemon PRT, Bruot BC: Menstrual cycle and exercise effects on protein catabolism. Med Sci Sports Exerc 19(2):106–110, 1987.

32. Lavoie M, Dionne N, Helie R, Brisson GR: Menstrual cycle phase dissociation of blood glucose homeostasis during exercise. J Appl Physiol 62:1084–1089, 1987.

33. Lebrun CM: Effect of the different phases of the menstrual cycle and oral contraceptives on athletic performance. Sports Med 16:400–430, 1993.

34. Lebrun CM, McKenzie DC, Prior JC, Taunton JE: Effects of menstrual cycle phase on athletic performance. (Submitted for publication 1994.)

35. Lebrun CM, McKenzie DC, Prior JC, Taunton JE: Effects of a triphasic oral contraceptive on athletic performance. (Submitted for publication 1994.)

36. Lehtovirta P, Kuikka J, Pyorala T: Hemodynamic effects of oral contraceptives during exercise. Int J Gynaecol Obstet 15:35–37, 1977.

37. Littler WA, Bojorges-Bueno R, Banks J: Cardiovascular dynamics in women during the menstrual cycle and oral contraceptive therapy. Thorax 29:567–570, 1974.

38. McNeill AW, Mozingo E: Changes in the metabolic cost of standardized work associated with the use of an oral contraceptive. J Sports Med 21:238–244, 1981.

39. Möller-Nielsen J, Hammar M: Women's soccer injuries in relation to the menstrual cycle and oral contraceptive use. Med Sci Sports Exerc 21(2):126–129, 1989.

40. Möller-Nielsen J, Hammar M: Sports injuries and oral contraceptive use: Is there a relationship? Sports Med 12(3):152–160, 1991.

41. Montes A, Lally D, Hale RW: The effects of oral contraceptives on respiration. Fertil Steril 39:515–519, 1983.

42. Nicklas BJ, Hackney AC, Sharp RL: The menstrual cycle and exercise: Peformance, muscle glycogen and substrate responses. Int J Sports Med 10:264–269, 1989.

43. Notelovitz M, Zauner C, McKenzie L, et al: The effect of low-dose contraceptives on cardiorespiratory function, coagulation, and lipids in exercising young women: A preliminary report. Am J Obstet Gynecol 156:591–598, 1987.

44. Petrofsky JS, Ledonne DM, Rinehart JS, Lind AR: Isometric strength and endurance during the menstrual cycle. Eur J Appl Physiol 35:1–10, 1976.

45. Pivarnik JM, Marichal CJ, Spillman T, Morrow JR Jr.: Menstrual cycle phase affects temperature regulation during endurance exercise. J Appl Physiol 72:543–548, 1992.

46. Prior JC, Vigna YM: Gonadal steroids in athletic women: Contraception, complications and performance. Sports Med 2:287–295, 1985.

47. Prior JC, Vigna YM, Sciarretta D, et al: Conditioning exercise decreases premenstrual symptoms: A prospective controlled six month trial Fertil Steril 47:402–408, 1987.

48. Quadagno D, Faquin L, Lim G-N, et al: The menstrual cycle: Does it affect athletic performance? Phys SportsMed 19(3):121–124, 1991.

49. Robertson LA, Higgs SL: Menstrual cycle variations in physical work capacity, postexercise blood lactate and perceived exertion [abstract]. Can J Appl Sports Sci 8:220, 1983.

50. Schelkun PH: Exercise and "the pill": Putting a rumor to rest. Phys SportsMed 19(3):143–152, 1991.

51. Schoene RB, Robertson HT, Pierson DJ, Peterson AP: Respiratory drives and exercise in menstrual cycles of athletic and nonathletic women. J Appl Physiol 50:1300–1305, 1981.

52. Shangold MM, Mirkin G (eds): Women and Exercise: Physiology and Sports Medicine, 2nd ed. Philadelphia, F.A. Davis Company, 1994.

53. Southam AL, Gonzaga FP: Systemic changes during the menstrual cycle. Am J Obstet Gynecol 91:142–165, 1965.

54. Stephenson LA, Kolka MA, Wilkerson JH: Perceived exertion and anaerobic threshold during the menstrual cycle. Med Sci Sports Exerc 14:218–222, 1982.

55. Stephenson LA, Kolka MA, Wilkerson JE: Metabolic and thermoregulatory responses to exercise during the human menstrual cycle. Med Sci Sports Exerc 14:270–275, 1982.

56. Tarnopolsky LJ, MacDougall JD, Atkinson SA, et al: Gender differences in substrate for endurance exercise. J Appl Physiol 68:302–308, 1990.

57. Walters WAW, Lim YL: Cardiovascular dynamics in women receiving oral contraceptive therapy. Lancet 2:879–881, 1969.
58. Wearing MP, Yuhosz MD, Campbell R, Love EJ: The effect of the menstrual cycle on tests of physical fitness. J Sports Med Phys Fitness 12:38–41, 1972.
59. Wells CL (ed): Women, Sport, and Performance: A Physiological Perspective, 2nd ed. Champaign, IL, Human Kinetics Publishers, 1991.
60. Wells CL, Horvath SM: Heat stress responses related to the menstrual cycle. J Appl Physiol 35:1–5, 1973.
61. Wells CL, Horvath SM: Responses to exercise in a hot environment as related to the menstrual cycle. J Appl Physiol 36:299–302, 1974.
62. Winget CM, DeRoshia CW, Holley DC: Circadian rhythms and athletic performance. Med Sci Sports Exerc 17(5):498–516, 1985.
63. Wirth JC, Lohman TG: The relationship of static muscle function to use of oral contraceptives. Med Sci Sports Exerc 14:16–20, 1982.
64. Zaharieva E: Survey of sportswomen at the Tokyo Olympics. J Sports Med Phys Fitness 5:215–219, 1965.

Chapter 12: Psychosocial Factors and the Developing Female Athlete

NANCY P. BARNETT, M.S.
PRISCILLA WRIGHT, Ph.D.

In this chapter we outline some of the fundamental issues related to the psychological experience of being female and an athlete. We include general information about female participation in sport, socialization, and the impact of external influences, such as the media, on the activities of young women. Information about the psychological characteristics of women athletes is provided, as are brief descriptions of a number of issues common to the experience of athletes in general and the female athlete in particular. An introduction to performance enhancement skills is also presented.

I. **FACTORS RELATED TO SPORT INVOLVEMENT FOR GIRLS**

   A. **Socialization:** The process by which children are taught the values and expectations of their culture, as well as the behavior that is deemed acceptable for their gender.

      1. **Socialization into sport:** Children are taught to select activities that are "appropriate" for their gender, and are discouraged, directly or indirectly, from engaging in activities deemed "inappropriate." Historically, sport has been considered a more appropriate activity for boys than girls; this sex-typed socialization tends to put girls at a disadvantage in that they typically do not receive the same kind of encouragement as boys to become athletes.

         a. **The "acceptability" problem:** Traditionally fewer sports have been considered "acceptable" for women—e.g., dance, tennis, gymnastics, and equestrian events. Some sports have been played in modified ways (e.g., six-player basketball), and others are played infrequently by girls and women (e.g., boxing, American football). Few, if any, sports are considered "unacceptable" for male participation.

         b. **Limited encouragement:** Encouragement to participate in sports may be limited by the encourager's own investment in sports, and by a relatively lower rate of involvement in sport by adult women. Participation may also be discouraged if it interferes with other "more appropriate" female sex-role activities.

            i. Participation rates: Girls do not participate in sports to the same degree as boys; they participate in substantially fewer numbers, even in the sports preferred by or acceptable for girls.

            ii. Attrition: When girls consider discontinuing their sport participation, they may not be encouraged (as often as boys are) to persist. Although girls are allowed to play, they may not be discouraged from quitting or, if they do quit, may not be redirected into other sports.

         c. **Cultural and socioeconomic differences:** Involvement in sport is related to social class; females from lower economic levels participate to a lesser degree than those from economically advantaged groups. Different ethnic groups also have different norms regarding sport participation.

      2. **Girls' sense of athletic competence:** Gender-typed expectations are reflected in girls' perceptions of themselves in that they tend to have a more negative assessment of their athletic competence than boys. A child's sense of competence in sport is predicted by the extent to which he or she sees sport as appropriate for his or her gender.

3. **Social support and modeling:** The family, as the primary agent of socialization, is especially influential. By encouraging girls to become involved in athletics, by providing the opportunity and social support necessary for participation in sport, and by serving as role models, parents can combat the effects of cultural attitudes.

4. **Media influence:** The media imparts an important cultural influence in that it communicates standards through the use of verbal and visual information and images.

   a. **Portrayal of women athletes:** Female athletes are frequently described in different terms than male athletes; they are often praised for being attractive and feminine rather than strong, fast, or athletic. This emphasis on appearance, femininity, and marital status rather than athletic expertise undermines and trivializes the female athletes' participation.

   b. **Lack of role models for girls:** The portrayal of athletic women is still fairly uncommon in both written and electronic media (with the exception of the Olympic games). The comparatively low visibility of female athletes in the media precludes young aspiring female athletes' exposure to same-gender role models, which is an important element of the social learning process.

B. **Stereotypes**

   1. **Negative stereotypes of the female athlete:** The characteristics of a good athlete (competitive, physically strong and fit, achievement oriented) are typically considered to be more "masculine" characteristics. A female athlete, especially one participating in what is seen as a more traditionally "masculine" type sport may suffer negative status or stereotyping by being labeled as manly, unattractive, or lesbian. If a woman fears this negative stereotyping, or if parents or peers who have similar concerns discourage her from pursuing athletics, she may modify her participation or dedication.

   2. **Adolescence:** Adolescents may be especially sensitive to stereotypes; at this age the socialization influence of the family declines, the peer group begins to play a more prominent role, and girls become more concerned about social evaluation. As "fitting in" becomes very important to the young teenager, an athletic female may not want to be more talented than her male peers. As might be expected, this is a time when attrition is the greatest for female sport participants.

   3. **Adult influence:** Teachers and coaches provide a significant socializing influence for teenage girls and can be effective in supporting the continued participation of girls by providing a variety of sport activities and access to female athlete peers, by increasing the visibility of local athletes who might serve as role models, and by actively discouraging negative stereotypes.

C. **Role conflict:** Role conflict occurs when a person, because of his or her gender and interests, experiences the conflicting demands of different roles.

   1. **Role conflict and the female athlete:** Since the traditional roles of female and athlete are contradictory, it has been thought that the female athlete might experience a psychological conflict regarding her participation. However, studies have consistently found that the majority of female athletes, even those athletes in more traditionally "masculine" sports, perceive and experience relatively low levels of role conflict. In other words, we must not assume that the female athlete internalizes negative stereotype images or that these images have a negative impact on her self-concept.

   2. **Androgyny:** It is possible that female athletes avoid the impact of role conflict by developing a self-schema in which being a female and being involved in sports are not contradictory. Indeed, psychological androgyny is more commonly seen in female athletes than nonathletes, and female athletes are more likely to endorse a masculine or androgynous sex role than feminine or undifferentiated. Individuals with androgynous orientations typically have a more broadly

defined area of acceptable behavior and will therefore be less likely to experience role conflict.

    a. **Self-esteem:** Women athletes who describe themselves as more androgynous or masculine in sex-role have higher self-esteem than stereotypic females.

D. **Conclusion:** Girls have vastly different socialization experiences, and the likelihood that an individual female will experience opposition to her involvement in sports, negative stereotypes, fear of masculinization, or role conflict will greatly depend upon the socializing influences in her life, including family, culture, and community, and the messages they impart about participation for women in general and her in particular.

II. PSYCHOLOGICAL PROFILE OF THE FEMALE ATHLETE

A. **Psychological characteristics:** Female athletes tend to be more intrinsically motivated, assertive, achievement oriented, independent, and self-sufficient than nonathletic women. Sporting experience in females is also related to greater self-concept, especially of physical ability but also including physical appearance and general self-esteem.

B. **Skill level differences:** Successful athletes tend to have higher levels of self-confidence, better concentration, lower levels of anxiety before and during competition, less preoccupation with thoughts of failure, and a greater ability to recover from errors than their less-successful counterparts.

C. **Mood states:** Athletes tend to show well-below-average levels of the negative mood states of tension, depression, anger, fatigue, and confusion, but well-above-average levels of vigor.

D. **Source of differences:** It is important to note that while there seem to be differences between athletes and nonathletes, it is unclear whether the athletic experience leads to the development of these characteristics or if people with these characteristics gravitate toward (or persist in) athletics. It is likely that both of these factors are at work; people with characteristics that are associated with success in sport will be more likely to pursue sport experience, while sport is likely to facilitate the development of these characteristics as well.

E. **Prediction of performance:** Numerous attempts have been made to predict sport performance on the basis of some of the personality characteristics described above. The use of psychological instruments alone to predict athletic outcome has had limited success. However, when used in conjunction with other measures of athletic competence, such as physiologic measures and coach evaluations of skill, these assessment instruments add another level of understanding of the athlete and may best be utilized in the identification of individual athletes' weaknesses which can then be targeted for change.

III. PSYCHOLOGICAL AND BEHAVIORAL PROBLEMS

In some cases experience in competitive athletics enhances a person's ability to cope with life events and stressors of everyday life, and in other instances the very qualities that contribute to an individual's athletic prowess may make her more prone to developing problems. Following are some difficulties that female athletes can experience.

A. **"Sport-only" identification:** For many athletes their sense of self revolves around their role as an athlete.

    1. **Risk factors**

        a. **Sacrifice:** In many instances, an athlete must put the other demands of life on hold until her athletic career is over. Athletes will frequently describe not having had typical growing experiences or a normal social life so that they could better focus on their skill development.

        b. **Lack of balance:** Athletes can become so focused on and identified with their sport that they do not develop other interests or the coping skills and support structure important for a balanced lifestyle.

    c. **Loss of the sport activity:** A "sport-only" identification is not necessarily problematic in and of itself, as it often provides the athlete with self-confidence, fitness, and a social support system. However, if this identification is threatened, e.g., by injury or a decline in performance, the athlete may suffer.

B. **Eating disorders:** The prevalence of disordered eating in female athletes, based on a number of small studies, has been reported in the 15–62% range and is more prevalent in "thin-build" sports such as gymnastics and long-distance running.

    1. **Demands of sport:** The expectation that an athlete will maintain a constant weight goal along with the immense pressure to perform may tax the athlete's coping abilities.

    2. **Personality:** Athletes are highly trained, competitive, achievement-oriented, disciplined, often perfectionistic individuals who have goals to perform to the best of their abilities. Although it is exactly these characteristics and desires that facilitate success in athletics, they are also characteristics commonly seen in women with eating disorders.

    3. **Cultural context:** In the context of Western culture's obsession with thinness, the personality disposition of the athlete may interact with the demands of the athlete's sport and can result in an athlete making an effort to acquire an extremely lean body in an attempt to gain a competitive edge.

C. **Competitive stress:** Often, athletes are under considerable pressure to succeed; the expectations of coaches, parents, teammates, and spectators can be overwhelming. A common response to the pressures of competition is to experience tension or anxiety.

    1. **Symptoms:** The anxiety reaction of the competitive athlete is very similar to psychological reactions to other situations, such as public speaking or test-taking.

        a. **Somatic:** Nervous stomach or "butterflies"; increased respiration, heart rate, and perspiration; frequent urination; dry mouth; or trembling.

        b. **Cognitive:** Mental distress; self-doubt about one's ability to perform at her best, worry about the competition itself, concern about other people's impressions, and a general sense of confusion.

    2. **Identifying the anxious athlete:** An athlete who experiences high competitive anxiety may or may not be easy to identify. Before competition she may seem more jittery or look more nervous than usual. She may verbalize her negative thinking about herself or the event. Over time certain patterns may emerge, such as the inability to perform as well in competition as in practice, or the report of physical complaints unrelated to a specific injury.

    3. **Impact of competitive anxiety:** An overaroused state can lead to poor or misdirected concentration, which may result in performance errors and "choking." Athletes who experience chronically high levels of competitive anxiety or are unable to cope well with their anxiety risk physical and psychological injury and may stop playing their sport because their participation has become too aversive.

    4. **Managing competitive stress:** Some athletes are better able than others to manage their responses to stressful competitive situations. Those athletes who effectively control their arousal, or more specifically are able to reach their optimal arousal level for the task to be performed, experience more success in their sport.

        a. **Techniques:** Several ways that an athlete can be taught to control her competitive anxiety include breathing exercises, relaxation or meditation techniques, and cognitive techniques such as thought-stoppage and changing negative or distorted thinking (*see* Section IV.B.2).

D. **Drug abuse:** There are indications that drug use is no less of a problem in athletic populations than in others. One investigation of female university athletes found that 40% of the women surveyed reported that others on their team took a drug that was illegal or banned from their sport. It is important to recognize the situational characteristics of competitive athletics that make the use of substances attractive, as well as the specific factors that place certain individuals at risk.

1. **Categories of drug use:** The objectives for drug use tend to fall into three categories: medicinal (e.g., pain relief, treatment of injury or illness), "recreational," and performance enhancement (e.g., stimulants, anabolic steroids).
2. **Reasons for drug use in athletes:** The following points pertain not to the use of drugs prescribed and monitored for illness or injury, but to the misuse of drugs by athletes for the purposes of mood or performance enhancement.
   a. **External factors**
      i. **Expectations:** The expectations of coaches, parents, fans, and the media and the rewards derived from doing "whatever it takes" to win can be great enough to make an athlete consider ingesting substances to improve her strength, endurance, reaction time, etc.
      ii. **Financial incentives:** Athletes whose financial status or future depends on their performance may be especially vulnerable to temptations to use performance-enhancing drugs such as steroids or stimulants.
      iii. **Peer pressure:** The effects of peer pressure should not be underestimated; athletes may use drugs as a way of gaining social acceptance from their friends or teammates.
   b. **Individual factors**
      i. **"Sports-only" identification:** Individuals who over-identify with their role as athletes may have a hard time imagining themselves not participating in their sport someday or may not believe that life after competition can be fulfilling. Young athletes may be particularly vulnerable, as they may be more likely to lose their perspective and develop a narrow focus on their sport.
      ii. **Esteem:** The esteem an athlete derives from her participation may lead her to believe that the glory is worth any negative after-effect.
      iii. **Feelings of invulnerability:** Athletes—young, healthy, and fit as they are—may feel as though they are invulnerable to the negative side-effects of drugs.
      iv. **Coping mechanism:** Like nonathletes, athletes use substances to manage stress or anxiety, to escape interpersonal problems, to overcome low self-confidence, or to avoid boredom. Athletes who have suffered an injury or who have been cut from their team may use alcohol or drugs to manage the stress of this transition.
E. **Injury:** Due to the physically stressful and sometimes dangerous nature of competitive sports, athletes are at a significant risk for injury. By the time an athlete has participated in a sport for 3–5 years, most have suffered an injury significant enough to make them miss a practice or event.
   1. **Risk factors:** Although many of the causal factors in sport injury are physical, specific psychological and psychosocial factors may contribute to an athlete's vulnerability to injury.
      a. **Depression:** Athletes who are depressed or have a poor sense of well-being may be more susceptible to injury or health problems.
      b. **Life events:** General stressful life events (e.g., death of a family member or changes in residence) and stressful events specific to sport (e.g., having problems with coaches and being demoted in player status) have been positively associated with increased risk of injury.
         i. Coping mechanisms and social support: The efficacy of an athlete's coping mechanisms (e.g., her ability to think clearly under stress and to use effective problem-solving strategies) and the quality of her social support system may be critical in moderating the impact of life stressors.
   2. **Consequences of injury**
      a. **Inability to practice or compete:** The injured athlete may be unable to practice at her preinjury level; she may be removed from the team's competitive

roster or from her normal routine altogether and shifted over to a routine of rehabilitation.

   b. **Emotional distress:** Initially, the athlete may respond with shock and confusion, followed by frustration, anger, or depression. If the injury lasts more than a few days, the athlete may begin to feel isolated or forgotten. She may fear losing her preinjury fitness or performance level or may develop a concern about reinjury or future new injuries. She may feel as if she has let her team down by becoming injured or may deny the seriousness of the injury to her coach, athletic trainer, and herself.

   c. **Self-image:** The process of rehabilitating an injury can be especially difficult for the athlete whose self-esteem is defined by her athletic status or her ability to perform. When an athlete loses control over her body, as in the case of injury, self-image decreases. As she regains control over her body, she will tend to feel better about herself.

   d. **The severely injured athlete:** Athletes who are unable to participate for longer periods of time show greater tension, depression, and anger and can develop a prolonged mood disturbance.

  3. **Individual differences:** Athletes with similar injuries will differ in the way they respond psychologically. An athlete's reaction will depend on her prior level of psychological functioning, the nature, location, severity, and duration of the injury, and the lifestyle changes it requires and how she perceives the meaning of the disability.

  4. **Treatment:** Recognizing the valid reactions of the injured athlete and treating her emotional needs may facilitate rehabilitation and improve the speed with which she is able to return to sports participation.

F. **Staleness and burnout:** The combination of high psychological and physical stress, a significant time commitment, and minimal time off can result in a sense of staleness, which can progress to burnout. This process has been conceptualized as a negative response to training stress.

  1. **Staleness:** When an athlete can no longer positively adapt to the psychological and physical demands of athletic competition, she may experience a loss of enthusiasm and desire to practice or improve, physical fatigue, and a performance plateau.

   a. **Inability to recover:** If an athlete is unable to "train through" the initial and highly common reaction of staleness and is continually exposed to training stress, she may experience more acute symptoms of depression, mental exhaustion, and an inability to prepare for competition.

  2. **Burnout:** The end-point of this stress process; it consists of a loss of interest or desire to participate, and extreme physical and emotional exhaustion. The experience of burnout is very common: 47% of collegiate athletes reported having experienced burnout, and these athletes believed it was the worst training response an athlete can have.

   a. **Sport withdrawal:** Athletes commonly resolve their experience of chronic stress by quitting their sport entirely. The experience of participating in an activity that was once the athlete's top priority has become so aversive that the athlete resolves the problem by dropping out.

  3. **Contributing factors**

   a. **Situational factors:** High amounts of training, lack of sufficient time to recover from practice or competition, and conflict with coaches are situational factors that can contribute to the development of burnout.

   b. **Individual characteristics:** Being perfectionistic and "other-oriented" and lacking assertive personal skills may also predispose athletes to burnout.

G. **Career termination:** Athletes typically receive a great deal from their participation in sports, such as a sense of accomplishment, positive self-image, and support system of teammates and coaches. Retiring from competitive athletics can mean losing some or all of these benefits and can be experienced as difficult.

1. **Emotional reactions:** Retiring athletes may experience emotions that resemble those of a grief reaction. This may include feelings of shock, confusion, denial, anger, and depression. After these initial normal reactions, the majority will adjust to the changes and will feel satisfied with their lives.
   a. **Individual differences:** How an athlete responds to career termination will depend on her overall adjustment and sense of self as well as resources, such as her personal coping skills, social support, and the availability of preretirement planning.

2. **Adjustment:** Retired athletes need to become accustomed to a new lifestyle. The graduating collegiate athlete, for example, whose life for so many years was dictated by practice and competition schedules, will be required to make important decisions about her future.
   a. **Positive transitions:** Some athletes adjust to the change by moving to a different level of competition, becoming involved in a different sport, refocusing their efforts on their academic or occupational goals, or developing new interests.
   b. **Difficult transitions:** A small proportion of athletes will have difficulty adjusting to new careers or redirecting their energies. Retirement can be expected to be more difficult for those athletes who have made greater investments of time and personal energy to their training and competing, as this can lead to an imbalance in the development of other interests, support systems, and coping strategies.
   c. **Importance of achievement:** Athletes who feel they have achieved their sport-related goals have a more positive adjustment to their retirement, while those who feel their retirement was due to a decline in performance experience more difficulties with self-confidence and loss of status.
   d. **Importance of social interaction:** Former athletes most frequently report missing the social aspect of their sport.

H. **Conclusion:** Athletes may be at a disadvantage in dealing with emotional, psychological or behavioral difficulties because the cultural expectations of athletes tend to not be compatible with having psychosocial problems. Having problems or being distressed may be seen as a sign of personal weakness, and those who seek help through counseling or therapy are often stigmatized. It is important to recognize when an athlete can benefit from additional help and to provide her with the necessary resources. Our recommendation is that, just as with nonathletes, professional consultation be sought if psychological treatment is deemed necessary.

IV. PERFORMANCE ENHANCEMENT

As noted earlier, people who are successful in athletics differ from their less-successful counterparts in a number of ways. Many of these differences can be described as better developed psychological skills or strategies rather than physical or technical ability.

A. **Importance of mental skills:** Mental training is an important adjunct to physical preparation, and often the athlete who is more "mentally tough" prevails in competition.

B. **Psychological techniques to improve performance**
   1. **Goal setting:** Goal setting has been shown to be an effective method for improving performance in work settings and in sports. The following are some principles of goal setting:
      a. **Performance goals:** Goals should be set for aspects of the sport that the athlete has control over (i.e., her performance) rather than for things that are largely affected by other players, officials, etc. (e.g., the outcome of the competition). For example, a *performance goal* for a swimmer would be to achieve a specific time for a race, while an *outcome goal* for that swimmer might be to win the race (something that is less under her control).

   b. **Specific goals:** Goals should be precise and measurable so that progress can be assessed.

   c. **Challenging goals:** Goals should be appropriately difficult. Goals that are too easy are not motivating, and goals that are unrealistic lead to discouragement.

     i. Revise unrealistic goals: Assess the appropriateness of goals that are not being achieved. It is sometimes difficult for athletes to lower their expectations by adjusting goals, but this is a more effective strategy than refusing to lower goals that are too difficult.

   d. **Short-term and long-term goals:** Setting short-term goals is an essential component of goal setting. They help maintain the athlete's focus on her ultimate objective and enhance motivation by providing evidence of improvement.

   e. **Feedback:** Goal setting will not be effective unless the athlete receives evaluative feedback about her progress toward her goals.

2. **Stress management:** Athletes often get overaroused, especially before competition. Anxiety is a common experience but can have negative effects (*see* Section III.C).

   a. **Identification of stress response:** Athlete stress responses vary; each athlete must identify situations in which she is likely to feel stress, precisely how she feels and what she thinks when she becomes overaroused, and how her stress response tends to affect her performance.

   b. **Techniques for controlling stress**

     i. **Relaxation:** Many types of relaxation programs exist; the goal of most is for the individual to learn to recognize signs of tension and replace those sensations with relaxation.

       (a) **Deep breathing:** Typically breathing is disrupted during periods of tension. Athletes may hold their breath, take shallow breaths, or hyperventilate. Taking deep, slow, complete breaths will frequently induce relaxation.

       (b) **Progressive relaxation:** This technique involves voluntarily tensing and relaxing of specific muscle groups and attending to the contrast between these states. The principle is that after training the individual will learn to notice when and where she is tense and will be able to induce relaxation before the tension becomes problematic.

       (c) **Meditation:** In meditation the athlete focuses her mind on repeating a mantra (a short sound or word) or looking at an object. During meditation the athlete adopts a passive attitude and lets any thoughts move through her mind without attending directly to them.

       (d) **Autogenic training:** A form of self-hypnosis in which the athlete learns to induce physical sensations of warmth and heaviness in her body.

     ii. **Thought control:** Athletes sometimes have difficulty controlling their negative or irrelevant thoughts. They may worry about how they are performing or how other people are evaluating them, or they may be preoccupied with aspects of their lives that are unrelated to their sport involvement. There are many ways that athletes can learn to think differently.

       (a) **Positive communication:** Persistent negative thinking can lead to emotional distress. Athletes can be taught to attend to their thoughts and to change their negative thoughts into neutral or positive thoughts which in turn will affect their emotional responses.

       (b) **Thought stoppage:** If an athlete is aware of having undesirable thoughts she can interrupt them by saying "Stop!" (to herself or aloud) or by using a physical motion such as a snap of the fingers. The athlete should then concentrate on a positive thought or focus on a specific aspect of what she is doing in the moment.

(c) **Use "do" statements:** Self-instructions or corrections should be worded effectively. Reminders about what *is* desired are better than imperatives that begin with "Don't . . ." For example, if a runner is trying to remember to keep her arms a certain way, it is better if she tells herself how she wants her arms to hang, rather than reminding herself of what she does not want to do.

3. **Imagery training:** Imagery is a mental technique that involves using all the senses to imagine or recreate an experience. An athlete can use imagery to "program" herself to respond effectively.

   a. **Uses for imagery**
      i. To practice a recently learned skill or strategy
     ii. To practice responding effectively to difficult situations. The athlete can imagine situations that are physically or emotionally challenging and can practice responding effectively.
    iii. To practice recovering from errors. Athletes who have difficulty recovering after they have made a mistake can use imagery to practice coping with errors and their reactions to these errors.

   b. **Principles of imagery training**
      i. **Vividness:** To make an imagined experience as realistic as possible, the athlete should include all the senses in her imagery and should try to imagine specific details of the situation (e.g., details of the sporting venue, equipment, etc.).
     ii. **Controllability:** Athletes can learn to willfully control their images. With practice, athletes can imagine themselves performing a difficult sport skill effectively.
    iii. **Internal perspective:** Imagery may be more effective if the athlete has an internal perspective (i.e., imagines what it looks and feels like from inside her body as opposed to what she looks like from someone else's perspective).

4. **Concentration/attention control:** Being able to recover from the inevitable distractions during a sport performance is an important skill.

   a. **Know what to concentrate on:** The athlete must learn what is relevant and irrelevant in the situation so that she knows what to concentrate on in that moment.
      i. **Triggers:** Words or actions that can be used to remind the athlete what to focus on. They should be meaningful to the individual athlete.

   b. **Focus on the present:** The athlete should attend to the skill she is going to execute in that moment. Focusing on what just happened the moment before, or what will happen in the future is distracting.
      i. **Following an error:** It is common for athletes to lose their concentration after they have made a mistake. Thinking or talking about the mistake, however, makes them more likely to make another similar mistake because they are training themselves to respond the same way. Instead athletes should identify how they could have responded more effectively and should imagine themselves performing in this way.

   c. **Using pre-event routines:** Having a set routine to follow before competition (or practice) helps reduce uncertainty and decrease distraction. Routines should include things that help the athlete prepare mentally and physically.

REFERENCES

1. Allison MT: Role conflict and the female athlete: Preoccupations with little grounding. J Appl Sport Psychol 3:49–60, 1991.
2. Anshel MH: Causes for drug abuse in sport: A survey of intercollegiate athletes. J Sport Behav 14:283–307, 1991.

3. Bramwell ST, Masuda M, Wagner NN, et al: Psychological factors in athletic injuries: Development and application of the Social and Athletic Readjustment Rating Scale. J Hum Stress 1:6–20, 1975.
4. Brownell KD, Rodin J: Prevalence of eating disorders in athletes. In Brownell KD, Rodin J, Wilmore JH (eds): Eating, Body Weight, and Performance in Athletes. Philadelphia, Lea & Febiger, 1992, p 128.
5. Chalip L, Villiger J, Duignan P: Sex-role identity in a selected sample of women field hockey players. Int J Sport Psychol 11:240–248, 1980.
6. Eccles J, Harold RD: Gender differences in sport involvement: Applying the Eccles' expectancy-value model. J Appl Sport Psychol 3:7–35, 1991.
7. Greendorfer SL: Shaping the female athlete: The impact of the family. In Boutilier MA, SanGiovanni L (eds): The Sporting Woman. Champaign, IL, Human Kinetics, 1983, p 135.
8. Higginson D: The influence of socializing agents in the female sport-participation process. Adolescence 20:73–82, 1985.
9. Jackson SA, Marsh HW: Athletic or antisocial? The female sport experience. J Sport Psychol 8:198–211, 1986.
10. May JR, Sieb GE: Athletic injuries: Psychosocial factors in the onset, sequelae, rehabilitation, and prevention. In May JR, Asken MJ (eds): Sport Psychology: The Psychological Health of the Athlete. New York, PMA, 1987, p 157.
11. Morgan WP, O'Connor PJ, Sparling PB, et al: Psychological characterization of the elite female distance runner. Int J Sports Med 8:124–131, 1987.
12. Orlick T, Partington J: Mental links to excellence. Sport Psychol 2:105–130, 1988.
13. Silva JM: An analysis of the training stress syndrome in competitive athletics. J Appl Sport Psychol 2:5–20, 1990.
14. Sinclair DA, Orlick T: Positive transitions from high performance sport. Sport Psychol 7:138–150, 1993.
15. Skrinar GS, Bullen BA, Cheek JM, et al: Effects of endurance training on body-consciousness in women. Percept Mot Skills 62:483–490, 1986.
16. Smith RE, Smoll FL: Sport performance anxiety. In Leitenberg H (ed): Handbook of Social and Evaluation Anxiety. New York, Plenum, 1990, p 417.
17. Smith RE, Smoll FL, Ptacek JT: Conjunctive moderator variables in vulnerability and resiliency research: Life stress, social support and coping skills, and adolescent sport injuries. J Pers Soc Psychol 58:360–370, 1990.
18. Theberge N: A content analysis of print media coverage of gender, women and physical activity. J Appl Sport Psychol 3:36–48, 1991.
19. Williams JM: Personality characteristics of the successful female athlete. In Straub WF (ed): Sport Psychology: An Analysis of Athlete Behavior. New York, Mouvement Publications, 1978, p 249.
20. Williams JM (ed): Applied Sport Psychology, 2nd ed. California, Mayfield, 1993.

Chapter 13: Differentiating Healthy from Unhealthy Behaviors in Active and Athletic Women

JENNIFER D. BOLEN, MD

Attempting to differentiate healthy from unhealthy behaviors is at best a biased undertaking. Limitations to clinical understanding of behavioral and cultural influences regarding diet and exercise affect the accuracy of assumptions. Making a distinction between behavior that is health-promoting and/or part of athletic conditioning and performing versus behavior that is detrimental to a woman's mental and physical health is often a judgment call.

The following chapter reviews three areas of suffering commonly seen in females—eating, anxiety, and affective disorders—and targets these disorders in relationship to diet and exercise.

I. **EATING DISORDERS**

Eating disorders are relatively ubiquitous in females and rare in males. The most common are reviewed here, as well as eating behavior that can sometimes be viewed as a precursor to an eating disorder. (*See also* Chapter 20.)

A. **DSM-III-R criteria**
  1. **Anorexia nervosa**
     a. Refusal to maintain body weight over a minimal weight for age and height
     b. Weight loss of >15% below that expected
     c. Failure to gain weight during growth, leading to body weight 15% below expected
     d. Fear of weight gain or becoming fat
     e. Fat phobic despite underweight status
     f. **Distorted body image**
     g. Three missed consecutive menstrual cycles
  2. **Bulimia nervosa**
     a. Recurrent binge eating
     b. Loss of control over eating during binges
     c. Self-induced vomiting, laxative or diuretic use, fasting, excess exercise to prevent weight gain
     d. Minimum of 2 binges/week for at least 3 months
     e. Overconcern with weight and shape

B. **General considerations**
  1. Prevalence figures are misleading for eating disorders since these illnesses often go undetected.
  2. Bulimia sufferers are of normal weight, and even when interviewed with specific questions regarding purges, laxative abuse, etc., they often will not report these behaviors because of shame and embarrassment.
  3. Western culture fosters significant weight consciousness in girls and women, so that recent surveys of *fourth-grade girls* reveal high percentages of these children are already becoming weight conscious and fat phobic. **Women and girls are often body-image and weight conscious beginning in early childhood.**
  4. Female athletes are subject to the cultural problems affecting women in general and also influenced by their particular sport demands.

 5. Male athletes (e.g., wrestlers) are more at risk for exhibiting unhealthy eating behaviors than nonathletic males, demonstrating the influence of external factors on an individual's behavior.
 6. Borgen et al.[3] showed that 20% of athletes in sports that emphasize leanness and 10% of all athletes had tendencies toward eating disorders versus 6% of similar-aged nonathletic women.

C. **Medical work-up, specific considerations**
 1. Include questions regarding eating behaviors, nutritional balance, past or current history of food restriction, binging, purging, laxative use, etc.
 2. The majority of women with problems in these areas suffer shame and embarrassment regarding their behavior, but most will respond honestly to direct and compassionate, nonjudgmental questioning.
 3. Examples of questions to ask:
    a. Do you ever go through bouts of not eating or severely restricting your intake of food?
    b. If so, for how long: days, weeks, months?
    c. Have you ever felt that you have lost control around food and eaten much more than you had wanted?
    d. Do you ever feel guilty after eating?
    e. Have you ever made yourself vomit?
    f. Have you ever used laxatives to lose weight?
    g. How many laxatives used per day and when?
    h. How comfortable are you eating with family or friends?
    i. Do your friends ever seem concerned with your body weight, food intake, etc.?
    j. How do you feel about your body?
    k. Do you see yourself as being about the right weight for your build?

D. **Pathogenic weight-control behavior in female athletes**
 1. In Rosen's excellent review of 182 college athletes,[17] about 32% practiced at least one unhealthy weight-control behavior.
    a. Included were self-induced vomiting, laxative use, diet-pill use, diuretic use, biweekly binges, and excess weight loss.
    b. The behavior was practiced daily for at least 1 month.
    c. An athlete at risk would be someone who feels she is currently overweight or in the past perceived herself to be overweight.
    d. Of the athletes engaging in these behaviors, 70% felt they *were harmless,* an attitude prevalent in adolescents regarding many high risk health behaviors, such as unprotected intercourse and drug use.
 2. **Distinguishing features** between truly eating-disordered women and athletic women[1,14]
    a. **Athletes** are goal-directed in their training with good exercise tolerance, well-developed muscles, unimpaired body image, fat stores in the normal range, and efficient energy metabolism.
    b. **Anorectics** have poor to decreasing exercise tolerance, low body fat stores, dry skin, cold intolerance, distorted body image, and engage in repetitive physical activity that is aimed at weight loss, i.e., running in place in their rooms.
 3. Is the active or athletic female more at risk for disordered eating behavior? There is some research that supports this view.

II. ANXIETY DISORDERS

Anxiety disorders more prevalent in women include panic disorder, generalized anxiety disorder and post-traumatic stress disorder. Obsessive-compulsive disorder seems to afflict males and females equally. Obsessive/compulsive traits are common in highly competitive athletes and often highly adaptive for maximal performance.

A. **DSM-III-R criteria**
  1. **Panic disorder**
     a. Spontaneous discrete periods of intense fear
     b. Four attacks in 4 weeks
     c. Four of the following symptoms associated with the attack:
        i. Shortness of breath
        ii. Dizziness
        iii. Palpitations
        iv. Trembling
        v. Sweating
        vi. Choking
        vii. Nausea or gastrointestinal distress
        viii. Feeling of unreality
        ix. Numbness
        x. Flushes
        xi. Chest pain
        xii. Fear of dying
        xiii. Fear of going crazy
     d. Organic factors ruled out
  2. **Post-traumatic stress disorder**
     a. History of major trauma such as childhood abuse or sexual assault, life-threatening event
     b. Persistent intrusive recollections of the trauma or traumatizer
     c. Recurrent dreams
     d. Reliving the traumatic events
     e. Distress at reexposure to reminders of the trauma
     f. Avoidance of reminders of the trauma
     g. Increased arousal autonomically and reactivity
     h. Hypervigilance
     i. One-month duration of symptoms
  3. **Generalized anxiety disorder**
     a. Worries a lot
     b. Six of the following symptoms:
        i. Motor tension such as restlessness, muscle tension, feeling shaky
        ii. Autonomic hyperactivity, such as palpitations, dry mouth, flushes, sweaty palms, frequent urination, lump in the throat
        iii. Vigilance and scanning, such as an exaggerated startle response
        iv. Difficulty concentrating, feeling keyed up or on edge
     c. Other disorders and conditions ruled out
B. **General considerations**
  1. Review papers or brief studies looking at the prevalence of anxiety disorders related to activity and/or athletic performance are not obvious in a literature search.
  2. These disturbances are probably not uncommon but might be difficult to delineate because of an overlap with **performance anxiety** (common in competing athletes).
  3. Regular training and exercise have also been reported to reduce anxiety which would mask the anxiety disturbance.
  4. Unmasking might occur in the context of injury, with an affected woman developing overt symptoms in the context of forced inactivity.
  5. Many women with chronic traumatic disorders find regular exercise helps them to modulate anger and high reactivity. Most importantly, motor movement gives a sense of psychological freedom counteracting the chronic sense of entrapment these patients feel.

III. **AFFECTIVE DISORDERS**

Depressive disorders are diagnosed twice as commonly in women as in men.

A. **DSM-III-R criteria**
 1. **Major depressive disorder**
  a. Five of the following symptoms experienced daily for >2 weeks' duration
   i. Depressed mood, diminished interest or pleasure in activities of daily living
   ii. Weight loss or gain, sleep disturbance, fatigue
   iii. Agitation or psychomotor slowing
   iv. Guilt and sense of worthlessness
   v. Decreased concentration
   vi. Recurrent suicidal thoughts
  b. Organic factors have been ruled out (such as hypo- or hyperthyroidism, multiple sclerosis, Cushing's disease, etc.)
 2. **Cyclothymic disorder**
  a. Mood swings for 2 years that are not severe enough to fulfill criteria for bipolar disorder
 3. **Dysthymic disorder**
  a. Depressed mood for ≥2 years that does not meet criteria for major depression
  b. Two of the following symptoms:
   i. Poor appetite or increased eating
   ii. Low energy or fatigue
   iii. Low self-esteem
   iv. Decreased concentration and trouble deciding
   v. Feeling of hopelessness
 4. **Adjustment reaction with depressed mood**
  a. Psychosocial stressor not more than 3 months preceding onset of symptoms
  b. Symptoms are in excess of a normal reaction
  c. Functioning is impaired
  d. History is not one of overreaction to stress
  e. Duration is <6 months
  f. Other mental disorders and uncomplicated bereavement have been ruled out

B. **General considerations**
One study done in Colorado by Gadpaille et al.[10] compared amenorrheic runners to regularly menstruating runners of similar weight, with the following findings:
 1. The amenorrheic group had major depression, eating disorders, and a high rate of family members suffering from affective illness.
 2. Eating disorders and depression are often comorbid.
 3. The presence of **amenorrhea** in an active or athletic woman ought to trigger a more extensive history for mood disturbance past or present and family history of depression.
 4. **Age of onset** for affective illness is highest in women between the ages of 24–44 so that younger women may not have experienced their first clinically significant index episode.
 5. **Dysthymic symptoms** may be self-treated to some extent by regular exercise.
 6. The presence of **irritability** rather than frank mood disturbance may be an important warning of an underlying depressive diasthesis.
 7. These patients are more commonly viewed as unpleasant people rather than as atypical depressives.

IV. **TREATMENT INTERVENTIONS**

 A. Take a **proactive, positive, nonjudgmental approach.**
 B. **Maladaptive eating behavior patterns in athletes** (*see also* Chapter 20)

1. **Recommend regular meals with teammates,** renormalizing dietary patterns, and education regarding long-term health benefits of good nutritional intake.
2. **Intervention with an overzealous coach** may be needed to eliminate major dysfunctional input from a clearly powerful source.
3. Longer duration of involvement in unhealthy eating patterns will require longer periods of time for renormalization.
4. Concern for bone density and bone growth during the teens, early 20s, and later make intervention regarding unhealthy eating patterns critically important, as lack of bone development and loss of bone may not be reversible.
5. Severe eating disorders require mental health referral and tend to be chronic.

C. **Maladaptive eating behavior patterns in nonathletic active women**
1. Provide education, dietary consultation.
2. Encourage renormalization.
3. Emphasize health-related benefits of good nutrition: i.e., bone density preservation, prepregnancy planning, optimal health.

D. **Anxiety-related illnesses**
1. May respond to simple reassurance and education.
2. Cognitive behaviorally oriented therapy, relaxation training, stress management, and autohypnosis are often helpful.
3. Medication management is needed in some patients.
4. Panic disorder is commonly treated with antidepressants or antianxiety agents, which may have an impact on activity and athletic performance:
   a. Antidepressants may increase heart rate and affect maximal cardiac performance (aerobic intolerance).
   b. Thermoregulatory dyscontrol such as excess sweating, piloerection, flushing, and/or heat intolerance
   c. Benzodiazepines may affect coordination.
   d. Antipsychotics may cause amenorrhea.

E. **Affective illnesses**
1. Best treated with cognitive behavioral or interpersonal therapy.
2. Antidepressants are indicated if the mood is markedly disturbed and associated with physical symptoms such as lethargy, insomnia, weight loss, psychomotor retardation, or agitation.
3. Use of chemotherapy is helpful for mood but often makes exercise less pleasant because of postural dizziness, increased heart rate, flushing, etc.
4. Prozac and the newer serotonin re-uptake inhibitors, Zoloft and Paxil, and Wellbutrin have much less cardiac and anticholinergic effect and seem better tolerated by regularly exercising women.
5. There have been some recent reports of bradycardia in women on Prozac. Given the normally slower heart rates in athletic women, an even further drop may pose some risks.
6. Studies done on compromised patients (i.e., geriatric, cardiac) on antidepressants show no negative inotropic effects in these patients when studied on treadmill.
7. Antidepressants exert complex sympathetic and parasympathetic effects that warrant more in-depth study especially during exercise.

V. CONCLUSIONS

Psychiatric referral is indicated for the more severely impaired athlete or active woman who meets DSM-III-R criteria for the disorders reviewed above. Difficulties will be found in the type of intervention most appropriate for patients exhibiting some disturbances behaviorally that put them at risk for more full-blown disorders but at the point of notice are still less than conclusive. The analogy might be made to alcoholism: An occasional experience of overdrinking may not flag anything more serious on the horizon for a given person. On the other hand, some occurrences, such as impairment at work, are a late feature.

Data and longitudinal studies are lacking that would help assign some weight to a variety of unhealthy behaviors engaged in during athletics. The ideal for women and girls involved in athletics and exercise-related activity is a boost in self-esteem and an amelioration of the cultural obsession with how female bodies look versus how they function. A lifelong commitment to well care of females could be readily enhanced and reinforced by participation in sports and exercise.

REFERENCES

1. Agostini R: Women in sports. In Mellion MB, Walsh JM, Shelton G (eds): The Team Physician's Handbook. Philadelphia, Hanley & Belfus, 1990, pp 179–188.
2. Benson JE, Allemann Y, Theintz HH: Eating problems and calorie intake levels in Swiss adolescent athletes. Int J Sports Med 11:249–252, 1990.
3. Borgen JS, Corbin CB: Eating disorders among female athletes. Phys SportsMed 15:89–95, 1987.
4. Brouns FJPH, Saris WHM, Ten Hoor F: Dietary problems in the case of strenuous exertion. J Sports Med 26:306–312, 1986.
5. Bulbulian R: Eating problems related to prolonged amenorrhea in athletes [letter]. Med Sci Sports Exerc 19:525–527, 1987.
6. Burckes-Miller M, Black DR: Eating disorders: A problem in athletics? Health Educ 19:22–25, 1988.
7. Carr DB, Bullen BA, Skrinar GS, et al: Physical conditioning facilitates the exercise-induced secretion of beta-endorphin and beta-lipotropin in women. N Engl J Med 305:560–562, 1981.
8. Davis C, Cowles M: A comparison of weight and diet concerns and personality factors among female athletes and non-athletes. J Psychosom Res 33:527–536, 1989.
9. Dishman RK: Medical psychology in exercise and sport. Med Clin North Am 69:123–143, 1985.
10. Gadpaille WJ, Sanborn CF, Wagner WW: Athletic amenorrhea, major affective disorders, and eating disorders. Am J Psychiatry 144:939–942, 1987.
11. Garner DM, Olmsted MP, Bohr Y, et al: The eating attitudes test: Psychometric features and clinical correlates. Psychol Med 12:871–878, 1982.
12. Mansfield MJ, Emans SJ: Anorexia nervosa, athletics, and amenorrhea. Pediatr Clin North Am 36:533–549, 1989.
13. McKay RJ: Excessive weight loss and food aversion in athletes simulating anorexia nervosa. Pediatrics 66:139–143, 1980.
14. McSherry JA: The diagnostic challenge of anorexia nervosa. Am Fam Phys 29:144, 1984.
15. Ossip-Klein DJ, Doyne EJ, Bowman ED, et al: Effects of running or weight lifting on self-concept in clinically depressed women. J Consult Clin Psychol 57:158–161, 1989.
16. Perron M, Endres J: Knowledge, attitudes, and dietary practices of female athletes. J Am Diet Assoc 85:573–576, 1985.
17. Rosen LW, McKeag B, Hough DO, et al: Pathogenic weight-control behavior in female athletes. Phys SportMed 14:79–86, 1986.
18. Rucinski A: Relationship of body image and dietary intake of competitive ice skaters. J Am Diet Assoc 89:98–100, 1989.
19. Sexton H, Maere A, Dahl NH: Exercise intensity and reduction in neurotic symptoms. Acta Psychiatr Scand 80:231–235, 1989.
20. Weight LM, Noakes TD: Is running an analog of anorexia?: A survey of the incidence of eating disorders in female distance runners. Med Sci Sports Exerc 19:213–217, 1987.
21. Yates A, Leehey K, Shisslak CM: Running—An analogue of anorexia? N Engl J Med 308:251–255, 1983.

Chapter 14: Alcohol Abuse and Prevention in Collegiate Women Athletes

LINDA A. DIMEFF, MS

G. ALAN MARLATT, PhD

A number of important gender differences result in different risk constellations for young women and men and may place women at greater risk for certain alcohol problems and other related negative consequences due to drinking. Such risks include differences in alcohol metabolism, sustained peak degree of intoxication for women due to hormonal factors, and societal perceptions about women who drink that increase vulnerability for unwanted sexual advances and rape. This chapter explores the prevalence and risks associated with use of alcohol among collegiate women athletes. In addition to examining drinking norms and risks among college drinking women, this outline provides a practical guide for practitioners for assessing risky use of alcohol and providing an effective, brief intervention to reduce these risks.

I. **SCOPE OF THE PROBLEM**
   A. **Pervasive heavy use of alcohol among college students**
      1. Estimates of prevalence of drinking among college students range from 73–98%.[38]
      2. National average quantity of drinking per week for college students: 3–4 drinks on 2 occasions weekly.
      3. A national survey found that over 20% of all college students drink 6 or more drinks per occasion at least weekly.[14]
      4. Consistent with other studies,[38] a recent survey of 1669 students at 14 colleges identified 35% of the women as "binge" drinkers, consuming more than 5 drinks in a row at least once in the past 2 weeks.[47]
      5. While consuming fewer drinks per occasion, college women typically reach comparable blood alcohol levels and degree of intoxication as men due to weight and metabolic differences.[12]
   B. **Common consequences associated with heavy drinking by college students**
      1. **Behavioral and health problems**
         a. Alcohol-related accidents remain the leading cause of death among young adults 16–24 years of age in the U.S.
         b. Diminishing academic performance
         c. Transmission of sexually transmitted diseases
         d. Vandalism and aggressive behaviors
         e. Unplanned pregnancies and risk of fetal alcohol syndrome
         f. Nonconsensual sex
         g. Disordered eating behaviors preceding and following drinking occasion (e.g., binging and purging)
         h. Compromised sports performance
      2. **Risk of future alcohol dependence**
   C. **Course of alcohol problems among heavy college drinkers**
      1. **Epidemiologic findings**[15]
         a. Approximately two-thirds of college student problem drinkers mature out of alcohol abuse by their mid to late 20s.
         b. Maturation out of problematic alcohol use occurs naturally and without treatment or intervention.

2. **Implications of epidemiologic findings**
   a. Excessive drinking during this period is largely influenced by developmental and environmental factors.
      i. Rite of passage into adulthood
      ii. First experience of autonomy and independence for persons living away from home
      iii. Last opportunity to be "carefree" prior to entering workforce and assuming increased financial and professional responsibilities
   b. Elevated chance of problems for the majority of college students is confined to a "window of risk," particularly for heavy drinkers.

II. SPECIAL ISSUES FOR COLLEGE WOMEN WHO DRINK

A. **Differential risk for women who drink**
   1. Physiologic differences in gender influence health risks for women.
      a. Total weight for typical woman is composed of less water (45–55%) than in men (55–65%). Therefore, alcohol is more diluted in absorption process for men than women and thus contributes to women obtaining higher blood alcohol levels per alcoholic beverage consumed (Table 1).
      b. Women typically weigh less than their male counterparts and therefore have less volume of blood, resulting in higher blood alcohol levels per alcohol dose.
      c. Men may contain greater levels of the enzyme alcohol dehydrogenase in their stomachs, which may assist in the metabolism of alcohol.[25,45,46]
      d. Increases in estrogen seem to result in a prolonged peak of intoxication. Hence, use of oral contraceptives and 1 week prior to menstruation are conditions that can extend the intoxication peak.

B. **Increased risk of sexual assault and rape**[1]
   1. 75% of men and 55% of women drink or take drugs prior to sexual assault.[24]
   2. Degree of intoxication impairs ability to perceive and evaluate "risky" situations and to communicate effectively or negotiate consensual sex.[42]
   3. Alcohol intoxication diminishes the woman's ability to physically resist the assault.
   4. In comparison with women who abstain from drinking alcohol, women who drink are perceived in a highly sexualized fashion,[18] including:
      a. More sexually disinhibited
      b. More likely to be seduced
      c. More willing to engage in foreplay
      d. Easier to initiate sexual activity with than a nondrinking women

C. **Increased risk of eating disorders and less severe, yet problematic patterns of eating** ("disordered eating")[22,50]
   1. **The relationship between alcohol abuse and eating disorders is well documented in the empirical literature.**
      a. Russel[37] noted that his bulimia-nervosa patients had a "particular propensity" to abuse drugs and alcohol.
      b. Stern et al.[43] found that 30% of 27 bulimic patients had "substance use disorders" compared with 4% in a matched control group.
      c. Mitchell et al.[30] reported that of their 275 bulimia subjects, 23% had histories of problem drinking.
      d. Bulik[5] compared alcohol use/abuse histories of 35 bulimic women with a "healthy" control group: 17 (49%) of the bulimic patients manifested symptoms consistent with alcohol abuse (compared with 23% of controls), and 3% met diagnostic criteria for alcohol dependence (compared with 0% of controls).
      e. Among a sample of women receiving treatment for alcohol problems, 22 (30.1%) met DSM-III-R criteria for an eating disorder; 25 of the 96% of women receiving treatment for eating disorders (26.9%) met DSM-III-R criteria for alcohol dependence.[19]

TABLE 1. Approximate Blood Alcohol Levels as a Function of Number of Drinks and Time Determined by Weight for Women*
* One drink equals 4 ozs. wine or 1 cooler, 12 ozs. beer, 1 shot, or 1 cocktail.

100 lb. Woman

Number of Drinks	Number of Hours							
	1	2	3	4	5	6	7	8
1	.029	.013	0	0	0	0	0	0
2	.074	.058	.042	.026	.010	0	0	0
3	.119	.103	.087	.071	.055	.039	.023	.007
4	.164	.148	.132	.116	.100	.084	.068	.052
5	.209	.193	.177	.161	.145	.129	.113	.097
6	.254	.238	.222	.206	.190	.174	.158	.142
7	.299	.283	.267	.251	.235	.219	.203	.187
8	.344	.328	.312	.296	.280	.264	.248	.232
9	.389	.373	.357	.341	.325	.309	.293	.277
10	.434	.418	.402	.386	.370	.354	.338	.322
11	.479	.463	.447	.431	.415	.399	.383	.367
12	.524	.508	.492	.476	.460	.444	.428	.412

120 lb. Woman

Number of Drinks	Number of Hours							
	1	2	3	4	5	6	7	8
1	.021	.005	0	0	0	0	0	0
2	.059	.043	.027	.011	0	0	0	0
3	.096	.080	.064	.048	.032	.016	0	0
4	.134	.118	.102	.086	.070	.054	.038	.022
5	.171	.155	.139	.123	.107	.091	.075	.059
6	.209	.193	.177	.161	.145	.129	.113	.097
7	.246	.230	.214	.198	.182	.166	.150	.134
8	.284	.268	.252	.236	.220	.204	.188	.172
9	.321	.305	.289	.273	.257	.241	.225	.209
10	.359	.343	.327	.311	.295	.279	.263	.247
11	.396	.380	.364	.348	.332	.316	.300	.284
12	.434	.418	.402	.386	.370	.354	.338	.322

140 lb. Woman

Number of Drinks	Number of Hours							
	1	2	3	4	5	6	7	8
1	.016	0	0	0	0	0	0	0
2	.048	.032	.016	0	0	0	0	0
3	.080	.064	.048	.032	.016	0	0	0
4	.112	.096	.080	.064	.048	.032	.016	0
5	.144	.128	.112	.096	.080	.064	.048	.032
6	.176	.160	.144	.128	.112	.096	.080	.064
7	.209	.193	.177	.161	.145	.129	.113	.097
8	.241	.225	.209	.193	.177	.161	.145	.129
9	.273	.257	.241	.225	.209	.193	.177	.161
10	.305	.289	.273	.257	.241	.225	.209	.193
11	.337	.321	.305	.289	.273	.257	.241	.225
12	.369	.353	.337	.321	.305	.289	.273	.257

160 lb. Woman

Number of Drinks	Number of Hours							
	1	2	3	4	5	6	7	8
1	.012	0	0	0	0	0	0	0
2	.040	.024	.008	0	0	0	0	0
3	.068	.052	.036	.020	.004	0	0	0
4	.096	.080	.064	.048	.032	.016	0	0
5	.124	.108	.092	.076	.060	.044	.028	.012
6	.152	.136	.120	.104	.088	.072	.056	.040
7	.180	.164	.148	.132	.116	.100	.084	.068
8	.209	.193	.177	.161	.145	.129	.113	.097
9	.237	.221	.205	.189	.173	.157	.141	.125
10	.265	.249	.233	.217	.201	.185	.169	.153
11	.293	.277	.261	.245	.229	.213	.197	.181
12	.321	.305	.289	.273	.257	.241	.225	.209

180 lb. Woman

Number of Drinks	Number of Hours							
	1	2	3	4	5	6	7	8
1	.009	0	0	0	0	0	0	0
2	.034	.018	.002	0	0	0	0	0
3	.059	.043	.027	.011	0	0	0	0
4	.084	.068	.052	.036	.020	.004	0	0
5	.109	.093	.077	.061	.045	.029	.013	0
6	.134	.118	.102	.086	.070	.054	.038	.022
7	.159	.143	.127	.111	.095	.079	.063	.047
8	.184	.168	.152	.136	.120	.104	.088	.072
9	.209	.193	.177	.161	.145	.129	.113	.097
10	.234	.218	.202	.186	.170	.154	.138	.122
11	.259	.243	.227	.211	.195	.179	.163	.147
12	.284	.268	.252	.236	.220	.204	.188	.172

200 lb. Woman

Number of Drinks	Number of Hours							
	1	2	3	4	5	6	7	8
1	.006	0	0	0	0	0	0	0
2	.029	.013	0	0	0	0	0	0
3	.051	.035	.019	.003	0	0	0	0
4	.074	.058	.042	.026	.010	0	0	0
5	.096	.080	.064	.048	.032	.016	0	0
6	.119	.103	.087	.071	.055	.039	.023	.007
7	.141	.125	.109	.093	.077	.061	.045	.029
8	.164	.148	.132	.116	.100	.084	.068	.052
9	.186	.170	.154	.138	.122	.106	.090	.074
10	.209	.193	.177	.161	.145	.129	.113	.097
11	.231	.215	.199	.183	.167	.151	.135	.119
12	.254	.238	.222	.206	.190	.174	.158	.142

TABLE 1. Approximate Blood Alcohol Levels as a Function of Number of Drinks and Time Determined by Weight for Men*

* One drink equals 4 ozs. wine or 1 cooler, 12 ozs. beer, 1 shot, or 1 cocktail.

120 lb. Man

Number of Drinks	Number of Hours			
	1	2	3	4
1	.015	0	0	0
2	.046	.030	.014	0
3	.077	.061	.045	.029
4	.109	.093	.077	.061
5	.140	.124	.108	.092
6	.171	.155	.139	.123
7	.202	.186	.170	.154
8	.234	.218	.202	.186
9	.265	.249	.233	.217
10	.296	.280	.264	.248
11	.327	.311	.295	.279
12	.359	.343	.327	.311

140 lb. Man

Number of Drinks	Number of Hours			
	1	2	3	4
1	.010	0	0	0
2	.037	.021	.005	0
3	.064	.048	.032	.016
4	.091	.075	.059	.043
5	.117	.101	.085	.069
6	.144	.128	.112	.096
7	.171	.155	.139	.123
8	.198	.182	.166	.150
9	.225	.209	.193	.177
10	.251	.235	.219	.203
11	.278	.262	.246	.230
12	.305	.289	.273	.257

160 lb. Man

Number of Drinks	Number of Hours							
	1	2	3	4	5	6	7	8
1	.007	0	0	0	0	0	0	0
2	.030	.014	0	0	0	0	0	0
3	.054	.038	.022	.006	0	0	0	0
4	.077	.061	.045	.029	.013	0	0	0
5	.101	.085	.069	.053	.037	.021	.005	0
6	.124	.108	.092	.076	.060	.044	.028	.012
7	.148	.132	.116	.100	.084	.068	.052	.036
8	.171	.155	.139	.123	.107	.091	.075	.059
9	.194	.178	.162	.146	.130	.114	.098	.082
10	.218	.202	.186	.170	.154	.138	.122	.106
11	.241	.225	.209	.193	.177	.161	.145	.129
12	.265	.249	.233	.217	.201	.185	.169	.153

180 lb. Man

Number of Drinks	Number of Hours							
	1	2	3	4	5	6	7	8
1	.004	0	0	0	0	0	0	0
2	.025	.009	0	0	0	0	0	0
3	.046	.030	.014	0	0	0	0	0
4	.067	.051	.035	.019	.003	0	0	0
5	.088	.072	.056	.040	.024	.008	0	0
6	.109	.093	.077	.061	.045	.029	.013	0
7	.129	.113	.097	.081	.065	.049	.033	.017
8	.150	.134	.118	.102	.086	.070	.054	.038
9	.171	.155	.139	.123	.107	.091	.075	.059
10	.192	.176	.160	.144	.128	.112	.096	.080
11	.213	.197	.181	.165	.149	.133	.117	.101
12	.234	.218	.202	.186	.170	.154	.138	.122

200 lb. Man

Number of Drinks	Number of Hours							
	1	2	3	4	5	6	7	8
1	.002	0	0	0	0	0	0	0
2	.021	.005	0	0	0	0	0	0
3	.040	.024	.008	0	0	0	0	0
4	.059	.043	.027	.011	0	0	0	0
5	.077	.061	.045	.029	.013	0	0	0
6	.096	.080	.064	.048	.032	.016	0	0
7	.115	.099	.083	.067	.051	.035	.019	.003
8	.134	.118	.102	.086	.070	.054	.038	.022
9	.152	.136	.120	.104	.088	.072	.056	.040
10	.171	.155	.139	.123	.107	.091	.075	.059
11	.190	.174	.158	.142	.126	.110	.094	.078
12	.209	.193	.177	.161	.145	.129	.113	.097

220 lb. Man

Number of Drinks	Number of Hours							
	1	2	3	4	5	6	7	8
1	.001	0	0	0	0	0	0	0
2	.018	.002	0	0	0	0	0	0
3	.035	.019	.003	0	0	0	0	0
4	.052	.036	.020	.004	0	0	0	0
5	.069	.053	.037	.021	.005	0	0	0
6	.086	.070	.054	.038	.022	.006	0	0
7	.103	.087	.071	.055	.039	.023	.007	0
8	.120	.104	.088	.072	.056	.040	.024	.008
9	.137	.121	.105	.089	.073	.057	.041	.025
10	.154	.138	.122	.106	.090	.074	.058	.042
11	.171	.155	.139	.123	.107	.091	.075	.059
12	.188	.172	.156	.140	.124	.108	.092	.076

2. **The relationship between alcohol abuse and less severe patterns of eating is well established empirically.**
   a. Severity of dieting and bulimia associated with increased frequency, quantity, and peak consumption patterns of alcohol use.[23]
   b. Significant differences in peak quantity of alcohol consumption between purgers and nonpurgers, with purgers averaging 36.5 drinks/week compared with an average of 24.5 drinks for the remaining sample.[28]

III. **LITERATURE REVIEW ON DRINKING PATTERNS OF COLLEGE WOMEN ATHLETES**

A. **Limitations of current body of literature**
   1. Dearth of rigorous, empirical studies on alcohol use among athletes
      a. Few studies use rigorous measures to assess drinking behavior; most studies examine drinking unidimensionally rather than multidimensionally.
      b. No study to date has examined patterns of alcohol use over time (e.g., on and off season) using longitudinal methods.
   2. Most studies are about male athletes; few studies on female athletes.

B. **Review of empirical findings**
   1. In general, no differences in drinking patterns are found between high school and collegiate women athletes and nonathlete women.[6,32,33]
   2. Male and female collegiate athletes may engage in more risky behavior in general, including driving while intoxicated, than college nonathletes.[32]
   3. High-risk behavior may be due to predisposing personality style that may also facilitate athlete's interest in high-risk sports.[32]
   4. Pattern of alcohol use may vary for athletes depending on sports season.
      a. Risk of heavier use of alcohol may increase during the off season.[40]
      b. Alcohol used more as a means to relax than to cope with competition.[40]
   5. Sex role conflict may heighten the risk for alcohol problems among female athletes.[48]
      a. Hypothesized conflict: The personal characteristics required to succeed as an athlete (e.g., competitiveness, aggressiveness, etc.) are often diametrically opposed to female socialization. Acquisition of these "masculine" skills while maintaining "feminine" identity can result in such conflict.
      b. Magnitude vs. direction of conflict: The magnitude of the sex-role conflict is of greater significance than the direction of the conflict (e.g., "too masculine" vs. "not masculine enough") with respect to increased risk for alcohol abuse.[39,48]

C. **College women athletes may experience more risky drinking situations (e.g., sports trips) and/or pressure from males to drink more.**
   1. A woman's drinking patterns and pace are often influenced by the drinking pace of her male counterpart, despite differences in size and weight.[8]
   2. Affiliation to a unified social group (e.g., sorority, athletic team, etc.) increases risk of heavy drinking.

IV. **ASSESSING ALCOHOL PROBLEMS AMONG COLLEGE WOMEN**

A. **DSM-III-R diagnostic criteria for alcohol abuse and alcohol dependence**[2]
   1. **Alcohol abuse:** Applies to the "maladaptive patterns of psychoactive substance use that have never met the criteria for dependence" (Table 2).
   2. **Alcohol dependence:** Characterized by a cluster of cognitive, behavioral, and physical dependence syndromes (e.g., tolerance and withdrawal) indicating that the individual has "impaired control of psychoactive substance use and continues use of the substance despite adverse consequences" (Table 2).
   3. The **distinction between abuse and dependence** is based on the premise that alcohol problems exist on a continuum (Fig. 1).

TABLE 2.   DSM-III-R Criteria for Psychoactive Substance Abuse and Dependence

Abuse

A. A maladaptive pattern of psychoactive substance use indicated by at least one of the following: (1) continued use despite knowledge of having a persistent or recurrent social, occupational, psychological, or physical problem that is caused or exacerbated by use of the psychoactive substance; and (2) recurrent use in situations in which use is physically hazardous (e.g., driving while intoxicated).

B. Some symptoms of the disturbance have persisted for at least one month, or have occurred repeatedly over a longer period of time.

C. Never met the criteria for Psychoactive Substance Dependence for this substance.

Dependence—At least three of the following:

1. Substance often taken in large amounts or over a longer period than the person intended.
2. Persistent desire or one or more unsuccessful efforts to cut down or control substance use.
3. A great deal of time in activities necessary to get the substance, taking the substance, or recovering from its efforts.
4. Frequent intoxication or withdrawal symptoms when expected to fulfill major role obligations at work, school, or home.
5. Important social, occupational, or recreational activities given up or reduced because of substance use.
6. Continued substance use despite knowledge of having a persistent or recurrent social, psychological, or physical problem that is caused or exacerbated by the use of the substance.
7. Marked tolerance: Need for markedly increased amounts of the substance in order to achieve intoxication or desired effects.
8. Characteristic withdrawal symptoms.
9. Substance often taken to relieve or avoid withdrawal symptoms.

From American Psychiatric Association: Diagnostic and Statistical Manual of Mental Disorders, III-R. Washington, D.C., American Psychiatric Press, 1987.

B. **Assess multiple dimensions of drinking**
   1. **Pattern of use**
      a. Typical weekly frequency and quantity
      b. Typical weekly peak degree of intoxication: When and how much?
      c. Peak degree of intoxication in the past month
      d. The most consumed in history of alcohol use
   2. **Assess how different social context and other situational factors affect the pattern of drinking (e.g., moderate, heavy, or binge drinking).**
      a. Who does the athlete drink with?
      b. Where does she drink?
      c. What mood is she in when she drinks?
      d. What kind of drink does she consume?
      e. Does she use other substances when drinking alcohol (drug potentiation)?
   3. **Methods of assessment**
      a. Interview athlete
      b. Athlete keeps track of daily drinking pattern (including abstinent days) for approximately 2 weeks.
      c. Measures
         i. Rutgers Alcohol Problems Inventory (RAPI): Common problems and consequences[49]
         ii. Comprehensive Effects of Alcohol (CEA): Beliefs and expectations about the effects of alcohol[16]
         iii. Alcohol Dependence Scale (ADS): Assesses degree of alcohol dependence
         iv. Eating Attitudes Test-26 (EAT-26): Assesses eating disorders in three dimensions (dieting, bulimia and food preoccupations, and oral control)[17]
   C. **Determine pattern of college student drinking**
   1. **Abstainer**
      a. Does not drink alcohol
      b. Approximately 10% of college student population
   2. **Moderate drinker**
      a. Drinks on several occasions weekly and several drinks per occasion
      b. Occasionally may drink to intoxication

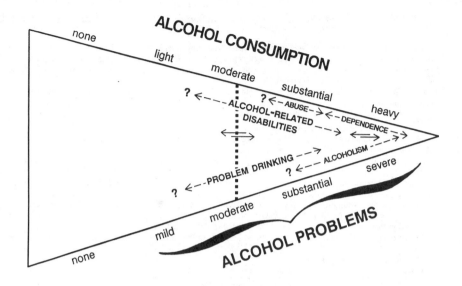

FIGURE 1.   Spectrum of drinkers.

3. **Heavy drinker**
   a. Drinks 4 or more times weekly, frequently reaching blood alcohol levels >0.1%.
   b. 15–25% of the college student population
4. **Binge drinkers**
   a. May not have a steady, heavy typical pattern of drinking
   b. When individual does drink, they drink quickly and to intoxication.
   c. Wechsler and Isaac found 35% of college women consumed more than 5 drinks in a row at least once in 2 weeks.[47]
D. **Determine alcohol use and associated problems along the above continuum.**

V. **PROFESSIONAL ADVICE: A BRIEF INTERVENTION APPROACH TO REDUCING HEALTH RISKS FROM ALCOHOL IN FEMALE ATHLETES**

   A. **Defining professional advice**
      1. **Brief** (1 session); not more than 45 minutes is typically needed.
         a. Minimal relationship found in the literature across populations between duration of treatment and treatment effectiveness.[3,21] (For a review of this literature, see Bien et al.[4])
            i. Minimal, or brief, intervention found more effective than no counseling.
            ii. Brief interventions are often as effective as more extensive treatment.
            iii. Brief interventions can also enhance the effectiveness of subsequent treatment.
      2. **Based on harm-reduction principles**
         a. Comprehensive model designed to reduce the harmful consequences of alcohol and other substance use as a primary goal.
         b. Methods of harm-reduction varied.
            i. Individual clinical treatment
            ii. Public health programs to promote changes in the environment (e.g., distribution of condoms in high schools, needle-exchange programs)
            iii. Public policy changes

3. **Stepped-care approach**
   a. Initially direct intervention at the minimal level appropriate to the individual's risks.
   b. Assess impact of intervention on reducing health risks.
   c. Increase level of intervention as needed until therapeutic effect is achieved.
   d. Approach stands in contrast to a standard model of care recommended for all patients regardless of history and severity of presenting problem (e.g., 28-day inpatient program for alcohol abusers, etc.)
4. **Focus on enhancing motivation to change risky behaviors**
   a. Motivational enhancement is the frame in which all content is embedded.
   b. Practitioner seeks to increase natural curiosity and interest in examining risks associated with alcohol use.
   c. Practitioner facilitates athlete's interest and motivation to change.
   d. Particularly important for individuals with elevated risk, but who perceive their risks as low
5. **Tailored to individual student's personal risks**
   a. Through interview and/or questionnaires, information is obtained about athlete's personal risk factors (e.g., drinking pattern, family history of problematic drinking, etc.).
   b. Feedback is tailored to presenting risks.
6. **Nonconfrontational and nonjudgmental**
   a. Moral judgments about the behavior are avoided.
   b. Examination of risks and behavior is provided in neutral, objective fashion.

B. **Essential elements of brief interventions—FRAMES**[29]
   1. *Feedback:* Provision of specific feedback about drinking
      a. Comparison of client's pattern of drinking to norms for age group or other meaningful cohort group
      b. Review of specific ways alcohol is compromising or impairing client's health
      c. Identification of personal risk factors (e.g., family history of alcohol problems, history of conduct disorder, etc.)
   2. *Responsibility:* Drinking pattern and other behaviors are emphasized as the client's responsibility as means to increase student's perceived control over her behavior.
      a. "What you do with this information is really up to you."
      b. "No one but you can make you change. What you decide to do with this information is really up to you."
   3. *Advice:* Explicit verbal and written advice in ways to reduce or stop drinking are typically provided.
      a. General tips
         i. Set a drinking limit prior to partying.
         ii. Keep track of your drinks.
         iii. Do not exceed more than x drinks per drinking occasion.
         iv. Alternate drinking nonalcoholic drinks and alcoholic drinks.
         v. If you choose to drink, drink beer and avoid hard alcohol.
      b. Specific advice
         i. "You may want to consider refraining from alcohol use prior to the game."
         ii. "I am concerned about the physical effects alcohol may be having on your liver and recommend that we do a (liver screening) blood work-up just to make sure."
   4. *Menu of options:* Multiple options are provided from which the client can choose depending on her level of interest and comfort.
      a. Quit drinking, or continue to abstain.
      b. Drink moderately and avoid intoxication.
      c. Seek out additional alcohol outpatient treatment.

       d. Attend meetings of Alcoholics Anonymous or Rational Recovery.

       e. If severely dependent, recommend inpatient treatment or detoxification program.

    5. **Empathy:** "The skillful *reflective* listening that *clarifies* and *amplifies* the client's own experiencing and meaning *without imposing* (one's) own motive."[29]

      a. Functional rationale for use of empathy

        i. Minimizes likelihood of evoking resistance or defensiveness.

        ii. Facilitates the student to continue talking and exploring the topic area.

        iii. Aids communication of respect and caring, and consequently facilitates building a working alliance between the student and professional.

        iv. Clarifies for the professional exactly what the student means.

      b. Empathy consistently viewed as single most important element.

      c. Confrontation and coercive approaches produce iatrogenic effects and have little overall impact on the targeted behavior.

    6. **Self-efficacy:** Focus on fostering client's abilities to change rather than client's perceived helplessness and powerlessness.

      a. Assist client in bolstering confidence to meet demands.

      b. Optimize and augment client's skill repertoire in deficit areas to establish self-efficacy.

VI. CLINICAL APPROACH RECOMMENDED IN PROFESSIONAL ADVICE

  A. **Understand influences on college student drinking and barriers to change.**

    1. Few heavy drinking students recognize their drinking as atypical or problematic.

    2. Many students often feel innundated with information about alcohol abuse and are often "numb" to additional information and feedback.[11]

    3. Many students expect to hear abstinence messages from adults and prepare themselves by "shutting down" or disengaging.

    4. Stigma associated with having alcohol problems remains high, especially for women; this often compromises interest and motivation to seek help.

  B. **Develop a positive health behaviors approach.**

    1. Avoid problem-focus, problem-phrases, and medical terminology or labels (e.g., "problem drinker," "alcoholic," "alcohol problems," "alcohol abuse," etc.)

    2. Cast a broader lifestyle behaviors frame (e.g., general diet, smoking, condom use and other safer sex practices, use of a helmet when riding a bike, etc.), then embed the alcohol assessment and feedback within this frame.

    3. Focus on minimizing risks associated with behavior.

      a. Allows for more valuefree, nonjudgmental discussion.

      b. Emphasizing risks associated with particular behavior can suggest behavioral alternatives that will reduce risk to promote health.

  C. **Establish trust and rapport.**

    1. Mandatory drug testing programs may compromise trust of women athletes, thereby limiting opportunity for useful intervention.

    2. Strategies to build trust

      a. Speak and behave in a nonjudgmental fashion.

      b. Make use of accurate empathy.

      c. Work with athlete in exploration of risks associated with drinking.

    3. Behaviors that compromise rapport building

      a. Use of "problem" labels or problem focus

      b. Use of confrontational strategies

      c. Pathologizing drinking behavior

    4. Many athletes view their sports medicine physicians as approachable and would seek out her or him regarding personal health concerns.[40]

  D. **Enhance athlete's interest and motivation to change behavior.**

    1. **Models for motivation and their implications for treatment**[29]

a. Motivation as a personality trait
   i. Static personality dimension—"You either have it or you don't."
   ii. Historical origins in psychoanalysis
   iii. Limits means and extent to which professional can help patient if the patient is "lacking" in this trait.
b. Motivation as a state
   i. A flexible, dynamic state of readiness that one can move into and out of
   ii. Origins in motivational psychology
   iii. Model more consistent with how addictive behaviors are typically changed
     (a) Smokers typically stop and start on average of four times before achieving long-term abstinence.
     (b) "Every slip or relapse brings you one step closer to recovery."
   iv. Enhances role of professional in facilitating behavior change.

2. **Assess state of readiness** using the States of Change model[34] and work to enhance motivation for change by actively facilitating forward movement along the change continuum.[29]

  a. **Precontemplative**
   i. Athlete is unaware of risks or problems associated with her present pattern of drinking.
   ii. Role of professional
     (a) Increase awareness of risk in athlete.
     (b) Raise doubt about normative nature of drinking and her high-risk situation.
     (c) Information and feedback comparing their use with normative data are often useful.

  b. **Contemplative**
   i. Athlete has begun to recognize risks and/or problems associated with her pattern of alcohol use and may vacillate between interest in changing pattern and maintaining status quo.
     (a) "I don't really think I have a problem; it's just what we do in the off-season."
     (b) "Maybe I'd be healthier if I did cut back, but I'm just not sure I'm ready."
   ii. Role of professional
     (a) Evoke and provide reasons for change.
     (b) Use open-ended questions to elicit from the athlete risks (short- and long-term) of not changing risky behavior.
     (c) Help tip the balance of ambivalence to change in favor of change.

  c. **Preparation**
   i. Athlete is ready to change the behavior, to move in the direction of action.
     (a) "I didn't realize things had become this bad. I've got to do something."
     (b) "I'm ready to try something else to change what I'm doing."
   ii. Role of professional
     (a) Help athlete find appropriate resources if needed.
     (b) Provide specific skills and strategies to reduce risks.

  d. **Action**
   i. Athlete has commenced with action steps (e.g., cut down, found a new peer group that drinks less, etc.).
   ii. Role of professional
     (a) Elicit from athlete how action steps are working to achieve their goals.
     (b) Problem-solve ways to improve action steps, if necessary.

        (c) Continue to provide praise and positive reinforcement of behavioral gains.
  e. **Maintenance**
     i. Once goals are met, athlete continues efforts to support and maintain her gains.
  f. **Relapse**
     i. Athlete may have "slipped" or relapsed from original goal.
     ii. Role of professional
        (a) Acknowledge and address athlete's feelings related to the relapse (e.g., discouragement, guilt, shame, sadness, anger, etc.)
        (b) Facilitate rebuilding of commitment to change and resuming tasks at athlete's state of change.
3. **Explore athlete's ambivalence to change.**
  a. What does the athlete stand to gain and lose in the short and long term by changing behavior?
  b. Attempt to tip the balance of ambivalence in the direction of change.[29]
4. **Pull for material during assessment that can help tip balance of ambivalence** in direction of change (e.g., increase athletic performance by not compromising REM sleep due to excessive alcohol use).
E. **Elicit self-motivational statements from the student.**
1. Encourage a process whereby the student provides the reasons to change her behavior.
2. Facilitate full examination of self-motivated reasons to change by providing prompts (e.g., "What else?" "Are there any other reasons that come to mind?")
F. **Build a case for change.**
1. Facilitate the athlete's recognition that the reasons to reduce heavy alcohol consumption outweigh the reasons to continue status quo pattern of heavy drinking.
2. Draw upon information about athlete's personal risks and pattern of drinking, accurate information about the effects of drinking and debunking myths about alcohol as means to build reasons to change risky behavior.

VII. **BUILDING THE CASE FOR CHANGE**

A. **Sleep, alcohol, and performance**
1. **Effects of acute alcohol intoxication on sleep** (blood alcohol concentration at approximately 0.10% at initiation of sleep)[7,20]
  a. Increases total sleep time (TST) first half of night; TST decreases second half of night.
  b. Decreases wakefulness after sleep onset (WASO) first half of night; increases WASO second half of night.
  c. Decrease in rapid eye movement (REM) first half of the night; REM rebound occurs in later portion of night following alcohol metabolism.
  d. Increase in delta sleep
  e. Physical effects vary depending on blood alcohol level. Greater levels may fully suppress REM sleep and prevent rebound until following night due to set metabolism rate (approximately 1 drink/hour).
2. **Psychological effects following sleep deprivation due to acute alcohol intoxication**
  a. Unrested and unrefreshed feeling
  b. Increased irritability
  c. Fatigue
  d. Cognitive dampening (e.g., less "sharp" or "quick" in thinking and responses)
  e. Diminished mental stamina
3. **Physical effects following sleep deprivation that compromise athletic performance**[31,35,44]

  a. Normal levels of prolactin, cortisol, and growth hormone (hGH) are suppressed.
  b. Plasma levels of thyroxine, triiodothyroine, and reverse triiodothyroine increase.
  c. VE/VO_2 ratios are greater at the submaximal (75% of the VO_2max) and maximal workload; oxygen consumption decreases at maximal workload. May suggest that sleep deprivation alters endurance performance by impairment of aerobic pathways.[31]
  d. Time to exhaustion decreases.
  e. Ratings of perceived exhaustion increase with sleep deprivation, but are not reliable assessments of athlete's ability to perform as perception does not correlate with cardiovascular changes.[44]
B. **Exposing the myth: alcohol outcome expectancies:**[27] Refers to the experiences (whether favorable or negative) one expects to have upon drinking alcohol and due to the alcohol. The extent to which these expectancies are positive influences the use and reliance on alcohol to achieve these effects.
  1. **Common myth:** Increased energy, confidence, sexual attractiveness, and sexual prowess are due to pharmacologic properties of alcohol.
  2. **Myth explored:** Laboratory ("balanced placebo design") studies to examine psychological and pharmacologic effects of alcohol have used 2×2 matrix designs to tease out contributions from both:
    a. Two dimensions
      i. Beverage type (vodka vs tonic water) the subject *expects* to receive
      ii. Beverage type the subject *actually* receives
    b. Four research conditions
      i. "Spiked drink": Expect tonic but receive vodka
      ii. Placebo: Expect vodka but receive tonic
      iii. Control: Expect vodka and receive vodka
      iv. Control: Expect tonic and receive tonic
    c. Results
      i. Women become less sexually aroused when drinking alcohol.
      ii. Women become more anxious in social situations when they believe they have had alcohol.
      iii. Men become more aggressive when they are drinking only tonic water but believe their drink contains vodka.
      iv. Men become relatively less aggressive when they think they are drinking only tonic water but their drink really contains vodka.
      v. Men become less anxious in social situations when they believe they have had alcohol, regardless of what drink they actually consumed.
      vi. Men become more sexually aroused when they believe they are drinking alcohol, even when they are not physiologically aroused.
  3. **Results** from these studies conclude that *many of the social effects commonly associated with the chemical properties of alcohol are significantly influenced by psychological expectations:* What one believes will occur when they drink ("mental set") and the psychological influence of the setting (e.g., dimly lit bar, soft music, neon signs, etc.).
C. **Alcohol myopia**[42]
  1. Alcohol intoxication creates a kind of cognitive near-sightedness (myopia) that reduces information processing and abstract reasoning to simple, immediate concrete cues.
    a. Alcohol reduces the range of what one can perceive and process.
    b. Perception and emotions are restricted to immediate cues while intoxicated; peripheral and subtle cues are typically not accessible to an intoxicated individual.
  2. The degree of myopia increases as the individual becomes more intoxicated.

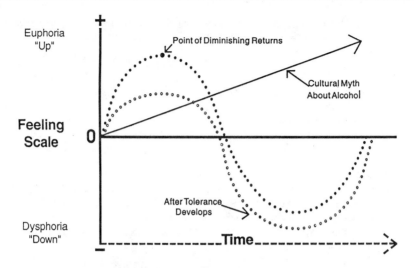

FIGURE 2. The biphasic response to alcohol. The *open circles* indicate the diminished initial response in drinkers who have developed tolerance.

    D. **The biphasic effect of alcohol:** Disspelling the myth of "more is better"
        1. Two separate phases of alcohol effect produce different experience and sensation (Fig. 2).
           a. Common effects during ascending blood alcohol level:
              i. Mild arousal
              ii. Excitement
              iii. Increased energy
           b. Common effects during descending blood alcohol level:
              i. Mild physical depression
              ii. Decreased energy
              iii. Tired and fatigue
        2. Studies using animal model have found a dampened effect in the initial arousal phase in animals with tolerance to alcohol.

VIII. **SUMMARY**

    A. **Moving past barriers to effective treatment and prevention of alcohol problems:** *The Institute of Medicine Report* recommendations:
        1. Broaden the base of treatment for alcohol problems to prevention and early intervention efforts for targeted at-risk groups.
        2. Match client to particular prevention or treatment program that is most likely to result in favorable outcome.
           a. All persons with alcohol problems are not alike.
           b. Different approaches may be optimal for different types of people.
           c. Some factors to consider in treatment matching
               i. Age
              ii. Severity of symptoms
              iii. Duration of abusive use
              iii. Beliefs about treatment
              iv. Client preference
    B. **Empirically derived results regarding the effectiveness of professional advice as a brief intervention harm-reduction strategy for college students**[3,21]
        1. Significant reduction of weekly frequency and quantity of use of alcohol

2. Significant reduction in peak blood alcohol levels
3. Significant reduction in negative consequences and/or problems associated with alcohol use.
4. Effects maintained throughout 1- and 2-year follow-up periods

C. **Rationale for targeting collegiate women athletes using physician-facilitated professional advice:**

1. College athletic women are a ready-made at-risk population for experiencing social, health, and behavioral problems due to effects of alcohol; therefore, suitable for professional advice.
2. Athletes have frequently established rapport with team physician and view this person as credible and trustworthy.
3. Professional advice can easily be incorporated into discussion of broader-based health concerns, as part of regular examination and consultation.
4. Because of highly flexible nature, professional advice can easily be tailored to the specific risks and needs of the woman athlete.
5. Professional advice is likely to produce a clinically significant therapeutic effect.

REFERENCES

1. Abbey A: Acquaintance rape and alcohol consumption on college campuses: How are they linked? J Am Coll Health 39:'165–169, 1991.
2. American Psychiatric Association: Diagnostic and Statistical Manual of Mental Disorders (3rd ed, rev.). Washington, DC, APA, 1987.
3. Baer JS, Marlatt GA, Kivlahan DR, et al: An experimental test of three methods of alcohol risk-reduction with young adults. J Consult Clin Psychol 60:974–979, 1993.
4. Bien TH, Miller WR, Tonigan JS: Brief interventions for alcohol problems: A review. Addiction 88:315–335, 1993.
5. Bulik CM: Drug and alcohol abuse by bulimic women and their families. Am J Psychiatry 144:1604–1606, 1987.
6. Carr CN, Kennedy SR, Dimick KM: Alcohol use among high school athletes: A comparison of alcohol use and intoxication in male and female high school athletes and nonathletes. J Alcohol Drug Educ 36:39–43, 1990.
7. Carskadon MA, Dement WC: Normal sleep and its variations. In Kryger MH, Roth T, Dement WC (eds): Principles and Practice of Sleep Medicine. Philadelpha, W.B Saunders, 1989.
8. Collins RL, Parks GA, Marlatt GA: Social determinants of alcohol consumption: The effects of social interaction and model status on the self-administration of alcohol. J Consult Clin Psychol 53:189–200, 1985.
9. Connors ME, Johnson CL: Epidemiology of bulimia and bulimic behaviors. Addictive Behav 12:165–179, 1987.
10. Crandall CS: Social contagion of binge eating. J Personality Soc Psychol 55:558–598, 1988.
11. Dees SM, Dansereau DF, Peel JL, et al: Using knowledge maps and scripted cooperation to inform college students about patterns of behavior related to recurring abuse of alcohol. Addictive Behav 17:307–318, 1992.
12. Dimeff LA, Baer JS, Kivlahan DR, Marlatt GA: Professional Advice Manual: A Brief Intervention for the Prevention of Alcohol Problems in College Students. (In press).
13. Dimeff LA, Baer JS, Larimer ME, et al: Differential blood alcohol levels and risks for college men and women. (In preparation).
14. Engs RC, Hanson DJ: University students' drinking patterns and problems: Examining the effects of raising the purchasing age. Public Health Rep 103:667–673, 1988.
15. Fillmore KM: Alcohol Use Across the Life Course. Toronto, Alcoholism and Drug Addiction Research Foundation, 1988.
16. Fromme KI, Strutt E, Kaplan D: Comprehensive effects of alcohol: Development and psychometrics of a new expectancy questionnaire. Psychol Assess 5:19–26, 1993.
17. Garner DM, Olmsted MP, Bohr Y, Garfinkel PE: The Eating Attitudes Test: Psychometric features and clinical correlates. Psychol Med 12:871–878, 1982.
18. George WH, Gournic SJ, McAfee MP: Perceptions of post-drinking female sexuality: Effects of gender, beverage choice and drink payment. J Appl Soc Psychol 18:1295–1317, 1988.
19. Goldbloom DS, Naranjo CA, Bremner KE, Hicks LK: Br J Addict 87:913–920, 1992.

20. Kay DC, Samiuddin Z: Sleep disorders associated with drug abuse and drugs of abuse. In Williams RL, Karacon I, Moore CA (eds): Sleep Disorders: Diagnosis and Treatment. New York, John Wiley & Sons, 1988.
21. Kivlahan DR, Marlatt GA, Fromme K, et al: Secondary prevention with college drinkers: Evaluation of an alcohol skills training program. J Consult Clin Psychol 58:805–810, 1990.
22. Krahn DD: The relationship of eating disorders and substance abuse. J Substance Abuse 3:239–253, 1991.
23. Krahn DD, Kurth C, Demitrack M, Drewnowski A: The relationship of dieting severity and bulimic behaviors to alcohol and other drug use in other women. J Substance Abuse 4:341–353, 1992.
24. Koss MP, Gidycz CA, Wisniewski N: The scope of rape: Incidence and prevalence of sexual aggression and victimization in a national sample of higher education students. J Clin Consult Psychol 55:162–170, 1987.
25. Lee L, Schmidt KL, Tornwall MS, Miller TA: Gender differences in ethanol oxidation and injury in the rat stomach. Alcohol 9:421–425, 1992.
26. Luce KH, DuBois HM, Dimeff LA, et al: Exploring the relationship between problematic eating and drinking behaviors among sorority women. Poster presented at the International Conference on the Treatment of Addictive Behaviors (ICTAB), January 1993.
27. Marlatt GA, Larimer ME, Baer JS, Quigley LA: Harm reduction for alcohol problems: Moving beyond the controlled drinking controversy. Behav Ther 24:461–504, 1993.
28. Meilman PW, von Hippel FA, Gaylor MS: Self-induced vomiting in college women: Its relation to eating, alcohol use, and Greek life. J Am Coll Health 40:39–41, 1991.
29. Miller WR, Rollnick S: Motivational interviewing: Preparing people for change. New York, Guilford Press, 1991.
30. Mitchell JE, Hatsukami D, Eckert ED, Pyle R: Characteristics of 275 patients with bulimia. Am J Psychiatry 142:482–485, 1985.
31. Mougin F, Davenne D, Simon RML, et al: Disturbance of sports performance after partial sleep deprivation. C.R. Seances Soc Biol 183:461–466, 1989.
32. Nattiv A, Puffer JC: Lifestyles and health risks of college athletes. J Fam Pract 33:585–590, 1991.
33. Overman SJ, Terry T: Alcohol use and attitudes: A comparison of college athletes and nonathletes. J Drug Educ 21:107–117, 1991.
34. Prochaska JO, DiClemente CC: Toward a comprehensive model of change. In Miller WR, Heather N (eds): Treating Addictive Behaviors. New York, Plenum Press, 1982.
35. Radomski MW, Hart LE, Goodman JM, Plyley MJ: Aerobic fitness and hormonal response to prolonged sleep deprivation and sustained mental work. Aviat Space Environ Med 63:101–106, 1992.
36. Rollnick S, Heather N, Bell A: Negotiating behaviour change in medical settings: The development of brief motivational interviewing. J Mental Health 1:25–37, 1992.
37. Russell GFM: Bulimia nervosa: An ominous variant of anorexia nervosa. Psychol Med 9:429–448, 1979.
38. Saltz R, Elandt D: College student drinking studies 1976–1985. Contemp Drug Probl 13:117–159, 1986.
39. Scida J, Vannicelli M: Sex role conflict and women's drinking. J Stud Alcohol 40:28–44, 1979.
40. Selby R, Weinstein HM, Bird TS: The health of university athletes: Attitudes, behaviors, and stressors. J Am Coll Health 39:11–18, 1990.
41. Skinner HA, Horn JL: Alcohol Dependence Scale (ADS) User's Guide. Toronto, Addiction Research Foundation, 1989.
42. Steele CM, Josephs RA: Alcohol myopia: Its prized and dangerous effects. Am Psychol 45:921–933, 1990.
43. Stern SL, Dixon KN, Nemzer E, et al: Affective disorder in the families of women with normal weight bulimia. Am J Psychiatry 141:1224–1227, 1984.
44. VanHelder T, Radomski MW: Sleep deprivation and the effect on exercise performance. Sports Med 7:235–247, 1989.
45. VanThiel DH, Gavaler JS: Ethanol metabolism and hepatotoxicity: Does sex make a difference? Rec Devel Alcohol 6:291–304, 1988.
46. VanThiel DH, Tarter RE, Rosenblum E, Gavales JS: Ethanol, its metabolism and gonadal effects: Does sex make a difference? Adv Alcohol Subst Abuse 7:131–169, 1988.
47. Weschler H, Issac N: "Binge" drinkers at Massachusetts colleges: Prevalence, drinking style, time trends, and associated problems. JAMA 267:2929–2931, 1992.
48. Wetzig DL: Sex-role conflict in female athletes: A possible marker for alcoholism. J Alcohol Drug Educ 35:45–53, 1990.
49. White HR, Labouvie EW: Towards the assessment of adolescent problem drinking. J Stud Alcohol 50:30–37, 1989.
50. Yeary JR, Heck CL: Dual diagnosis: Eating disorders and psychoactive substance dependence. J Psychoactive Drugs 19:239–349, 1982.

Chapter 15: Personal Safety and Exercise

JULIE WENTWORTH COLLITON, MD

Women are assuming increasingly active and visible roles in today's society. Unfortunately, today's society is not entirely safe for any of its members. In this country, someone becomes the victim of a violent crime every 17 seconds. How violent crime and abuse impact on women is hard to quantitate because of underreporting of these crimes by victims. Fifty percent of rapes in this country go unreported, and it is estimated that every minute in America 1.3 rapes of adult women occur. The percentage of these assaults that target the active, athletic female population is not known. However, because of the magnitude and devastating consequences which result from these crimes, it is imperative that all women assume an active role in their personal safety.

I. BACKGROUND INFORMATION

A. **Statistics** regarding women and abuse are inaccurate because of the under-reporting of these types of crimes. Approximately 50% of rapes in this country go unreported.

B. Every 17 seconds, someone becomes a victim of **violent crime.**

C. Every minute in America, 1.3 rapes of adult women occur.

II. PROTECTIVE DEVICES

A. Self-defense spray

1. **Active ingredients**
   a. Pepper gas and tear gas are most commonly used.
   b. UV marker is also contained, to be used in identification of the attacker.

2. **Mode of action**
   a. Causes pain in attacker's eyes, including animals, which incapacitates the attacker.
   b. No permanent damage results.
   c. Acts immediately.

3. **Operation**
   a. A small canister weighing a few ounces is easy to carry.
   b. It is quick and easy to use; the victim is able to spray her attacker before the attacker is able to gain access to the victim.
   c. **It should be carried visibly,** to display one's weapon of aggression.
   d. Directons for use should be understood and followed carefully.
   e. Testing should be done initially to determine effectiveness: administer a small amount on a paper napkin and then dab on finger and rub gently approximately 1 inch below eye. Effectiveness is confirmed by slight burning around the eye.
   f. The spray and distance of the stream should be tested in an open space to become familiar with these characteristics. Most sprays extend approximately 8 feet.

4. **Legality**
   a. Local police departments can advise about laws in their area.
   b. Illinois: One must be 18 or older to possess the spray.
   c. California: The purchase must be registered.
   d. Wisconsin: It is illegal to enter the state with self-defense spray.
   e. New York: It is legal to bring self-defense spray into the state, but illegal in New York City.
   f. Self-defense spray may not be brought on commercial airlines.

   5. **Availability**
      a. Mail order, sporting good stores, hardware stores
      b. 0.5-oz size is on a key ring and easy to carry. Approximate cost is $15.00.
      c. 2-oz size is in a larger canister and more cumbersome. Approximate cost is $20.00.
B. **Personal alarms**
   1. **Mode of action**
      a. Alerts attention to oneself with a loud siren.
      b. Startles attacker, causing him to flee.
      c. User must be in a populated area in order to be heard by others.
   2. **Operation**
      a. They are small, approximately the size of a matchbook.
      b. Weighs a few ounces; easy to carry.
      c. Works by pressing a button to sound alarm.
      d. It should be tested periodically to ensure batteries are working.
   3. **Availability**
      a. Mail order, sporting goods, hardware stores
C. **Whistle**
   1. **Mode of action**
      a. Alerts attention to oneself.
      b. Unlikely to startle attacker, as victim is witnessed bringing whistle to the mouth.
      c. User must be in a populated area in order to be heard.
   2. **Operation**
      a. Requires bringing the whistle to one's mouth and then generating a forceful expiration to produce sound. This is both time-consuming and involves multiple steps, making the whistle less effective than personal alarms.
   3. **Availability**
      a. Multiple locations and very inexpensive
D. **Dog**
   1. The dog represents an unknown entity to the attacker. The attacker does not know what the animal is capable of or how protective the animal is of its master.

III. **SELF-DEFENSE CLASSES**

A. **A self-defense class should be used for sport, not for personal protection.**
   1. During an attack, there is only approximately 2 seconds in which to act. There is not enough time for a lot of self-defense options.
   2. One should become familiar with a few basic moves and kicks and be able to call on them quickly. This can be accomplished through an **inexpensive clinic** as opposed to an expensive and time-consuming self-defense class.
   3. In general, a woman does not have enough upper-body strength to keep a man away from her. She should concentrate on using her legs to kick the attacker.
   4. If grabbed by an attacker, the victim should grab the attacker's thumb and abduct it **forcefully.** If done forcefully, it is very painful and will incapacitate the attacker and result in releasing the grip on the victim.

IV. **SAFETY TIPS WHILE EXERCISING**

A. **Carry some change in case a phone call must be made.**
B. **Carry identification.**
C. **Headphones**
   1. They reduce awareness of one's environment.
   2. The victim is less likely to hear an attacker approaching and forfeits the 3–4 yard head start needed to escape being abducted.

D. **Time**
1. **Early morning is the safest time to run.** It is thought that attackers are more likely to be sleeping at this time.
2. Sexual assaults are most common at approximately 6:00 p.m.

E. **Clothing**
1. Tight revealing clothing may attract attention to oneself.
2. In order to be safe while exercising, one should **dress to look secure** and confident, not vulnerable.

F. **Location**
1. It is safest to exercise where there are people and activities around.
2. Exercise route and exact time of exercise should be varied so that it will be difficult to track the exerciser predictably.

G. **Clubs**
1. It is safest to exercise with others.
2. Clubs are a good way to find someone who matches both one's ability and exercise schedule.

V. GENERAL SAFETY TIPS

A. **Guidelines**
1. Remember, **tough targets do not get selected.**
2. **Predators** walk with head up, aware of their environment.
3. **Prey** walk with head down, making themselves vulnerable to attack.
4. **Attackers like to ask questions to test their potential victim's response.** Is the response meek and timid or self-assured and strong.
5. **Flee vs fighting:** Fighting is good, but if one has the opportunity to flee, **fleeing is better.**
6. **An attacker has the least control initially, making immediate protective measures crucial.**
7. **If attacked, one should yell,** even if no one is around. This not only draws attention to oneself, but also startles and confuses the attacker. Yelling "fire" tends to be more effective than yelling "help." This is because fire affects the safety of many persons, but yelling "help" is a request for someone to get involved.
8. **Cars** are used by attackers to take victims to secondary crime scenes where the attacker has more control. Fatality in crimes involving an attacker with a car approaches 100%. **At all costs, getting into an attacker's vehicle should be avoided.**
9. **If an attacker has a gun,** it is still safer to fight and flee than it is to comply with the attacker. Statistically, the risk of being shot and hit is 50%; of being seriously wounded by the shot, 25%; and of being killed, 12.5%. The real figures from the Department of Justice are even lower, with a 5% risk of being killed.

B. **Hand bags and brief cases**
1. Shoulder straps secure the bag to the owner more effectively than handles.
2. A more secure bag is less appealing to an attacker.
3. The shoulder strap should be worn across the chest with the bag secured in front of the body with one's hands. Better, the bag should be under a coat so as not to be visible to an attacker.
4. If someone is after a hand bag or brief case, give it up. It is a small price to pay for a life.

C. **Elevators**
1. Always try to stand next to the buttons.
2. If one is alone in an elevator with a stranger and for any reason feels uncomfortable or threatened, one should quickly jump out or press the button for the next floor, then get out.

3. If attacked in an elevator, press as many of the buttons as possible. Each floor at which the elevator stops at is an opportunity for help. At all costs, do not let the attacker press the red emergency stop button.

D. **Stairwells**
   1. Less safe then elevators
   2. Because stairwells are required to be fireproof, they are also soundproof, making them an excellent location for an attacker to strike.

E. **Cars**
   1. Keep all valuables out of sight.
   2. After getting out of a car, do not immediately put keys away; keep them handy in case one has to get back into the car quickly because of a potential threatening situation.
   3. If involved in an accident, there is no obligation to get out of the car. Information can be exchanged through the window. If the car is able to be driven, there is no obligation to remain at the scene after information has been exchanged.
   4. If involved in an accident and the car is not able to be driven, there is still no reason to get out of the car. A sign should be made and placed in the window asking for someone to notify the police.
   5. Car phones are extremely valuable in case of emergency.

F. **Banks**
   1. Transaction slips should be filled out away from windows and other people, as potential attackers may be watching from inside or outside the bank.

G. **Bus and subway**
   1. Sit near the driver, who has access to a radio to call for help quickly if needed. A victim sitting in the back of the bus or subway may go unnoticed by the driver until it is too late.

H. **Taxi**
   1. Always say the number of the cab so the driver can hear in a nonthreatening way. This ensures that the driver is aware that he will be able to be identified at a future date.

VI. **SAFETY TIPS TO TEACH CHILDREN**

A. **Under no circumstances should they talk to strangers.**
   1. Teach them that even people who look like nice people may be potentially harmful.
   2. Teach them that people in uniforms are still strangers and may not really be who they are dressed up to be.

B. **Determine an escape plan**
   1. They should be taught to run to a predetermined location if threatened by a stranger.
   2. They should be aware that it is all right to drop their school books or other materials to make a safe escape.

C. **Cars**
   1. Explain that they should never get into a car with a stranger.
   2. They should be taught to flee to a predetermined location rather than getting into a car.

VII. **APPLYING SAFETY TIPS**

A. **A stranger approaching a woman**
   1. The woman should not look away or down, because this is a sign of weakness or vulnerability.
   2. She should look at strangers and meet their gaze; this gives a message of power and strong self-image.

B. **A stranger begins to run with a woman.**

1. It is all right to talk to and run with the stranger if the woman feels comfortable and other people are around.
2. If the runner feels threatened, then she should assert her desire to be left alone and use her spray or personal alarm.
3. Never leave one's normal exercise route when with a stranger.

C. **A woman suspects she is being followed**
   1. She should not ignore her instincts; they do not lie.
   2. Do not confront the person.
   3. Get to a more populated area as soon as possible.

D. **An attacker grabs a woman.**
   1. She should attempt at all costs to flee.
   2. Use self-defense spray, sound personal alarm, or yell.
   3. Initially is the time of least control for the attacker.
   4. Grab the attacker's thumb and abduct it forcefully.
   5. She should never get on her knees during a struggle. This allows the attacker to get his victim in a choke hold, which gives the attacker optimum control.
   6. If the attacker has hold of clothing only, the woman should get out of the clothing and flee.

E. **A stranger asks for money.**
   1. Keep some money on a money clip, easily accessible and ready just for this situation.
   2. Take out the money clip to show the stranger and say, "This is all I have."
   3. Then throw the money in one direction and run yelling in the other direction. The stranger is most likely to go after the quiet guarantee and get the money as opposed to pursuing the victim.

F. **An attacker assures the victim that she will be let go if she meets his demands.**
   1. She should not believe the attacker; statistically this is a lie.
   2. The reason the victim is likely to believe the attacker is because she wants so badly for the lie to be true.
   3. In this situation, she is much more likely to survive if she attempts to fight and flee.

G. **A woman is attacked and raped.**
   1. Get medical attention as soon as possible.
   2. She should resist the urge to bathe before seeking medical attention. After bathing, DNA analysis is not possible.

VIII. CONCLUSION

In all threatening situations, there are no absolutes. All threats should be evaluated on their own merits and responded to in a manner appropriate to an individual's preference. For more information write to:

> The National Crime Prevention Council
> 1700 K Street NW, Second Floor
> Washington, DC 20006

Ask for packet F-1.

RECOMMENDED READING

1. Miller L: Street smarts. Runner's World June 1993, pp 58–65.

Chapter 16: Sports Medicine and the Law

ELIZABETH M. GALLUP, MD, JD

Liability in the area of sports medicine is one of the most rapidly evolving areas of law. As sports medicine becomes a more well-defined specialty in medicine, the standard of care to which team physicians are held also becomes more defined. This chapter discusses the law as it relates to the sports medicine practitioner.

I. **LEGAL BASIS OF LIABILITY**
   A. The legal basis of liability for team physicians, in general, falls under the **theory of negligence**.
   B. For a physician to be found to be negligent, all four elements of negligence must be demonstrated:
      1. **Duty**
         a. The physician has a duty to care for the athlete in a nonnegligent manner.
         b. The team physician must have acted in the same manner as a minimally competent team physician would in the same or similar circumstances.
      2. **Breach**
         a. To be found negligent, the physician must have breached, or not fulfilled his or her duty to act in a nonnegligent manner.
      3. **Causation**
         a. The physician's breach of duty must be the cause of the patient's damages.
         b. This is often the turning point of a medical negligence case. Did the breach of duty cause the patient's damages, or were the damages caused by some other factor?
      4. **Damages**
         a. The patient must have suffered some sort of measurable damages.
         b. Damages are not necessarily relegated to physical injury, but may be mental and emotional distress, loss of earnings, or loss of career potential.

II. **STANDARD OF CARE**
   A. The standard of care is one of the most difficult-to-define concepts in the area of law and sports medicine:
      1. There are no universally accepted standards in sports medicine.
      2. Athletes with the same injury participating in different sports may be treated differently.
      3. Standards of care are, more often than not, simply "opinions" of different practitioners.
         a. In the courtroom, standards are determined by the testimony of expert witnesses for the plaintiff (athlete) and defendant (physician).
         b. Many states have laws that govern expert witnesses, requiring them to be:
            i. in the same specialty as the defendant physician
            ii. practicing clinical medicine a certain percentage of the time
         c. Some organizations, such as the American Academy of Pediatrics, publish guidelines for sports medicine that can possibly be labeled as "standards" by attorneys.
      4. Background and training of team physicians vary widely.
         a. Some team physicians have completed fellowships in sports medicine. Fellowships are available for family physicians, pediatricians, and orthopedic surgeons.

      b. Some team physicians have extensive CME training in sports medicine, while others have little.

      c. Some team physicians are primary care physicians, others orthopedic surgeons, and others subspecialists in other disciplines.

      d. The American Board of Family Practice and American Board of Pediatrics offer a Certificate of Added Qualification for physicians who pass a competency examination in sports medicine.

B. In general, there are some well-accepted attributes of the standard of care for team physicians. The team physician should:

  1. Understand the sport that is being attended.

      a. Know the types of injuries most common in the sport.

      b. Know how to counsel both athletes and coaches on injury prevention.

         i. Proper conditioning

        ii. Proper stretching

       iii. Prevention of heat and cold injury

      c. Know how to foresee injuries in a particular sport.

  2. Know how to diagnose, acutely treat, and rehabilitate common sports-related injuries.

      a. Know your individual limitations and when to refer.

      b. Know how to apply splints and other equipment commonly used to treat and prevent injuries in athletes.

  3. Ascertain that the athlete for whom you have prescribed equipment designed to prevent injury knows how to apply that equipment.

      a. Do not just hand the athlete a splint; make sure that either you or your designee teaches the athlete proper equipment application.

      b. Explain what the equipment is designed to do and why it is essential to wear and apply it correctly.

  4. Understand the prudence (or possible lack of prudence) of the coaches and athletes.

      a. Coaches, in general, prioritize winning; athletes, in general, prioritize playing. Therefore, it is up to you to keep a clear head about the medical condition of the athlete and how it affects her ability to participate.

  5. Understand that your allegiance is to the athlete, not the team, the coach, or the parents.

      a. This may be a potential conflict.

      b. Place the athlete's interest first.

      c. Treat a first-string athlete the same as you would a bench sitter.

      d. Informed consent is very important.

III. GOOD SAMARITAN STATUTES

A. A statute designed to increase the number of physicians who are team physicians by protecting them from lawsuits.

B. Instead of being held to the negligence standard, a physician is liable only for committing **"wanton and willful"** acts, acts so bad as to shock the public conscience.

C. Although state laws vary, to be protected by the statute, a physician must:

  1. Be acting at the scene of the athletic event.

  2. Be a team physician for an activity which must be at a school-related event, usually high school, junior high, and grade school.

  3. Receive no remuneration for services as team physician.

      a. You can charge for seeing athletes in the office or hospital or for such things as preparticipation examinations.

      b. For showing up and being on the sidelines during a practice or game, you receive no compensation.

IV. INFORMED CONSENT, ASSUMPTION OF RISK, EXCULPATORY WAIVERS

A. **Informed consent** is the process of informing the athlete of the risks and benefits of participating in an athletic event.
   1. At the beginning of the season, have all the parents and participants attend a meeting where the sport is discussed as well as the risks of injury in that sport. In this way, all parents understand.
   2. Inform the athlete and parents of the risks of returning to participation after sustaining an injury.
   3. If the athlete is a minor, you must also inform the parents.
   4. Document that you informed and the information you transmitted.

B. **Assumption of risk** is where the individual, fully informed of the risks, assumes the risks and elects to participate in an activity which may cause injury.

C. **Exculpatory waiver** is based on assumption of risk and is a release executed by a patient or her guardian which relieves a physician from liability for negligence.
   1. Use of these waivers in sports medicine is controversial.
   2. Some courts have found them to be against public policy and therefore invalid.
   3. Minors cannot execute exculpatory waivers because these are a form of a contract.
   4. A conservative recommendation would be not to use the waivers.

V. DOCUMENTATION IN SPORTS MEDICINE

A. One simple rule, **document everything.** Your records are your biggest ally in a lawsuit.
B. General recommendations for **good record-keeping**:
   1. Document what you conveyed to parents in the preseason.
   2. Document the athlete's name, nature of injury, acute treatment, rehabilitation and recommendations for continuing treatment, ongoing care, and follow-up.
   3. Date all entries.
   4. If you treat an athlete from an opposing team, document the same as you would for your own athletes.

REFERENCES

1. Brandt EA: Good samaritan laws–legal dismay: An update. Mercer Law Rev 38:1447, 1987.
2. Brandt EA: Good samaritan laws—The legal placebo: A current analysis. Akron Law Rev 17-1 (summer):303, 1983.
3. Davis JE: Fixing the standard of care: Motivated athletes and medical malpractice. Am J Trial Advocacy 12-2(fall):218, 1988.
4. Hawkins JD: Sports medicine recordkeeping: The key to effective documentation. Sports Med Standards Malpractice Reporter 1-2(4):31, 1989.
5. Herbert DL: Record retention: How long is enough? Sports Med Standards Malpractice Reporter 2-3(6):51, 1990.
6. Herbert DL: Express assumption of risk and decisions to exclude from play. Sports Med Standards Malpractice Reporter 2-1(1):1, 1990.
7. Herbert DL: Express assumption of risk and decisions to exclude from play: The sports medicine dilemma. Sports Med Standards Malpractice Reporter 2-1(1):5, 1990.
8. Herbert DL: The use of exculpatory language in a medical setting including rehabilitative and some exercise programs. Exerc Standards Malpractice Reporter 5:75, 1987.
9. Herbert DL: The use of prospective releases containing exculpatory language in exercise and fitness programs. Exerc Standards Malpractice Reporter 1-6(10):90, 1987.
10. Herbert DL: Who will judge sports medicine in court. Sports Med Standards Malpractice Reporter 1-1(1):6, 1989.
11. Immunity of medical practitioner or registered nurse volunteering services to school athletic program. Ohio Revised Code, Sect 2305.23.1 and Sect 2305.231.
12. King JH: The duty and standard of care for team physicians. Houston Law Rev 18-4(5):693, 1981.
13. Mellion M, Walsh W, Shelton G: The Team Physician's Handbook. Philadelphia, Hanley & Belfus, 1990, pp 480–481.
14. Prosser W: Law of Torts. St. Paul, MN, West Publishing, 1982, p 150.
15. Russell CV: Legal and ethical conflicts arising from the team physician's dual obligations to the athlete and management. Seton Hall Leg J 10-2:301, 1987.
16. Taraska JM: Legal Guide for Physicians. New York, Matthew Bender, 1990, p 501:5-2.

Chapter 17: Sexual Harassment in Women's Sports

ELIZABETH M. GALLUP, MD, JD

Sexual harassment permeates society at all levels. Unfortunately, it is very prevalent in women's sports. Anita Hill's testimony at Clarence Thomas's Supreme Court confirmation hearings brought the issue to a more conscious level for the American public. Since the hearings, more cases have been filed at a faster rate than ever before. This chapter defines sexual harassment and examines it in the environment of women's sports.

I. **DEFINITION**

   A. Courts recognize two types of sexual harassment:
   1. *"Quid pro quo"* **sexual harassment**
      a. **Strict liability,** where the sue-er (plaintiff, usually a woman) just has to show that the sue-ee (defendant, usually a man) acted. If the action occurred, the defendant is liable.
      b. An example is where a supervisor (coach, teacher) extorts sexual favors from a subordinate in exchange for job (team) and athletic benefits and then retaliates if she demurs.
   2. **"Hostile environment" sexual harassment**
      a. Employer's (coaches, teachers) knowledge that the situation is occurring is generally required.
      b. An example is a situation where harassing conduct, either by a supervisor or coworkers (coaches, teachers), has the effect of "unreasonably interfering with an individual's work performance or creating an intimidating, hostile, or offensive work environment."
      c. Conduct must be such that a "reasonable *woman*" would find it to be interfering, intimidating, hostile, or offensive.

   B. **Establishing a** *prima facie* **case of sexual harassment:** *Prima facie* case means "the elements necessary to establish that something has occurred."
   1. Under Title VII (*see* below), five elements must be met:
      a. Plaintiff belongs to a protected class (e.g., female).
      b. She was subject to unwelcome harassment.
      c. The harassment was based on sex.
      d. The harassment affected a term, condition, or privilege of employment (team participation).
      e. The employer (coach, teacher, school official) knew or should have known of the harassment and failed to take prompt remedial action.

   C. **Burden of proof**
   1. The plaintiff always bears the burden of proof (the plaintiff has to show the elements outlined).
   2. Once a *prima facie* case is established, the defendant then carries the "burden of production" to present a legitimate, nondiscriminatory reason for his or her conduct, that this conduct was not intended to be discriminatory, and rather that it had a legitimate intent.
   3. Plaintiff then must persuade the court that the proffered reason was merely pretextual.

II. APPLICABLE FEDERAL LAW

A. Statutory

1. **Title VII of the Civil Rights Act of 1964**
   a. Title VII prohibits organizations of five or more workers from discriminating in hiring, promotion, and firing procedures.
   b. School systems obviously are employers and thus covered under Title VII.
2. Title VII established the **Equal Employment Opportunities Commission** (EEOC).
   a. EEOC was given the power to investigate complaints of discrimination and attempt conciliation.
   b. Under **EEOC guidelines:**
      i. Sexual harassment is defined as unwelcome sexual advancements, requests for sexual favors, and other verbal or physical conduct of a sexual nature.
      ii. Submission to such conduct is either made, explicitly or implicitly, a term or condition of an individual's employment (team participation).
      iii. Submission to or rejection of such conduct by such individual is used as a basis for an employment (team) decision's affecting such individuals
      iv. Such conduct has a purpose or effect of interfering with an individual's work performance or creating an intimidating, hostile, or offensive working environment.

III. COMMON LAW CLAIMS

Some claims may be filed by a plaintiff against a defendant in civil court for damages (i.e., money). These claims may be varied by state laws. They are as follows:

A. **Intentional infliction of emotional stress**

1. Conduct by the defendant is extreme or outrageous.
2. Taken in an intentional or reckless manner.
3. Results in severe emotional distress which is "medically diagnosable" and "medically significant."

B. **Negligent infliction of emotional distress**

1. Defendant should have known or realized his or her conduct involved unreasonable risk of causing the plaintiff emotional distress.
2. Emotional distress is "medically diagnosable" and "medically significant."
3. In some states, the emotional distress must also manifest itself in physical illness or bodily harm.

C. **Invasion of privacy or intrusion upon seclusion**

1. The existence of a secret and private subject matter.
2. Plaintiff's right to keep that subject matter private.
3. The defendant's obtainment of information about that subject matter through methods objectionable to the reasonable woman.

D. **Interference with contractual or business relationship**

1. The existence of a valid business relationship or expectancy.
2. Knowledge of that relationship or expectancy by the defendant.
3. Intentional interference with relationship or expectancy—e.g., inducing or causing a breach or termination of the relationship or expectancy—by the defendants.
4. Absence of justification for defendant's conduct.
5. Resultant damage to party whose relationship or expectancy is disrupted.

E. **Assault and battery**

1. **Assault:** An intentional unlawful offer to touch a person in a rude or angry manner under such circumstances as to create in the mind of the party alleging the assault a well-founded fear of an imminent battery, coupled with the apparent present ability to effectuate the attempt (e.g., to intentionally make someone feel afraid that they are going to be harmed or touched inappropriately).
2. **Battery:** The willful, unwelcome touching of a person.

F. **Breach of contract or wrongful discharge**
  1. **Contract employee:** Possibly applicable when sexual harassment culminates in the dismissal or "forced quitting" of the victimized employee.
  2. **At-will employee:** May have a claim if dismissal was made in bad faith or in violation of "public policy."
  3. May also be classified as "breach of implied covenant of good faith and fair dealing."

IV. **SUPREME COURT**

In a recent supreme court case regarding sexual harassment, *Franklin vs Gwinnett County Public Schools,* the Court found sexual harassment had occurred and stated that Title IX authorizes an award of damages.

REFERENCE

1. Duvall DP, Shaney MJF: Sexual Harassment Issues for the Professional Woman. University of Missouri Kansas City Continuing Legal Education Lecture Series, February 1992.

Chapter 18: Women's Sports Equipment: Is It a Marketing Ploy?

ROBYN STUHR, MA

For many years, women have used sports equipment and clothing designed by men, for men. Only recently have some industries become more responsive to the women's market and made functional design adaptations to meet the needs of a female clientele. Equipment targeted to women is frequently a standard "man's model" hidden by pastel colors or feminine graphics.

I. **BICYCLES**

    A. **Factors to be considered.** Compared to men, the average female is:
        1. Shorter
        2. Longer legs, shorter arms and torso
        3. Center of gravity lower by 1 inch
        4. Higher percentage of body fat and less lean muscle mass
        5. Smaller hands and feet
        6. Narrower shoulders
        7. Pelvic shape differences

    B. **Design features for a woman's bike:**
        1. Shorter reach (stem length plus top tube length)
        2. Smaller frame size
        3. Narrower handlebars
        4. Smaller brake levers, toe clips
        5. Shorter crank arms

    C. **Proper fit is key to comfortable and efficient cycling.**
        1. Bike manufacturers are not yet making women's bikes easily available.
        2. Bike should be custom fitted to adapt to a woman's body dimensions.
        3. Professional bike shop can use "fit kit" or customize bike.
        4. Mixte, step-through frames and smaller front wheel are less-than-ideal designs for women's bikes.

    D. **Guidelines for proper fit**
        1. **Standover height**
            a. 1 inch for road bike
            b. 2–3 inches for mountain bike
        2. **Fore-aft position and height** (Fig. 1)
            a. Sit with feet in pedals at 3 and 9 o'clock positions.
            b. Plumbline should drop through bottom of patella, ball of foot, and axle of pedal.
            c. Adjust seat position accordingly.
        3. **Seat height:** 20° knee flexion on downstroke (with slight foot dorsiflexion)
        4. **Reach to handlebars** should be comfortable; not locked elbows.

    E. **Saddle tilt** should be level; only slight up or downward tilt if necessary for comfort.

    F. **Saddle design**
        1. Women's saddles are typically wider everywhere, which may not be the best design. More research is needed.
        2. Cover saddle and ride for a week before purchase.

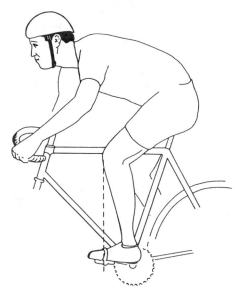

FIGURE 1. Fore and aft saddle position. With the rider in the saddle and the pedals at the 3 and 9 o'clock positions, the seat should be adjusted so that a plumb line dropped from the tibial tubercle would intercept the axle of the forward pedal. (From Mellion MB, Hill JW: Bicycling. In Mellion MB, Walsh WM, Shelton GL (eds): The Team Physician's Handbook. Philadelphia, Hanley & Belfus, 1990; with permission.)

II. SKIS

A. **Factors affecting choice of ski**
   1. Body weight
   2. Ability level
   3. Style of skiing (aggressive vs cautious)
   4. Type of snow conditions
   5. Slalom vs grand slalom

B. **Characteristics common to women that may affect ski choice**
   1. Typically lighter than males
   2. Center of gravity 1 inch lower
   3. Wider pelvis
   4. Shorter height
   5. Less strength

C. **Flex pattern**
   1. **Definition:** Ratio of stiffness between ski's shovel and tail. Flex pattern is a key design feature that affects the performance of the ski.
   2. Soft flex pattern makes ski easier to turn.
   3. "Women's pastel" skis are usually very soft; this would be appropriate for beginner or intermediate skier, less than 130 lbs, in powder.
   4. Performance skis with soft shovel and stiff tail are easy to start a turn and do not skid on the way out.
   5. Women with less leg strength cannot handle too stiff a tail or get through the turn.
   6. Look for balance in flex pattern.
   7. Flex pattern for women's skis is for any person 130 lbs or lighter.

III. WIND SURFING

A. Equipment changes have only recently provided options for the lighter, smaller person (female). There is not a big enough market for a specific women's line, a professional salesperson should be able to suggest appropriate models.
   1. **Mast:** Becoming lighter so it is easier to lift out of water.
   2. **Harnesses:** Lower in bottom and different off-center hook attachment to boom to accommodate women's leverage.
   3. **Diameter of boom:** Smaller for small hands.

IV. ATHLETIC CLOTHING

A. **Factors to be considered:** Female is typically:
1. Smaller and shorter
2. Smaller thorax and larger abdominal cavity
3. Narrower shoulders
4. Shorter limbs relative to body length
5. Protection of sex-specific organs
   a. Breast support
   b. Prevention of vaginitis
6. Thermoregulation differences: women have more vasoconstriction of extremities in cold.
7. Smaller body has lower thermal mass.
8. Larger ratio of surface area/mass allows for more rapid heat loss/gain in cold/heat.

B. **Athletic clothes with functional considerations**
1. Bras
2. Athletic tights and biking shorts
3. Aerobic dance wear
4. Shoes
5. Swimwear

C. **Bras**
1. Two types:
   a. **Encapsulation:** Smaller mass is easier to control.
   b. **Compression:** Press breasts flat against the body.
2. Many bras advertised as "sports" bras offer little support for the larger woman.
3. **Important features:**
   a. Control of breast motion
   b. Reduce chafing
   c. Allow for evaporation of sweat
4. **Feature designs:**
   a. Judicious placement of seams
   b. Wide nonelastic shoulder straps
   c. Breathable fabrics (mesh, cotton/poly blend)
   d. Seamless cups
   e. Ample armholes
   f. Covered hooks or fasteners (if present)
   g. Little vertical stretch compared with horizontal stretch (for dressing/comfort)
5. **Larger-breasted women** do not have the choice of bra designs. Usually the encapsulation model is the only style feasible.
6. **For painful breasts prior to menstruation,** an option is to wear two bras, preferably one from each design theory.

D. **Athletic clothing:** A few manufacturers pay special attention to design features that enhance comfort, performance, fit, and hygiene concerns of women.
1. **Athletic tights:** Unisex can work because of lycra stretch. Women's models have longer crotch-to-waist dimensions and cotton crotch.
2. **Biking shorts:** Attention should be paid to seam placement in the crotch to avoid chafing. Women's models have cotton panels.
3. **Running shorts:** Can be designed with more buttocks coverage and cut allowing for hip width and waist-to-crotch length.
4. **Tank tops** with snaps to keep bra straps hidden and secure.

V. SUMMARY

As women's sports participation increases, manufacturers and retailers will respond to that market segment. More women-owned and operated businesses are making design changes for the woman athlete. The problem is that the athlete often has trouble finding these products in sufficient quantity or selection, and often, the athlete is not even aware that she can be more comfortable or efficient in her sport with well-fitting, gender-sensitive equipment and clothing. So, she makes do with a man's model or derivation. Women are establishing records and expanding the horizons of achievement and artistry in sports. Hopefully, the sports equipment and clothing industry will follow suit.

REFERENCES

1. Cycling for women. Bicycling Magazine (Published by Rodale Press, Emmaus, PA), 1989.
2. Women's Sports and Fitness Magazine, Boulder, CO:
    - McCloy M, Masia S: Ladies' choice. 12:38–45, Oct. 1990.
    - Tilin A: If the bike fits, ride it. 13:27–38, Apr. 1991.
    - McCloy M: Alpine skis. 14:56–58, Oct. 1992.
    - Banks L: The lowdown on mountain bikes and accessories. 15:68–73, 1993.

Chapter 19: Women's Athletic Shoes

KATRINA SULLIVAN, DPM, ATC, MS

Never have active women had so many excellent athletic shoes to choose from. However, this can present a perplexing problem: Which shoe to choose? Does one pick a sports-specific shoe, a shoe designed exclusively for women, or an all-around shoe?

I. **HISTORY**
  A. 1600s—In England, a felt shoe intended for tennis was created.
  B. 1700s—Leather shoes with a spike were developed for running events.
  C. 1868—Charles Goodyear invented vulcanized rubber, and the early sneaker as we know it was born. It was, however, cost prohibitive for the general public at $6 a pair.
  D. Late 1800s—Keds® came into mass production and were worn by the masses for gym class and most athletic activities.
  E. 1917—Marquis M. Converse introduced the Converse All-Star® basketball shoe, giving birth to the sport-specific shoe.
  F. 1960s—Shoe manufacturers began paying professional athletes to wear their products.
  G. 1970s—The running boom sparked the rapid development and application of advanced technology in the running shoe. Shoes for other applications also benefited.
  H. 1980s—The sport-specific shoe, or specialty shoe, came into its own. Motion-control devices became prevalent, and enhanced cushioning was developed with encapsulation of special materials (air and gel) to improve the shoe's performance and fit.
  I. 1990s—The sneaker, or multipurpose athletic shoe, has returned, incorporating the benefits of advanced technology yet the versatility of the much-beloved Keds®.

II. **SHOE-FIT GUIDELINES**
  A. **Women's vs men's shoes**
    1. Research has shown that a woman's foot has a different shape, not just size, from a man's foot. Differences also exist in average size and shape between groups of elite women athletes—e.g., long-distance runners vs basketball players.
    2. Today's women's shoes are not just scaled-down versions of the men's models. Many specific biomechanical differences are taken into account.
    3. Women who wear larger sizes or have particularly wide feet may still find that a men's shoe offers a better fit. The opposite is true for men with small, narrow feet.
  B. **Straight vs curved last:** The last is the model upon which the shoe manufacturer builds the shoe. Lasts come in three basic shapes: straight, curved, and semicurved. This refers to the overall shape of the shoe. A **straight lasted shoe** is filled in under the medial arch, whereas a **curve lasted shoe** is flared medially at the ball of the foot.
    1. A pronated, flat foot requiring extra medial support tends to do better in a straight lasted shoe.
    2. The high-arched foot or in-toed foot often fits better into a curve lasted shoe.
    3. The rectus, or straight foot, can fit into most shoes despite the shape of the last.
  C. **Break-in period**
    1. Today's athletic shoes do not require a break-in period. They should feel comfortable right out of the box.

III. **SHOE FEATURES**
  A. **Heel counters** need to be firm enough to provide stability. These can be extended toward the midfoot for added support.

138

B. **Midsoles** can offer motion control and protective cushioning.
  1. Encapsulated air or gel, cantilever construction, and carbon-kelvar plates all increase the shoes' ability to provide protection from shock.
  2. Forefoot protection is very important.
C. **Lateral forefoot support**
  1. A frequently undersupported area for people who run or perform activities on the ball of their foot.

IV. **SPORT-SPECIFIC GUIDELINES**
Specialty shoes are often designed for a reason, due in part to the particular demands of a sport. Substitution of an inappropriate shoe can increase the risk of injury, either traumatic or overuse.
A. **Running**
  1. A running-specific shoe is recommended for:
     a. Distance >3 miles/run
     b. Frequency >3 times/week
     c. Known running-related injuries
     d. Structural abnormalities of the foot or leg
  2. Shoe should have good shock absorption, rigid heel control, good flexibility at midfoot break, provide good traction, and protect the foot.
  3. Snug fit, but provide for expansion during running.
B. **Aerobics**
  1. An aerobic-specific shoe is recommended for:
     a. Exercise duration = 60+ min/session
     b. Frequency >3 times/week
     c. Known aerobic or running injuries
  2. Demands firm heel counters, forefoot support, midsole cushioning, full leather upper.
C. **Indoor court sports**
  1. A court-style shoe is recommended for:
     a. Frequency >3 times/week
     b. Known sport-related injuries
  2. Not recommended for this activity are
     a. Running shoes (insufficient lateral stability)
     b. Carbon outsole shoes (marks the court floor)
     c. Overly soft leather shoes (insufficient support)
  3. Recommended features
     a. Cup-sole shoes that provide a stable base for foot that moves forward and side-to-side
     b. For hardwood floors, a rubber or rubber blend sole provides best traction.
     c. Synthetic surfaces tend to grab, and a polyurethane/rubber blend sole is appropriate.
  4. High-tops provide added ankle support for basketball or volleyball. Leather or canvas (nylon stretches).
D. **Outdoor court sports**
  1. A court shoe performs best for:
     a. Frequency >3 times/week
     b. Known sport-related injuries
  2. Not recommended for this activity are:
     a. Running shoes or overly soft shoes
     b. Gum rubber shoes (lack durability)
  3. Recommended are:
     a. Rubber blend base is preferred for playing tennis on grass.
     b. Polyurethane outsole and midsole for abrasive surfaces

  E. **Field sports**
1. A sport-specific cleat or tread is recommended.
2. Match the cleat to playing surface, conditions, and sport. There is a high likelihood of injury with incorrect shoe gear.
   a. Soccer: Soft shoe allows the foot to "feel" the ball but with toughness for kicking.
3. Artificial playing surfaces need a stiffer-soled shoe.

  F. **Bicycling**
1. A stiff midsoled cycling shoe distributes the force of pedalling over the entire foot and will reduce injury when:
   a. Distance >20 miles/day
   b. Frequency >3 days/week
   c. Added weight on the bike (i.e., commuting or touring)
   d. Intensity >20 mph
2. Even a touring shoe will dramatically improve efficiency—e.g., a cycling shoe provides 30% increase in efficiency over soft-soled running shoes.
3. Racing shoes connect to pedals via cleats or toe clips.
   a. Cleat adjustment is critical to ensure smooth pedalling and to prevent overuse injury. Adjustments can be made with a Fit Kit.

  G. **Hiking:** A lightweight boot is sufficient for:
1. Day hike or overnight hike up to intermediate distance
2. Carrying loads <30 lbs
3. Greater demands require additional ankle and midfoot support
4. Patellofemoral pain patients

  H. **Cross-training:** A multipurpose shoe can be adequate for:
1. Running short distances infrequently
2. Occasional aerobic classes or court play
3. General fitness training, especially when traveling
4. Casual wear. Here, it surpasses specialty shoes.

  I. **Golf.** A golf shoe is recommended for:
1. Frequent participants. It improves traction for swings and walking the course.

V. OBTAIN HELP

Many of the specialty athletic shoe stores employ knowledgable staff with good technical support from the shoe companies. Develop a working relationship with a good store in your location; they are happy to share information and assist in special shoe requirements. The store staff will also know the shoes currently available, as new or updated models are introduced every 6–12 months.

REFERENCES

1. Bednarski KN: Marketing athletic footwear to women. NGSA Sports Retailer (Oct), 1987.
2. Bednarski KN: Foot morphology of women athletes: Implications for foot development [masters thesis]. Current address: Nike, Inc., One Bowerman Drive, Beaverton, OR 97005.
3. Cavanagh PR: History of the running shoe. In Cavanagh PR (ed): The Running Shoe Book. Mountain View, CA, Anderson World, 1980.
4. Swann JN: Sports Shoes. Northampton, Central Museum, 1988. Reprinted by Lizabeth Holloway, Center for History of Foot Care and Foot Wear, Philadelphia, PA, 1990

PART III
MEDICAL AND ORTHOPEDIC CONDITIONS

Chapter 20: Disordered Eating

MIMI D. JOHNSON, MD

Under pressure to excel at their sport, some women athletes attempt to lose weight or body fat by restricting food intake, bingeing, or purging. In recent years, studies have shown these practices of disordered eating to be more prevalent among athletes than previously thought. This article reviews the psychologic, nutritional, and medical considerations in the athlete involved in disordered eating, discusses recognition and screening of the athlete, and offers guidelines for a treatment approach.

I. **GENERAL PRINCIPLES**
   A. The spectrum of eating disorders ranges from mild to severe.
   B. The severe form of this behavior results in the clinically recognized diagnoses of **anorexia nervosa** (Table 1) or **bulimia nervosa** (Table 2).
   C. Most athletes display disordered eating behavior to a lesser degree, but some do meet these diagnostic criteria.
   D. Disordered eating of any degree can have adverse health effects, with morbidity and risk of mortality increasing as the severity of disordered eating behavior increases.
   E. Athletes with disordered eating of any degree are at risk for progressing to an eating disorder, and their behavior should be addressed.

II. **PREVALENCE OF DISORDERED EATING**
   A. **General population**
      1. 0.5–1% of adolescent and young adult women have anorexia nervosa.
      2. 2–4% of adolescent and young adult women have bulimia nervosa.
      3. Rates of anorexia and bulimia in men are 10% of those in women (0.05% and 0.1%, respectively).
   B. **Female athletes**
      1. 32% (58 of 182) of women collegiate athletes practiced one form of disordered eating (vomiting, laxative use, excessive weight loss, or diuretic or diet pill use) daily for at least 1 month. At least 1 athlete was identified from each sport surveyed.
      2. 62% (26 of 42) of female college gymnasts used at least one method of disordered eating twice weekly over 3 or more months.
         a. Methods used included
            i. 26% vomiting
            ii. 24% diet pill use
            iii. 24% fasting
            iv. 12% diuretic use
            v. 7% laxative use
         b. 28 of these 42 gymnasts had been told by their coach that they were too heavy, and 21 (75%) of them exhibited disordered eating behaviors, suggesting that coaches may unknowingly influence these behaviors in athletes.

TABLE 1. Diagnostic Criteria for Anorexia Nervosa

A. Refusal to maintain body weight at or above a minimally normal weight for age and height (e.g., weight loss leading to maintenance of body weight <85% of that expected; or failure to make expected weight gain during period of growth, leading to body weight <85% of that expected).

B. Intense fear of gaining weight or becoming fat, even though underweight.

C. Disturbance in the way in which one's body weight or shape is experienced; undue influence of body weight or shape on self-evaluation; or denial of the seriousness of the current low body weight.

D. In postmenarchal females, amenorrhea, i.e., the absence of at least 3 consecutive menstrual cycles. (A woman is considered to have amenorrhea if her periods occur only following hormone [e.g., estrogen] administration.)

Specify type:
Restricting type: During the episode of anorexia nervosa, the person does not regularly engage in binge eating or purging behavior (i.e., self-induced vomiting or the misuse of laxatives or diuretics).
Binge eating/purging type: During the episode of anorexia nervosa, the person regularly engages in binge eating or purging behavior (i.e., self-induced vomiting or the misuse of laxatives or diuretics).

From Task Force on DSM-IV: DSM-IV Draft Criteria. Washington, DC, American Psychiatric Association, 1993, pp 1–2.

TABLE 2. Diagnostic Criteria for Bulimia Nervosa

A. Recurrent episodes of binge eating. An episode of binge eating is characterized by both of the following:
 1. Eating, in a discrete period of time (e.g., within any 2-hour period), an amount of food that is definitely larger than most people would eat during a similar period of time and under similar circumstances, *and,*
 2. A sense of lack of control over eating during the episode (e.g., a feeling that one cannot stop eating or control what or how much one is eating.

B. Recurrent inappropriate compensatory behavior in order to prevent weight gain, such as: self-induced vomiting; misuse of laxatives, diuretics or other medications; fasting; or excessive exercise.

C. The binge eating and inappropriate compensatory behaviors both occur, on average, at least twice a week for 3 months.

D. Self-evaluation is unduly influenced by body shape and weight.

E. The disturbance does not occur exclusively during episodes of anorexia nervosa.

Specify type:
Purging type: The person regularly engages in self-induced vomiting or the misuse of laxatives or diuretics.
Nonpurging type: The person uses other inappropriate compensatory behaviors, such as fasting or excessive exercise, but does not regularly engage in self-induced vomiting or the misuse of laxatives or diuretics.

From Task Force on DSM-IV: DSM-IV Draft Criteria. Washington, DC, American Psychiatric Association, 1993, pp 1–2.

  3. 15.4% (75 of 487) of female elite swimmers, aged 9–18 years, engaged in disordered eating patterns:
   a. 12.7% vomiting
   b. 1.5% diuretic use
   c. 2.5% laxative use
   d. 62–77% were skipping meals or eating smaller meals.

III. RISK FACTORS IN ATHLETICS

 A. **Stress, personality, and competitive drive**
  1. Pressure and desire to **optimize performance** may lead an athlete to attempt weight loss, often inappropriately.
  2. Pressure to meet **weight or body fat goals,** particularly in a short period of time and without appropriate guidance, can force an athlete to develop disordered eating behavior.

3. Athletes often have **heightened body awareness,** which may make them more prone to body image concerns.

4. **Personality traits,** such as perfectionism, compulsiveness, and expectations of high achievement, are felt to be advantageous for the high-level athlete, but are also commonly associated with development of an eating disorder.

5. The athlete has learned to **block distractions,** even pain, to train, and she may use this ability to block hunger and other feelings associated with disordered eating.

6. The athlete's drive for sport excellence may possibly be channeled into her disordered eating.

7. In high levels of competition, the stakes are higher (e.g., maintaining a college scholarship, winning a gold medal), and the possibility is greater that the athlete may be willing to take unnecessary risks.

B. **Sports at highest risk:** Disordered eating may be seen in all sports, although some sports place the athlete at higher risk.

1. Sports emphasizing lean appearance or in which judging evaluates physical appearance: gymnastics, diving, figure skating, dance, synchronized swimming.

2. Sports emphasizing body leanness for optimal performance: long-distance running, swimming, cross-country skiing.

3. Sports utilizing weight classifications: rowing, weight-lifting, martial arts (judo, taekwondo).

IV. FACTORS CONTRIBUTING TO DEVELOPMENT OF DISORDERED EATING

A. **Sociocultural factors**

1. The desire to be thin is perpetuated by sociocultural norms in Western culture.

2. Behaviors to achieve thinness that contribute to the development of disordered eating (e.g., dieting) have become normative for girls and women.

3. Thinness is equated with control, success, goodness, power, and beauty.

B. **Biologic factors**

1. Gender: There is a 10 to 1 ratio of eating disorders in females as compared to males.

2. Imbalances in the neurotransmitters serotonin and norepinephrine, and more recently melatonin, have been postulated as a possible etiologic factor.

3. Active bulimics have decreased secretion of cholecystokinin, which can decrease the sense of satiety. Starvation itself can result in loss of cues for satiety.

C. **Psychological factors**

1. **Family**

a. Families of women who develop eating disorders may not provide them with appropriate coping skills to deal with stress. These families may have difficulty in resolving conflict, expressing or tolerating negative emotions, and regulating distance and intimacy among family members, particularly in times of stress.

b. Women in these families often derive much of their sense of self-worth from others' responses to them, particularly their appearance or performance.

2. **Victimization**

a. 20–35% of persons with eating disorders report sexual abuse.

b. 67% of bulimics report sexual and/or physical abuse.

c. These etiologies may not be common among athletes but should be considered.

3. **Poor coping skills**

a. Disordered eating is often an unhealthy attempt to deal with stress. Many of these athletes lack assertiveness skills. The athlete may feel overwhelmed and out of control because of academic demands, injury, perceived poor sports performance, social relationships, financial concerns, or family issues.

b. Instead of managing her problems in a healthy way, she instead may try to manage her weight as a way of feeling a sense of control.

    4. **Low self-esteem**
        a. Common among athletes with disordered eating
        b. The athlete who derives her sense of self from external feedback (e.g., from a coach or sports performance) is at risk of a fluctuating sense of self-esteem.
        c. Her sense of self-esteem may be a reflection of how she feels about her sports performance or other areas of her life.
    5. **Lack of identity**
        a. An athlete may lack a sense of identity outside of being an athlete. She has developed her sense of "who she is" around sports, failing to develop other areas of her life.
        b. This can become a difficult issue when nearing the end of her athletic career.

V. RESTRICTIVE EATING BEHAVIOR IN ATHLETES

Restrictive eating behavior may range from inadvertently failing to meet basal caloric needs or poor nutrition, to voluntary starvation coupled with extreme exercise regimens. Most athletes who restrict eating do not meet the criteria for anorexia nervosa.

  A. **Development of disordered eating patterns**
    1. The athlete often begins by restricting food intake, such as eliminating red meat or sweets from her diet.
    2. Her list of acceptable foods typically narrows over time.
    3. She often overexercises, performing aerobic exercise outside of her routine workouts.
    4. She becomes more obsessive and compulsive about her other daily activities.
    5. She may begin to criticize teammates about eating patterns and often becomes increasingly socially isolated.
  B. **Physical signs and symptoms of restrictive eating behavior**
    1. Associated with weight loss and fluid/electrolyte imbalance
    2. **Common physical symptoms**
        a. Cold intolerance
        b. Amenorrhea, delayed menarche
        c. Lightheadedness
        d. Constipation
        e. Abdominal bloating
        f. Fatigue
        g. Decreased ability to concentrate
    3. **Common physical signs**
        a. Dry skin, brittle hair and nails
        b. Decreased subcutaneous fat and muscle
        c. Hypothermia
        d. Bradycardia
        e. Lanugo (fine, baby hair)
        f. Orthostatic blood pressure changes (due to dehydration)
        g. Cold and discolored hands and feet
    4. **Common laboratory findings**
        a. Normal follicle-stimulating hormone (FSH) and low normal luteinizing hormone (LH)
        b. Thyroxine (T4) and thyroid-stimulating hormone (TSH) are normal but triiodothyronine (T3) is low to low-normal, most likely due to decreased peripheral conversion of T3 to T4 resulting from malnutrition (medical treatment is not warranted).
        c. Blood urea nitrogen (BUN) is sometimes elevated.
        d. Serum carotene is sometimes elevated.
        e. Cholesterol and serum transaminases may be elevated, due to starvation.
        f. Pyuria, hematuria, proteinuria, elevated urine pH sometimes present.
        g. Leukopenia, anemia, thrombocytopenia may be seen.
        h. Hyponatremia (seen in women who are fluid overloading)

5. **Electrocardiographic changes**
   a. Bradycardia ($\leq$60 beats/min)
   b. Low voltage
   c. Low or inverted T-waves
   d. Prolonged QT interval (rarely)
   e. Reduction of maximal aerobic capacity with low maximal heart rate during exercise (in anorexics)
   f. Echocardiographic changes also reported
6. **Bone density changes**
   a. Bone loss seen in oligomenorrheic and amenorrheic athletes (*see* Chapters 21 and 22)

VI. BINGE-PURGE BEHAVIOR IN ATHLETES

Binge-purge behavior in the athlete may vary in frequency (continuous, cyclic, or episodic). Some athletes may binge and purge only occasionally, and others, multiple times a day.

A. **Development of binge-purge patterns**
   1. The binge-purge cycle begins with a "diet" or food restriction. The resulting hunger causes a binge, which is followed by guilt and purging.
   2. The binge often takes place in the evening following a day of restriction. Typically, a large amount of food is eaten quickly, followed by purging behavior.
   3. Some athletes may purge after small meals, which they may perceive as a binge.
B. **Methods of purging**
   1. **Vomiting**
      a. Usually does not remove all calories eaten
      b. Results in fluid and electrolyte loss
      c. Does not relieve hunger, making future binge likely
   2. **Laxative use**
      a. Acts on large intestines
      b. Result in fluid and electrolyte loss
      c. Does not affect calories absorbed
   3. **Diuretic use**
      a. Acts on the kidneys
      b. Causes fluid and electrolyte loss
      c. Has no effect on calorie absorption
   4. **Excessive exercise** may be used instead of purging.
C. **Signs and symptoms of binge-purge behavior** (Table 2)
   1. Associated with fluid and electrolyte imbalance and the purging method itself
   2. **Common symptoms**
      a. Fatigue
      b. Constipation/diarrhea
      c. Irregular menses
      d. Sore throat and chest pain
      e. Bloating, abdominal pain
      f. Face and extremity edema (due to rebound fluid retention or secondary hyperaldosteronism)
      g. Depression
   3. **Common signs**
      a. Parotid gland enlargement
      b. Erosion of dental enamel
      c. Calluses on dorsum of hand (Russell's sign, results from inducing gag response)
      d. Orthostatic blood pressure changes (due to dehydration)
      e. Rarely, esophagitis and Mallory-Weiss tears

4. **Common laboratory findings**
   a. Hypokalemia, hypochloremic alkalosis (vomiting), acidosis (laxatives)
   b. Elevated urine pH, pyuria, proteinuria
   c. Elevated blood urea nitrogen
   d. Hypocalcemia sometimes seen
5. **Electrocardiographic changes reported**

VII. EFFECTS OF DISORDERED EATING ON ATHLETIC PERFORMANCE

A. **Impaired performance and increased risk of injury**
   1. Decreased caloric intake and fluid/electrolyte imbalances can result in decreased endurance, strength, speed, and ability to concentrate, and increased reaction time.
   2. The body initially adapts to the metabolic changes, so a decrease in performance may not be evident for some time.

VIII. EVALUATION AND TREATMENT

A. **Multidisciplinary team**
   1. **Physician** monitors medical status and athletic participation, as well as coordinates care.
   2. **Nutritionist** provides appropriate nutritional guidance.
   3. **Mental health professional** addresses psychological issues.
   4. **Coach, trainer, or exercise physiologist** can help as ancillary team members.
   5. **Family** involvement is often necessary for the younger athlete living at home.
B. **Intervention**
   1. An athlete with disordered eating may be identified in various ways: the physician may suspect it during the preparticipation physical examination; parents may call with concerns; coaches, teammates, or trainers may note suspicious behavior; the athlete may seek help from a nutritionist (for a diet plan) or, occasionally, will recognize the problem and seek help directly.
   2. The athlete suspected of disordered eating should be approached gently, not accusingly.
   3. Present evidence of disordered eating behavior, along with expressions of concern about her health and well-being.
C. **Screening during the preparticipation examination** (*see also* Chapter 6)
   1. **Menstrual history**
      a. Age of menarche
      b. Frequency and duration of menstrual periods
      c. Date of last menstrual period
      d. Use of hormonal therapy
   2. **Nutritional screen**
      a. 24-hour recall
      b. Number of daily meals and snacks
      c. List of forbidden foods (e.g., meat or sweets)
   3. **Body weight**
      a. Highest and lowest weights since menarche offer a picture of eating patterns.
      b. Is she satisfied with her present weight?
      c. What does she feel her ideal weight should be?
      d. Has she ever tried to control her weight using vomiting, laxatives, or diuretics?
   4. **Further testing or referral**
      a. An athlete suspected of disordered eating can be seen later for an in-depth evaluation by the physician or referred to a nutritionist for screening.
      b. The nutritionist can screen more completely for disordered eating as well as provide guidelines on healthy nutrition and caloric intake.
      c. If the athlete is oligomenorrheic or amenorrheic or has clear signs of an eating disorder, she should be referred for an in-depth medical evaluation.

D. **Medical evaluation**
 1. **History**
   a. Menstrual history
   b. Nutritional screen
   c. Exercise history
    i. Athlete's sports participation
    ii. Hours spent training per week
     (a) Aerobic and anaerobic training
     (b) Time spent exercising outside of normal training regimen (e.g., Stairmaster, calisthenics)
    iii. If the athlete engages in aerobic exercise outside of her aerobic training regimen, suspicions should be raised.
   d. Family history, including if possible weight history of family members
   e. Brief psychological history
    i. Particular stresses in her life (e.g., social, academic, sports, or family)
    ii. General mood, body image, self-esteem
   f. Past medical history (any chronic diseases, infections, previous surgery, medications, stress fractures)
 2. **Systems review**
   a. Cover symptoms of starvation and purging (*see above*)
 3. **Physical examination**
   a. Evaluate for signs of starvation and purging.
   b. Check blood pressure for orthostatic changes.
   c. Pelvic examination if athlete has irregular or absent menses
   d. Consider differential diagnoses for an eating disorder
    i. Metabolic disease
    ii. Malignancy
    iii. Inflammatory bowel disease
    iv. Achalasia (difficulty swallowing)
    v. Infection
 4. **Laboratory examination**
   a. Urinalysis (evaluate for pH, specific gravity, signs of infection)
   b. Complete blood count and sedimentation rate
   c. Chemistry panel (electrolytes, calcium, magnesium, potassium)
   d. Kidney, thyroid, and liver function tests
   e. If menses irregular or absent, pregnancy test and possibly FSH, LH, and prolactin
 5. **Electrocardiography**
   a. Appropriate if pulse is <50 beats/min, electrolyte abnormality is present, or there is frequent purging.
   b. Note for findings of bradycardia, low voltage, low or inverted T-waves, or (most important) prolonged QT interval.
 6. **Positive evaluation**
   a. If evaluation is positive for disordered eating or an eating disorder, the physician should determine sport or exercise participation.
    i. If the athlete is losing weight, prepare a verbal or written contract with sports participation dependent on weight gain (e.g., ½ lb/week).
    ii. Electrolyte abnormalities: Limit exercise until corrected.
    iii. ECG abnormalities: Limit exercise until corrected.
   b. Monitor physical status and laboratory values as needed.
   c. Encourage hormone replacement in amenorrheic or oligomenorrheic athletes if there is no other etiology for menstrual dysfunction. Consider bone densitometry.
   d. Refer athlete to a nutritionist and mental health professional.

E. **Nutritional evaluation and treatment**
   1. The nutritionist should be a registered dietician who has experience in managing eating disorders and understands sports participation.
   2. **Initial evaluation**
      a. Detailed food and weight/height history
      b. Exercise history
      c. 3-day food diary to assess caloric, carbohydrate, protein, and nutrient intake
      d. Body composition measurements
         i. Arm circumference and triceps skinfold thickness to assess lean muscle mass
         ii. 3- or 7-site skinfold thickness to estimate percent body fat
      e. Estimate caloric intake, caloric needs, and healthy weight range (25–50%).
      f. Educate athlete on appropriate weight range, percent body fat, and lean muscle mass.
      g. Emphasize the effects of starvation on body composition and loss of muscle mass.
   3. **Follow-up visits**
      a. Educate athlete on how to adequately fuel the body and avoid binges by eating regular meals and snacks.
      b. Recommendations must be individualized, helping the athlete to schedule meals and snacks around practices and competitions and, for college athletes, how to cook healthily and efficiently or to select healthy foods from cafeterias.
      c. Provide guidelines on how to make gradual changes in caloric and nutrient intake.
      d. Measure body composition every 1–2 months for feedback and evaluation of change.
F. **Psychological evaluation and treatment**
   1. The mental health practitioner needs to have expertise in the management of eating disorders and some undestanding of sports activities.
   2. **Initial evaluation**
      a. Identify stresses in the athlete's life, both in and out of sport:
         i. Academic pressure
         ii. Relationships with teammates and coaches
         iii. Social contacts and family
         iv. Her perception of her sports performance
      b. How does the athlete perceive that she deals with stress?
      c. How does she define her eating patterns?
      d. Consider the need for individual vs group therapy (or both).
   3. **Follow-up treatment**
      a. Help the athlete develop an awareness of her stressors and work on healthy coping strategies, identity issues, self-esteem issues, and assertiveness skills (Fig. 1).
      b. A support group limited to other women athletes can help athletes identify stressors (which are often common among the group), recognize how these stressors affect their eating, and develop coping skills.
G. **Criteria for hospitalization**
   1. Weight loss >30% of normal
   2. Cardiac compromise
   3. Hypotension or dehydration
   4. Electrolyte abnormalities
   5. Failing outpatient treatment (failure to improve or symptoms worsening after 3 months of therapy)

IX. **PROGNOSIS**
   A. Long-term studies of athletes with disordered eating are not published.
      1. It is unknown how often disordered eating patterns subside after college or competitive athletics end.

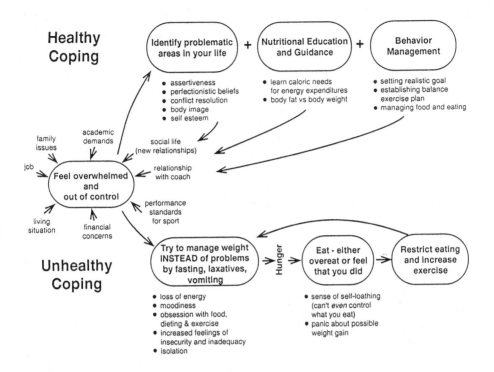

Healthy Coping

Identify problematic areas in your life
- assertiveness
- perfectionistic beliefs
- conflict resolution
- body image
- self esteem

+

Nutritional Education and Guidance
- learn caloric needs for energy expenditures
- body fat vs body weight

+

Behavior Management
- setting realistic goal
- establishing balance exercise plan
- managing food and eating

family issues

academic demands

social life (new relationships)

job

Feel overwhelmed and out of control

relationship with coach

living situation

financial concerns

performance standards for sport

Unhealthy Coping

Try to manage weight INSTEAD of problems by fasting, laxatives, vomiting
- loss of energy
- moodiness
- obsession with food, dieting & exercise
- increased feelings of insecurity and inadequacy
- isolation

Hunger

Eat - either overeat or feel that you did
- sense of self-loathing (can't *even* control what you eat)
- panic about possible weight gain

Restrict eating and increase exercise

FIGURE 1. A conceptual model of unhealthy coping mechanisms used by the athlete with disordered eating and the therapeutic process used in the development of healthy coping skills. (Courtesy of Priscilla Wright, PhD.)

    2. Many athletes continue to struggle with concerns about weight control and eating patterns after their athletic careers are over.
- B. In nonathletes treated for an eating disorder, the prognosis is as follows:
  - 1. 50% do well.
  - 2. 30% improve but struggle with weight control, body image, and relapses.
  - 3. 20% do poorly.
- C. Causes of death include suicide, cardiovascular collapse or arrest, sepsis, and gastric or intestinal perforation.

X. PREVENTION

Prevention is the key to addressing this problem, and education is the necessary first step.

- A. **Athletes, parents, coaches, athletic administrators, training staff, and physicians need to be educated about the risks and warning signs of disordered eating** (Table 3).
  - 1. Athletes should be educated on physiologic, psychological, nutritional, and performance effects of disordered eating; counseling should address appropriate methods of weight control, ways to avoid disordered eating, and available local resources.
  - 2. Coaches should be educated on ways they may influence the development of disordered eating in their athletes.
  - 3. The National Collegiate Athletic Association (NCAA) offers an educational videotape on eating disorders in athletes (contact: Karol Video, PO Box 7600, Wilkes-Barre, PA 18773-7600; telephone 800-526-4773).

TABLE 3.   Signs of Disordered Eating

1. A preoccupation with food, calories, and weight
2. Repeatedly expressed concerns about being or feeling fat, even when weight is average or below average
3. Increasing criticism of one's body
4. Secretly eating or stealing food
5. Eating large meals, then disappearing or making trips to the bathroom
6. Consumption of large amounts of food not consistent with the athlete's weight
7. Bloodshot eyes, especially after trips to the bathroom
8. Swollen parotid glands at the angle of the jaw, giving a chipmunk-like appearance
9. Vomitus, or odor of vomitus in bathroom
10. Wide fluctuations in weight over short periods of time
11. Periods of severe calorie restriction
12. Excessive laxative use
13. Compulsive, excessive exercise that is not part of the athlete's training regimen
14. Unwillingness to eat in front of others (e.g., teammates on road trips)
15. Expression of self-deprecating thoughts following eating
16. Wearing baggy or layered clothing
17. Mood swings
18. Appearing preoccupied with the eating behavior of others
19. Continuous drinking of diet soda or water

4. The preparticipation examination is an excellent opportunity for screening as well as advising the athlete about healthy nutrition and appropriate methods of weight control.
5. The physician should become familiar with the medical evaluation for disordered eating as well as the concept of the treatment team.
6. The physician should be a resource person for educating other physicians as well as trainers, coaches, parents, and athletes.

REFERENCES

1. Arden MR, Budow L, Bunnell DW, et al: Alkaline urine is associated with eating disorders. Am J Dis Child 145:28–30, 1991.
2. Amrein PC, Friedman R, Kosinski K, et al: Hematologic changes in anorexia nervosa. JAMA 24:2190–2191, 1979.
3. Bhanji S, Mattingly D: Anorexia nervosa: Some observations on "dieters" and "vomiters," cholesterol and carotene. Br J Psychiatry 139:238, 1981.
4. Bowers TK, Eckert E: Leukopenia in anorexia nervosa: Lack of increased risk of infection. Arch Intern Med 138:1520, 1978.
5. Drinkwater BL, Nilson K, Chesnut CH III, et al: Bone mineral content of amenorrheic and eumenorrheic athletes. N Engl J Med 311:277–281, 1984.
6. Dubois A, Gross HA, Ebert MH, et al: Altered gastric emptying and secretion in primary anorexia nervosa. Gastroenterology 77:319, 1979.
7. Dummer GM, Rosen LW, Heusner WW, et al: Pathogenic weight-control behaviors of young competitive swimmers. Phys SportsMed 15:75–86, 1987.
8. Fohlin L: Body composition, cardiovascular and renal function in adolescent patients with anorexia nervosa. Acta Paediatr Scand 268:1–20, 1977.
9. Fohlin L, Freyschuss U, Barke B, et al: Function and dimensions of the circulatory system in anorexia nervosa. Acta Paediatr Scand 66:11–16, 1978.
10. Garfinkel PE, Moldofsky H, Garner DM, et al: Body awareness in anorexia nervosa: Disturbances in "body image" and "satiety." Psychosom Med 40:487, 1978.
11. Goldberg SJ, Comerci GD, Feldman L: Cardiac output and regional myocardial contraction in anorexia nervosa. J Adolesc Health Care 7:15–21, 1988.
12. Harris RT: Bulimarexia and related serious eating disorders with medical complications. Ann Intern Med 99:800–807, 1983.
13. Hurd HP, Palumbo PJ, Gharid H: Hypothalamic-endocrine dysfunction in anorexia nervosa. Mayo Clin Proc 52:711–716, 1977.
14. Isner JM, Roberts WC, Heymsfield SB, et al: Anorexia nervosa and sudden death. Ann Intern Med 102:49–52, 1985.

15. Kaye WH, Weltzin TE: Neurochemistry of bulimia nervosa. J Clin Psychol 52:21–28, 1991.
16. Kennedy S: Melatonin disregulation in anorexia nervosa and bulimia nervosa. Int J Eating Dis (in press).
17. Keys A, Henschel A, Taylor HL: The size and function of the human heart at rest in semi-starvation and in subsequent rehabilitation. Am Heart J 55:584–602, 1948.
18. Kreipe RE, Harris JP: Myocardial impairment resulting from eating disorders. Pediatr Ann 21:760–768, 1992.
19. Levin PA, Falko JM, Dixon K, et al: Benign parotid enlargement in bulimia. Ann Intern Med 93:827–829, 1980.
20. Milner MR, McAnarney ER, Klish WJ: Metabolic abnormalities in adolescent patients with anorexia nervosa. J Adolesc Health Care 6:191–195, 1985.
21. Palla B, Litt IF: Medical complications of eating disorders in adolescents. Pediatrics 81:613–623, 1988.
22. Polivy J, Herman CP: Diagnosis and treatment of normal eating. J Consult Clin Psychol 55:635–644, 1987.
23. Pomeroy C, Mitchell JE: Medical issues in the eating disorders. In Brownell KD, Rodin J, Wilmore JH (eds): Eating, Body Weight and Performance in Athletes: Disorders of Modern Society. Philadelphia, Lea & Febiger, 1992.
24. Roberts MW, Li S-H: Oral findings in anorexia nervosa and bulimia nervosa: A study of 47 cases. J Am Dent Assoc 115:407, 1987.
25. Root MPP: Persistent, disordered eating as a gender-specific, post-traumatic stress response to sexual assault. Psychotherapy 28:96–102, 1991.
26. Rosen LW, Mckeag DB, Hough DO, et al: Pathogenic weight-control behavior in female athletes. Phys SportsMed 14:79–86, 1986.
27. Rosen LW, Hough DO: Pathogenic weight-control behaviors of female college gymnasts. Phys SportsMed 16:141–146, 1988.
28. Russell G: Bulimia nervosa: An ominous variant of anorexia nervosa. Psychol Med 9:429–448, 1979.
29. Silverstein B, Perdup L: The relationship between role concern, preferences for slimness, and symptoms of eating problems among college women. Sex Roles 18:101–106, 1988.
30. Steinhausen H, Rauss-Mason C, Seidel R: Follow-up studies of anorexia nervosa: A review of four decades of outcome research. Psychol Med 21:447–454, 1991.
31. Striegel-Moore RH, Silberstein LR, Rodin J: Toward an understanding of risk factors for bulimia. Am Psychol 41:246–263, 1986.
32. Vigersky RA, Anderson AE, Thompson RH, et al: Hypothalamic dysfunction in secondary amenorrhea associated with simple weight loss. N Engl J Med 297:1141–1145, 1977.
33. Warren MP, VandeWiele RL: Clinical and metabolic features of anorexia. Am J Obstet Gynecol 117:435, 1973.
34. Yates A: Biologic considerations in the etiology of eating disorders. Pediatr Ann 21:739–744, 1992.

Chapter 21: Clinical Evaluation of Amenorrhea

LORNA A. MARSHALL, MD

Disorders of menstrual function occur more frequently in female athletes than in the general population. The most extreme menstrual dysfunction, amenorrhea, is associated with vigorous exercise in women throughout the range of reproductive ages. This topic has recently drawn more attention as part of the "female athletic triad"—disordered eating, amenorrhea, and osteoporosis. Disordered eating and osteoporosis are dealt with more extensively in other chapters of this text.

This chapter is intended to guide the clinician's approach to the active or athletic woman who presents with amenorrhea. Although the diagnosis of "exercise-associated" or "athletic" amenorrhea can eventually be assigned to many of these women, it is important to recognize that this is a **diagnosis of exclusion**. Other causes of amenorrhea occur with the same frequency in athletic women as in sedentary women. The role of the clinician is to exclude these other causes of amenorrhea.

I. DEFINITION

A. **Amenorrhea** means "absence of menstrual bleeding" and is defined as:
1. The absence of menstrual bleeding for 6 months or for a length of time equivalent to a total of at least three of her previous cycle lengths in a woman who has established menstrual cycles.
2. No menstrual bleeding by age 16 or by age 14 in the absence of sexual development.
3. One period or less per year as defined by the International Olympic Committee.
B. **Primary amenorrhea:** Women who have never had menstrual bleeding.
C. **Secondary amenorrhea:** Women who have had at least one episode of menstrual bleeding before amenorrhea.

II. PREVALENCE

A. Up to 5% of the general population, excluding pregnant women. In an unselected adolescent population, this may be as high as 8.5%.
B. 10–20% of vigorously exercising women
C. As high as 40–50% of elite runners and professional ballet dancers

III. PHYSIOLOGY OF THE MENSTRUAL CYCLE

Amenorrhea can result from abnormalities at the genital organs, ovaries, pituitary gland, or hypothalamus. Requirements for normal cyclic menstrual bleeding include:
A. **Reproductive tract**
1. A uterus, normal endometrial lining and a tract connecting the uterine cavity with the external genitalia must be present for menstrual bleeding to be observed.
2. A normal uterus with an obstructed outflow tract may result in a uterus, vagina, and peritoneal cavity distended with menstrual blood, and amenorrhea will be reported.
B. **Ovaries must produce estrogen and progesterone** in a sequential manner (Fig. 1).
1. Estrogen stimulates the endometrium to develop, and the withdrawal of both estrogen and progesterone results in menstrual shedding. When there is estrogen but no progesterone (as in chronic anovulation and polycystic ovarian disease), the endometrium will build up but will usually bleed erratically and infrequently.
2. The production of estrogen and progesterone by the ovaries depends on the presence of oocytes (eggs), their maturation, and the appropriate development of a corpus luteum after ovulation.

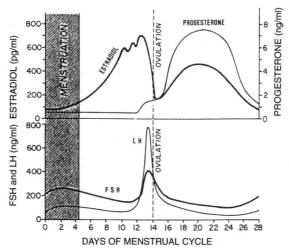

FIGURE 1. Plasma concentrations of the gonadotropins and ovarian hormones during the normal menstrual cycle. (From Guyton AC: Textbook of Medical Physiology, 7th ed. Philadelphia, W.B. Saunders, 1986, with permission.)

   3. Ovarian failure means that there are few or no functional oocytes remaining, and despite normal pituitary and hypothalamic function, the ovary cannot produce significant estrogen or progesterone.
C. The cells in the **pituitary gland** that produce **luteinizing hormone** (LH) and **follicle-stimulating hormone** (FSH) must be intact and functional.
   1. LH and FSH are necessary to initiate the maturation of the egg, stimulate ovulation, and support the corpus luteum after ovulation.
   2. Large pituitary tumors or ischemia may compromise or destroy these cells.
   3. Prolactin is also secreted by the pituitary gland; when prolactin levels are high from any cause, LH and FSH production falls, and amenorrhea may follow.
D. **Gonadotropin-releasing hormone** (GnRH) must be produced by the **hypothalamus** in sufficient quantity, and it must be secreted in a regular, pulsatile pattern.
   1. It is released into the portal vessels through which it travels down the pituitary stalk to affect the LH- and FSH-producing cells in the pituitary gland.
   2. The GnRH-producing cells in the hypothalamus can be damaged or congenitally deficient or the pituitary stalk can be traumatized, causing GnRH pulses reaching the pituitary gland to decrease below a critical frequency; amenorrhea will result.
   3. There are many neurohormones including endorphins and catecholamines that modulate the GnRH-producing centers. Physical and emotional stresses are believed to result in "hypothalamic amenorrhea" by affecting these or other neurohormones.

IV. ETIOLOGY OF AMENORRHEA

Although the majority of athletic women with amenorrhea will have a subtype of hypothalamic amenorrhea, all other causes for amenorrhea should be considered (Table 1). "Exercise-related" or "athletic" amenorrhea is a diagnosis of exclusion. Causes for amenorrhea include:
A. **Pregnancy**: This is the most common cause of amenorrhea and *must* be excluded in all sexually active women.
B. **Abnormalities of the reproductive tract**
   1. **Asherman's syndrome:** Severe scarring of the endometrial cavity from a uterine curettage, particularly after a pregnancy, may result in amenorrhea in women who have previously had normal menses.

TABLE 1. Causes of Amenorrhea

Pregnancy	Hypothalamic amenorrhea
Abnormalities of the reproductive tract	Chronic anovulation
Ovarian failure	Polycystic ovarian disease
Pituitary tumors or abnormalities	Exercise-associated amenorrhea

     a. A suspicious history, normal hormonal evaluation, and failure to bleed after an estrogen/progestin challenge suggest the diagnosis.

     b. A hysterosalpingogram will suggest and hysteroscopy will confirm the diagnosis.

  2. **Developmental abnormalities of the genital tract:** Discontinuities of the female genital tract, or müllerian system, can occur and should be considered when a woman presents with primary amenorrhea and normal sexual development.

     a. When the uterus and endometrium are present, but there is an **obstruction** due to an imperforate hymen or absent vagina, the woman will present with amenorrhea and pelvic pain from blood in the uterus, peritoneal cavity, and/or vagina.

     b. It is possible for both the uterus and vagina to be absent (**müllerian agenesis**); on examination, there is a short vaginal pouch with no cervix. A karyotype should be performed in müllerian agenesis to exclude complete androgen insensitivity.

     c. Some müllerian abnormalities are associated with urinary tract developmental abnormalities.

  3. **Complete androgen insensitivity** (testicular feminization): This diagnosis should be considered when a patient has primary amenorrhea and an absent uterus.

     a. Breasts are large but with small nipples, pubic and axillary hair is scant or absent, and inguinal hernias containing testes are sometimes present.

     b. The karyotype is XY, but androgen receptors are insensitive to normal levels of testosterone.

     c. These patients are phenotypically female and are always reared as females.

     d. The care of these patients involves many sensitive issues and should be referred to a specialist.

C. **Ovarian failure:** This can occur before the first menstrual period or at any time after the menstrual cycle has been initiated. At any age, it is characterized by low estrogen levels and elevated FSH levels. Estrogen production by the ovary normally feeds back to the pituitary gland to keep FSH levels low. If hypothalamic and pituitary function is normal, a high FSH specifically reflects diminished or absent oocytes in the ovary, and the consequent failure of the ovaries to produce estrogen. Most women who have ovarian failure after establishing normal menses will experience vasomotor symptoms, or hot flashes.

  1. **Normal menopause:** The average age of menopause is 51, but it is considered normal to have ovarian failure anytime after age 40. Normal menopause should be high on the differential list of women 40 or over who present with amenorrhea.

  2. **Premature ovarian failure:** Women less than 40 may have secondary amenorrhea associated with a high FSH level. In general, this disorder reflects early destruction of oocytes.

     a. Possible etiologies include autoimmune destruction, chemotherapy or radiation therapy, genetic abnormalities, or rarely galactosemia.

     b. Chromosomal abnormalities such as Turner mosaicism may be associated with normal menarche and premature ovarian failure, so chromosomal studies should be performed in all women under age 30 who have ovarian failure.

     c. Autoimmune ovarian failure is associated with other organ-specific autoimmune disorders. Because the understanding of autoimmune ovarian failure is limited and there is not yet an adequate diagnostic test, all women with premature ovarian failure should undergo testing to exclude other autoimmune disorders.

3. **Gonadal failure secondary to chromosomal abnormality.** Women with primary amenorrhea and a high FSH level often have a chromosomal abnormality and need karyotype evaluation. The presence of a Y chromosome mandates gonadectomy to prevent malignancy.

D. **Pituitary tumors or abnormalities**
  1. **Prolactin-secreting pituitary tumor**
     a. This is the most common pituitary tumor
        i. Microadenoma (<1 cm)
        ii. Macroadenoma (≥1 cm)
     b. Elevated prolactin levels suggest the diagnosis. Magnetic resonance imaging (MRI) is the best imaging test to detect microadenomas.
     c. Micro- and macroadenomas are usually treated medically with the dopamine agonist bromocriptine.
     d. Galactorrhea occurs in only one-third of women with elevated prolactin levels, so its absence does not exclude the diagnosis.
  2. **Other tumors**: Less commonly, nonsecreting pituitary tumors or tumors secreting other hormones may result in amenorrhea by compressing the LH- and FSH-producing cells or by compressing the pituitary stalk and causing elevated prolactin levels. These tumors are usually large (>2 cm).
  3. **Other causes of hyperprolactinemia:**
     a. Damage to the pituitary stalk may prevent delivery of dopamine (which keeps prolactin levels low) to the pituitary gland and result in elevated prolactin levels.
     b. Breast trauma, hypothyroidism, and many medications such as phenothiazine and metachlopromide can cause elevated prolactin levels and amenorrhea.

E. **Hypothalamic amenorrhea:** This is the most common cause of secondary amenorrhea (except for pregnancy) and can also be a cause of primary amenorrhea or delayed menarche. **Exercise-associated amenorrhea** is generally considered a subset of hypothalamic amenorrhea amd accounts for the higher prevalence of amenorrhea in athletes than in the general population of women.
  1. **Pulsatile GnRH** produced by the hypothalamus is deficient, absent, or inappropriately secreted in hypothalamic amenorrhea. Causes include:
     a. Psychological or physical stress affecting neurohormones that modulate GnRH.
     b. Congenital abnormalities that affect the GnRH-producing nuclei.
     c. Rarely, a destructive process such as trauma or tumor may affect GnRH secretion.
  2. Patients may have **hypoestrogenic changes in the genital tract** but do not generally have hot flashes. They have normal prolactin levels, normal or low LH and FSH levels, low estrogen levels, and no withdrawal bleeding after a progestin challenge. Changes in GnRH secretion cannot be determined by peripheral blood sampling, and so are indirectly demonstrated by the tests listed above.
  3. **Pituitary tumor** should be excluded to confirm the diagnosis. Some reproductive endocrinologists recommend **pituitary imaging** in all women with the profile of hypothalamic amenorrhea. **We carefully consider pituitary imaging in all such women** but do not always perform testing in women for whom the relationship between the onset of amenorrhea and abrupt weight loss or a profoundly stressful event is unequivocal.
  4. When **physical or psychological stress** is implicated as the cause, the onset of amenorrhea may be abrupt or gradual.
     a. A period of oligomenorrhea (menstrual interval >35 days) may precede the amenorrhea.
     b. Recovery from amenorrhea is much more prolonged than its onset, and it may be months or years after the stress is relieved before normal menses resume.

5. Examples of hypothalamic amenorrhea are:
   a. **Isolated gonadotropin deficiency** (a similar disorder in the male is called Kallmann's syndrome) is associated with a developmental defect in the hypothalamic olfactory centers and GnRH-producing centers. It is characterized by lack of sexual development, primary amenorrhea, low LH and FSH levels, normal female karyotype, and sometimes, an undeveloped sense of smell.
   b. **Weight-loss amenorrhea:** Acute weight loss may result in hypothalamic amenorrhea. It has been proposed that a critical weight, and perhaps a critical percentage of body fat, is necessary for the initiation and maintenance of reproductive function. Anorexia nervosa is invariably associated with amenorrhea, presumably from the profound weight loss. In addition, marked weight fluctuations ($>$10 lb loss and regain), especially in adolescents, have been associated with amenorrhera.
   c. **Psychogenic amenorrhea:** Stressful life situations such as moving away to college, divorce, or death of a family member can result in a variable period of amenorrhea. An individual's perception of such events, her coping skills, and perhaps her individual reproductive system will determine whether or not menstrual dysfunction will occur.
   d. **Exercise-induced amenorrhea:** This is usually considered to be a subset of hypothalamic amenorrhea, but is discussed separately below.
F. **Chronic anovulation** and **polycystic ovarian disease:** Some women have abnormal feedback mechanisms which result in failure to ovulate and produce **progesterone**. These women often have high estrogen levels from the conversion of excess androgens to estrogens in fat cells. They usually present with irregular or infrequent menses since menarche but may present with primary or secondary amenorrhea.

V. EXERCISE-ASSOCIATED OR ATHLETIC AMENORRHEA

Exercise is often considered one cause of hypothalamic dysfunction leading to amenorrhea. Whether it is an entity separate from weight loss or psychogenic amenorrhea is controversial. Here, exercise-induced amenorrhea is discussed as a separate entity. As with other classes of hypothalamic amenorrhea, the diagnosis can be made only after the exclusion of other causes for amenorrhea.

A. **Profile of women with exercise-induced amenorrhea**
   1. Adolescent with primary amenorrhea or adult with secondary amenorrhea
   2. Competitive long-distance runners, gymnasts, and professional ballet dancers at highest risk; cyclists, swimmers also at risk; menstrual disorders also documented in recreational weight-lifters and competitive body-builders.
   3. Low weight plus loss of weight after training initiated
   4. Low body fat for weight
   5. If weight stable, total calorie intake may be less than for eumenorrheic athletes and inadequate to meet energy demands.
   6. Decreased percentage of protein in diet
   7. "Anorectic reaction" is common, with deliberate attempts to decrease weight. Eating disorders are especially common in adolescents and highly competitive athletes. Major affective disorders are sometimes associated with eating disorders in athletes.
   8. High incidence of menstrual abnormalities prior to vigorous training. Athletes with secondary amenorrhea have a higher incidence of delayed menarche, even if they were not training as adolescents.
   9. Amenorrheic athletes associate a higher level of stress with training than do athletes with normal menses.
   10. Some have return of menses during intervals of rest, even without weight gain or change in body fat.
   11. More likely to have begun training at an earlier age. Overall, amenorrheic runners have been running longer than eumenorrheic runners.

12. Exercise intensity is high and is more likely to have been increased rapidly. Runners with a weekly training mileage >30 miles are at increased risk of amenorrhea.
13. Hormonal profile:
    a. LH and FSH levels normal or low
    b. Estradiol levels are low; no withdrawal bleeding after a progestin challenge
    c. Prolactin normal
    d. Androgens, testosterone, and dehydroepiandrosterone sulfate (DHEAS) normal
    e. Thyroid hormone levels are usually in the normal range, although thyroxine (T_4), triiodothyronine (T_3), free T_4 and free T_3 are often lower than the mean. Thyroid-stimulating hormone is normal.
    f. Cortisol, both daytime and nocturnal, is slightly elevated.
B. **Pathophysiology:** Probably complex, involving hypothalamic dysfunction. The entity of athletic amenorrhea is heterogenous, with varied contributions of weight loss, lowered body fat, emotional stress, and physical stress involved. Not all thin, competitive runners become amenorrheic, suggesting individual variations in the resiliency of the reproductive system. Most theories agree that hypothalamic secretion of GnRH is diminished, resulting in decreased pulsatile LH and FSH, and therefore minimal production of estrogen by the ovaries.
    1. **Reproductive potential is suspended** to preserve an individual with inadequate energy stores to support a fetus. Somehow, the hypothalamus senses the inadequate weight, body fat, and nutritional intake for the activity of that individual.
    2. **Increased endogenous opioids from a "runner's high"** directly suppress the frequency and amplitude of GnRH pulses. Beta-endorphins have been most widely discussed as the involved opioid. Opioid antagonists such as naltrexone or naloxone have been shown, in some cases, to restore normal gonadotropin pulses and even ovulation and menses.
    3. **Hypercortisolism**, occurring as a result of the stress of exercise, inhibits GnRH pulsatile secretion, either through cortisol or corticotropin-releasing factor.
    4. **Lowered estrogen production by fat cells** results in abnormal feedback to the hypothalamus and resulting amenorrhea.
    5. **Another neurohormone**, such as melatonin or dopamine, is elevated with aerobic training and suppresses GnRH pulsatile secretion.

VI. EVALUATION OF AMENORRHEA

All exercising women need a complete evaluation for the etiology of amenorrhea, no matter how clearly exercise seems by history to be the causative factor.
A. **History:** A careful interview should address all of the following areas:
    1. **Menstrual history**
       a. Age at menarche (first menstrual period)
       b. Previous menstrual pattern, when not using oral contraceptives
       c. Previous episodes of amenorrhea
       d. Transition to amenorrhea
    2. **Development of secondary sexual characteristics** (important in primary amenorrhea)
       a. Breast development
       b. Growth spurt
       c. Axillary and pubic hair development
    3. **Sexual activity:** At risk for pregnancy?
    4. **Pregnancy history**
       a. Uterine curettage for pregnancy loss, termination, or postpartum bleeding
       b. Postpartum endometritis
    5. **Birth control**
       a. Women on birth control pills may stop having withdrawal bleeding and *do not* need to be evaluated for amenorrhea if pregnancy has been excluded.

b. If menstrual periods do not resume within 6 months of discontinuing birth control pills, an evaluation should be initiated. "Post-pill amenorrhea" is no longer felt to be a separate entity.

6. **Nutritional history**
   a. Weight gain or loss in the year prior to onset of symptoms as well as a careful history to determine fluctuations in weight
   b. Vegetarian diet has been associated with amenorrhea.
   c. History suggestive of eating disorder: self-induced vomiting, use of laxatives or diet pills, periods of fasting, marked weight fluctuations

7. **Physical activity**
   a. Daily frequency
   b. Intensity
   c. Duration of training
   d. Any changes in above

8. **Conflicts and support systems**
   a. Home
   b. Work
   c. Social

9. **Coping skills**

10. **Symptoms of estrogen deficiency**
    a. Vaginal dryness, dyspareunia
    b. Vasomotor symptoms (hot flashes) usually suggest menopause or premature ovarian failure.

11. **Symptoms of androgen excess:** In polycystic ovarian syndrome, these symptoms are usually present since menarche; a rapid onset of symptoms mandates evaluation.
    a. Coarse facial, chest, or abdominal hair. Elicit history because many women control with waxing or electrolysis.
    b. Acne
    c. Temporal balding

12. **Other symptoms**
    a. Galactorrhea: spontaneous secretion of milk
    b. Headaches
    c. Decreased sense of smell

13. **Other medical history**
    a. Chemotherapy or radiation therapy
    b. Stress fractures
    c. Low bone density

14. **Medications:** Many **psychotropic medications** are dopamine antagonists and may result in prolactin levels high enough to cause amenorrhea.

15. **Family history**
    a. Age of menopause may have familial component.
    b. Sexual immaturity associated with decreased smell may suggest isolated gonadotropin deficiency.
    c. Polycystic ovarian syndrome has genetic component.

B. **Physical examination**
   1. **Height, weight, general examination:** Skeletal proportions and stigmata of syndromes such as Turner's should be evaluated in women with primary amenorrhea.
   2. **Body fat** is usually estimated rather than formally measured in a clinical setting.
   3. **Hair distribution**
      a. Tanner staging of pubic hair
         Stage 1—preadolescent; no pubic hair
         Stage 2—sparse growth of downy hair along labia

Stage 3—coarser hair, but spread sparsely
Stage 4—adult-type hair, but not spread to inner thighs
Stage 5—adult hair pattern in inverse triangle, with spread to inner thighs

   b. Axillary hair: Absence of both axillary and pubic hair suggests complete androgen insensitivity.

   c. Excessive and coarse facial or chest hair; presence of hair along linea alba or above inverse triangle suggests androgen excess.

4. **Thyroid**
5. **Breasts**
   a. Tanner staging
     Stage 1—preadolescent, elevation of papilla only
     Stage 2—breast bud stage
     Stage 3—further enlargement of breast and papilla, with no separation of contours
     Stage 4—projection of areola and papilla to form a mound above level of breast
     Stage 5—mature, projection of papilla
   b. Galactorrhea: White secretions which microscopically are fat globules; present in one-third of women with elevated prolactin level.

6. **Pelvis**
   a. Normal **clitoris** should measure <1 cm.
   b. **Vaginal**
     i. Note moisture, presence of rugae.
     ii. Vaginal smear for maturation index can give estimate of estrogenic status.
   c. **Cervix:** Its presence almost always suggests there is a uterus; pap smears should be done yearly once women are sexually active or over age 20.
   d. **Uterus:** A normal-sized uterus on examination does not absolutely exclude pregnancy.
   e. **Adnexa:** Rarely, ovarian tumors are associated with amenorrhea.

C. **Laboratory evaluation**
1. **Pregnancy test:** Order liberally.
2. **Thyroid-stimulating hormone (TSH):** Hypothyroidism is not frequently a cause of amenorrhea, but screening of all patients is recommended.
3. **Prolactin:** The test is most accurate when blood is drawn midmorning after fasting or a low-protein breakfast. Sleep, large protein meals, a recent breast exam may all result in falsely high prolactin levels. Pregnancy also elevates prolactin.
4. **FSH:** Recommended in all women with primary or secondary amenorrhea. If elevated (>40 IU/L), it should be repeated at least once before the diagnosis of ovarian failure is made.
5. **Karyotype**
   a. All women under age 30 with an elevated FSH level and amenorrhea
   b. All women with absent uterus
6. **Estrogen level:** Measurement of estradiol is rarely helpful in diagnosing amenorrheic patients.
   a. It can be used instead of a progestin challenge to help determine whether estrogen replacement should be advised.
   b. If estradiol is consistently <50 pg/ml, she may benefit from estrogen replacement.
7. **Other hormonal measurements**
   a. **LH:** Not routinely necessary in evaluation of amenorrhea; ratio of LH/FSH is elevated in polycystic ovarian syndrome.
   b. **Androgens:** Testosterone and dehydroepiandrosterone sulfate (DHEAS) should be measured in women with signs of androgen excess to exclude ovarian and adrenal androgen-producing tumors.

8. **Endometrial biopsy**
   a. Women with normal to high levels of estrogen and anovulation (usually polycystic ovarian syndrome) do not produce enough progesterone to prevent the continued proliferation of the endometrium.
   b. If they are 30 years or older and amenorrheic, an endometrial biopsy should be done to exclude endometrial hyperplasia/malignancy prior to initiating treatment.
   c. Hypoestrogenic women usually have an atrophic endometrium and do not need endometrial sampling.

D. **Indirect tests: role of hormonal challenges**
   1. **Progestin challenge:** Useful test to assess the amount of endogenous estrogens and the normalcy of the genital outflow tract.
      a. Medroxyprogesterone acetate (Provera), 10 mg orally for 5 days; *or* progesterone-in-oil, 100–200 mg intramuscularly, single dose.
      b. Pregnancy test must be confirmed as negative prior to progestin administration.
      c. A positive response to hormonal challenge is any vaginal bleeding within 10 days of the injection or last pill; it suggests that the uterine lining is present and sufficiently prepared by endogenous estrogens and that the genital outflow tract is present and unobstructed.
      d. Negative response is usually consistent with an abnormal or obstructed outflow tract, hypoestrogenemia from any cause, pregnancy, or occasionally, normal estrogens with excessive androgen effect on the endometrium.
   2. **Estrogen/progestin challenge:** This test is performed after a failed progestin challenge to demonstrate an intact system in women with primary amenorrhea and to exclude Asherman's syndrome in women with secondary amenorrhea.
      a. Conjugated estrogens, 1.25–2.5 mg, or micronized estradiol, 2–4 mg, are given for 25 days, plus 10 mg of medroxyprogesterone acetate for the last 5 days.
      b. If a negative response, the test should be repeated.

E. **Imaging tests**
   1. **Pituitary:** If LH and FSH levels are both <5 IU/L and no withdrawal bleeding occurs after a progestin challenge, pituitary imaging should be carefully considered.
      a. **Lateral coned-down view of the sella** will pick up a large pituitary lesion and is sufficient to exclude a tumor in most amenorrheic women with a normal prolacting level. Many institutions no longer perform this test because of its low sensitivity.
      b. **Computerized tomography** (CT) is our procedure of choice when the prolactin level is normal; it is less expensive than MRI.
      c. **Magnetic resonance imaging** (MRI) of the pituitary is our procedure of choice to evaluate the pituitary when the prolactin level is elevated.
   2. **Pelvis**
      a. **Sonography** is a good screening test to affirm the presence or absence of a uterus and ovaries when the pelvic examination is unsatisfactory in the adolescent female; generally this mode is inadequate to assess the nature of müllerian abnormalities.
      b. **MRI** of the pelvis is a promising but incompletely tested, modality to define müllerian abnormalities.
      c. **Hysterosalpingogram** involves injecting radioopaque dye into the uterus to outline intrauterine adhesions significant enough to cause amenorrhea.
   3. **Bone age determinations** should be done when pubertal development as well as menarche is delayed.
   4. **Bone mineral density determinations** are helpful to determine risk for osteoporosis when hypoestrogenic amenorrhea has been prolonged. Normal ranges for adolescents are not well established. It is sometimes useful when the amenorrheic woman is resisting estrogen therapy.

VII. **TREATMENT**

A. Detailed discussion of treatment options for categories besides athletic amenorrhea is beyond the scope of this chapter, and consultation with a gynecologist or reproductive endocrinologist should be arranged.

    1. **Amenorrhea associated with hypoestrogenism** (hypothalamic amenorrhea, ovarian failure):

        a. Estrogen replacement is advised to prevent osteoporosis and possibly to lower the risk of coronary artery disease.

        b. Estrogen administration may sometimes stimulate the growth of prolactinomas or further elevate prolactin levels..

        c. **Bromocriptine** administration to lower prolactin levels, restore normal menses, and increase estrogen production is the treatment of choice for amenorrheic women with hyperprolactinemia.

    2. **Amenorrhea associated with normal to high levels of estrogen and anovulation** (polycystic ovarian syndrome): Progestins should be administered (medroxyprogesterone acetate 10 mg × 10 days every 1–3 months) to prevent endometrial hyperplasia and malignancy.

B. **Athletic amenorrhea**

    1. **Adult female who does not currently desire conception:**

        a. Optimize nutritional intake

        b. Increase calcium to 1500 mg daily; there is no evidence that weight-bearing exercise plus calcium alone prevents osteoporosis in the absence of estrogen.

        c. If the patient is sexually active, advise her to use contraception; the first ovulation after amenorrhea often occurs prior to the first episode of menstrual bleeding.

        d. Encourage decrease in exercise intensity and/or 2–3% increase in body weight. Weight as well as amenorrhea is important in determining bone mineral density.

        e. Recommend use of estrogen and dispel myths associated with its use. Maximum bone loss probably occurs in early phase of amenorrhea, so treatment soon after the diagnosis is made is recommended.

            i. If the patient is sexually active, **oral contraceptives** are a good choice. Advise that they do not correct the problem and that amenorrhea will likely resume after they are discontinued. For athletes who find it desirable to avoid menses, monophasic oral contraceptives can sometimes be given without the usual placebo week; the benefits of estrogen are achieved and vaginal bleeding is usually avoided.

            ii. **Cyclic estrogen/progestin administration** is another option; it has the advantage of not suppressing the hypothalamic-pituitary axis; recovery from amenorrhea is suspected when bleeding is erratic.

            iii. Symptoms of normal estrogen levels are transitory but occasionally marked in these women used to the hypoestrogenic state; they include breast tenderness and bloating.

        f. Bone mineral density examination at 1–2 year intervals if estrogen is refused.

        g. Suggest reassessment every 3–6 months.

    2. **Adult female who desires conception:**

        a. The reproductive effects of athletic amenorrhea are reversible.

        b. Optimize nutritional intake including calcium.

        c. *Very strongly* advise a decrease in exercise intensity.

        d. Exclude other causes of infertility with semen analysis on partner and possibly evaluation of tubal function wiht hysterosalpingogram.

        e. Ovulation induction

            i. **Clomiphene citrate** may be successful if any bleeding occurs after progestin challenge; sometimes 25 mg rather than the standard 50-mg dose is more successful.

      ii. **Pulsatile GnRH** administered via infusion pump results in ovulation in >90% of women with hypothalamic amenorrhea.

      iii. **Human menopausal gonadotropins** (Pergonal) are also very successful in achieving ovulation, but these are associated with a higher chance of multiple pregnancies than the GnRH pump.

3. **Adolescent female:** May have delayed menarche or amenorrhea after one or more menstrual periods.

    a. Optimize nutritional intake including calcium; follow carefully to ensure that anorexia nervosa was not missed at original assessment.

    b. Consider modifying training program.

    c. Usually delay estrogen until age 16–18 unless there is a history of stress fractures or if 2 or more years of amenorrhea have occurred after menarche. The appropriate time to initiate estrogen therapy remains controversial; further studies on bone mineral density and longer follow-up are needed to determine if estrogen therapy should be prescribed more aggressively in this age group.

    d. Discuss contraception.

    e. Long-term consequences of adolescent amenorrhea remain to be determined.

    f. Reassessment at least every 3–6 months to ensure that training and diet modifications are being followed.

REFERENCES

1. American Academy of Pediatrics, Committee on Sports Medicine: Amenorrhea in adolescent athletes. Pediatrics 84:394–395, 1989.
2. Baer JT, Taper LJ: Amenorrheic and eumenorrheic adolescent runners: Dietary intake and exercise training status. J Am Diet Assoc 92:89–91, 1992.
3. Bullen BA, Skrinar GS, Beitins IZ, et al: Induction of menstrual disorders in untrained women by strenuous exercise. N Engl J Med 312:1349–1353, 1985.
4. Carr DB, Bullen BA, Skrinar GS, et al: Physical conditioning facilitates the exercise-induced secretion of beta-endorphin and beta-lipoprotein in women. N Engl J Med 305:560–563, 1981.
5. Cumming DC, Vickovic MM, Wall SR, et al: The effect of acute exercise on pulsatile release of luteinizing hormone in women runners. Am J Obstet Gynecol 153:482–485, 1985.
6. Davies M, Hall M, Jacobs H: Bone mineral loss in young women with amenorrhera. BMJ 301:790–793, 1990.
7. DeCree C: Endogenous opioid peptides in the control of the normal menstrual cycle and their possible role in athletic menstrual irregularities. Obstet Gynecol Surv 44:720–732, 1989.
8. DeSouza MJ, Metzger DA: Reproductive dysfunction in amenorrheic athletes and anorexic patients: A review. Med Sci Sports Exerc 23:995–1007, 1991.
9. Drinkwater BL, Nilson K, Chestnut CH, et al: Bone mineral content of amenorrheic and eumenorrheic athletes. N Engl J Med 311:277–281, 1984.
10. Emans SJ, Grace E, Hoffer FA, et al: Estrogen deficiency in adolescents and young adults: Impact on bone mineral content and effects of estrogen replacement therapy. Obstet Gynecol 76:585, 1990.
11. Frisch RE, Gotz-Welbergen AV, McArthur JW, et al: Delayed menarche and amenorrhea of college athletes in relation to age of onset of training. JAMA 246:1559–1563, 1981.
12. Frisch RE, McArthur JW: Menstrual cycles: Fatness as a determinant of minimum weight for height necessary for their maintenance or onset. Science 185:949–951, 1974.
13. Frisch RE, Wyshak G, Vincent L: Delayed menarche and amenorrhea in ballet dancers. N Engl J Med 303:17–19, 1980.
14. Gadpaille WJ, Sanborn CF, Wagner WW: Athletic amenorrhea, major affective disorders, and eating disorders. Am J Psychiatry 14:939–942, 1987.
15. Glass AR, Deuster PA, Kyle SB, et al: Amenorrhea in Olympic marathon runners. Fertil Steril 48:740–745, 1987.
16. Johnson J, Whitaker AH: Adolescent smoking, weight changes, and binge-purge behavior: Association with secondary amenorrhea. Am J Public Health 82:47–54, 1992.
17. Laughlin GA, Loucks AB, Yen SSC: Marked augmentation of nocturnal melatonin secretion in amenorrheic athletes, but not in cycling athletes: Unaltered by opioidergic or dopaminergic blockade. J Clin Endocrinol Metab 73:1321–1326, 1991.
18. Liu JH: Hypothalamic amenorrhea: Clinical perspectives, pathophysiology, and management. Am J Obstet Gynecol 163:1732–1736, 1990.

19. Lloyd T, Triantafyllou SJ, Baker ER, et al: Women athletes with menstrual irregularity have increased musculoskeletal injuries. Med Sci Sports Exerc 18:374–379, 1986.
20. Loucks AB, Horvath SM: Athletic amenorrhea: A review. Med Sci Sports Exerc 17:56–72, 1985.
21. Loucks AB, Horvath SM: Exercise-induced stress responses of amenorrheic and eumenorrheic runners. J Clin Endocrinol Metab 59:1109–1120, 1984.
22. Loucks AB, Laughlin GA, Mortola JF, et al: Hypothalamic-pituitary-thyroidal function in eumenorrheic and amenorrheic athletes. J Clin Endocrinol Metab 75:514–518, 1992.
23. Loucks AB, Mortola JF, Girton L, et al: Alterations in the hypothalamic-pituitary-ovarian and hypothalamic-pituitary-adrenal axes in athletic women. J Clin Endocrinol Metab 68:402–411, 1989.
24. Malina RM: Menarche in athletes: A synthesis and hypothesis. Ann Hum Biol 10:1–24, 1983.
25. Malina R, Spirduso W, Tate C: Age at menarche and selected menstrual characteristics in athletes at different competitive levels and in different sports. Med Sci Sports Exerc 10:218–222, 1978.
26. Marcus R, Cann C, Madvig P, et al: Menstrual function and bone mass in elite women distance runners: Endocrine and metabolic features. Ann Intern Med 102:158–163, 1985.
27. Rebar RW: Exercise and the menstrual cycle. In Soules MR (ed): Controversies in Reproductive Endocrinology and Infertility. New York, Elsevier Science Publishing Co., 1989, pp 41–58.
28. Samuels MH, Sanborn CF, Hofeldt F, Robbins R: The role of endogenous opiates in athletic amenorrhea. Fertil Steril 55:507–512, 1991.
29. Sanborn CF, Albrecht BH, Wagner WW Jr: Athletic amenorrhea: Lack of association with body fat. Med Sci Sports Exerc 19:207–212, 1987.
30. Sanborn CF, Martin BJ, Wagner WW: Is athletic amenorrhea specific to runners: Am J Obstet Gynecol 142:859–861, 1982.
31. Schwartz B, Cumming DC, Riordan E, et al: Exercise-associated amenorrhea: A distinct entity? Am J Obstet Gynecol 141:662–670, 1981.
32. Shangold MM, Levine HS: The effect of marathon training upon menstrual function. Am J Obstet Gynecol 143:862–869, 1982.
33. Shangold M, Rebar RW, Wentz AC, Schiff I: Evaluation and management of menstrual dysfunction in athletes. JAMA 263:1665–1669, 1990.
34. Speroff L, Glass RH, Kase NG: Clinical Gynecologic Endocrinology and Infertility, 4th ed. Baltimore, Williams & Wilkins, 1989.
35. Veldhuis JD, Evans WS, Demers LM, et al: Altered neuroendocrine regulation of gonadotropin secretion in women distance runners. J Clin Endocrinol Metab 61:557–563, 1985.
36. Walberg JL, Johnston CS: Menstrual function and eating behavior in female recreational weight lifters and competitive body builders. Med Sci Sports Exerc 23:30–36, 1991.
37. Warren MP: Clinical Review 40: Amenorrhea in endurance runners. J Clin Endocrinol Metab 75:1393–1397, 1992.
38. Warren MP: The effect of exercise on pubertal progression and reproductive function in girls. J Clin Endocrinol Metab 51:1150–1157, 1980.
39. Warren MP, Brooks-Gunn J, Hamilton LH, et al: Scoliosis and fractures in young ballet dancers. N Engl J Med 314:1348–1353, 1986.
40. Weight LM, Noakes TD: Is running an analog of anorexia? A survey of the incidence of eating disorders in female distance runners. Med Sci Sports Exerc 19:213–217, 1987.
41. White CM, Hergenroeder AC: Amenorrhea, osteopenia, and the female athlete. Pediatr Clin North Am 37:1125–1141, 1990.
42. Wildt L, Leyendecker G: Induction of ovulation by the chronic administration of naltrexone in hypothalamic amenorrhea. J Clin Endocrinol Metab 64:1334–1335, 1987.
43. Wilmore JH, Wambsgans KC, Brenner M, et al: Is there energy conservation in amenorrheic compared with eumenorrheic distance runners. J Appl Physiol 72:15–22, 1992.
44. Yen SSC, Jaffe RB: Reproductive Endocrinology, 2nd ed. Philadelphia, W.B. Saunders, 1986.

Chapter 22: Athletic Amenorrhea and Bone Health

CHRISTINE SNOW-HARTER, PhD

For years, it has been known that competitive female athletes have a higher incidence of menstrual cycle irregularities than nonathletic women. Changes in reproductive endocrine function leading to irregular menses range from 2–51% among athletes compared with 2–5% in nonathletes. "Irregularity" is defined as amenorrhea (0–2 periods/year) and oligomenorrhea (3–9 periods/year) (*see* Chapter 21). In many ways, the reproductive endocrine profile of these women is very similar to that of postmenopausal women in that they also exhibit low levels of the hormones estrogen and progesterone. This phenomenon has led researchers to hypothesize that bone mass in these athletes is also reduced as a result of the hormone changes. Over the past 10 years, studies have reported that amenorrheic and oligomenorrheic athletes have bone mass values that are significantly lower than those of other women athletes and nonathletes. This chapter serves to provide background information, highlight specific studies, and present additional supporting information and recommendations.

I. THE MENSTRUAL CYCLE AND ENDOCRINE PROFILE OF THE AMENORRHEIC ATHLETE

A normal menstrual cycle varies between 23–35 days. The cycle is regulated by the hypothalamus, which releases gonadotropin-releasing hormone (GnRH) to stimulate pituitary hormones. It is important to note that the hypothalamus is affected by other endocrine organs (i.e., the adrenal and thyroid glands) as well as external stimuli and stressors.

A. **Follicular phase** of the cycle is characterized by an increase in follicle-stimulating hormone (FSH), which results in the production of estrogen during the first half of the menstrual cycle. These hormones stimulate the formation of the primary follicle and proliferative growth of the uterine lining. Length of the follicular phase is variable.

B. The **luteal phase** is marked by a surge in luteinizing hormone (LH), which is triggered by rising levels of estrogen. A resultant rise in progesterone stimulates maturation of the follicle and ovulation. A normal luteal phase is 14 ± 2 days.

C. If fertilization does not occur, luteal function decreases and menstruation follows an abrupt decline in estrogen and progesterone.

D. The amenorrheic athlete exhibits decreased levels of gonadotropic hormones (FSH, LH), estrogen, and progesterone. This contrasts with the profile of the postmenopausal women whose levels of gonadotropic hormones are elevated.

II. MENSTRUAL IRREGULARITIES ASSOCIATED WITH STRENUOUS EXERCISE TRAINING

Menstrual cycle irregularities associated with exercise training vary.

A. **Amenorrhea** ($\leq$2 menstrual cycles/year)
  1. Accompanied by very low levels of reproductive hormones (estrogen and progesterone)
  2. Skeletal health is greatly compromised as a result, and values for spine bone mineral density (BMD) are often similar to those in postmenopausal women.

B. **Oligomenorrhea** (3–9 menstrual cycles/year)
   1. Accompanied by levels of reproductive hormones that are lower than eumenorrheic women
   2. Women with sporadic periods can lose bone mass due to chronically low levels of estrogen and progesterone.
C. **Menarche** (first menstrual cycle, marks adolescence)
   1. During adolescence, 48% of skeletal mass and 15% of adult height are attained.
   2. Delayed menarche accompanied by hypoestrogenism can have profound negative effect on skeletal development.[1]
D. **Luteal phase deficiency**
   1. Shortened luteal phase and inadequate production of progesterone
   2. Women typically have no symptoms, as menstrual cycle length is usually normal.
   3. There is one report that luteal phase deficiency reduces vertebral bone mass.[18] This remains quite controversial.
E. **Anovulation** (lack of ovulation)
   1. Accompanied by very low levels of progesterone
   2. Women with this problem may have very short (<21 days) or long cycle length (35–150 days).
   3. Anovulation has been associated with reduced bone mass in preliminary investigation.[18] These data are not conclusive.

III. **ETIOLOGY**

Athletic amenorrhea has a multifactorial etiology. In the case of most athletes, no one cause can be singled out.
A. **High-volume, intense training regimens** and **abrupt changes** in training may result in menstrual irregularity.
B. **Decreased caloric consumption** which may lead to an energy deficit appears to be related to menstrual irregularities and possible alteration in metabolism.[22]
C. **Low body weight** may reduce mechanical loading to the skeleton and also the conversion of androgens to estrone, which requires adequate levels of body fat.
D. **Higher cortisol levels** as a result of exercise and stress may impair the hypothalamic-pituitary-ovarian axis.
   1. Increased cortisol may reduce bone mineral density.
   2. Ding et al.[3] reported higher cortisol and lower BMD in amenorrheic versus eumenorrheic athletes.
E. **Athletes at greatest risk** for developing menstrual cycle irregularities are those who begin training early (i.e., prior to age of normal menarche, 12–16 years), adhere to the most intense training regimens, consume the fewest calories, and have the lowest body weight.

IV. **SKELETAL COMPOSITION**

The skeleton is organized into two primary parts, each having different proportions of **cortical bone** (plates of bone that are tightly compacted) and **trabecular bone** (a "spongy" bone with a honeycomb-type network).
A. The **peripheral skeleton**, the long bones, is comprised primarily of cortical bone which is tightly compacted and less susceptible than trabecular bone to alterations in reproductive hormones. Eighty percent of the skeleton is cortical bone.
B. The **axial skeleton** (the vertebral column, pelvis, and ends of long bones) is comprised of a large proportion of trabecular bone, which is highly susceptible to alterations in reproductive hormones.
C. **After peak bone mass is achieved at about the age of 18 years, there is a window of approximately 12 years during which bone mass *may* be gained.** The aging **trabecular** skeleton begins to lose bone early in the fourth decade, and in cyclic women, this loss is accelerated at menopause.

V. EVALUATION OF BONE MINERAL DENSITY BY DUAL ENERGY X-RAY ABSORPTIOMETRY

A. Bone mineral density (bone mineral content/area or volume of bone in the site of measurement) is most precisely measured *indirectly* by dual energy x-ray absorptiometry (DEXA).

B. DEXA uses x-rays that emit two different energies in order to separate bone from surrounding soft tissue. During the assessment, the subject lies quietly on a table for 10–15 minutes while a picture of the bones being scanned is reconstructed on a computer screen and data are collected.

C. The amount of x-ray dose to the subject is <5 mrem/scan. This value can be compared with that of a chest x-ray at 20–60 mrem or a full dental x-ray at 300 mrem.

D. In addition to the value of bone mass measurements for assessing skeletal status in research settings, many intervention strategies for osteoporosis depend upon accurate bone mass measurements. Because osteoporotic fractures are due, at least in part, to low bone mineral density, evaluation by DEXA can help to estimate fracture risk and to make sound clinical decisions.[9]

VI. BONE MINERAL DENSITY AND MENSTRUAL STATUS IN ATHLETES

A. **Vertebral BMD is lower in amenorrheic athletes than in controls.**
   1. In the past 10 years, Drinkwater et al.,[4] Cann et al.,[2] Lindberg et al.,[10] and Linnell et al.[12] reported significantly lower vertebral BMD in amenorrheic athletes when compared with eumenorrheic women, suggesting osteopenia (lower-than-normal bone mass) in this population.
   2. Marcus et al.[13] reported vertebral BMD to be 20% lower in amenorrheic athletes than in cyclic athletes and 10% lower than in nonathletic cyclic women of similar age.
      a. Athletes were matched for aerobic capacity, percent body fat, exercise intensity, and age of menarche.
      b. Radial (cortical) BMD did not significantly differ between groups.

B. **Menstrual history as a determinant of BMD**
   1. Drinkwater et al.[6] observed vertebral BMD to be significantly lower in athletes with lifetime histories of irregular menses.
   2. Findings support earlier data that menstrual history is a primary determinant of trabecular BMD.
      a. Subjects with lowest values were characterized by lower estradiol, progesterone, and body weight and by later menarche.
      b. Subjects with lowest values began training earliest, trained the greater number of miles per week, and were youngest.

C. **Peripheral bone mass is lower in amenorrheic athletes.**
   1. Drinkwater et al.[6] reported lower femur mid-shaft BMD in athletes with menstrual irregularities since menarche compared with cyclic women or women with episodic irregularities.
   2. Myburgh et al.[15] found femoral-neck and whole-body BMD significantly lower in amenorrheic athletes than in controls.

VII. RISK FACTOR ASSESSMENT

A. **All groups of competitive athletes with menstrual cycle irregularities may *not* be at risk for developing low bone mass.**
   1. Recent work investigating two groups of athletes (gymnasts and runners) produced results that contradict the notion that all athletes with menstrual cycle irregularities have bone mass values that are lower than eumenorrheic controls.
   2. Robinson et al.[19] have reported that competitive female **gymnasts** experiencing the same incidence of menstrual cycle irregularities as competitive female **runners** have bone mass values for the hip and lumbar spine **well above the mean for their age.**

3. This suggests either that gymnasts produce other systemic or local factors that offset low levels of estrogen and progesterone or that the high mechanical forces of the sport can override the negative influence of low hormone levels.

B. **Hypoestrogenism and possibly low progesterone** diminish an athlete's ability to fully *develop* skeletal mass, *attain* peak bone mass, and *maintain* bone mass. This may increase an athlete's risk of stress fractures and premature osteoporotic fractures.

   1. **Stress fractures:** Evidence generally supports a higher incidence of stress fractures in amenorrheic athletes, particularly those with late menarche.[13,14,20] Late menarche in some athletes may seriously alter skeletal mass development during adolescence and reduce peak bone mass.

   2. **Premature osteoporotic fractures:** Reduced bone mass as a result of menstrual cycle irregularities may predispose athletes to early osteoporotic fractures. A premature osteoporotic fracture of the femur resulting from the lower BMD values has been reported in an amenorrheic athlete with a history of menstrual cycle irregularity.[8] Additionally, many athletes with menstrual cycle irregularity have lumbar spine bone mass values that are similar to those of postmenopausal women.

VIII. REVERSIBILITY OF BONE LOSS

Reversibility of bone loss among athletes with menstrual cycle irregularities is not well studied. Two studies indicate that lumbar spine BMD can be partially restored upon resumption of menses but still remains lower than in eumenorrheic athletes.

A. Lindbergh et al.[11] evaluated 7 runners with athletic amenorrhea over a 15-month period. Four runners with low vertebral bone mass took supplemental calcium and reduced weekly running distance by 43%, which resulted in a 5% increase in body weight, normal periods, and increased estradiol levels. Bone mass increased an average of 6.7%. The remaining 3 runners did not change their exercise levels and remained amenorrheic with low estradiol levels and no change in bone mass, despite supplemental calcium.

B. Drinkwater et al.[5] studied 9 amenorrheic runners for 15.5 months. Seven runners who had decreased training mileage and intensity and increased body weight had regained their menses. Vertebral bone mass was increased by 6.3% in these women, while the 2 runners who remained amenorrheic lost 3.4%.

C. Two recent studies investigating increased calcium intake (1500 mg/day) have shown no change in BMD at the proximal femur or lumbar spine after 12 and 24 months of intervention.[7,21] However, Drinkwater et al.[7] did observe an increase in tibial BMD in the high-calcium amenorrheic group, indicating a site specificity.

IX. RECOMMENDATIONS FOR FEMALE ATHLETES

A. **Complete, thorough histories** on all female athletes is recommended. Additionally, it is necessary to maintain a close relationship wiht athletes and query them regarding menstrual cycle irregularities.

B. **Bone mass evaluation** may be indicated to assess skeletal status of an athlete with menstrual cycle irregularity. Recommendations for treatment can be based, in part, upon these results. Currently, the most accurate method of bone mass evaluation is DEXA.

C. For athletes experiencing menstrual cycle irregularities accompanied by low bone mass, **a decrease in training intensity and volume** may be indicated. For runners, a reduction of 16–32 km/week has been recommended.

D. **An increase in total calories and calcium intake** (1200–1500 mg/day) is suggested. Both could be accomplished by adding 3 glasses of skim milk to the daily dietary patterns.

E. **Estrogen replacement therapy** (ERT) may be indicated for women who are not willing to make changes in exercise or dietary patterns. While there are currently no controlled trials which examine the efficacy of ERT for treating these athletes, it is assumed that the doses prescribed to postmenopausal women would be adequate for reducing bone loss among amenorrheic athletes.

REFERENCES

1. Bachrach LK, Katzman DK, Litt LF, et al: Recovery from osteopenia in adolescent girls with anorexia nervosa. J Clin Endocrinol Metab 72:602–606, 1991.
2. Cann CE, Martin MC, Genant HK, Jaffe RR: Decreased spinal mineral content in amenorrheic women. JAMA 251:626–629, 1984.
3. Ding J, Checkter CB, Drinkwater BL, et al: High serum cortisol levels in exercise-associated amenorrhea. Ann Intern Med 108:530–534, 1988.
4. Drinkwater BL, Milson K, Chesnut CH III, et al: Bone mineral content of amenorrheic and eumenorrheic athletes. N Engl J Med 311:277–281, 1984.
5. Drinkwater BL, Bruemer B, Chesnut CH III: Bone mineral density after resumption of menses in amenorrheic athletes. JAMA 256:380–382, 1986.
6. Drinkwater BL, Bruemer B, Chesnut CH III: Menstrual history as a determinant of current bone density in young athletes. JAMA 263:545–548, 1990.
7. Drinkwater BL, Chesnut CH III: Site specific skeletal response to increased calcium in amenorrheic athletes. Med Sci Sport Exerc 24(5):S45, 1992.
8. Dugowson CE, Drinkwater BL, Clark J: Nontraumatic femur fracture in an oligomenorrheic athlete. Med Sci Sport Exerc 23:1323–1325, 1991.
9. Johnston CC Jr, Melton LJ III: Bone density measurement and management of osteoporosis. In Favus MJ (ed): Primer on the Metabolic Bone Diseases and Disorders of Mineral Metabolism, 2nd ed. New York, Raven Press, 1993.
10. Lindberg JS, Fears WB, Hunt MM, et al: Exercise-induced amenorrhea and bone density. Ann Intern Med 101:647–648, 1984.
11. Lindberg JS, Powell MR, Hunt MM, et al: Increased vertebral bone mineral in response to reduced exercise in amenorrheic runners. West J Med 146:39–42, 1987.
12. Linnell SI, Stager JM, Blue PW, et al: Bone mineral content and menstrual irregularity in female runners. Med Sci Sport Exerc 16:343–348, 1984.
13. Marcus R, Cann C, Madvig P, et al: Menstrual function and bone mass in elite women distance runners: Endocrine metabolic features. Ann Intern Med 102:158–163, 1985.
14. Myburgh K, Hutchins J, Fataar AB, et al: Low bone density is an etiologic factor for stress fractures in athletes. Ann Intern Med 113:754–759, 1990.
15. Myburgh K, Bachrach LK, Lewis B, et al: Low bone mineral density at axial and appendicular sites in amenorrheic athletes. Med Sci Sport Exerc 25:1197–1202, 1993.
16. Myerson M, Gutin B, Warren MP, et al: Total body bone density in amenorrheic runners. Obstet Gynecol 79(6):973–978, 1992.
17. Nelson ME, Fisher EC, Castos PD, et al: Diet and bone status in amenorrheic runners. Am J Clin Nutr 43:910–916, 1986.
18. Prior JC, Vigna YM, Martin RN, et al: Spinal bone loss and ovulatory disturbances. N Engl J Med 323:1221–1227, 1990.
19. Robinson T, Snow-Harter C, Gillis D, Shaw J: Bone mineral density and menstrual cycle status in competitive female runners and gymnasts. Med Sci Sport Exerc 25(Suppl):S49, 1993.
20. Warren MP, Brooks-Gunn J, Fox RP, et al: Lack of bone accretion and amenorrhea: Evidence for a relative osteopenia in weight-bearing bones. J Clin Endocrinol Metab 72:847–853, 1991.
21. Weltman A, Snead DB, Weltman JY, et al: Effects of calcium supplementation on bone mineral density (BMD) in premenopausal women. Med Sci Sport Exerc 24(5):S12, 1992.
22. Wilmore JH, Wambsgans KC, Brenner M, et al: Is there energy conservation in amenorrheic compared with eumenorrheic distance runners? J Appl Physiol 72:15–22, 1992.

Chapter 23: The Female Athlete Triad

AURELIA NATTIV, MD
KIMBERLY YEAGER, MD, MPH
BARBARA DRINKWATER, PhD
ROSEMARY AGOSTINI, MD

Although the increased participation of women in physical activity has led, for the most part, to significant health benefits and to improved physical fitness and well-being, some women face a risk for the development of one or more of a triad of medical disorders, collectively known as the *female athlete triad*.[1,30] Each of these disorders is examined individually in other chapters.

I. GENERAL CONSIDERATIONS

A. **The *female athlete triad* refers to the interrelatedness of three medical disorders:**
   1. Disordered eating
   2. Amenorrhea
   3. Osteoporosis
B. **Etiology**
   1. The female athlete feels pressure to fit a specific athletic image (e.g., leanness, low percent body fat, or lower weight) in order to reach her performance goals; to control her weight, she may develop a pattern of **disordered eating.**[3,30]
   2. Disordered eating may lead to **menstrual dysfunction.**[3,6,14,17,25]
   3. Amenorrhea or oligomenorrhea, in turn, leads to premature **osteoporosis.**[7,26]
C. **Each disorder is of significant medical concern** in its own right, but collectively, there is a potential for serious health effects and risk of mortality.[18,19]
   1. **Mortality** among *treated* anorectic women (nonathletes) is 10–18%. In addition, there may be lifelong psychological problems and severe health problems due to any one of the triad disorders.
   2. The emphasis must be on identifying women at risk and on **prevention and early treatment.**
D. **Federal legislation** in the form of the Women's Health Equity Act of 1993 recognizes eating disorders as a priority item regarding women's health and, through an incorporated bill, the Eating Disorders Act of 1993, provides information and education to the public on prevention and treatment of eating disorders.

II. COMPONENT DISORDERS

A. **Disordered eating** (*see* Chapter 20)
   1. Refers to the spectrum of abnormal patterns of eating:
      a. **Behaviors**
         i. Binging with or without purging
         ii. Food restriction
         iii. Prolonged fasting
         iv. Purging by use of diet pills, laxatives, diuretics, self-induced vomiting, and/or excessive exercise
         v. Loss of control over eating
      b. **Thought patterns**
         i. Preoccupation with food
         ii. Dissatisfaction with one's body
         iii. Fear of becoming fat

      iv. Distorted body image

      v. Overconcern with body shape and weight

    c. **Anorexia nervosa** and **bulimia nervosa** are at the extreme end of the spectrum of disordered eating.

    d. Although most athletes do not meet the strict clinical criteria for anorexia or bulimia nervosa,[2] many exhibit similar behaviors and thought patterns which place them at significant risk for developing eating disorders and their sequelae.

B. **Amenorrhea** (*see* Chapter 21)

  1. **Secondary amenorrhea:** Defined as the absence of at least 3–6 consecutive menstrual cycles in a woman who has already begun menstruating.

  2. **Primary amenorrhea:** Female athletes who begin training before puberty may experience **delayed menarche**, defined as no menstrual periods by age 16 years.

  3. **Menstrual irregularities** seen in female athletes may also fall along a spectrum and range from the extreme of **hypoestrogenic amenorrhea** to periods of **oligomenorrhea** (menstrual cycles >36 days) and includes luteal suppression.

    a. **Oligomenorrhea** may result from anovulation, in which estrogen is produced but there is no basal body temperature rise and low levels of progesterone, or from low levels of estrogen and progesterone.[25]

    b. **Luteal suppression** may occur in athletes[14,17] and is manifested by a shortened luteal phase and inadequate production of progesterone. These women often present with irregular menses, although some have normal menses. Luteal phase suppression may be an early stage of menstrual dysfunction[24] or may represent an athletic training response.[14,17]

C. **Osteoporosis** (*see* Chapters 22 and 24)

  1. In young athletes, it refers to premature bone loss and inadequate bone formation, resulting in low bone mass, microarchitectural deterioration, increased skeletal fragility, and increased risk for fracture.[16,30]

  2. **Premature osteoporosis** may occur in the young female athlete[8] and may be irreversible, even with calcium supplementation, resumption of menses, or estrogen replacement therapy.[5,9]

  3. **Acceleration of trabecular bone mass** occurs in the immediate postmenopausal period as well as in women undergoing oophorectomy, presumably due to the hypoestrogenic state.[11,26] If this pattern is also true in young athletes, early intervention to maintain skeletal integrity becomes very important.

III. PREVALENCE

There is a lack of data or exact numbers with regard to the female athlete triad, in part due to the secretive nature of disordered eating as well as the denial and minimizing of symptoms by affected persons. Self-report questionnaires probably underreport the true prevalence.

A. In the general female population, using the strict DSM-IV criteria,[2] the prevalence of **anorexia nervosa** is 1% and **bulimia nervosa** is 1–3%.

  1. Some studies of disordered eating patterns in young female athletes [22,23] report rates of 15–62%.

  2. Prevalence of disordered eating in athletes and nonathletes is higher in adolescent and younger women, those with higher socioeconomic status, and those with a family history of disordered eating.

B. **Amenorrhea** occurs more commonly in athletes (3.4–66%) than in the general female population (2–5%) and has been reported to be higher in certain sports.[17,24]

C. The prevalence of **premature osteoporosis** in young females, athletic or nonathletic, is not known. Lower bone age has been reported in some young athletes with delayed menarche, and increased risk of stress fractures and scoliosis has been noted in ballet dancers with delayed menarche.[28]

D. On the other hand, some researchers have demonstrated that **high-intensity exercise may increase bone mineral density (BMD) at specific skeletal sites that are maximally stressed,**[15] even in amenorrheic and oligomenorrheic athletes.[26,27,29] In some studies, female gymnasts, elite rowers, and elite young figure skaters with amenorrhea and oligomenorrhea have had greater BMD in the upper and lower extremities, lumbar spine, and pelvis and legs, respectively, than nonathlete controls.

1. **Greater mechanical loading forces** generated at specific skeletal sites in certain sports may provide more effective osteogenic stimulus compared to lower, more evenly distributed loads seen in other sports or nonathletes and may partially offset the adverse effects of amenorrhea on BMD at these sites.
2. It cannot be concluded that amenorrheic female athletes in these sports do not experience premature osteoporosis.
3. Recommended preventive strategies and treatments should be implemented in all female athletes with disordered eating and menstrual irregularities until more research has been conducted.

IV. RISK PROFILE

A. Sports in which low body weight and lean physique are considered advantageous place athletes at greater risk, **especially those athletes at elite or highly competitive levels**:
   1. Gymnastics, figure skating, ballet dancing, distance running
   2. Judging for some sports may be subjective and influenced by esthetics, height, weight, age, and body type.
B. **Individual sports** seem to place athletes more at risk than team sports, because pressure is on the athlete to fit a certain pattern or body type.
C. Sports focusing on **ideal body weight or optimal percent body fat** confer increased risk. In distance running or gymnastics, for example, low percent body fat or weight is often believed by athletes to be associated with improved performance, despite little evidence to support this perception.
D. A **sport-athlete mismatch** can place an athlete at risk, when an athlete may not have the genetic capability to attain the presumed ideal body type for the sport.
E. During **adolescence and young adulthood,** there is significant risk, due to psychological and societal pressures as well as biologic factors. Skeletal integrity is a key risk because of the rapid growth and development occurring at this time.
F. Females are at greater risk than males to develop disordered eating (female-to-male ratio = 9:1), but **some male sports** such as wrestling place athletes at greater risk because of pressure to "make weight." Premature osteoporosis has been seen in males with delayed puberty, anorexia and nutritional disorders, as well as long-distance runners;[10,12,20] although the pathophysiology is unclear, parallels may be drawn to the female triad.

V. PREDISPOSING FACTORS

A. **Internal factors**
   1. **Focus on thinness or an ideal body type and weight:** Often the initial impetus to the development of disordered eating patterns and subsequent triad disorders. The proposed mechanisms for athletic amenorrhea include:
      a. Caloric intake insufficient for energy expenditure in exercise training results in an **energy drain**, leading to a decrease in basal metabolic rate and subsequent hypothalamic dysfunction[14,17]; *or*
      b. Inhibition of the hypothalamic gonadotropin-releasing hormone pulse (decreasing luteinizing hormone and follicle-stimulating hormone) by activation of the adrenal axis in strenuously exercising athletes.[4,6,14]
   2. **Life stressors, abrupt changes in body composition, nulliparity, and previous history of delayed menarche, and/or menstrual irregularity:** May also predispose

athletes to menstrual dysfunction and a hypoestrogenic state.[3,14,17] There is probably no single factor sufficient to explain exercise-associated amenorrhea. The etiology and pathophysiology seem to be multifactorial.

  B. **External factors**
    1. **"Win at all costs" mentality:** Coaches and parents can place incredible pressure on young athletes and inadvertently make a psychological impact. Pressure to excel and the emphasis on low body weight/thinness can place the athlete at risk for the triad disorders.
    2. **Harmful training techniques and strict weight standards:** Coaching strategies involving daily or frequent "weigh-ins" are common themes in athletes with disordered eating histories. Also, **punitive measures** or **negative reinforcement** for weight gain or poor performance are common predisposing factors to disordered eating patterns.
    3. **Overly controlling coach or parent:** The athlete who perceives no control over her environment often compensates by controlling her food intake. These highly perfectionistic, competitive athletes perceive the need for more control over their highly structured lives and manifest it in excessive exercise, food restriction, or pathogenic behaviors.
    4. **Social isolation:** Lack of a social support system with peers may predispose athletes to disordered eating. Many of these athletes have fairly narrow goals and life interests that focus on their sport and winning, incorporating extremely regimented diets and minimal socializing.
    5. **Family history:** Disordered eating is more common in athletes with a family history of these disorders and may predispose these women to subsequent triad disorders.
    6. **Societal influences:** Schools and universities which rely on athletic success for notoriety and financial support often overpraise successful athletes or those who fit the image of what an athlete should look like, thus inadvertently contributing to the development of triad disorders in female athletes. Society also promotes stereotyped images of the small, thin, petite female athlete (e.g., gymnasts).

VI. **SCREENING**
  A. The team physician, primary-care physician, and other members of the athlete's health care team should have an increased awareness of the problem and its presenting signs and symptoms. **All female athletes should be evaluated carefully.**[3,13,30]
  B. **Following the screening history and physical examination,** the athlete identified as at risk should be scheduled for follow-up visits with the physician for a thorough diagnostic work-up and more detailed history and physical examination, as well as a pelvic examination if menstrual dysfunction is present.
    1. The multidisciplinary team, including a nutritionist and psychologist familiar with the triad, may need to be consulted.
    2. Educating the athlete about potential short-term and long-term consequences of the triad disorders is of paramount importance.
  C. The **preparticipation physical examination** offers an ideal opportunity for screening the athlete.
    1. Information should be requested on:
      a. Disordered eating behaviors
      b. Amenorrhea or a history of menstrual irregularity and delayed menarche
      c. History of stress fractures or potentially pathologic fractures
      d. Life stressors
      e. Depressive symptoms
      f. Dissatisfaction with weight or body shape
      g. Training intensity
      h. Pressures from coach, parents, peers to excel and/or lose weight.

2. The athlete will usually not bring such personal issues to the attention of the physician unless specifically asked.

3. In the athlete with menstrual irregularities, eliminate other potential causes of menstrual dysfunction before attributing it to sports and exercise.

VII. PREVENTION AND TREATMENT

A. **Treatment relies on prevention,** which ultimately depends on widespread educational efforts to reach the athlete.

B. **"Calls to Action":** The American College of Sports Medicine Ad Hoc Task Force on Women's Issues in Sports Medicine has developed an action plan that addresses strategies for future prevention and treatment of the triad disorders:[1]

1. **Prevention**
   a. Develop health advisories and educational modules.
   b. Promote safe weight-training techniques.
   c. Evaluate all women with changes in menstruation and weight.
   d. Promote positive and realistic images of active women.
   e. Include screening and evaluation for triad disorders in preparticipation physicals.

2. **Research**
   a. Facilitate and support research in areas of body composition, weight loss, disordered eating, menstrual function, and osteoporosis.

3. **Health consequences**
   a. Increase awareness of the triad's existence.
   b. Develop multidisciplinary teams to evaluate and treat triad disorders, provide support services, remove contributing factors, and develop risk profiles.
   c. Define parameters for percentage of lean mass, strength, etc., compatible with optimal performance and health.
   d. Better describe and quantify the morbidity and the risk of mortality of triad disorders.

4. **Medical care**
   a. Increase awareness through medical advisories or publications to remove "at-risk" athletes from competition.
   b. Develop guidelines for hormonal nutritional treatment and bone mass assessment.

5. **Education**
   a. Facilitate the development of educational materials.
   b. Develop a Triad Coalition.
   c. Identify newsletters already in existence and disseminate.
   d. Provide public service announcements on triad disorders.
   e. Propose a scientific symposium at the International Olympic Committee's Sports Medicine Conference at the 1996 Olympics.
   f. Develop a speakers' bureau and engage other physician groups.

6. **Agency and administration responsibilities**
   a. Better describe and convey the administration's role and responsibility in perpetuating conditions that facilitate the development of triad disorders and in preventing the conditon.
   b. Provide information and speakers to conferences at high school, college, and club administrative meetings.

REFERENCES

1. American College of Sports Medicine: The female athlete triad: Disordered eating, amenorrhea, osteoporosis: Call to action. Sports Med Bull 27(4), 1992.
2. American Psychiatric Association: Diagnostic and Statistical Manual of Mental Disorders–IV. Washington, DC, American Psychiatric Press, 1994.

3. Brownell KD, Rodin J, Wilmore JH (eds): Eating, Body Weight and Performance in Athletes. Philadelphia, Lea & Febiger, 1992.
4. Bullen BA, Skrinar GS, et al: Induction of menstrual disorders by strenuous exercise in untrained women. N Engl J Med 312:1349, 1985.
5. Cann CE, Martin MC, Genant HK, et al: Decreased spinal mineral content in amenorrheic women. JAMA 251:626, 1984.
6. De Souza MJ, Metzger DA: Reproductive dysfunction in amenorrheic athletes and anorexic patients: A review. Med Sci Sports Exerc 23(9):995, 1991.
7. Drinkwater BL, Bruemmer B, Chestnut CH III: Menstrual history as a determinant of current bone density in young athletes. JAMA 263:545, 1990.
8. Drinkwater BL, Nilson K, Chestnut CH III, et al: Bone mineral content of amenorrheic and eumenorrheic athletes. N Engl J Med 311:277, 1984.
9. Drinkwater BL, Nilson K, Chestnut CH III, et al: Bone mineral density after resumption of menses in amenorrheic athletes. JAMA 256:380, 1986.
10. Finkelstein JS, Neer RM, Beverly MK, et al: Osteopenia in men with a history of delayed puberty. N Engl J Med 326:600, 1992.
11. Gallagher JC, Goldgar D, Moy A: Total bone calcium in normal women: Effect of age and menopause status. J Bone Miner Res 2:491, 1987.
12. Hetland ML, Haarbo J, Christiansen C: Low bone mass and high bone turnover in male long distance runners. J Clin Endocrinol Metab 77:770, 1993.
13. Johnson MD: Tailoring the preparticipation exam to female athletes. Phys Sportsmed 20(7):61, 1992.
14. Loucks AB: Effects of exercise training on the menstrual cycle: Existence and mechanisms. Med Sci Sports Exerc 22:275, 1990.
15. Marcus R, Drinkwater B, Dalsky G, et al: Osteoporosis and exercise in women. Med Sci Sports Exer 24(suppl 6):S301, 1992.
16. Myburgh K, Hutchins J, Fataar AB, et al: Low bone density is an etiologic factor for stress fractures in athletes. Ann Intern Med 113:754, 1990.
17. Otis CL: Exercise-associated amenorrhea. Clin Sports Med 11:351, 1992.
18. Palla B, Litt IF: Medical complications of eating disorders in adolescents. Pediatr 81:613, 1988.
19. Ratnasuriya RH, Eisler I, Szmukler GI, et al: Anorexia nervosa: Outcome and prognostic factors after 20 years: Brit J Psych 158:495, 1991.
20. Rigotti NA, Neer RM, Jameson L: Osteopenia and bone fractures in a man with anorexia nervosa and hypogonadism. JAMA 256:385, 1986.
21. Rigotti NA, Neer RM, Skates SJ, et al: The clinical course of osteoporosis in anorexia nervosa: A longitudinal study of cortical bone mass. JAMA 265:1133, 1991.
22. Rosen LW, Hough DO: Pathogenic weight control behaviors of female college gymnasts. Physician Sportsmed 16(9):141, 1988.
23. Rosen LW, McKeag DB, Hough DO, et al: Pathogenic weight control behaviors of female college athletes. Physician Sportsmed 14(1):79, 1986.
24. Shangold M: Menstruation. In Shangold M, Mirkin G (eds): Women and Exercise. Philadelphia, F.A. Davis, 1988, pp 129–145.
25. Shangold M, Rebar RW, Wentz AC, et al: Evaluation and management of menstrual dysfunction in athletes. JAMA 263:1665, 1990.
26. Slemenda CW, Johnston CC: High intensity activities in young women: Site specific bone mass effects among female figure skaters. Bone Miner 20:125, 1993.
27. Snow-Harter C, Bouxsein M, Lewis B, et al: Effects of resistance and endurance exercise on bone mineral status of young women: A randomized exercise intervention trial. J Bone Miner Res 7:761, 1992.
28. Warren MP, Brooks-Gunn J, Hamilton WG: Scoliosis and fractures in young ballet dancers: Relation to delayed menarche and secondary amenorrhea. N Engl J Med 314:1348, 1986.
29. Wolman RL, Clark P, McNally E, et al: Menstrual state and exercise as determinants of spinal trabecular bone density in female athletes. Br Med J 301:516, 1990.
30. Yeager KK, Agostini R, Nattiv A Drinkwater B: The female athlete triad: Disordered eating, amenorrhea, osteoporosis [commentary]. Med Sci Sports Exerc 25:775, 1993.

Chapter 24: Osteoporosis and Menopause

DAWN P. LEMCKE, MD

Osteoporosis is a significant cause of morbidity and mortality, particularly in the postmenopausal woman. The current state-of-the art treatment of osteoporosis continues to be in flux as new treatments and data are revisited. At present, prevention of osteoporosis is clearly the most efficacious in decreasing morbidity and mortality from fractures. The current mainstays of prevention are estrogen replacement therapy, calcium supplementation, vitamin D, and appropriate exercise.

I. SCOPE OF THE PROBLEM

   A. Osteoporosis represents a major public health problem in the U.S., affecting 15–20 million persons/year, mostly postmenopausal women. It accounts for 1.3 million fractures/year.
   B. **Major manifestations are:**
   1. Proximal hip fractures (250,000/year)
   2. Distal forearm and Colles' fracture (250,000/year)
   3. Vertebral fractures (500,000/year)
   4. All of the above fractures cost over $10 billion annually (in 1986 dollars).
   C. 15% of white women will fracture a hip in their lifetime, with a mortality of 5–20% higher in the year following the fracture than is expected for age-matched controls. 15% of white women over age 50 will have a wrist fracture in their lifetime.
   D. With the increase in the elderly population, over the next 30 years there may be 350,000 hip fractures/year at an annual cost of $31–62 billion.
   E. For many, it means the end of independent life with an additional cost and decreased quality of life.
   F. To reduce the number of fractures, prevention is the key, rather than improving methods of treating the subsequent fractures.

II. PATHOPHYSIOLOGY OF OSTEOPOROSIS

   A. **Definition:** Osteoporosis is characterized by low bone mass, microarchitectural deterioration of bone tissue leading to bone fragility, and consequent increase in fracture risk.
   1. **Bone mass peaks** shortly after puberty at the end of the growth period, about age 17. Small gains in bone mass may be achieved to age 30, followed by progressive loss of bone mass.
   2. **Biphasic pattern in bone loss:** slow protracted phase in both men and women, and an accelerated phase which is transient and affects only menopausal women.
   3. The **accelerated phase** generally occurs after menopause and lasts 5–10 years, at which time a woman may have lost 30–40% of her total bone mass.
   4. Most women do not lose further bone mass after age 70.
   B. **Pathophysiology**
   1. **Slow protracted phase** of osteoporosis is related to decreased bone formation. There is continued activity of osteoclasts, but osteoblasts fail to re-create bone, which leads to decreased overall total bone mass (uncoupling).
   2. **Accelerated phase** of osteoporosis in women shows a marked increase in osteoclastic activity with continued activity in the osteoblasts which cannot keep up with osteoclast activity.

175

3. **Calcium absorption from the gastrointestinal tract** mediated by 1,25-dihy-droxyvitamin D increases until age 65, then decreases. There also appears to be decreased responsiveness of the intestine to 1,25-dihydroxyvitamin D, with subsequent decrease in absorption of calcium.
4. **Elevated parathyroid hormone** (PTH), due to decreased calcium levels, stimulates bone turnover, thus decreasing overall bone density.
5. **Decreasing vitamin D stores.** With age, there is decreased synthesis in the skin of vitamin D and decreased absorption of vitamin D through intestines, thus leading to osteomalacia and increased fracture risk.
6. **Estrogen loss.** The primary effect of estrogen is to decrease bone turnover by decreasing osteoclast activity, which is actually a direct effect of estrogen on bone. A major contribution to accelerated bone loss in postmenopausal women is their loss of intrinsic estrogen. The usual duration of accelerated bone loss is 5–10 years, but even in postmenopausal women more than 10 years after menopause, estrogen replacement can decrease bone resorption and stabilize bone loss.

III. RISK FACTORS

Risk factors fail to identify up to 30% of women at high risk for osteoporosis and subsequent fracture.

A. **Definite risk factors**
   1. **Age**
   2. **Female sex**
   3. **White race** (bone density lowest in whites, then Asians, then blacks and Hispanics)
   4. **Slim body build:** Increasing weight and fat stores lead to increased estrogen and decreased risk of osteoporosis. Increasing weight and muscle mass may also place increased strain on bone which increases overall bone mass.
   5. **Decreased muscle strength**
   6. **Bilateral oophorectomy** prior to age 50
   7. **Heavy alcohol use:** Alcohol impairs bone remodeling. Alcoholics have lower bone mass and increased incidence of falls and thus more fractures. One or more drinks/day in a woman correlates with a 15–40% increased risk of hip fracture.
   8. **Medications:** Corticosteroids, thyroid hormone over-replacement, prolonged heparin use
   9. **Family history:** Daughters of women with vertebral fractures have a slightly lower bone density than age-matched controls.
   10. **Lack of physical activity:** Very sedentary lifestyle (as in prolonged bedrest) markedly reduces bone density. Conversely, professional athletes have somewhat greater bone mass due to increased physical activity.
B. **Controversial risk factors**
   1. **Calcium intake**
      a. In women who had been menopausal for >6 years and had calcium intake <400 mg/day, bone mass became stable when calcium intake was increased and supplemented to 500 mg/day.[11] Only calcium in the form of calcium maleate had that effect when compared with calcium carbonate.
      b. The recommended dose of calcium in postmenopausal women is 1500 mg.
   2. **Caffeine consumption:** Increased amounts may cause urinary loss of calcium.
   3. **Dietary phosphorus:** Increases calcium loss.
   4. **Dietary protein:** Increased amounts may cause urinary loss of calcium.
   5. **Smoking:** May result in decreased bone mass.
   6. **Age of natural menopause**
   7. **Sedentary lifestyle**
C. **Causes of secondary osteoporosis**
   1. **Hyperparathyroidism:** Increased PTH, with subsequent increased osteoclastic activity, means decreasing bone mass.

2. **Hyperthyroidism** (also, over-replacement with thyroid supplementation): The new super-sensitive thyroid-stimulating hormone (TSH) provides excellent ways of monitoring to ensure adequate replacement but not over-physiologic replacement in patients on thyroid medication.

3. **Multiple myeloma**

4. **Chronic steroid use:** As little as the equivalent of 10 mg/day of prednisone markedly accelerates trabecular bone loss, with subsequent increased risk in vertebral fracture.

5. **Amenorrhea:** Can be multifactorial and all cause decreased estrogen levels (e.g., hypothalamic amenorrhea, exercise-induced amenorrhea, anorexia nervosa, and prolatinoma).

   a. Recent evidence shows that even if an anorexic female reached 80% of ideal body weight and uses estrogen or calcium supplementation, she fails to regain normal bone mass.

   b. In the same study, anorexic females who did not attain 80% of ideal body weight had bone loss similar to those who did attain 80% of ideal body weight.

IV. SCREENING FOR OSTEOPOROSIS

A. Methods for measuring bone density

1. **Single-photon absorptiometry**

   a. Limited to peripheral sites and cannot be used to measure spine and hip bone mineral density.

   b. Short scan time of 10–20 minutes

   c. Costs approximately $35–120 a test

   d. 4–5% accuracy with a precision error of 1–2%. May be beneficial in states such as hyperparathyroidism where cortical bone is reduced more than trabecular bone.

2. **Dual-photon absorptiometry**

   a. Can be used for spine and hip measurements.

   b. Scan time is longer, from 20–60 minutes.

   c. Cost generally over $100

   d. 3–6% accuracy with a precision error of 2–4%

3. **Dual-energy x-ray absorptiometry (DEXA)**

   a. Newer technique which replaces an isotope source with an x-ray source.

   b. Short scan time of 10 minutes

   c. Cost approximately $100

   d. 3–6% accuracy with a precision error of <1%, which makes it an excellent test for following a patient over time, to monitor either therapy or ongoing losses.

4. **Quantitative computed tomography (QCT)**

   a. Can be used at any area of the bony skeleton

   b. Scan time 15 minutes

   c. Costs $100–400

   d. 5–10% accuracy with precision error of 4%

B. Who should be screened?

1. **Mass screening** of all women at risk for osteoporosis. Screening in this sense would be defined as the application of tests to measure bone mass in unselected persons who have no apparent signs or symptoms of osteoporosis and who are not seeking care for osteoporosis.

   a. This has not been the approach used to present, perhaps because there is no clearcut guideline as to when to begin treatment.

   b. If this strategy were employed, one study[18] predicts the proportion of women receiving estrogen replacement therapy would increase from 15–19% and lifetime hip fracture risk would fall from 10% to 8%.

    c. At present, none of the major health organizations recommend routine screening for osteoporosis.

    d. If specific programs or protocols were developed with clear guidelines for treatment, then this approach may be justified.

    e. Cost-effectiveness is undetermined.

2. **Selective screening approach** (adapted from Scientific Advisory Board of the National Osteoporosis Foundation[16])

    a. **Indications for bone mass measurement**

       i. Estrogen-deficient women, to diagnose significantly low bone mass in order to make decisions regarding estrogen replacement therapy

       ii. Patients with vertebral abnormalities or radiographic osteopenia, to diagnose spinal osteoporosis in order to make decisions about further diagnostic evaluations and therapy

       iii. Patients receiving glucocorticoid therapy, to diagnose low bone mass in order to adjust therapy

       iv. Patients with primary symptomatic hyperparathyroidism, to diagnose low bone mass in order to identify those at risk for severe skeletal disease who may be candidates for surgical intervention

    b. **Potential indications for bone mass measurement**

       i. Universal screening for osteoporosis prophylaxis

       ii. Monitoring bone mass to assess therapy efficacy. Current methods may not have enough precision to make these useful measurements unless large changes in bone mass are anticipated. DEXA may be useful in following patients (it has a precision error of $<1\%$).

       iii. Identifying "fast losers" of bone for more aggressive therapy

       iv. Evaluating high-risk patients for osteoporosis (amenorrhea, anticonvulsant therapy, thyroid replacement, anorexia nervosa, alcoholism, disuse, multiple atraumatic fractures, breast cancer)

C. **Who should *not* be screened?**

1. If the decision to treat will *not* be affected by bone mass measurement (e.g., if a woman were placed on estrogen therapy for reasons other than osteoporosis or if she would not comply with treatment regardless of the finding, then bone mass measurement is not indicated).

2. If bone mass measurements cannot be performed reliably.

D. **When should bone mass be measured?**

1. No clear consensus exists, but **most recommend that bone mass measurement be performed in the perimenopausal period** (i.e., amenorrhea for >6 months).

    a. Some argue that only one measurement is needed in the perimenopausal period and that treatment decisions be based on that measurement.[1]

    b. Some argue that bone mass might change over time and thus subsequent measurements may be necessary, particularly if the patient's initial measurement falls into a borderline category.

2. **National Osteoporosis Foundation recommendations**[16]

    a. Women who are amenorrheic and who have a bone mass 1 SD below the mean for young normals should be strongly considered for estrogen replacement therapy. This level approximates the fracture threshold of approximately $1.0g/cm^2$ in the proximal femur.

    b. Women whose bone mass is >1 SD above the mean for young normals are protected against osteoporosis and have a low risk of fracture, but may benefit from re-measurement in 5 years if there is any concern about changing bone mineral density.

    c. Women with intermediate values should have bone mineral density re-measured in 2–5 years to look for further bone loss and to guide therapeutic decisions.

E. **Rationale for measuring bone mineral density**
   1. **Several studies now show good correlation between bone mineral density (bone mass) and fracture risk.** Using bone mass measurements in the radius, os calcis, or spine predicts risks for fracture at all sites, and now the availability of methods of measuring hip density allows site-specific measurements for risk of hip fracture.
   2. **Fracture risk** has been shown to be negligible with bone mass measured $>1g/cm^2$. Fracture risk increases as bone mineral density decreases. In general, osteopenia is defined as bone density 1 SD below normal age-matched population mean.
   3. With each $0.1g/cm^2$ decrease in bone mass, fracture risk increases 1.5 times for all sites and 1.9 times for hip.

V. **PREVENTION AND TREATMENT OF OSTEOPOROSIS**
   A. **Estrogen** is the only therapy shown to effectively maintain bone mass and effectively reduce fractures.
      1. The **mechanism** is most likely by decreasing the effect of PTH on bone and the direct effect on decreasing bone resorption.
      2. **Effective dose** necessary to prevent bone loss is 0.625 mg/day of conjugated estrogen (as in Premarin), 2 mg/day of 17β-estradiol (as in Estrace), and/or 50–100 μg/day of transdermal estrogen.
      3. Recent evidence shows that **smokers** who take oral estrogen preparations were not afforded protection against hip fracture as in nonsmoking women who take estrogen. Smoking may decrease the effect of oral estrogens by increasing the activity of hepatic mixed function oxidase systems, which increase the metabolism of sex hormones. This may mean that in women who smoke and wish to take estrogen for prevention of osteoporosis, the percutaneous route of estrogen may be better. Ideally, they should quit smoking.
      4. Estrogen's effect of maintaining bone mass lasts as long as therapy continues, and a positive effect of estrogen has been shown up to age 70.
      5. 50% decrease in hip and wrist fractures and a 90% decrease in vertebral fractures with estrogen therapy
      6. **Risks of estrogen therapy**
         a. Endometrial cancer: The risk is negligible if a progestational agent is added for at least 10 days of the month with cyclic therapy or daily with continuous therapy.
         b. Breast cancer: No clear consensus on the risk, but there does not appear to be a consistent increase in the risk of breast cancer for ever-users of estrogen. A slight increase may occur in long-term users of >10 years, in those using higher doses of estrogen, and in patients with a positive family history of breast cancer.
      7. **Estrogen therapy should begin as soon as possible after menopause,** generally within 3–5 years, which are the times of accelerated bone loss.
      8. Recent trials[7] show elderly women with established osteoporosis also benefited from transdermal estrogen with an increase in bone mineral density or steady-state bone mineral density. This clearly would broaden the indications for estrogen replacement therapy and mean that even elderly women and women with established osteoporosis may benefit from estrogen.
   B. **Diphosphonates–etidronate**
      1. Prospective, randomized, double-blind study[19] has shown 2 years of intermittent etidronate, 400 mg/day for 2 weeks out of every 3 months, successfully increased bone mineral density in the spine, the greater trochanter and femoral neck, and decreased the incidence of new vertebral fractures by 50%. The study included only patients with previously diagnosed osteoporosis.
      2. Inhibits osteoclast-mediated bone resorption.
      3. After 4–5 years, the effect of etidronate may not be sustained, and in 10 patients now followed for 5 years on therapy, they began showing decreasing bone mineral

density and increasing fracture rate. Because of this, the FDA has not approved etidronate for treatment of osteoporosis.
4. Recent evidence and more analysis of data continue to show benefit with increasing bone mineral density and decreased fracture risk with etidronate-treated group compared with placebo.

C. **Calcium**
1. Effectiveness of calcium in preventing osteoporosis is inconclusive and variable from study to study and from skeletal site to skeletal site.
2. Some evidence shows that women menopausal for >5 years with average calcium intake of <400 mg/day benefit from calcium supplementation to 800 mg/day. These patients may stabilize bone mineral density in spine, hip, and radius with calcium supplementation.
   a. Effect seen only with calcium citrate maleate, not with calcium carbonate.
   b. Early menopausal women in the accelerated bone loss phase from 2–5 years of menopause show no benefit from calcium supplementation.
3. In a recent study,[11] 120 women who were >3 years menopausal and had mean calcium intakes of 750 mg/day were given either calcium supplementation (calcium lactate gluconate, 1000 mg/day) or placebo. Over 2 years, bone mineral densities determined by DEXA at 6-month intervals improved in the supplementation group and bone loss actually slowed by 43%. While no significant differences were seen in rates of bone loss in all skeletal sites, it was significant in the lumbosacral spine.
4. In light of this study, it is reasonable (despite previous controversial studies) to include adequate calcium intake in both treating and preventing osteoporosis.
5. It is important that young, premenopausal women have adequate calcium intake to improve bone stores of calcium and improve peak bone mineral density in adolescence.
6. **Recommended amounts are 1000–1500 mg/day of elemental calcium:** 1200 mg/day in adolescence, and 1500–1600 mg/day in pregnancy, perimenopause, and menopause.

D. **Vitamin D**
1. Perimenopausal women may have relative vitamin D deficiency due to decreased gastrointestinal absorption and decreased synthesis of vitamin D by skin. This plus relative vitamin D deficiency during winter may accelerate bone loss.
2. In winter months, perimenopausal women in general lose bone mineral density and in summer regain it to a small degree. Diets supplemented with 400 IU/day of vitamin D lead to slower wintertime loss of bone mineral density in spine compared with placebo and a small but significant net increase in bone mineral density through the year.[2]
   a. All women in this study were supplemented with calcium citrate maleate to a total intake of 800 mg/day.
   b. This study was done in Boston at 42° latitude, and its results may not be significant closer to the equator.

E. **Exercise**
1. Some claim **moderate exercise** (consisting of 1 weekly exercise class led by a physiotherapist plus 2 brisk 30-minute walks/week) is effective at slowing bone loss, but in a recent comparative study, this exercise regimen showed a rate of bone loss similar to that in the placebo-treated group; exercise plus calcium slowed bone loss somewhat, but exercise plus estrogen was most effective.
2. **Therefore, exercise *alone* is not a good treatment or prophylaxis for osteoporosis.**

F. **Calcitonin**
1. Works in preventing osteoporosis by inhibiting osteoclastic activity.
2. Synthetic salmon calcitonin has been shown to stabilize bone mineral density over 2–3 years but has not been proved to decrease fracture risk, although this appears a reasonable assumption.

3. Calcitonin has analgesic properties which may be useful in acute osteoporotic fracture. Mechanism for analgesia may be stimulated release of beta-endorphins.
4. Disadvantages:
    a. Subcutaneous or intramuscular injection with patient inconvenience
    b. Cost is approximately $2000/year for 100-U/day dosage.
    c. Patients may develop antibodies to the preparation which neutralize the calcitonin activity. This effect may be decreased by giving salmon calcitonin every other day, giving lower doses, or giving intranasally (currently not available in U.S.).
G. **Sodium fluoride**
    1. A 4-year study in 135 women showed increased bone mineral density in cancellous bone in those given sodium fluoride but a decrease in bone mineral density in cortical bone. Patients showed no decrease in vertebral fractures but a marked increase in nonvertebral fractures.[13]
    2. Major side effects include gastrointestinal upset and lower extremity pain.
    3. Thus **fluoride is *not* effective treatment for osteoporosis.** Although bone mineral density increases, resulting bone has abnormally decreased strength.
H. **Tamoxifen**
    1. Both antiestrogenic and estrogen agonist-like properties at different body sites. On bone, it acts as an estrogen agonist and therefore **may be beneficial in treatment of osteoporosis.**
    2. In a recent study,[6] 140 postmenopausal women with breast cancer received tamoxifen, 10 mg orally, twice daily for 1 year. Tamoxifen-treated patients showed a 61% increase in bone mineral density of the lumbar spine, but similar values in radius compared with placebo.
    3. Fracture risk does not appear to decrease overall.
    4. These data may indicate that women on tamoxifen for breast cancer may be protected against osteoporosis despite their inability to take estrogen.

REFERENCES

1. Cummings SR, Browner WS, Grady D, Eddinger B: Should prescription of postmenopausal hormone therapy be based on the results of bone densitometry [editorial]? Ann Intern Med 113:565–567, 1990.
2. Dawson-Hughes B, Dallal GE, Krall, et aL: Effective vitamin D supplementation on wintertime and overall bone loss in healthy postmenopausal women. Ann Intern Med 115:505–512, 1991.
3. Dawson-Hughes B, Dallal GE, Krall, et al: A controlled trial of the effect of calcium supplementation on bone density in post menopausal women. N Engl J Med 323:878–883, 1990.
4. Eddinger B, Genant HK, Cann CE: Long-term estrogen replacement therapy prevents bone loss and fractures. Ann Intern Med 102:319–324, 1985.
5. Kiel DP, Baron JA, Anderson JJ, et al: Smoking eliminates the protective effect of oral estrogens on the risk for hip fracture among women. Ann Intern Med 116:716–721, 1992.
6. Love RR, Mazess RB, Barden HS, et al: Effects of tamoxifen on bone mineral density in postmenopausal women with breast cancer. N Engl J Med 326:852–856, 1992.
7. Lufkin EG, Wahner HW, O'Fallon WM, et al: Treatment of post-menopausal osteoporosis with transdermal estrogen. Ann Intern Med 117:1–9, 1992.
8. Marcus R: Understanding osteoporosis. West J Med 155:53–60, 1991.
9. Melton LJ III, Eddy DN, Johnston CC: Screening for osteoporosis. Ann Intern Med 112:516–528, 1990.
10. Prince RL, Smith M, Dick IM, et al: Prevention of post-menopausal osteoporosis: A comparative study of exercise, calcium supplementation, and hormone-replacement therapy. N Engl J Med 325:1189–1195, 1991.
11. Reid IR, Ames RW, Evans MC, et al: Effective calcium supplementation on bone loss in postmenopausal women. N Engl J Med 328:460–464, 1993.
12. Riggs BL: Overview of osteoporosis. West J Med 154:63–77, 1991.
13. Riggs BL, Hodgson SF, O'Fallon WM, et al: Effect of fluoride treatment on the fracture rate in postmenopausal women with osteoporosis. N Engl J Med 322:802–809, 1990.
14. Riggs BL, Melton LJ III: The prevention and treatment of osteoporosis. N Engl J Med 327:620–627, 1992.

15. Rigotti NA, Neer RM, Skates SJ, et al: The clinical course of osteoporosis in anorexia nervosa: A longitudinal study of cortical bone mass. JAMA 265:1133–1138, 1991.
16. Scientific Advisory Board of the National Osteoporosis Foundation: Clinical indications for bone mass measurement. J Bone Miner Res 4(2):1–28, 1989.
17. Slemenda CW, Hui SL, Long CC, et al: Predictors of bone mass in perimenopausal women: A prospective study of clinical data using photon absorptiometry. Ann Intern Med 112:96–101, 1990.
18. Tosteson ANA, Rosenthal DI, Melton LJ II, Weinstein NC: Cost effectiveness of screening perimenopausal white women for osteoporosis: Bone densitometry and hormone replacement therapy. Ann Intern Med 113:594–603, 1990.
19. Watts NB, Harris ST, Genant HK, et al: Intermittent cyclical etidronate treatment of post-menopausal osteoporosis. N Engl J Med 323:73–79, 1990.

Chapter 25: Hormone Replacement Therapy

JULIE PATTISON, MD

Estrogen deficiency related to menopause can be a significant cause of morbidity and mortality for active women. Initially, vasomotor symptoms, insomnia, and decreased concentration can impair athletic performance. A few years after menopause, genitourinary atrophy may result in urinary incontinence and frequent urinary tract infections. At 5–10 years postmenopausally, osteoporosis and coronary heart disease can result in greatly diminished capacity for activity and even in death. Prevention of these complications with hormonal replacement is an area of intense research. Management of replacement hormones in the perimenopausal women is facilitated by knowledge of hormonal risks and benefits, indications, regimens, and follow-up.

I. OVERVIEW OF MENOPAUSE

A. **Menopause is the end result of the gradual demise of ovarian follicles** and the subsequent decline in ovarian hormone production.

1. In the years surrounding the menopause, or **perimenopause**, menstrual cycles may shorten and many are anovulatory, resulting in missed menses, irregular bleeding, and vasomotor symptoms.

2. **Average age of natural menopause is 51 years.** Diagnosis is made by detection of increased levels of follicle-stimulating hormone (FSH).

B. **Consequences of estrogen deficiency**

1. **Vasomotor symptoms:** Hot flashes occur in 75% of women. May be more severe in thin women. If untreated, they may last several years.

2. **Insomnia and problems with concentration:** Depression may result from these side effects but is not felt to be caused by estrogen deficiency alone. In some studies, depression is correlated with a woman's former mental health and other life stressors common to this age group.

3. **Genitourinary atrophy:** Within 2–3 years, symptoms such as vulvar and vaginal pruritus, dyspareunia, and urinary incontinence occur, as well as more frequent urinary tract infections.

4. **Osteoporosis:** Accelerated bone loss begins in the perimenopausal years. Within 5–10 years, osteoporosis may result with complications of chronic bone pain and fractures.

5. **Coronary heart disease:** Premenopausal cardiovascular protection from estrogen is lost after menopause. Ten years postmenopausally, a woman's cardiovascular morbidity and mortality rate approaches that of a man's.

II. RISKS AND BENEFITS OF HORMONAL REPLACEMENT

A. **Risks**

1. **Endometrial cancer**

a. 2.6% lifetime probability of developing endometrial cancer in the average perimenopausal woman on no hormones. Usually curable; only 0.3% lifetime probability of dying of endometrial cancer.

b. **Estrogen and endometrial cancer**

i. **Risk increases with increasing dose and duration of unopposed estrogen use.** Relative risk is 2–6 times higher in ever-users and 7–12 times higher in long-term users, but exact risk associated with the commonly recommended dose of 0.625 mg of conjugated estrogen is unknown (due to small studies on this dosage).

   ii. **Cyclic use** of estrogen alone (e.g., 25 days monthly) does not reduce the risk.

   iii. At the time of diagnosis, endometrial cancer in women who have used estrogen is generally pathologically of lower grade and earlier stage with **better survival potential than in nonusers** (adjusted 5-year survival of 94% compared with 81% for nonusers). This may be due to closer surveillance of women on hormones, resulting in detection at an earlier stage.

c. **Combination therapy and endometrial cancer**

   i. **The addition of a progestin to estrogen therapy** significantly reduces the risk of development of endometrial cancer, perhaps to lower than in women who use no hormones at all.

   ii. **Endometrial hyperplasia**, which may be a precursor to endometrial cancer, occurs in 20–40% of women on unopposed estrogens and can be prevented by adding a progestin to the estrogen regimen.

   iii. Studies show no increased development for endometrial hyperplasia when 10 mg of **medroxyprogesterone acetate** (MPA) is given daily for 10–14 days each month. Cyclic regimens using 5 mg of MPA also appear to be protective, though there is less evidence. Continuous regimens using 2.5 mg of MPA daily with estrogen have also been shown to prevent endometrial hyperplasia. Further study investigating the minimal dose and frequency of progestin administration to protect the endometrium is needed.

2. **Breast cancer**

   a. 10% lifetime probability of developing and 3% probability of dying from breast cancer in the average perimenopausal woman on no hormones.

   b. **Estrogen and breast cancer**

      i. Results of observational studies are inconsistent. **Appears to be no increased risk for short-term use of estrogen, but there may be a slight risk for long-term use** (1.2–1.3 relative risk). Studies are flawed by small numbers, failure to control for other risk factors such as age and estrogen dosage, and variable endpoints. Any increased risk may be secondary to observational bias, such that breast cancer is detected earlier secondary to increased surveillance while on hormonal therapy. Randomized prospective trial needed to eliminate bias.

      ii. Risk in women with a **family history** of breast cancer is not known and might be higher.

   c. **Combination therapy and breast cancer**

      i. Limited studies with inconsistent results make evaluation of risk difficult.

3. **Other diseases**

   a. **Stroke:** A few studies show a slightly increased risk, and a few show a slightly decreased risk. Studies that have evaluated risk of death from stroke have shown a decreased risk among estrogen users. No data for combined hormonal replacement exist.

   b. **Hypertension:** Does not change or may be slightly improved with estrogen replacement. Few data exist on combination therapy.

   c. **Thrombosis:** No evidence that estrogen therapy at standard doses increases risk for thrombosis. Few data exist for combination therapy.

   d. **Gallbladder disease:** Twofold increased risk for disease with estrogen replacement, but few data available for combination therapy.

B. **Benefits**

1. **Coronary heart diseaase** (CHD)

   a. Leading cause of death in women in the U.S. Average postmenopausal woman has a 46% lifetime probability of developing and 31% probability of dying from CHD. Epidemiologic data suggest that endogenous estrogen is protective against CHD.

b. **Estrogen and CHD**

   i. Multiple and consistent observational studies have shown a **protective effect of exogenous oral estrogen in postmenopausal women,** with most showing a relative risk of 0.55–0.65 for development of CHD and 0.50–0.63 for death from CHD. Selection bias may play some role, but it is unlikely to explain the consistency and magnitude of the risk reduction.

   ii. Some evidence suggests that the protective effect is greater in women who already have CHD.

   iii. **Effect of estrogen** on CHD risk is probably multifactorial. Estrogen therapy reduces low-density lipoprotein (LDL) and increases high-density lipoprotein (HDL). Oral conjugated estrogen of 0.625 mg daily decreases LDL by 10–15% and increases HDL by 10–15%. Only about 25–50% of the reduction in deaths can be attributed to changes in the lipoproteins. There is increasing evidence that estrogen may exert some of its protective effects directly on the blood vessel wall as well as on hemostatic factors.

   iv. **Dose of estrogen** in most studies was equivalent to 0.625–1.25 mg of oral conjugated estrogen daily, but numbers are too small to predict dose-response relationship. Duration of therapy to achieve CHD benefit may be prolonged, but data are not yet sufficient to determine. Transdermal estrogen has a less favorable effect on LDL reduction and probably a less favorable HDL increase than oral estrogen.

c. **Combination therapy and CHD**

   i. **Progestins may reverse some of the beneficial effects on lipids and therefore some of the CHD benefit.** Effects of the most commonly prescribed progestin in the U.S., MPA, are less pronounced than with the more androgenic progestins (e.g., noresthisterone or levonorgestrel). Cyclic combined regimens using 5 mg of MPA show a reduction in the estrogen-related HDL increase. Continuous low-dose combination regimens using MPA also show a similar reduction in some studies. Micronized progesterone, not yet available for use in the U.S., may have less adverse impact on lipoproteins. The frequency and duration of progestin use may also affect lipoproteins.

   ii. Data are inadequate to fully assess the effects of progestins on lipoproteins as studies are small, of short duration and have not compared combination therapy to estrogen therapy alone.

   iii. Effects of combination therapy may not be fully mediated through effect on lipids. One study in monkeys showed as protective effect against development of atherosclerosis with combined therapy as with estrogen therapy despite an adverse effect on lipoproteins. Human data also suggest a significant reduction in CHD in women on combination therapy, but the degree of benefit is not yet known.

2. **Osteoporosis**

a. An average postmenopausal woman has a 15% lifetime probability of a hip fracture and a 1.5% probability of death from a hip fracture. Most estrogen-sensitive bone loss occurs within the first 5–10 years after menopause. It is not possible to predict risk of development of osteoporosis solely on a woman's risk factors.

b. **Estrogen and osteoporosis**

   i. Several studies have shown a **reduction in risk for hip fracture in estrogen users** compared with nonusers, with a relative risk of 0.50–0.75. Relative risk of vertebral fractures is 0.10. Risk for wrist fracture is also reduced.

    ii. **Dose:** Most studies have shown protection with use of 0.625 mg of conjugated estrogen daily. Data are insufficient to judge dose-response. Increased duration of use may provide more protection .

    iii. **Smokers** on estrogen therapy benefit less than nonsmokers with respect to hip fracture risk.

    iv. With **discontinuation of estrogen**, bone loss occurs at the accelerated early menopausal rate and risk for hip or forearm fracture may return to baseline within 6 years. This suggests that estrogen be continued for a prolonged period to reduce risk for osteoporosis.

    v. Elderly women with osteoporosis also benefit from **transdermal estrogen** with an increase in bone density.

  c. **Combination therapy and osteoporosis**

    i. Several studies show prevention of bone loss and possibly promotion of new bone formation with combination therapy, but no studies have yet been done on the effect on osteoporotic fractures. Combination therapy is probably as effective as estrogen therapy alone.

3. **Genitourinary atrophy and sexual dysfunction**

  a. **Estrogen effects**

    i. Urinary incontinence, frequency, and urgency are improved with estrogen (oral or vaginal).

    ii. Effect on sexual function is not consistent.

  b. **Combination therapy effects**

    i. Few data on urinary symptoms

    ii. One study has suggested that adding progestins may decrease any beneficial side effects of estrogen on sexual function.

4. **Mortality**

  a. Estrogen therapy has been shown to decrease overall mortality

  b. Data on combination therapy are not yet available.

III. INDICATIONS AND CONTRAINDICATIONS

A. **Indications**

1. **Short-term use** (1–2 years): All perimenopausal women with vasomotor symptoms.

2. **Long-term use:** All women should consider long-term preventive hormone therapy.

  a. Women who have had a hysterectomy have the potential for the greatest benefit.

  b. Women who have increased risk for or known CHD are likely to benefit.

  c. Woman who have decreased bone mineral density or osteoporosis are likely to benefit.

  d. In women who have an increased risk for breast cancer but not for CHD and who do not have decreased bone mineral density, potential risks from therapy may outweight benefits.

  e. Recommendations for women with no increased risks or a combination of risks must be individualized.

B. **Contraindications**

1. Personal history of breast cancer or other estrogen-dependent tumor, such as recent endometrial cancer.

2. Undiagnosed vaginal bleeding

3. Undiagnosed breast mass

4. History of deep vein thrombosis not considered a contraindication

5. Women who are not able to take hormonal replacement should be offered other options for symptomatic treatment of vasomotor symptoms and for prevention of CHD and osteoporosis.

IV. **HORMONE REGIMENS**

A. **Estrogens**
1. Generic forms are not recommended due to variable bioavailability
2. Estrogens should be prescribed continuously rather than cyclically.
   a. There is no benefit to the endometrium of cyclic estrogen use.
   b. Cyclic estrogen use is asssociated with estrogen-deficiency symtpoms such as hot flashes and insomnia during the period off estrogen.
   c. Cyclic regimens are also more complex and difficult to follow.
3. **Oral estrogen** replacement is preferred.
   a. Conjugated equine estrogen (e.g., Premarin) is usually prescribed in a dose of 0.625 mg daily.
   b. 17β-estradiol (e.g., Estrace) is usually prescribed in a dose of 1 mg daily.
   c. An advantage of using 17β-estradiol is that it is possible to measure etradiol levels if necessary to monitor absorption and compliance.
4. **Transdermal estrogen** (e.g., Estraderm patch) is usually prescribed as 0.05 μg twice weekly.
   a. Advantages include avoidance of first-pass effect of the liver and continuous delivery.
   b. Disadvantages are the less beneficial effect on lipoproteins and occasional allergic reaction to the patch material.
5. **Vaginal estrogen cream** is effective in treating genitourinary atrophy and preventing recurrent urinary tract infections.
6. **Side effects** of oral or transdermal estrogens occur in 5–10% of women and include mild bloating and breast tenderness.

B. **Progestins**
1. Generic progestins are adequate.
2. Progestins may be prescribed continuously or cyclically.
3. Less androgenic progestins, such as medroxyprogesterone acetate (MPA), are preferable to androgenic preparations, such as norethindrone and levonorgestrel.
4. Women who have had a hysterectomy have no reason to be placed on a progestin.
5. The lowest dose effective to protect the endometrium should be used.
6. **Side effects** vary with progestin dose and type and can include bloating, breast tenderness, and irritability. They appear to be less common in women on low-dose continuous regimens and in women on natural progesterone.

C. **Therapeutic regimens**
1. **Unopposed estrogen**
   a. Indications
      i. Prior hysterectomies
      ii. Vasomotor symptoms (short-term use, 1–2 years)
      iii. Women who decline combination therapy due to side effects of the progestin.
      iv. Known CHD or familial hyperlipidemias: The potential adverse lipid effects may be sufficient also to warrant unopposed estrogen use.
   b. A woman with an intact uterus who decides to go on unopposed estrogen should have endometrial sampling prior to starting estrogen and yearly thereafter while on unopposed estrogen.
2. **Estrogen and progestin**
   a. **Continuous estrogen plus cyclic progestin**
      i. Progestin (such as MPA) in dose of 5–10 mg daily for the first 10–14 days of each month
      ii. Advantages: Predictable withdrawal bleeding, ease of monitoring, reduced dysfunctional bleeding in the perimenopausal period compared with continuous combined regimen.

          iii. Bleeding is usually lighter, briefer, and without usual menstrual symptoms associated with usual menses.
- b. **Continuous combined estrogen plus progestin**
  - i. Progestin (such as MPA) in dose of 2.5 mg daily
  - ii. Advantages: No cyclic withdrawal bleeding and possibly less adverse effect on lipoproteins.
  - iii. Bleeding occurs in 50–80% of women in the first postmenopausal year, which may discourage a woman from using replacement, unless she knows to expect it. Less frequent bleeding if given after a few years of cyclic combined replacement or several years postmenopausally.

3. **Initiation and duration of therapy**
   - a. **Initiation** at onset of menopause is preferable. Beginning treatment in older women may also be beneficial.
   - b. **Duration:** Benefits in reducing risk for CHD and osteoporosis are most likely to be achieved with long-term preventive therapy (decades).

4. **Follow-up**
   - a. Initial follow-up 2–3 months after starting hormonal replacement therapy (HRT) is important to ensure compliance, to detect problems requiring further follow-up or evaluation, and to discuss side effects and make minor dosage adjustments.
   - b. Annual visits for appropriate health screening evaluations, including breast and pelvic examinations and mammography as indicated, are necessary for continuation of HRT. Discussion of bleeding pattern or any difficulties is important, and endometrial sampling should be done as indicated.
   - c. Patient's clinical symptoms and signs are the appropriate way to monitor HRT. The FSH test is only appropriate for diagnosing menopause, not following HRT.

5. **Management of bleeding**
   - a. **Unopposed estrogen**
     - i. Baseline endometrial sampling recommended.
     - ii. Women should be told to report any vaginal bleeding and endometrial sampling should be performed if one has not been done recently.
     - iii. If no bleeding occurs, yearly endometrial sampling should probably be done, though the optimal interval for sampling has not been determined.
   - b. **Cyclic combined HRT**
     - i. Baseline and routine endometrial sampling not required.
     - ii. When the progestin is added to the continuous estrogen for the first 12 days of the month, withdrawal bleeding beginning prior to day 10 or after day 17 correlates with unfavorable endometrial histology. Endometrial sampling should be performed if this bleeding pattern occurs for three cycles.
     - iii. Endometrial sampling should also be performed if bleeding is very heavy, occurs between cycles, or lasts for more than 10 days.
   - c. **Continuous combined HRT**
     - i. Baseline and routine endometrial sampling not required.
     - ii. Endometrial sampling is recommended if bleeding is heavy, spotting continues past 5–6 months (unless it resolves with increased progestin dose, such as 5.0 mg MPA, or patient switches to cyclic combined HRT with normal bleeding pattern), or bleeding recurs after achieving a period of amenorrhea.

6. **Endometrial evaluation**
   - a. Office-based biopsy is the standard. It is usually accurate and well-tolerated, except in women with cervical stenosis.
   - b. Transvaginal ultrasound can be used to determine which women should be sampled. Endometrial thickness >4 mm correlates with abnormal pathology

and tissue sampling should be done. Ultrasound is usually accurate and well-tolerated and may be helpful in women with cervical stenosis.
   c. Dilation and curettage may be necessary if office-based biopsy is not possible and endometrial thickness is >4 mm. It is usually accurate but can be painful and expensive and may require sedation and anesthesia.
   d. Favorable pathology on an adequate sample includes atrophic endometrium, secretory endometrium, or insufficient tissue.
   e. Proliferative endometrium indicates the need for a longer duration and/or higher dosage of progestin. Additionally, if the patient is using more estrogen than 0.625 mg conjugated estrogen equivalent, the dose of estrogen could be reduced.
   f. More aggressive treatment and consideration of gynecologic referral should occur with results of hyperplasia, focal glandular crowding, atypia, and malignancy.
   g. Referral to a gynecologist should also occur for an inability to obtain an adequate sample or in a patient with continued abnormal vaginal beeding despite normal endometrial sampling pathology.

V. PATIENT INFORMATION AND EDUCATION

   A. Patient participation in informed decision is crucial.
   B. Menopause is the appropriate time to review risk status for diseases such as CHD, osteoporosis, and breast cancer and to provide counseling on risk reduction. Increased calcium requirements should be discussed.
   C. Review of likely changes in her risk of disease, current disease, and life expectancy due to HRT is recommended.
   D. Baseline bone density study (e.g., dual-energy x-ray absorptiometry) once may be recommended if patient would only start HRT if she had decreased bone mineral density.
   E. Risks, benefits, and potential side effects of HRT, different regimens available, monitoring required, expected bleeding patterns, and potential need for endometrial sampling should all be reviewed.
   F. Contraception needed for the perimenopausal period and for at least 1–2 years after menopause. HRT doses are not adequate for contraception.

VI. MANAGEMENT DECISION

   Recommendations by provider should be based on expected effects of the selected HRT regimen individualized to each women's diseases, risk for disease development, proximity to menopause, and expected tolerance of side effects and endometrial monitoring. Each woman's individual preference concerning the risks and benefits of therapy should be incorporated into the management decision and will greatly affect compliance.

VII. FUTURE STUDY

   Current recommendations are based primarily on observational data. The Women's Health Initiative, a large multicenter prospective controlled study begun in 1993 which will have long-term follow-up of women on HRT with endpoints of CHD, breast cancer, and osteoporosis, will provide more definitive data for better recommendations in the future.

REFERENCES

1. American College of Physicians: Guidelines for counseling postmenopausal women about preventive hormonal therapy. Ann Intern Med 117:1038–1041, 1992.
2. Barrett-Connor E, Bush TL: Estrogren and coronary heart disease in women. JAMA 265:1861–1867, 1991.
3. Bergkvist L, et al: Prognosis after breast cancer diagnosis in women exposed to estrogen and estrogen-progestogen replacement therapy. Am J Epidemiol 130:221–228, 1989.

4. Dupont WD, Page DL: Menopausal estrogen replacement therapy and breast cancer. Arch Intern Med 151:67–72, 1991.
5. Grady D, Rubin SM, Petitti DB, et al: Hormone therapy to prevent disease and prolong life in postmenopausal women. Ann Intern Med 117:1016–1037, 1992.
6. Harder DR, Coulson PB: Estrogen receptors and effects of estrogen on membrane electrical properties of coronary vascular smooth muscle. J Cell Physiol 100:375–382, 1979.
7. Henderson BE, Paganini-Hill A, Ross RK: Decreased mortality in users of estrogen replacement therapy. Arch Intern Med 151:75–78, 1991.
8. Nabulsi AA, et al: Association of hormone-replacement therapy with various cardiovascular risk factors in postmenopausal women. N Engl J Med 328:1069–1075, 1993.
9. Padwick ML, Pryse-Davies J, Whitehead MI: A simple method for determining the optimal dosage of progestin in postmenopausal women receiving estrogens. N Engl J Med 315:930–934, 1986.
10. Stampfer MJ, Coldlitz GA: Estrogen replacement therapy and cardiovascular disease: A quantitative assessment of the epidemiologic evidence. Prev Med 20:47–63, 1991.
11. Stampfer MJ, Coldlitz GA: Postmenopasual estrogen therapy and cardiovascular disease. N Engl J Med 325:756–762, 1991.
12. Wood H, Wang-Cheng R, Nattinger A: Postmenopausal hormone replacement: Are two hormones better than one? J Gen Int Med 8:451–458, 1993.

Chapter 26: Exercise During Pregnancy and Post Partum

PATTY KULPA, MD

In general, women of all ages are trying to become more physically active in their daily lifestyles. Exercising women of reproductive age should be encouraged to continue this physical activity during their pregnancies. Exercise guidelines during pregnancy should relate to the individual and be continually reevaluated during the pregnancy and post partum.

I. **EXERCISE BENEFITS AND CONCERNS**
   A. The **major concern** for the pregnant exercising woman is the **safe level of exercise**. Each individual has an optimal zone for exercise quantity and quality.
   B. The **major goal** is to **maintain maternal/fetal physiologic reserve** while enjoying the benefits of exercise during the pregnancy and avoiding the risks.
      1. **Exercise benefits during pregnancy**
         a. Increase or maintain aerobic fitness
         b. Increase cardiopulmonary reserve
         c. Reduce the risk of gestational diabetes
         d. Potentially easier pregnancy and shorter labor[8]
         e. Promote faster recovery from labor
         f. Reduce postdate deliveries
         g. Improve psychological aspects of pregnancy (mood, body image, self-esteem) and reduce postpartum depression
         h. Promote good posture
         i. Improve muscle tone
         j. Improve sleep (irrelevant during late pregnancy)
         k. Prevent low back pain
         l. Prevent excessive "fat" weight gain
      2. **Exercise concerns during pregnancy**
         a. Acute fetal hypoxia (fetal distress, intrauterine growth retardation)
         b. Acute fetal hyperthermia (potential risk of neural tube defects, risk of preterm labor)
         c. Preterm labor
         d. Reduced birth weight (neonatal thermoregulation problems)
         e. Maternal acute hypoglycemia
         f. Maternal chronic fatigue
         g. Maternal musculoskeletal injury

II. **INDIVIDUALIZED EXERCISE PROGRAM**
   Guidelines for patients need to be tailored to each particular pregnancy at its specific gestational age and continually reevaluated throughout the pregnancy. Clinicians need to review the following areas before providing exercise guidelines to their pregnant patients:
   A. **Obstetrical and medical history:** Medical clearance is necessary when the woman initially finds out she is pregnant. Previous health and prenatal obstetrical risks need to be reviewed. Medical diseases that prohibit aerobic exercise in the nonpregnant state also apply to the pregnant state. Regardless of her level of

physical activity and fitness, certain obstetrical conditions may develop that disallow her to continue to exercise safely during the pregnancy. A healthy pregnancy reflects an intact maternal-fetal-placental unit. A compromised placenta lacks the physiologic reserve to tolerate any physiologic stress, including labor or exercise.

1. **Absolute contraindications to aerobic exercise:**
   a. Ruptured membranes (risk of prolapsed cord)
   b. Premature labor
   c. Undiagnosed vaginal bleeding (may be indicative of a placental abruption, placenta previa, impending abortion, or cervical dilatation)
   d. Suspected fetal distress
   e. Intrauterine growth retardation (this condition already has a compromised maternal-fetal-placental unit)
   f. Severe maternal heart disease (significant valvular or ischemic heart disease). The hypervolemic pregnant state along with the exercise load could cause cardiac failure.
   g. Multiple pregnancies (i.e, triplets)
   h. Acute infection
   i. Incompetent cervix (may exercise after surgically corrected)
   j. Pregnancy-induced hypertension, preeclampsia
2. **Relative contraindications to aerobic exercise:** These require closer medical supervision of the pregnant woman during exercise.
   a. Hypertension
   b. Anemia (moderate to severe)
   c. Uncontrolled, brittle diabetes
   d. Overweight (body mass index >25)
   e. Extremely malnourished or underweight
   f. Heavy smoker (>20 cigarettes/day)
   g. History of preterm labor, intrauterine growth retardation, or preeclampsia
   h. Significant pulmonary disease (i.e., exercise-induced asthma)
   i. Twin pregnancies after 24 weeks or term fundal height measurement reached (risk of preterm labor increased due to uterine distention)
   j. Breech presentation (higher risk of prolapse cord if membranes ruptured)
   k. Mild valvular heart disease or significant cardiac arrhythmais in maternal heart
   l. Previously sedentary lifestyle
3. **Warning signs to stop exercising while pregnant:**
   a. Shortness of breath
   b. Dizziness
   c. Headache (may be early sign of preeclampsia or pregnancy-induced hypertension)
   d. Chest pain
   e. Muscle weakness
   f. Calf pain or swelling (need to rule out thrombophlebitis)
   g. Regular good-quality contractions that change the cervix (true labor, not Braxton-Hicks contractions)
   h. Decreased fetal movement
   i. Amnionitic fluid leakage (unengaged fetal head or a malpresentation increases the risk of a cord prolapse)
   j. Generalized swelling (early sign of preeclampsia)
   k. Pain of hips, back, or pubis symphysis
B. **Lifestyle and social habits:** Social habits involving one or multiple substance abuses can increase obstetrical risks in themselves. They may be dangerous when in use in combination with exercise.

1. **Alcohol intake:** The lower limit of teratogenic potential is unknown. Alcohol use during pregnancy has been associated with high-risk obstetrical complications:
   a. Intrauterine growth retardation
   b. Preterm labor
   c. Stillbirths
   d. Fetal alcohol syndrome
2. **Caffeine use:** Athletes should avoid caffeine as an ergogenic aid. Its use (>150 mg/day) during pregnancy may present the following increased risks:
   a. Late spontaneous miscarriage
   b. Stillbirths
   c. Preterm births
   d. Low-birth-weight infants
3. **Smoking:** Smoking and exercise can be a harmful combination in pregnant women. Smoking causes fetal hypoxia due to the reduction in maternal oxyhemo-globin, uteroplacental constriction, and presumably a reduction in placental oxygen transfer to the fetus. It would be comparable to an anemic pregnant woman exercising vigorously. Smoking increases the following risks:
   a. Early spontaneous miscarriage ($1.7 \times$ greater risk)
   b. Premature delivery ($1.36 \times$)
   c. Perinatal death ($1.25 \times$)
   d. Full-term low birth weights ($1.98 \times$)
   e. Premature rupture of membranes
   f. Placental disorders (placental previa, abruptio, and infarcts)
   g. Fetal tobacco syndrome (decrease in infant's lean body mass)
4. **Cocaine use**: Its usage increases the circulatory level of catecholamines (norepine-phine) that can cause placental vasoconstriction and increased uterine contractility in a pregnant woman. Theoretically, cocaine use and exercise during pregnancy is an extremely dangerous combination. Cocaine use increases the following risks:
   a. Abruptio placenta (cocaine-induced hypertension)
   b. Stillbirths (cocaine-induced hypertension)
   c. Cardiac arrests (cocaine-induced hyperthermia and increased heart rate)
   d. Hyperthermia
5. **Marijuana usage:** There is no documented teratogenic effects during pregnancy, but its usage during pregnancy is not recommended.
C. **Nutrition:** The woman brings to her pregnancy all of her previous nutritional knowledge and dietary patterns (i.e., eating behaviors, use of vitamins and medications, cultural habits, medical conditions, and prepregnant nutritional risks).
   1. Markers of **nutritional risk** include:
      a. Obstetric history of high parity
      b. Young maternal age
      c. Previous low-birth-weight infants
      d. Short intervals between births
   2. **Loss of body image and body control** may be an issue with a pregnant athlete who can no longer control her body with diet and exercise. Her nutritional health should be supervised by a physician and nutritionist trained in the needs of pregnancy and eating disorders.
      a. Appropriate weight gain depends on the pregnancy weight, gestational age, and individual nutritional risks. One of the best indicators of the infant's future health is its birth weight. Maternal weight gain and prepregnant weight are independent factors contributing to the newborn weight. Low prepregnant weight and inadequate weight gain are dominant contributors to intrauterine growth retardation and low birth weights. Emphasis should be on the rate of weight gain as well as the total weight gain. Exercise may control the rate of weight gain and reduce the risk of gestational diabetes.

    i. Body mass index (BMI): Defined as weight/height (kg/cm^2). This is a good indicator of nutritional status.

    ii. Recommendations by the Committee on Nutritional Status During Pregnancy on target weight gain:

       (a) **Underweight women** (BMI <19.8): 28–40 lb at 40 weeks with a gain of 2 lbs/week during second and third trimesters

       (b) **Normal-weight woman** (BMI 19.8–26.0): 25–35 lb at 40 weeks with a gain of 1 lb/week during second and third trimesters

       (c) **Overweight women** (BMI >26): 15–25 lbs at 40 weeks with a gain of 0.5–0.75 lb/week during second and third trimesters

3. **Caloric intake:** Consider not only the total energy intake but also the source of the calories. Pregnancy is *not* the time to go on a calorie-reduction diet.

    a. Recommended additional calories for pregnancy alone is 300 kcal/day.

    b. Daily caloric needs are directly proportional to the frequency, duration, and intensity of exercise activity (2000–2400 kcal/day in nonexercising pregnant women vs 2500–3000 kcal/day in exercising pregnant women).

    c. Recommended daily total caloric mix for pregnant women:

       i. 50–60% carbohydrates (complex, high fiber)

       ii. 20–24% protein

       iii. 10–20% fat (<10% saturated fats)

       iv. Dietary fiber should be at least 40–50 g/day.

    d. Use the RDA nutritional requirements during pregnancy for both exercising and nonexercising women, except for the increased caloric need during exercise. This should be achieved with an increase in the amount of complex carbohydrates in her diet.

4. **Sepcial concerns for the pregnant athlete**

    a. **Type of diet**

       i. If she is a **lactovegetarian**, she may need vitamin supplementation.

       ii. If a strict vegetarian, she may need calories, protein, vitamin B12, iron, zinc, calcium, vitamin D, and riboflavin.

       iii. Vitamin and mineral supplements are recommended when the diet is not balanced.

    b. **Excessive vitamin use** should be avoided. Some fat-soluble vitamin excesses and deficiencies can cause birth defects. When megadoses of a fat-soluble vitamin are taken, it may cause a deficiency in another fat-soluble vitamin.

       i. Deficiency of vitamin D: Fetal rickets, infant tooth enamel hypoplasia

       ii. Deficiency of vitamin A: Eye abnormalities, impaired vision

       iii. Excess of vitamin D: Supravalvular aortic stenosis with mental retardation

       iv. Excess of vitamin A: Congenital renal anomalies, central nervous system malformations

    c. **Risks of hypoglycemia** during prolonged bouts of exercise or high-intensity workouts should be avoided. The athlete needs to increase her complex carbohydrate intake. Physical training blunts the degree of ketosis and hypoglycemia. **Avoid exercise if blood glucose is 60 mg/dl or less, 250 mg/dl or greater, or ketonuria is present.** In late pregnancy, woman have limited anaerobic capacity to exercise (lower respiratory ratio and a reduced ability to utilize carbohydrates).

    d. **Adequate hydration** is needed before, during, and after exercise (risk of hyperthermia increases).

    e. **Dietary habits:** Anorectic eating patterns and bulemic practices need to be addressed *early* by the physician.

    f. **Risk of iron-deficiency anemia:** Prepregnant reduced iron stores may exist in athletes due to low iron intake, low caloric intake, and vegetarian diets. Additional iron supplements (60–120 mg/day) are needed if the athlete is already anemic (hemoglobin <11 g in first and third trimester; <10.5 g in second trimester). Once anemia is corrected, prenatal vitamins should suffice.

g. **Avoid high-protein diet.** Use the same recommendations as for nonexercising pregnant women (60 mg/day).

h. **Body fat composition:** Educate the woman that an increase in fat stores during pregnancy is a normal physiologic adjustment (maximal levels during the second trimester). Avoid body fat measurements during pregnancy. All methods are invalid during pregnancy and need more research.

D. **Environment**

1. **Air pollution:** No studies are available on maternal and fetal effects of exercise in polluted environments during pregnancy. Avoidance during the worst periods of pollution or altogether may be advisable.

   a. Carbon monoxide (i.e., car fumes) can impair oxygen delivery, causing tissue hypoxia, potential fetal hypoxia, and decreased exercise performance.

2. **Altitude:** Advice for exercising at high altitude (8,000–10,000 ft) warrants individualization.

   a. With increasing altitude, placental insufficiency can occur with a subsequently higher occurrence of pregnancy-induced hypertension, intrauterine growth retardation, and placental abnormalities (previa, infarcts).

   b. Pregnant women with other hypoxic conditions (e.g., anemia, smoking intrauterine growth retardation) should be cautioned about traveling to high-altitude places and exercising there.

   c. Maternal acclimatization will determine what altitude may be safe and tolerable for exercise during pregnancy. As the elevation increases, exercise should be reduced. An unacclimated pregnant woman should avoid intense exercise during the first 3–4 days after gaining altitude (>6500 ft) and be aware of acute mountain sickness symptoms.

   d. A woman untrained in sports at altitudes >8000 ft (mountain climbing, hiking, skiing) should avoid them during pregnancy.

   e. An experienced hiker/athlete who is pregnant needs to avoid altitude sickness. The best prevention is to ascend slowly to allow her body to acclimatize to the higher altitudes. Adjust the schedule as to average no more than 1000 ft of elevation gain/day above 10,000 ft.

   f. Mild altitude illness may occur above 8000 ft. Symptoms include headache, difficult sleeping, easy fatigue, loss of appetite, and nausea. Typically, this begins on the second day after reaching high altitude. Proper treatment includes descending to an altitude where the symptoms resolve.

3. **Hyperthermia:** There is no evidence with prospective studies to show that induced hyperthermia causes fetal problems.

   a. With moderate aerobic exercise, the mother is able to dissipate heat effectively. Increased blood volume and skin blood flow from pregnancy allow better heat dissipation during pregnancy. Adequate hydration is necessary prior, during, and after exercise. Conditioned athletes are more efficient in heat dissipation.

   b. Caution should be made for other environmental factors (hydration, previous acclimatization, ambient temperature and humidity) that alter thermoregulation. Dehydration will cause uterine irritability and preterm labor during late pregnancy.

   c. Sport type, improper clothing, and vigorous or long endurance exercise can compromise thermoregulation.

   d. Water exercises may be more heat-tolerable than land exercises. Avoid untreated standing water of rivers and ponds, where natural microbial contaminants may pose an infectious risk. During the summer months, avoid public swimming pools in the third trimester where there may be a risk of an enterovirus epidemic. Avoid improperly treated pools.

4. **Hypothermia:** There is a higher risk of cold exposure due to improper clothing while exercising during pregnancy in winter sports. Avoid extremely hazardous outdoor conditions (i.e., subzero chill factor, icy conditions). Check wind chill readings prior to exercising outdoors. Adequate hydration is also important.

E. **Occupation**

1. **Prolonged-standing jobs** place women at risk of preterm deliveries, intrauterine growth retardation, and placental infarcts. The type of work she continues to do during pregnancy is another factor when counseling for her caloric requirements and exercise regimens.

2. **Increased risk of preterm births** is related to the degree of occupational fatigue. Posture, physical exertion, mental stress, working environment, work with industrial machinery, and commuting all contribute to occupational fatigue. During the third trimester, avoid repetitive heavy lifting, prolonged standing, and strenuous work.

F. **Exercise history**

1. **Prepregnant level of physical fitness** (novice, recreational athlete, elite)
   a. Physical activity is not the same as physical fitness (ability to perform daily tasks without experiencing undue fatigue).
   b. The degree of physical activity (inactive, very light, moderate, very, and exceptionally active) is important when determining the amount of exercise during pregnancy.
   c. Assessment of physical fitness (heart rate reduction, body fat reduction) during pregnancy is difficult due to the superimposed physiologic changes of pregnancy.
   d. Emphasis should be on promoting maternal and fetal well-being rather than increasing maternal oxygen consumption (VO_2max) or changing body composition.

2. **Specific sport:** Athlete may need to change, modify, or crosstrain in various sports.
   a. Body movements required by each sport may determine the safety of the sport.
   b. Each sport has various types of motion (walking, running, jumping, kicking, throwing, and stance). During the first two trimesters, sports with high requirements of stance (maintenance of particular posture), walking, and running are safe. Muscle strain and fatigue may develop if these are carried out during late pregnancy. Sports requiring agility, balance, and strength may increase likelihood of musculoskeletal injury after the first trimester.
   c. Gestational age determines the safety of the sport during pregnancy. Movement performance may be impaired by weight, fetal activity, and fetal position during late pregnancy despite physical fitness and motor activity level of the pregnant woman. Motion may be slowed by increasing mass, altered upright posture, and fluid retention. Increasing weight of pregnancy will require more physical work (weight × distance) to complete a given task. During the third trimester, an individualized approach is needed to the pregnant woman.
   d. Avoid high-injury sports involving the following components:
      i. High-impact acceleration and high loads (i.e., sky dive, stock car racing, body-building)
      ii. Unpredictable terrains (i.e., rock scrambling, hiking, horseback riding, competitive downhill skiing)
      iii. Risks of falls and collision (i.e., competitive soccer, rugby, gymnastics, using the beam and rings, speed skating, roller-blading)
      iv. Jumping from heights (i.e., ballet jumps, pool high dive)
      v. Sudden twisting or quick turns (i.e., dance, competitive racquet sports)
      vi. Ballistic movements (i.e., poor technique of calisthenics)

e. Musculoskeletal adjustments to pregnancy will dictate continuance of certain sports. The biomechanic changes associated with pregnancy increase muscular effort for simple tasks. The following guidelines may prevent potential injury:

   i. Encourage activities involving rhythmic motion of large muscle groups.
   ii. Teach the pregnant woman early about proper body mechanics of posture and lifting to reduce and prevent low back pain and strains.
   iii. Consult with a local physical therapist. He or she may provide the proper safe instructions on the muscle strengthening and flexibility exercises for the pregnant woman, along with educating her in her biomechanical changes of pregnancy.
   iv. Strength training of the upper and lower extremities may offset additional musculoskeletal loads during pregnancy and be helpful post partum. Concentrate more on form and control rather than frequency of each set of repetition. Do more repetition than increasing loads.
   v. Strength training of the abdominal and hip extensors (hamstring muscle) and stretching of the erector spine and hip flexors (rectus femoris) will reduce low back pain. Use of the maternity belts is a poor substitute for muscle tone and strength. Maternity belts may provide more abdominal support and decrease pubic discomfort for the pregnant runner.
   vi. Water aerobic activities have musculoskeletal benefits for the pregnant woman (less stress on joints, diuresis of fluid retention).

3. **Exercise guidelines.** There is no single exercise regimen to meet the needs of all women. The American College of Obstetrics and Gynecology (ACOG) guidelines provide the following:
   a. Meet the needs of the previously sedentary woman now pregnant.
   b. Provide framework to start a home exercise program during pregnancy.
   c. Ignore the needs of the previously recreational and performance female athlete now pregnant.
   d. Controversial issues
      i. Exercising in supine position after midpregnancy
      ii. Avoiding bouncing movement
      iii. Exercise prescription—target heart rate, duration, and frequency

4. **Duration, intensity, and frequency of exercise**
   a. **Duration:** 15–60 minutes
      i. Avoid anaerobic workouts. Interval exercise is preferable over continuous exercise (reduces risk of hyperthermia).
      ii. Avoid reaching levels of exhaustion. If there is a need for postexercise rest, the exercise is excessive.
   b. **Intensity:** 60–75% maximal heart rate is probably a safe range. The following problems exist in determining target heart rate during pregnancy:
      i. Cardiovascular changes during pregnancy interfere with the interpretation of heart rate and dominate over cardiovascular changes with physical conditioning.
      ii. Unreliable indicators during pregnancy include target heart rate, talk test, postexercise fatigue, role of rate of perceived exertion (RPE%), measured VO_2max.
      iii. If starting exercise, heart rate of approximately 140 beats/min
      iv. If previously exercising, heart rate of approximately 160 beats/min
      v. Encourage constant-intensity level workouts or gradually increasing intensity levels.
      vi. Heart rate >140 beats/min may unmask an organic disease (mitral valve prolapse), and exercise may be dangerous.

    c. **Frequency:** Avoid "athlete weekend" workouts. May want to exercise 3–4 times/week. More frequently during late pregnancy, but of shorter duration and lesser intensity.

III. **POSTPARTUM EXERCISE GUIDELINES**

A. **Length of time for postpartum physiologic changes to revert** to nonpregnant state:
1. Uterus involution: 6 weeks
2. Lochia discharge: 3 weeks
3. Episitomy/vaginal laceration: heal 1–2 weeks
4. Healed perineum: 6 weeks
5. Urinary tract: 8 weeks
6. Hormonal changes (i.e., breast): 4 weeks
7. Musculoskeletal
    a. Abdominal wall tone: 6 weeks
    b. Joint and ligament laxity: 12 weeks
8. Cardiovascular: 2 weeks

B. **Special considerations to exercise during postpartum period**
1. Type of delivery: vaginal vs cesarean
2. Breast-feeding vs bottle-feeding
    a. Feeding schedule demands
    b. Supportive bra for exercising
    c. Adequate nutrition/hydration: Optimal milk production requires a total of at least 1800 cal/day.
    d. Urinary incontinence
3. Infant sleep patterns vs adequate maternal sleep
4. Postpartum depression: role of exercise (stress relief vs stress provoking)

C. **Guidelines**
1. Avoid moderately strenuous activities if excessive vaginal bleeding is present or you have soreness of the episiotomy.
2. Correct any anemia: Stop exercising if it increases vaginal bleeding or bright-red blood appears.
3. Avoid water sports if persistent heavy lochia discharge and unhealed episiotomy/laceration.
4. Encourage Kegel exercises (squeeze and start-and-stop) to help control urinary incontinence and improve pelvic wall floor.
5. Use the same precautions as in pregnancy when considering workouts and type of sport relative to musculoskeletal injury risks.
6. Use proper biomechanics in daily tasks of child-rearing (lifting, carrying, bending) as well as during exercise.
7. Avoid competition during postpartum period. Gradual training for competition is recommended.
8. Expect to return to your prepregnant weight given appropriate exercise and diet post partum with or without breast-feeding. On average, a woman will weigh 2 lb above her prepregnant weight 1 year after the pregnancy.
9. Nursing will not accelerate weight loss. Severe caloric restriction will jeopardize milk production. Expect a gradual rate of weight loss in the first 6 months post partum in the lactating woman.
10. A brassiere that provides good support should be worn during postpartum exercise, especially by nursing women. Avoid chafing of the nipples.
11. Nursing women should feed the infant prior to exercising in order to avoid the discomfort of engorged breasts (hot, heavy, hard, and tender). Infrequent expression of engorged breasts predisposes to plugged ducts and eventual mastitis.

12. There are no good data to suggest that exercise has detrimental effects on the quality of milk or its production. However, proper nutrition, hydration, adequate rest, and a functional letdown reflex are essential to lactation.

REFERENCES

1. American College of Obstetrics and Gynecology: Exercise during pregnancy and the postnatal period. (ACOG Home Exercise Program). Washington, DC, American College of Obstetrics and Gynecology, 1985, p 4.
2. American College of Obstetrics and Gynecology: Nutrition during Pregnancy. ACOG technical bulletin no. 179. Washington, DC, American College of Obstetrics and Gynecology, 1993.
3. Artal A, Masaki D: Exercise in gestational diabetes: A new therapeutic approach. Pract Diabet (March/April):1989.
4. Artal R, Wiswell RA, Drinkwater B: Exercise in Pregnancy, 2nd ed. Baltimore, Williams & Wilkins, 1989.
5. Bottil JJ, Jones RL: Aerobic conditioning, nutrition and pregnancy. Clin Nutr 4:14–17, 1985.
6. Buschsbaum HJ: Trauma in pregnancy. In Nicholas JA (ed): Sports Injuries. Philadelphia, W.B. Saunders, 1979, pp 179–183.
7. Clapp JF: Exercise in pregnancy—Good, bad or indifferent (unpublished).
8. Clapp JF: Exercise in pregnancy: A brief clinical review. Fetal Med Rev 2:89–101, 1990.
9. Kulpa P: Exercise during pregnancy. Fam Pract Res J 11:35–36, 1989.
10. Mamelle N, Laumon B, Lazar P: Prematurity and occupational activity during pregnancy. Am J Epidemiol 119:309, 1984.
11. Nieman DC: Benefits and precautions in physical activity. An introduction. In Fitness and Sports Medicine. Palo Alto, CA, Bull Publ Co., 1990, pp 273–316.
12. Pritchard J, MacDonald P, Gant N: Williams Obstetrics, 17th ed. Norwalk, CT, Appleton-Century-Crofts, 1985, pp 367–379.
13. Sady SP, Carpenter MW: Aerobic exercise during pregnancy: Special considerations. Sports Med 7:357–375, 1989.
14. Wolfe LA, Hall P, Webb KA, et al: Prescription of aerobic exercise during pregnancy. Sports Med 8:273–301, 1989.
15. Worthington-Roberts B, Vermeersch J, Williams S: Nutrition in Pregnancy and Lactation, 1985, pp 61–131.

Chapter 27: Pelvic Floor Muscle Dysfunction and Its Behavioral Treatment

KATHE WALLACE, PT

The effects and benefits of exercise on the pelvic floor muscles and the urogenital system have received little attention in past decades. Recent research, however, indicates that pelvic floor muscle dysfunction can contribute to a variety of medical conditions, including urinary stress incontinence, fecal incontinence, sexual dysfunction, pelvic relaxation, and levator ani syndrome. These problems are commonly underreported, embarrassing, and undertreated[32] and may limit a woman's ability to function in daily activities and perform in an exercise program.

Urogynecologic dysfunctions have complex and multifactorial etiologies and require complete medical evaluations. When an evaluation indicates muscle dysfunction, it is the health care provider's role to increase women's awareness of this musculature and make therapeutic recommendations. This chapter reviews anatomy, specific muscle functions and dysfunctions, evaluation, and behavioral treatment options. It is intended to guide practitioners to a clearer understanding of pelvic floor muscle function and current rehabilitation strategies, so that they can incorporate this knowledge into practice.

I. FUNCTION OF THE PELVIC FLOOR

A properly maintained pelvic floor performs three important functions.

A. **Provides support of the pelvic viscera** through a group of structures which include bones, muscles, smooth muscles, and connective tissue.

B. **Sphincteric functions** aid the control of the perineal openings.
1. Muscles contribute to urethral closing pressure and maintenance of continence.
2. Aid in the constriction of the vagina during coitus and provide tone for the vaginal walls.
3. Muscles work to control flatus and relax for defecation.

C. **Sexual function**
1. Decreased pubococcygeal strength and awareness lead to poor sexual response.[13,20]
2. The muscles of the pelvic diaphragm form a reflex arc in the pudendal nerve pathway: stimulation of the clitoris causes reflex contraction of the pelvic diaphragm muscles (pubococcygeus) during orgasm.[12]

II. SCOPE AND PREVALENCE

The medical and economic consequences of lack of attention to the pelvic floor are unknown. The magnitude of pelvic floor-related urogynecologic dysfunctions can begin to be appreciated by a review of the scope and prevalence of a few problems.

A. **Urinary incontinence**
1. **Definition**: The Agency for Health Care Policy and Research (AHCPR)[41] defines urinary incontinence as the involuntary loss of urine which is sufficient to be a problem. Involuntary loss of urine during physical exertion is called **stress urinary incontinence**. The U.S. Public Health Service's guidelines for urinary incontinence[41] include pelvic muscle exercises (also called Kegel exercises) as a behavioral treatment for incontinence.
2. The **scope** of the incontinence problem
   a. Women are twice as likely as men to be incontinent.
   b. Incontinence affects between 10–11 million people of all ages.

    c. As many as 30% of men and women over age 60 living at home experience bladder control problems.

    d. Incontinence is associated with nursing-home admission with an estimated cost of $10 billion annually.

3. **Attitudes about incontinence**

    a. Most people do not understand the causes or treatment options.

    b. Denial is common, as the average person waits 7–9 years to seek help.

    c. Many feel it is an inevitable result of childbirth and aging.

    d. A lack of questioning about incontinence by health professionals is common.

4. **Impact on exercise**

    a. Nygaard et al.[30] surveyed 326 women regularly exercising women (mean age = 38.5 years).

    b. 47% reported some degree of incontinence.

    c. Incontinence correlated positively with number of vaginal deliveries. (However, 22% of the subjects were nulliparous women noting incontinence.)

    d. Exercises with high impact resulted in more episodes of incontinence (Table 1).

    e. Exercise modifications due to incontinence included stopping exercise, changing exercises or technique, or wearing a protective pad (Fig 1).

B. **Fecal incontinence**

  1. **Etiology** is multifactorial[14,25] but damage to the pelvic floor from obstetric trauma is felt to be a major cause.

C. **Pelvic relaxation or genital prolapse**

  1. Pelvic relaxation results from changes in pelvic support.

  2. Genital prolapse is descent of the pelvic organ from its normal position.

  3. **Causes:**

    a. Congenital or developmental weakness of the supportive stuctures

    b. Muscles, nerves, and fascia are damaged in pregnancy and vaginal delivery.

    c. The fascia and support structures are influenced by menopause and aging.

D. **Vaginismus**

  1. Definition: the recurrent or persistent involuntary muscle spasm of the musculature of the outer one-third of the vagina that interferes with coitus[23] and sexual function.

  2. The disturbance can have both physical and psychiatric etiologies.

  3. The prevalence in clinical samples has been estimated to be between 12–17%.[37]

E. **Chronic pelvic pain**

  1. It is the second most common complaint in gynecologic practice.

  2. Musculoskeletal etiologies are a component [22] and can lead to levator ani syndrome.

TABLE 1.   Association Between Various Exercises and Incontinence

Activity	No. Participating	No. Incontinent During Activity
Running	99	38 (38%)
High-impact aerobics	94	34 (36%)
Tennis	37	10 (27%)
Low-impact aerobics	134	29 (22%)
Walking	164	34 (21%)
Golf	38	7 (18%)
Bicycling	81	13 (16%)
Racquetball	31	4 (13%)
Swimming	87	10 (12%)
Weight lifting	54	4 (7%)

From Nygaard et al: Exercise and incontinence. Obstet Gynecol 75:848–851, 1990; with permission.

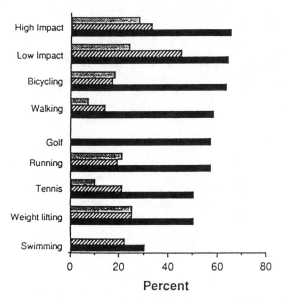

FIGURE 1. Adaptive mechanisms used by incontinent exercisers. Shaded bars = percent who stop; striped bars = percent who change; black bars = percent who wear pad. (Reprinted with permission from the American College of Obstetricians and Gynecologists. From Nygaard et al: Exercise and incontinence. Obstet Gynecol 75:848–851, 1990.)

III. ANATOMY OF THE PELVIC FLOOR

The entire pelvic floor complex consists of muscles, ligaments, and fascia forming a multi-layer hammock in the inferior pelvis. The most common terminology used is the **"levator ani"** or **"pelvic diaphragm complex."** The anatomy of the pelvic floor is described differently by the surgeon than the anatomist. Because multiple nomenclature is used for the same muscle, descriptions can be confusing. A functional approach is presented here.

A. **There is controversy over what specific muscle fiber types make up the pelvic floor.**[1,11]
 1. The urethral closure mechanism and the external anal sphincters are primarily type II, fast twitch to facilitate rapid sphincter closure.
 2. The pelvic diaphragm is primarily type I slow twitch for maintenance of tone and support.

B. **Muscles and fascia of the pelvic floor and urogenital system**
 1. **Pelvic diaphragm** (Fig. 2)
 a. Consists of the endopelvic fascial floor and the smooth muscle diaphragm in the base of the broad ligament.
 b. Muscles include pubococcygeus, puborectalis, pubovaginalis, and iliococcygeus.
 c. This is the deepest layer of striated muscles which are not visible by observation of the perineum.
 d. Coccygeus (ischiococcygeus) lies posterior to the levator ani group.
 e. The pelvic diaphragm is laterally bordered by the tendinous arch. The piriformis muscle and the obturator internus muscle and fascia are continuous with the pelvic diaphragm.
 2. **Urogenital diaphragm** region, or the perineal membrane region, is more anterior and superficial to, and oriented transversely with, the fascia and the muscle that spans from the ischiopubic rami bilaterally. It consists of the urethral sphincter (proximal one-third of the urethra), compressor urethrae, and urethrovaginal sphincter muscles.[27]

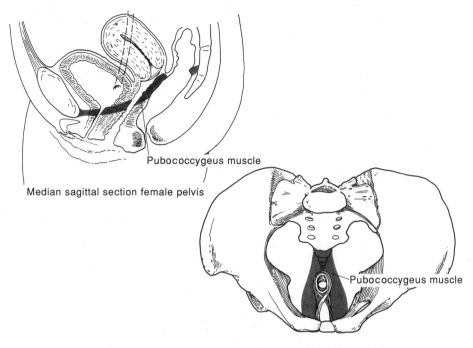

Pubococcygeus muscle

Median sagittal section female pelvis

Pubococcygeus muscle

Superior view female pelvis

FIGURE 2.   Pelvic floor muscles in the female. (Reprinted with permission form Govier FE: Stress urinary incontinence in the female. Virginia Mason Clinic Bulletin 45:17–24, 1991.)

3. **Female urethral sphincters**
    a. **Proximal urethral sphincter**, or the internal sphincter at the bladder neck, is composed of smooth muscle and innervated via the sympathetic system.
    b. **The distal urethral sphincters**
        i. The intrinsic urethral sphincter (striated rhabdosphincter) is composed of type I (slow-twitch) striated muscle and innervated by both the pudendal and sympathetic nerves.
        ii. The external urethral sphincter (striated muscle) is composed of type II (fast-twitch) striated muscle. Innervation is either by the perineal branches of the pudendal nerve or by the pelvic nerve.
4. **Superficial external genital muscles** include the external anal sphincter, transverse perineal, bulbocavernosus, and ischiocavernosus.
5. **Nerve supply**
    a. Sympathetic: hypogastric nerve
    b. Parasympathetic:
        i. Pudendal from S2–5, with inferior rectal and perineal branches
        ii. Direct branches of the sacral plexus S3–4

IV. **PELVIC FLOOR MUSCLE EVALUATION TECHNIQUES**

Techniques for evaluating the pelvic floor muscles include a self-administered functional test and medically directed evaluation techniques.
    A. **Functional stop test** of the pelvic floor musculature[4,24]: This technique is used for *evaluation only* and **should not be performed as an exercise** because of its potential to disrupt the normal voiding reflexes.
        1. The test should be performed while sitting on a toilet after the bladder has been partially emptied.

a. If the client is unable to deflect the flow or slow the stream of urine, her grade is *zero* (0).

b. Partial deflection of the urine stream that cannot be maintained is graded as *trace* (1).

c. Maintenance of a deflection in the flow of urine is graded as *poor* (2).

d. Ability to stop the flow of urine is graded as *fair* (3).

e. *Good* (4) and *normal* (5) strength are difficult to assess with this functional testing.

2. A grade of *fair* (3) or less for strength requires rehabilitation efforts. A woman should seek help from a health care provider. She would likely benefit from physical therapy for neuromuscular re-education and therapeutic exercise to the pelvic floor.

3. A woman with a grade of *good* (4) or *normal* (5) should be encouraged to maintain this strength through an exercise program for the pelvic floor muscles.

B. **Medically directed evaluations** of the pelvic floor musculature should be performed on all women for prevention and education.

1. **Visual inspection of the perineum** for accuracy of muscle contraction and relaxation

   a. To assure that contraction creates a lift of the perineum, not bearing down.

   b. To eliminate other muscle contractions of the gluteal, abdominal, or adductor muscles.

   c. To assess the degree and sequelae of pelvic relaxation

2. **Palpation of muscle contraction and relaxation**

   a. **External palpation techniques**

      i. Palpate for a muscle contraction at the perineal body and at points along the muscle insertions, i.e., coccyx, ischiopubic rami, and pubic symphysis.

   b. **Manual muscle testing for the pelvic floor**[24]

      i. This testing incorporates standard muscle assessment scales, differentiates between the state of the fast- and slow-twitch muscle components, and helps formulate an individual exercise program based on the evaluation.

      ii. Digital internal palpation techniques require the patient to contract the pelvic floor muscles around an examining finger inserted vaginally.[19,21]

      iii. The evaluator tests for muscle symmetry, tone, sensation, and muscle atrophy in anterior, posterior, left, and right middle-third of the vagina at the depth of the finger PIP joint. It is important to also feel for the ability to relax after a contraction.

      iv. Muscle grading scale as described by physical therapists Chiarelli and Laycock:[8,24]

         0 = no contraction
         1 = flicker, only with the muscles stretched
         2 = a weak squeeze, 2-second hold
         3 = a fair squeeze, definite "lift" (where the contraction can be felt to move in an upward direction)
         4 = a good squeeze, good hold with lift. The contraction must be able to be repeated a few times.
         5 = a strong squeeze, good lift, repeatable

3. **Pressure perineometers** are biofeedback devices. A vaginal probe uses the changes in pressure of air exerted on it to sense the strength of the pelvic floor muscles.

4. **Surface electromyographic (EMG) biofeedback**[16]

   a. Kasman describes surface EMG as an evaluation tool that provides feedback on muscle events (not single motor units) and assesses the magnitude and timing of overall muscle contraction and relaxation with the objective of restoring normal physical function to a muscle. It can be computer-assisted. It does not stand alone as an evaluation or treatment tool for muscle dysfunction.

    b. Its benefits include:[16a]

        i. The technique is noninvasive, painless, and relatively easy to perform.

        ii. The patient is not limited to a fixed testing position (i.e., supine) but may be evaluated in a functional position.

        iii. The recordings are sensitive to small changes in muscle activity that otherwise may not be perceived by the patient or health care practitioner.

        iv. Specific vaginal or anal electrodes allow for (within limits) the isolation of a specific muscle or muscle group.[7]

        v. Surface EMG is an excellent adjunct to a comprehensive rehabilitation program as it can improve motivation and provide feedback modes that best match the client's learning style.

    c. Surface EMG biofeedback evaluation produces a profile of muscle events with the ability to document responses in microvolts. Specific suggestions for pelvic floor surface EMG analysis:

        i. Baseline resting EMG looks at resting tension.

        ii. Peak EMG amplitude with a muscle contraction

        iii. The ability to sustain a contraction (endurance)

        iv. Muscle recruitment patterns (i.e., the rate of muscle responses)

        v. Positional differences in muscle response (i.e., supine or standing with rest and muscle contraction)

        vi. Muscle response to exercise and functional activities

        vii. Psychophysiologic stress profile through evaluation of muscle response to stressful situations

V. PELVIC FLOOR MUSCLE DYSFUNCTIONS

  A. **Disuse dysfunction** of the pelvic floor may be asymptomatic or contribute to problems with urogynecologic systems. Primary disuse occurs when a woman has no cognitive knowledge of the pelvic floor muscles or their functions. Prevention of some pelvic floor problems can begin if emphasis is placed on education of the muscle functions rather than on the rehabilitation of problems only after they occur. Females with disuse dysfunction may be asymptomatic. Promoting pelvic floor muscle awareness is important in women's health.

    1. **Promoting awareness of the pelvic floor** can be accomplished in several existing opportunities:

      a. During childhood bladder training, teach children that muscles help to control urine flow.

      b. Females involved in high-impact sports, such as gymnastics or basketball, should be taught to use the pelvic floor muscles on impact.

      c. Use health and sex education classes to teach females about pelvic floor muscle function.

      d. Adult fitness classes could incorporate pelvic floor exercises into exercise regimens.

      e. During routine pelvic examination, women could ask for a pelvic muscle assessment.

    2. Health care providers and exercise fitness personnel can begin asking their clients more questions about pelvic floor function. Routine screening and awareness questions include:

      a. Do you ever unintentionally lose urine?

      b. While laughing, sneezing, coughing, jumping, or exercising, do you have trouble maintaining urine control?

      c. Are pelvic floor exercises (Kegel) included in your regular exercise regimen? (Be sure to assess whether they are being performed correctly.)

      d. Do you have trouble controlling flatus?

      e. Are you aware of excess tension or holding of the pelvic floor muscles?

       f. Are you aware of diminished sexual feelings in the vagina, especially after childbirth?

B. **Supportive dysfunction** arises from loss of strength and integrity of connective tissue and muscular fibers of the pelvic floor.[29] It can occur with congenital weakness,[18] lack of hormonal balance, or loss of nerve, muscle, and fascial integrity.

  1. Supportive structure (musculoskeletal) injury in pregnancy and childbirth
    a. Muscle function can be impaired by partial denervation of pudendal nerve by traction or compression nerve injuries.[35,36]
    b. Can result from stretch weakness of muscles and ligaments after vaginal delivery.
    c. Inhibition of muscle function can result from pain of episiotomy or tearing of perineum.
    d. Scar tissue formation can cause changes in muscle contractility.
    e. Can occur from hormonal changes of decreased estrogen during pregnancy and breast-feeding.
  2. Influence of menopause on pelvic organs
  3. Obesity and repetitive heavy lifting can cause excessive stress on the pelvic floor muscles.
  4. Severe and persistent constipation sets up a pattern of intractable straining, perineal descent, stretch-induced sphincter denervation, and anorectal incontinence.[39]
  5. **Symptoms**
    a. Back pain and pelvic heaviness
    b. Sensation of suprapubic pressure
    c. Lack of sexual orgasmic appreciation
    d. Heaviness or a "falling out" feeling in perineum
    e. Urination difficulties
    f. Constipation or bowel elimination difficulties[38]
    g. Recurrent urinary tract infections, urinary frequency
  6. **Diagnoses** associated with supportive dysfunctions include:
    a. Urinary stress and/or urge incontinence
    b. Fecal incontinence
    c. Cystocele or rectocele, herniations of the bladder or rectum into the vaginal wall
    d. Uterine prolapse
    e. Urinary or fecal incontinence
  7. **Treatment options** are either surgical, pharmacologic, or behavioral. Current behavioral treatments for incontinence include:
    a. Pelvic muscle (Kegel) exercise
    b. Biofeedback with Kegel exercise as indices of pelvic floor muscle activity
    c. Femina vaginal cones: a set of 5 progressive vaginally-placed weights (20–70 g) of equal shape and volume used for a home program of resistive exercise training.
      i. They can be used to determine pelvic floor muscle strength. This is the weight in grams of the heaviest cone retained in standing and walking for 1 minute.
      ii. Research shows significant improvement in strength of the pelvic floor muscles and high correlations between decreased urine loss and increase in retaining cone weights.[31]
    d. Electrical stimulation can be used for neuromuscular re-education and reflexogenic stimulation of the pelvic floor muscles.[10,26]

C. **Hypertonus dysfunctions** of the musculoskeletal and urogynecologic systems are most often referred to as **levator ani syndromes**.

  1. **Its primary symptom is pain.** Symptoms are usually poorly localized in the perivaginal, perirectal, lower abdominal quadrants, and pelvis. Pain can also be located in suprapubic or coccyx regions and possibly down the posterior thigh.

Specific vulvar or clitoral burning can be present. Symptoms are usually reproduced by a vaginal or rectal examination.

2. These dysfunctions can be grouped into two basic categories based on etiology:
   a. **Muscle hypertonus** disorders can be caused by direct trauma in and of the pelvis, dysfunctional use patterns, or psychogenic factors. These cause a pain/tension cycle in the pelvic floor muscles.
      i. Pelvic inflammation, infection, or disease
      ii. Vaginal delivery and episiotomy
      iii. Surgeries with urogenital or rectal approaches
      iv. Sexual abuse[42]
      v. Musculoskeletal injuries of the coccyx or pelvis
      vi. Lifestyle and stress issues causing physiologic muscle tension held in the pelvic floor
      vii. Learned abnormal use of pelvic floor muscles
      viii. Habitual abnormal postures and holding patterns
   b. **Musculoskeletal dysfunction**[1a,15]
      i. Joint malalignment of S1–L5 region, coccyx, pubic symphysis
      ii. History of pelvic or coccyx fracture
      iii. Posture dysfunction[21]
      iv. Myofascial pain syndromes create pain, tenderness, and autonomic phenomena from myofascial trigger points. The specific muscles that cause symptoms in the pelvic floor region are identified by Travell and Simons.[40]
         (a) Pelvic pain—coccygeus, levator ani, obturator internus, adductor magnus, piriformis, oblique abdominals
         (b) Iliosacral pain—levator ani and coccygeus, gluteus medius, quadratus lumborum, gluteus maximus, multifudi, rectus abdominis, soleus

3. **Specific symptoms** include:
   a. Chronic pelvic pain, dysmenorrhea
   b. Dyspareunia and sexual dysfunction
   c. Constipation or voiding dysfunction
   d. Frequency and urgency of urination

4. **Tension myalgia of the pelvic floor** is a consolidation diagnosis of various syndromes of the pelvic musculature (piriformis syndrome, levator ani syndrome, levator spasm syndrome, coccygodynia, vaginismus).[33,34] Vaginismus and proctalgia fugax are specifically related to muscle spasm. Other diagnoses that may have a component of hypertonus dysfunction include:
   a. Chronic low back pain, endometriosis, chronic pelvic pain with negative laparoscopy
   b. Interstitial cystitis, urethral syndrome, sphincter dyssynergia

5. **Evaluation** of the pelvic floor in hypertonus dysfunctions usually reproduces pain.
   a. Pelvic floor muscle examination done externally or internally
   b. Specific musculoskeletal examination of sacroiliac joint and pelvic articulations
   c. Surface EMG biofeedback evaluation is useful and can be performed with a vaginal or rectal electrode.
      i. Specific pelvic floor EMG analysis
         (a) Baseline resting muscle activity
         (b) Positional differences
         (c) Exercise and functional activities
         (d) Psychophysiologic-stress profile

6. **Treatment for hypertonus dysfunction/levator ani syndromes**
   a. **Musculoskeletal dysfunction** is best treated with a combination of physical therapy including manual therapy, myofascial release, posture education, and biofeedback-assisted pelvic floor exercise.

b. **Hypertonus dysfunction** responds well to biofeedback for muscle identification, awareness, and relaxation techniques.
   i. A therapeutic exercise program can include strengthening exercises of antagonist musculature, aerobic exercise regimen, and specific pelvic floor exercises.
   ii. Relaxation exercises and training are recommended.
   iii. Physical therapy modalities of heat and cold

D. **Incoordination dysfunction** of the pelvic floor muscles can occur from improper muscle contraction, inappropriate use of the muscles, or neurologic disease. Many women do not perform pelvic floor exercises correctly.[5]

1. **Several etiologies** can independently or concurrently contribute to this problem. Incoordination problems may be a component of other pelvic floor dysfunctions.
   a. Improper exercise technique causes bearing down (as in delivering a child) rather than a lifting contraction of the pelvic floor muscles.[8] Concurrently, with this Valsalva technique, the abdominal muscles create an increase in intraabdominal pressure, making it more difficult for the pelvic floor to work correctly.
   b. Muscle strength imbalances of the gluteals, adductors, and abdominals can mask the weak contraction of the pelvic floor muscles.
   c. Myofascial or scar tissue formation can restrict the contractility of the pelvic floor muscles.
   d. Central nervous system disorders or peripheral nerve damage can create neuropathy[2] with sensory and motor deficits. This condition makes muscle contraction difficult or dyssynergic.
      i. Neurologic diseases most commonly causing symptoms are stroke, multiple sclerosis, or supraspinal cord (conus medullaris) lesions.
      ii. Damage to the pudendal nerve or pelvic plexus can result from childbirth.

2. **Symptoms**
   a. Voiding dysfunctions
   b. Urge incontinence
   c. Bearing down rather than proper muscle contraction

3. **Signs of sphincter dyssynergia** and incoordination can be recognized during urodynamic testing, EMG, or with observation of the pelvic floor muscle contraction.

4. **Treatment**
   a. Medications for neurologic etiologies
   b. Coordination and re-education of the pelvic floor muscles
      i. Breathing training—exhale on effort of pelvic floor muscle contraction
      ii. Facilitation of automatic pelvic floor muscle contraction with activities that increase intraabdominal pressure.
      iii. Elimination of unnecessary Valsalva during muscle contraction and functional activities
      iv. Learning pelvic floor contraction vs Valsalva
         (a) Surface EMG biofeedback for the pelvic floor muscles may assist coordination efforts.
         (b) Bladder pressure biofeedback[6] has also been effective.
         (c) Electrical stimulation for neuromuscular re-education

VI. TEACHING PELVIC FLOOR MUSCLE EXERCISE AND AWARENESS

A. **The neuromuscular and social aspects** of the pelvic floor muscles pose special challenges to teaching pelvic floor exercises.
1. Lack of a woman's awareness and knowledge about the muscles
2. Modesty level and preconceived ideas about the perineum

       3. Psychosocial effects of previous abuse or trauma

       4. Length of time of disuse

       5. Lack of proprioception during contraction

       6. Scar tissue limiting contractile properties of skin and muscles

       7. Pain inhibiting muscle contraction

  B. **Precede all exercise instruction with education about muscle location and functions.**

  C. **The specific language of the exercise technique** is very important. The concept of **lifting or "drawing in"** the anal sphincter and perivaginal muscles must be understood. Use descriptive language and imagery.

       1. Use action words to describe the contraction: e.g., "tighten," "squeeze," "pull up and in," "lift and hold the entire pelvic floor."

       2. Do an RV (rectal-vaginal) squeezing/lifting exercise.

          a. Have your patient visualize a circle closing as the muscles tighten, and then opening as they relax.

          b. Suggest that your patient imagine a sagging hammock being pulled taut at each end.[28]

       3. Group exercise instruction techniques include defining the perineum into the front passage (vaginal and urethral openings) and back passage (anal opening) and encouraging the contraction and lift of both passages.

  D. **Coordinate breathing with pelvic floor excercise.**

       1. The pelvic floor muscles should be prevented from working against increased intraabdominal pressure.

       2. The general rule of "exhale on effort" (pelvic floor muscle contraction) allows the breathing diaphragm to work synchronously with the pelvic floor.

       3. Functionally forced expiration (abdominal muscle contraction or cough) should be accompanied by a pelvic floor contraction to help prevent stress incontinence.

VII. **EXERCISE PRINCIPLES AND TREATMENT**

  A. Dr. Arnold Kegel, an American obstetrician and gynecologist, first described and promoted exercises for the pelvic floor in the late 1940s and early 1950s (**Kegel exercises**).[17]

       1. Kegel exercises were performed with the use of a vaginal perineometer. The perineometer is a pressure-sensing device inserted into the vagina that provides visual and proprioceptive feedback of muscle contractions to women performing the exercises.

       2. The exercises were promoted for problems with urinary stress incontinence, pelvic relaxation, and lack of sexual orgasm.

  B. The **type of exercise** prescribed depends on the evaluation of strength, sensation, and proper contraction ability.

       1. Cortical awareness, muscle length and fiber type, and proper functioning of the central and peripheral nervous system are factors affecting muscle contraction.

       2. Three types of exercises for the pelvic floor:

          a. **Concentric contraction** where the muscle creates a lift of the perineum. This can be demonstrated by the cranial and anterior movement of a pressure or EMG perineometer.[3]

          b. **Eccentric contraction** where the lengthening load is greater than the tension, as in a "descending elevator" pelvic floor exercise.[28]

          c. **Isometric contraction** where the tension equals the load, as in a contraction of pelvic floor muscles against a solid probe.[4]

  C. **Exercise prescription guidelines**

       1. Components of a complete exercise program include short- and long-duration exercises that are prescribed on the basis of evaluation as well as application of exercises to functional activities.

       2. Exercise type I and type II muscle fibers with overload strategies.

a. Train and strengthen quick response of the muscle (type II) with brief rapid contract-relax exercises of 1–2 second duration.

b. Facilitate endurance of antigravity muscles (type I, slow twitch) by performing prolonged holds (>5 seconds) progressing to 10–15 seconds.

c. A hold-to-relax ratio of at least 1:1.

3. Frequency and repetitions of exercise are best established by muscle assessment.

a. A daily or twice-a-day regimen of increasing repetitions—to fatigue. Based on muscle assessment, this could be between 3–30 repetitions.

b. Caution is recommended to avoid excessive overload and unrealistic repetition expectations.

4. Progression

a. Start in positions that eliminate gravity, especially when muscle grades are 3 or below.

b. Advance to upright and functional positions.

5. Specificity: working only on the muscle group you want to relax or strengthen

a. Reinforce muscle isolation within pelvis.

b. Initially discourage use of accessory muscles such as adductors, gluteals, and abdominals.

D. **Postulated changes in pelvic floor muscles after initiating a therapeutic exercise program.**

1. Short term (1–4 weeks)

a. Increased motor recruitment abilities

b. Improved muscle isolation techniques

c. An understanding of the difference between a relaxed and contracted pelvic floor muscle

d. Mobilization of soft tissue and fascia to promote normal tissue tone and function

e. Inhibition of unwanted muscle co-contraction.

2. Long-term (4–16 weeks)

a. Muscle hypertrophy from strength and endurance exercise programs

b. Acquisition of normal resting tone

c. Coordination and re-education of muscles

i. Facilitation of automatic pelvic floor muscle contraction with activities that increase intraabdominal pressure

ii. Elimination of unnecessary Valsalva during functional activities

d. Acquisition of the good supportive, sphincteric, and sexual function

VIII. RESEARCH NEEDS

A. Underreporting and lack of health care provider inquiry lead to underestimates in numbers of active women with pelvic floor dysfunction.

B. Research on normal pelvic floor musculature is limited, but more is clearly needed to help guide clinicians in rehabilitation strategies. There is a need to establish the optimum frequency, duration, and type of exercise necessary to maintain or improve strength, endurance, and coordination of the pelvic floor muscles.

C. The efficacy of treating muscle dysfunction components of urogynecologic problems needs further evaluation.

XI. SUMMARY

The emphasis on pelvic floor exercise should be preventative rather than rehabilitative. Health care providers, health educators, and fitness personnel need to ask women more questions about pelvic floor function. Only then will the magnitude and prevalence of pelvic floor muscle dysfunctions receive the attention that is needed.

Pelvic floor muscle contraction is an acquired function, not innate. Therapeutic exercise requires specificity training and dedication to an exercise program. Exercise programs should be specific to the type of pelvic floor muscle dysfunction and its etiology. Behavioral treatment options focus on traditional physical therapy techniques of muscle education, therapeutic exercise, and the use of physical modalities.

ACKNOWLEDGMENT

The author wishes to thank the medical center physicians and staff, medical library, and Department of Physical Therapy of Virginia Mason Medical Center in Seattle, Washington for their support in the development of physical therapy treatment programs for pelvic floor muscle dysfunctions.

REFERENCES

1a. Baker PK: Musculoskeletal origins of chronic pelvic pain: Diagnosis and treatment. Obstet Gynecol Clin North Am 20:719–742, 1993.

1. Benson JT (ed): Female Pelvic Floor Disorders: Investigation and Management. New York, W.W. Norton, 1992.

2. Benson JT: Pelvic floor neuropathy. In Benson JT (ed): Female Pelvic Floor Disorders: Investigation and Management. New York, W.W. Norton, 1992.

3. Bø K, et al: Pelvis floor muscle exercise for the treatment of female stress urinary incontinence: I. Reliability of vaginal pressure measurements of pelvic floor muscle strength. Neurourol Urodyn 9:471–477, 1990.

4. Brubaker L, Kotarinos R: Pelvic floor rehabilitation: The role of muscle training. Uro-Gynecol Soc Q Rep 11(2):1–4, 1993.

5. Bump RC, et al: Assessment of Kegel pelvic muscle exercise performance after brief verbal instruction. Am J Obstet Gynecol 165:322–329, 1991.

6. Burgio K: Biofeedback therapy. In Benson JT (ed): Female Pelvic Floor Disorders: Investigation and Management. New York, W.W. Norton, 1992.

7. Burns PA, et al: Kegel's exercises with biofeedback therapy for treatment of stress incontinence. Nurse Pract 10(2):28, 33–34, 46, 1985.

8. Chiarelli P: Incontinence: The pelvic floor function. Aust Fam Physician 18:943–949, 1989.

9. DeLancey J, Richardson AC: Anatomy of genital support. In Benson JT (ed): Female Pelvic Floor Disorders: Investigation and Management. New York, W.W. Norton, 1992.

10. Fall M, Lindstrom S: Electrical stimulation, evaluation, and treatment of urinary incontinence. Urol Clin North Am 18:393–407, 1991.

11. Gilpin SA, Gossling JA, Smith ARB, Warrell DW: The pathogenesis of genitourinary prolapse and stress incontinence of urine: A histological and histochemical study. Br J Obstet Gynaecol 96:15–23, 1989.

12. Graber B: Circumvaginal Musculature and Sexual Function. New York, Karger, 1982.

13. Graber B, Kline-Graber G: Female orgasm: Role of pubococcygeus muscle. J Clin Psychiatry 40(Aug):348–351, 1979.

14. Henry MM: Pathogenesis and management of fecal incontinence in the adult. Gastroenterol Clin North Am 16:35–45, 1987.

15. Herman H: Urogenital Dysfunction: Clinics in Physical Therapy (Vol 20, Obstetric and Gynecologic Physical Therapy). New York, Churchill-Livingstone, 1988.

16. Kasman G: Use of integrated electromyography for the assessment and treatment of musculoskeletal pain: Guidelines for physical medicine practitioners. In Cram JR (ed): Surface EMG for Clinical Recordings, Vol 2. Nevada City, Clinical Resources, 1990, pp 255–302.

16a. Kasman G: Surface EMG in Physical Therapy [Seminar]. Denver, Colorado, October 16–17, 1993.

17. Kegel AH: Progressive resistance exercise in the functional restoration of the perineal muscles. Am J Obstet Gynecol 56:238–248, 1948.

18. Kegel AH: The physiologic treatment of poor tone and function of the genital muscles and of urinary stress incontinence. West J Surg Obstet Gynecol 57:527–535, 1949.

19. Kegel AH: Active Exercise of the Pubococcygeus Muscle (Progress in Gynecology). New York, Grune & Stratton, 1950.

20. Kegel AH: Sexual functions of the pubococcygeus muscle West J Surg Obstet Gynecol 60:521–524, 1952.

21. Kegel AH: Early genital relaxation: New technic of diagnosis and nonsurgical treatment. Obstet Gynecol 8:545–550, 1956.

22. King PM, et al: Musculoskeletal factors in chronic pelvic pain. J Psychosom Obstet Gynecol 12(Suppl):87–98, 1991.

23. Klock SC: Female sexuality and sexual counseling. Curr Probl Obstet Gynecol Fertil 16:107–139, 1993.

24. Laycock J: Assessment and treatment of pelvic floor dysfunction [doctoral thesis]. Postgraduate School of Biomedical Sciences, University of Bradford, Bradford, UK, 1992.

25. McClellan E: Fecal incontinence: Social and economic factors. In Benson JT (ed): Female Pelvic Floor Disorders: Investigation and Management. New York, W.W. Norton, 1992.
26. Mills P, Deakin M, Kiff ES: Percutaneous electrical stimulation for ano-rectal incontinence. Physiotherapy 76:433–438, 1990.
27. Mostwin J: Current concepts of female pelvic anatomy and physiology. Urol Clin North Am 18:175–195, 1991.
28. Noble E: Essential Exercises for the Childbearing Year. Boston, Houghton Mifflin, 1988.
29. Norton PA: Histology and biochemical studies. In Benson JT (ed): Female Pelvic Floor Disorders: Investigation and Management. New York, W.W. Norton, 1992.
29a. Norton PA: Pelvic floor disorders: The role of fascia and ligaments. Clin Obstet Gynecol 36:926–938, 1993.
30. Nygaard I, et al: Exercise and incontinence. Obstet Gynecol 75:848–851, 1990.
31. Peattie AB, et al: Vaginal cones: A conservative method of treating genuine stress incontinence. Br J Obstet Gynaecol 95:1049–1053, 1989.
32. Physicians hear about incontinence. JAMA 264:2381–2382, 1990.
33. Salvati E: The levator syndrome and its variant. Gastroenterol Clin North Am 16:71–78, 1987.
34. Sinaki M, Merrit J, Stillwell GK: Tension myalgia of the pelvic floor. Mayo Clin Proc 52:717–722, 1977.
35. Smith ARB, Hosker GL, Warrell DW: The role of pudendal nerve damage in the etiology of genuine stress incontinence in women. Br J Obstet Gynaecol 96:29–32, 1989.
36. Snooks S, Swash M, Henry MM, et al: Risk factors in childbirth causing damage to the pelvic floor innervation. Br J Surg 72:S15–S17, 1985.
37. Spector I, Carey M: Incidence and prevalence of sexual dysfunction: A critical review of the empirical literature. Arch Sex Behav 19:389–408, 1990.
38. Spence-Jones C, et al: Bowel dysfunction: A pathogenic factor in uterovaginal prolapse and urinary stress incontinence. Neurourol Urodyn 11:313–314, 1992.
39. Swash M: New concepts in the prevention of incontinence. Practitioner 229:895–899, 1985.
40. Travell J, Simons D: Myofascial Pain and Dysfunction: The Trigger Point Manual, vol. 2. Baltimore, Williams & Wilkins, 1992.
41. Urinary Incontinence in Adults: Clinical Practice Guideline. Rockville, MD, Agency for Health Care Policy and Research, Public Health Service, U.S. Department of Health and Human Services, March 1992 [AHCPR pub no. 93-0038].
42. Walker E, et al: Relationship of chronic pelvic pain to psychiatric diagnoses and childhood sexual abuse. Am J Psychiatry 145:75–80, 1991.

Chapter 28: Depression

JENNIFER D. BOLEN, MD

Women are increasingly involved in active daily exercise, organized sports, and competitive athletics, as well as strenuous physically oriented occupations. The impact of exercise on mood has been actively studied over the recent years with positive benefits noted. Little is known about prevalence rates of depression in active and/or athletic women as compared with sedentary women. Clinicians might expect to see the same rates reflected in active and athletic women, but on the other hand, exercise may mask or even prevent the clinical expression of a mood disorder. All humans have the potential for depressed mood, and a variety of factors such as age, family history, gender, life events, and physical and mental status influence the likelihood of being at risk. Exercise may be a significant factor in protecting women from depressive illness. Just as diabetes mellitus can be brought on by obesity or pregnancy, but resuppress with weight loss or delivery, exercise may keep the depression threshold at a higher level.

The following outline covers some aspects of depression in active and athletic women, but in-depth studies in this area are lacking. The term *depression* will be used interchangeably with the descriptors *mood disorder* and *affective illness,* though these clinical terms are more encompassing of the broader range of mood disturbance which includes elevated mood states, i.e., mania and hypomania.

I. **DEPRESSION DEFINED**

   A. **DSM-III-R diagnostic criteria for various depression types**[1]

      1. **Major Depressive Episodes:** Five of the following symptoms must have been present during the same 2-week period and represent a change from previous functioning, at least one of the symptoms is either depressed mood or loss of interest or pleasure.

        a. Depressed or irritable mood

        b. Markedly diminished interest or pleasure in all, or almost all, activities most of the day

        c. Significant weight loss or weight gain when not dieting, or change in appetite

        d. Insomnia or hypersomnia

        e. Psychomotor agitation or retardation

        f. Fatigue or loss of energy

        g. Feelings of worthlessness

        h. Diminished concentration

        i. Recurrent thoughts of death, suicide

        j. Organic factors ruled out

      2. Major depression can be a single episode or recurrent.

      3. **Dysthymia:** Depressed mood for most of the day, more days than not, for at least 2 years.

        a. Presence of at least two of the above symptoms

      4. **Adjustment disorder with depressed mood:** A reaction to an identifiable psychosocial stressor (or multiple stressors) that occurs within 3 months of onset of the stressor(s). The reaction is severe enough to cause impairment in occupational or social functioning and the symptoms are in excess of a normal and expectable reaction to the stressor.

        a. Duration <6 months

        b. Mood disturbance is the predominant feature.

5. Other depressions include the following:
   a. Seasonal affective disorder (SAD): 3 episodes of depression in 3 separate years occurring within a particular 60-day period, e.g., fall, and lifting in another period, e.g., spring
   b. Rapid cycling bipolar disorder: more common in women especially towards midlife, associated with frequent mood swings from depressed to elevated mood or from depressed to more depressed mood.
   c. Post-partum depression
   d. Premenstrual mood drop, known as PMS, or late luteal phase dysphoric disorder

II. PREVALENCE OF AFFECTIVE DISORDERS

A. Incidence over a 6-month period
   1. Females = 7.5%
   2. Males = 4%
B. Lifetime incidence:
   1. Females = 14%
   2. Males = 7%
C. The lifetime prevalence rate for major depression is highest in the age group 25–44.
D. Rates of depression go up in ambulatory care settings versus the population at large.

III. FACTORS INFLUENCING MOOD STATES: BIOPSYCHOSOCIAL INFLUENCES

A. **Biology** usually implies a positive family history of affective illness. Individuals often at greatest risk have a first-degree relative with a past or present history for a mood disorder.
B. **Psychological** implies the frame of mind a person holds, attitudes, cognitive style, psychodynamic factors.
C. **Social** impacts include poverty, abuse, discrimination, loss.

IV. EXERCISE IS ASSOCIATED WITH GOOD MENTAL HEALTH IN SEVERAL STUDIES

A. Master athletes and female masters scored lower on tension, depression, anger, fatigue, and confusion and higher on vigor when compared to a college sample of nonactive females.[7]
B. **Psychological benefits of exercise** noted in several studies[4]
   1. Enhanced mental performance and concentration
   2. Improved self-image and feelings of confidence and well-being
   3. Perceived improvement in sleep quality, energy level, mood and tension, and stress levels
   4. Decreased anxiety, depression, and hostility
C. Symptoms of depression have been shown to abate with regular exercise, and exercise was superior to relaxation or pleasant activities in terms of a positive impact on mood.[6]
D. Aerobic and nonaerobic forms of exercise have been shown to benefit depression.[5]
E. The risk of depression may be lowered by high levels of physical activity and increased by low levels of physical activity.[2]
F. In moderately depressed elderly persons, exercise was associated with decreased somatic symptoms.

V. EVALUATION AND MEDICAL WORK-UP OF DEPRESSION

A. **A careful history of the present** episode would include:
   1. Detail the degree and severity of the mood disturbance
   2. Duration

3. Associated physical symptoms of depression, e.g., sleep problems, energy drop, concentration and memory impairment
4. Additional psychiatric symptoms associated with the depression, such as eating-disordered behavior, anxiety, obsessive-compulsive behaviors, suicidal ideation, pain symptoms
5. Impact of the disturbance on the individual's level of functioning
6. Current health, review of systems, and physical examination
7. Current laboratory work—complete blood count, liver function test, electrolytes, blood urea nitrogen, thyroid-stimulating hormone, urinalysis
8. Mental status examination
9. Beck depression inventory
10. Family history of psychiatric problems
11. Substance use, alcohol and street drugs
12. Over-the-counter drugs and any current prescription medications
13. Past psychiatric history, prior history of mood swings
14. Assess life-change events, recent and current stressors, losses, quality of work, and home environment and relationships

VI. CONSEQUENCES OF NONTREATMENT

A. Risk of suicide in depressed patients is high.
B. Patient suffers significantly with, at times, divorce, poor parenting, job loss, low self-esteem, vulnerability to other medical problems, and self-medicating with alcohol.

VII. TREATMENT OPTIONS FOR DEPRESSION

A. Chemotherapy with antidepressants, mood stabilizers, or both
B. Psychotherapy
C. A combination of chemotherapy and psychotherapy
D. 70% of depressed patients will respond to chemotherapy for depression.
E. Rates of positive response to cognitive-behavioral therapy for milder depression are in the same range as for antidepressants.
F. Continue or encourage regular daily activity or exercise.
G. Phototherapy is an option for SADS. In one study of SADS patients, 1 hour of walking at midday was as effective as phototherapy.
H. Side effects of chemotherapy with antidepressants:
1. **Tricyclics:**
   a. Include 10 beat/min heart rate increase noticed by many athletes, dry mouth, flushing, constipation, sedation and postural blood pressure drop.
   b. Nortriptyline (Pamelor) has lower effect on postural blood pressure.
   c. Desipramine (Norpramin) has lesser anticholinergic side effects and nonsedating properties.
2. **Prozac:**
   a. Some reports of bradycardia; lightens sleep cycles; causes jitteriness during the initiating phase of treatment in some individuals.
   b. In starting Prozac in someone with high levels of anxiety or panic, initiate with the elixir at a geriatric dose, 1–5 mg/day.
3. **Wellbutrin, Zoloft, and Anafranil:** These newer antidepressants have yet to be prescribed in large enough numbers of patients that their compatibility with exercise and activity is not well known.
4. **Mood stabilizers:**
   a. Include lithium, carbamazine and valproic acid and are used primarily in bipolar or rapidly cycling patients.
   b. With active aerobic conditioning or major activities such as cycling, running, etc., pay special attention to hydration status, since volume loss can be associated with a rise in lithium levels into the toxic range.

5. In younger women and adolescents and/or in competitive athletes, psychotherapy is the better first treatment choice.

VIII. **IS DEPRESSION MASKED OR PARTIALLY TREATED BY REGULAR EXERCISE?**

A. No studies have examined this possibility in depth.

B. One study of elite female runners noted that **amenorrhea was significantly associated with high rates of affective illness in first-degree family members or in the runners themselves.** The amenorrhea furthermore was correlated with a high rate of eating disorders, a condition not uncommonly seen in female athletes and frequently comorbid with depression. Since depression and eating disorders share some similarities in genetic markers, disturbed endocrine function and neurotransmitters, and EEG sleep changes, the presence of eating disordered behavior or amenorrhea should be a red flag for further evaluation for depression.[3]

C. Given the positive effect of exercise on mood, it seems reasonable to assume that **affective illness may be masked or partially treated in active and athletic women.** This group of women could be at risk for expression of their mood disturbance if inactivity were suddenly experienced due to an injury, lifestyle change, or chronic illness.

D. **Depression may present in less classic ways in active and athletic women.** For example, children often present with irritability and social or school failure when depressed. Athletes might present with increased numbers of injuries, lower vigor, burn-out for competition rather than with classic anhedonia.

REFERENCES

1. American Psychiatric Association: Diagnostic and Statistical Manual of Mental Disorders, 3rd ed., revised. Washington, DC, American Psychiatric Association, 1987.
2. Camacho TC, Roberts FE, Lazarus NB, et al: Physical activity and depression: Evidence from Alameda County Study. Am J Epidemiol 134:220–231, 1991.
3. Gadpaille WJ, Sanborn CF, Wagner WW: Athletic amenorrhea, major affective disorders, and eating disorders. Am J Psychiatry 144:939–942, 1987.
4. King AC, Taylor CD, Haskell WL, et al: Influence of regular aerobic exercise on psychological health: A randomized, controlled trial of healthy middle-aged adults. Health Psychol 8:305–324, 1989.
5. Martinsen EW, Hoffart A, Solberg O: Comparing aerobic with nonaerobic forms of exercise in the treatment of clinical depression: A randomized trial. Compr Psychiatry 30:324–331, 1989.
6. North TC, McCullagh P, Tran ZV: Effect of exercise on depression. Exerc Sport Sci Rev 18:379–415, 1990.
7. Ungerleider S, Golding JM, Porter K: Mood profile of masters track and field athletes. Percept Mot Skills 68:607–617, 1989.

Chapter 29: Dermatologic Issues

KELLI R. ARNTZEN, MD

Physical activity has become increasingly popular among women over the past few decades, and because of these physical pursuits, the skin is subjected to many hazards. Besides direct trauma, it can be injured from environmental insults, and many preexisting dermatoses may be exacerbated by sports activities.[10] The aspects of dermatology that are associated with physical activity are discussed in the following review.

I. **DIRECT TRAUMA**

   A. **Blisters**

      1. Probably the most common injuries

      2. Caused by shearing forces which create a split in the malpighian layer of the epidermis

      3. **Prevention:** The best therapy is prevention, such as properly fitted shoes, socks, and the use of talc powder.

      4. **Treatment:** Drain the fluid of the blister with a sterile needle within the first 24 hours and apply antibiotic cream such as Bacitracin ointment. **Do not de-roof blister.**[2] If you drain the area in the first 24 hours, the top has the greatest chance of reattachment to the base, which decreases pain.

   B. **Subungual hematomas**

      1. Caused by the foot sliding forward in shoes and meeting resistance (Fig. 1)

      2. They may be painful.

      3. **Prevention** may be difficult in sports with quick starts and stops (e.g., tennis).

      4. **Treatment:** None if asymptomatic. If symptomatic, a radiograph should be performed to rule out fracture.[10] Persistent pigmentation should alert to the possibility of subungual melanoma.

         a. Drain hematoma with "drill technique" or hot paper-clip technique.

         b. Drill technique: Using a 20-gauge needle placed over the hematoma, rotate the needle like a drill until it passes through the nail plate.

   C. **Black heel (talon noir)**

      1. Punctate hemorrhages are located on heels but can also occur on palmar surfaces (Fig. 2).[8]

      2. Most commonly seen in sports with frequent starts and stops.

      3. Most commonly seen in adolescents and young adults.[10]

      4. Shearing forces cause intraepidermal hemorrhage.

      5. **Treatment:** None; they resolve spontaneously.

   D. **Calluses:** In many sports, these are valued (e.g., gymnastics).

      1. Repeated rubbing causes the skin to attempt to protect itself by becoming hyperkeratotic.

      2. Occasionally these may be tender. There are two types of calluses, hard and soft (Fig. 3).

      3. It is important to distinguish calluses from warts (*see* Fig. 18). Warts commonly have punctate hemorrhages present and cause deviation of the skin lines, which calluses do not.

      4. **Prevention:** Remove cause of friction.

      5. **Treatment:** Paring or keratolytics.[1]

   E. **Jogger's nipples**

      1. Present as painful erythema with desquamation and fissures of the areolar area.

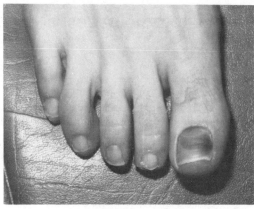

FIGURE 1. Subungual hematoma.

2. Occur in females who do not wear brassieres (or in men who wear shirts made of hard fabrics such as cotton).[1]
3. **Prevention:** Women should wear a sports bra (men should wear a semisynthetic or silk undershirt). Application of petrolatum or covering the area with tape is also effective.
4. **Treatment:** Emollients; may need mild topical steroids.
5. In females, especially those with unilateral involvement, consider the diagnosis of Paget's disease which may be associated with an underlying breast malignancy.
F. **Striae distensae (stretch marks)**
  1. Bands of thin wrinkled skin that are at first red, evolving to purple, then white.
  2. Occur most commonly over the anterior shoulders, lower back, and thighs.
  3. Weight-lifters, gymnasts, and growing teenagers are the most susceptible.
  4. These striae lie perpendicular to the direction of skin tension.[8]
  5. **Treatment:** Recently, tretinoin (Retin-A) has been shown to benefit striae.
G. **Piezogenic papules**
  1. Herniations of fat into the skin; these most commonly occur on the sides of the heel, causing pain[10] (Fig. 4).
  2. These are only visible when weight is placed on the area.
  3. **Prevention** and **treatment:** None known.

II. ENVIRONMENTAL INSULTS

A. **Sunlight**
  1. The damage ultraviolet light can do to skin is well known. Our sun exposure is unfortunately cumulative; we therefore need to protect ourselves as much as possible.
  2. Sun exposure can cause acute problems, such as sunburn and phototoxic reactions, and chronic problems, such as actinic damage and skin cancers (Fig. 5).
     a. Basal cell carcinomas are the most common malignant neoplasm in humans.

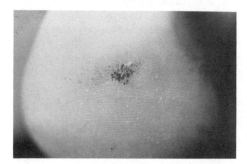

FIGURE 2. Black heel (photograph courtesy of Allan Kayne, MD).

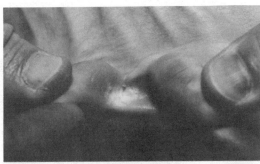

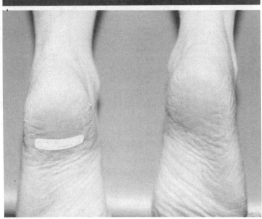

FIGURE 3. Calluses: Soft corn (*top*) and hard heel callus (*bottom*).

     b. Squamous cell carcinomas are second.

     c. Malignant melanoma the third most common. Malignant melanoma is on the rise, and it is predicted that by the year 2000, lifetime risk for a malignant melanoma will be 1 in 90.

  3. **Prevention:**

     a. Avoid activities in the sun between 10 AM and 3 PM.

     b. Daily use of sunscreens (SPF 15) with reapplication after swimming or sweating.

        i. **Physical sunscreens** include zinc oxide and titanium dioxide which block both long and short ultraviolet light.

        ii. Chemical sunscreens work by absorbing a specific portion of ultraviolet light.

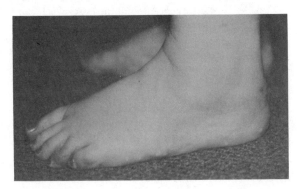

FIGURE 4. Piezogenic papules.

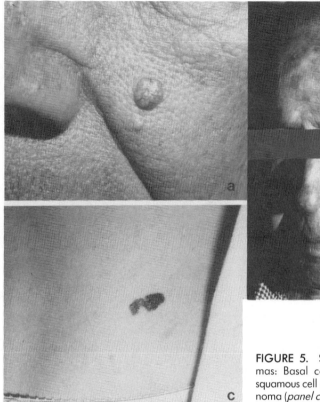
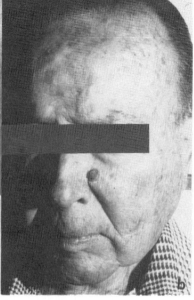

FIGURE 5. Sunlight-related carcinomas: Basal cell carcinoma (*panel a*); squamous cell carcinoma (*panel b*); melanoma (*panel c*) (photographs courtesy of LAC/USC Medical Center).

   (a) UVB absorbers (290–320 nm) include PABA, PABA esters, and cinnamates.
   (b) UVA absorbers (320–400 nm) include Parsol 1789, benzophenones, and anthralaites.
   c. It is best to use a broad-spectrum sunscreen to block both UVA and UVB.
   d. "Waterproof" means that the sunscreen is effective for 80 minutes in the water and then needs to be reapplied.
   e. Active patients often complain of a "stinging" sensation when applying sunscreens around the eyes, which can be avoided by using the "stick" type sunscreens around these areas.
   f. Start sunscreen use in small children; however, those under 6 months of age should not be allowed in the sun.[11]
   4. **Treatment:** For acute sunburns, use cool compresses and nonsteroidal antiinflammatory drugs (NSAIDs). Occasionally, systemic steroids may be needed.
B. **Heat**
   1. **Cholinergic urticaria**
      a. These develop as small erythematous papules 2–20 minutes after general body overheating and last for minutes to hours. These generally occur over the trunk and extremities (Fig. 6).
      b. These are acetylcholine-mediated.
      c. Test for these by having the patient exercise for 10–15 minutes and then observing for 1 hour.

FIGURE 6. Heat-induced papular urticaria (photograph courtesy of Allan Kayne, MD).

    d. **Prevention:** Avoid heat and exertion.

    e. **Treatment:** Antihistamines are generally not very useful,[8] but hydroxyzine, 25 mg 1 hour before exercise, may be of some benefit.

  2. **Miliaria**

    a. There are three types, depending upon the location of the blockage of the eccrine sweat duct:

       i. **Miliaria crystallina:** Very fragile small vesicles caused by blockage high in the stratum corneum (most commonly seen after sunburns).[9]

      ii. **Miliaria rubra** ("prickly heat"): Minute red papules that give a stinging or "prickly" sensation, caused by intraepidermal blockage.[9]

     iii. **Miliaria profunda:** Noninflammatory flesh-colored papules seen in repeated cases of miliaria rubra, caused by dermal blockage.[9]

    b. **Prevention:** Wear loose, well-ventilated clothing.

    c. **Treatment:** Stay in a cool, well-ventilated environment. Treatment is otherwise symptomatic.

  3. **Erythema ab igne**

    a. Persistent reticulated erythema and hyperpigmentation caused by the application of prolonged heat to a specific area.[10] A transient reticulated erythema is noted initially. With time and continued exposure, the erythema becomes more intense and persists between exposures with the appearance of the pigmentation (Fig. 7).

    b. There may be an increased risk of skin cancer developing in these areas.[9]

    c. **Prevention:** Avoid prolonged exposure to heating pads, etc.

C. **Cold**

  1. **Frost nip or frostbite**

    a. Frost nip is superficial frostbite.

       i. In frost nip, the skin appears waxy or white; after rewarming, it becomes numb with a mottled appearance, then swells, stings, and burns. Blisters develop in 24–36 hours and resolve in 2 weeks.[4]

      ii. In frostbite, the skin appears waxy or white and is anesthetic. The swelling and blister formation may take 3 days to 1 week to develop. After the first 24–48 hours, the affected area becomes painful, which may last 2–8 weeks.[4]

    b. The patient may have increased sensitivity to cold for many months after and may have complaints of pruritus and hyperhidrosis for >6 months.[10]

    c. **Prevention:** Multiple layers of loose-fitting clothing. If an area becomes anesthetic or white, find a warm environment immediately. Avoid washing

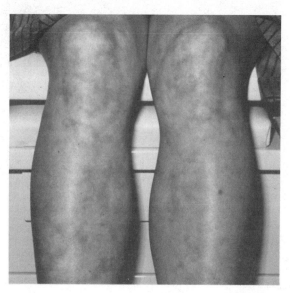

FIGURE 7. Erythema ab igne (photograph courtesy of LAC/USC Medical Center).

the face or shaving prior to cold exposure, since sebum gives some protection, or apply petrolatum or a creamy sunscreen to protect the face.

    d. **Treatment:** Rapid rewarming, preferably in a warm water bath not warmer than 44°C for 20 minutes. **Do not rub the frozen part.**[10]

2. **Pernio** (chilblain)

    a. Edematous reddish-blue plaques that are tender after exposure to cold, wet environments[8] (Fig. 8).

    b. Most commonly seen over the digits.

    c. Young females seem to be more susceptible.

    d. **Prevention and treatment:** Keep the affected area warm and dry; wool socks are helpful; avoid constriction by shoes that are too tight. Nitroglycerin paste may be helpful.

3. **Cold urticaria**

    a. There are two types:

      i. **Familial:** Autosomal-dominant inheritance pattern. They have their onset early in life and are rare. There are two types:

        (a) **Immediate:** urticarial lesions within 3 hours after exposure.

        (b) **Delayed:** urticarial lesions 9–18 hours after exposure.

      ii. **Acquired:** Two types:

        (a) **Primary** is the most common.

        (b) **Secondary** may be associated with cryoproteins; check for underlying diseases, such as collagen vascular disease, dysglobulinemias, leukemia, liver disease, malignancy, and infections.

        (c) The mean age of onset is 18–25 years, and the urticarial lesions occur after rewarming.[6]

    b. Patients may have severe reactions to cold environments (such as cold water), resulting in anaphylaxis and death.

    c. **Prevention and treatment:** Decrease exposure to cold environments. Cyproheptadine, 2 mg orally twice daily, and doxepin, 10 mg once to three times daily, are helpful.[6]

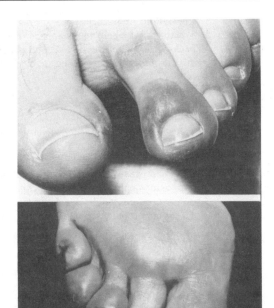

FIGURE 8. Pernio (photographs courtesy of Allan Kayne, MD, and Charles Hammer, MD).

D. **Contact dermatitis**
   1. **Plants:** poison oak, poison ivy, poison sumac
      a. "Leaves of three, leave them be."
      b. Exposure to the broken plant is necessary to react.
   2. **Rubber products:** Mercaptobenzathiazole and accelerators may be leached out by sweating.[8]
   3. **Leather products:** Potassium dichromate may be leached out by sweating[8] (Fig. 9).
   4. **Topical medications:** Antibiotics (neomycin), anesthetics (benzocaines), liniments and rubbing compounds, lanolin moisturizers.[8]

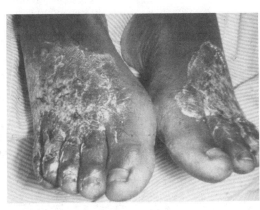

FIGURE 9. Shoe contact dermatitis (photograph courtesy of LAC/USC Medical Center, Department of Dermatology).

     5. **Prevention:** Avoidance.

     6. **Treatment:** Use cool soaks, topical or systemic steroids. **Do not use steroid dose packs**—they taper too quickly and patients will often flare after these have been discontinued. Taper systemic steroids over 2–3 weeks.

E. **Insects**

    1. **Mosquitoes**

      a. Prefer dark to light skin, warm over cool skin, sweet smelling over nonperfumed, those on birth control pills or hormones over nonmedicated.[3]

      b. **Prevention:** Use insect repellants containing DEET (N,N-diethyl-*m*-toluamide); wear long sleeves and pants in light colors.[3]

    2. **Bees and Wasps**

      a. Do not wear perfumes, scented lotions, or shampoos.[3]

      b. Do not wear brightly colored clothes; wear tan, white, light green, or khaki.[3]

      c. Do not wear jewelry, suede, or leather.[3]

      d. Do not go barefoot.[3]

F. **Water hazards**

    1. **Green hair:** occurs in blond, white, or gray-haired individuals after swimming in pools.

      a. Caused by the deposit of copper in the hair matrix.

      b. **Prevention:** Shampoo immediately after leaving the water. It can be prevented by stabilizing the pH of the pool water between 7.4–7.6.

      c. **Treatment:** 3% hydrogen peroxide applied to the hair for 2–3 hours or the application of a chelating agent (EDTA) for 30 minutes.[5]

    2. **Chlorine effects**

      a. Dry skin and hair: Due to the degreasing effects of chemically treated water.

      b. Bleaching of hair: More common in lighter-haired individuals.

      c. **Treatment:** After swimming, shower or bathe and shampoo hair; use a conditioner on the scalp and apply a moisturizer to the skin.

    3. **Swimmer's ear (otitis externa)**

      a. Acute bacterial infection of the external ear canal caused by maceration secondary to water trapped in the ear canal.[7] Prolonged exposure to the water also removes the earwax and changes the acid-base balance of the ear canal.

      b. **Treatment:** Keep water out of the ear; culture for isolation and sensitivity. For those with recurrent disease, petroleum-coated earplugs can be used, or the prophylactic use of Vosol (2% acetic acid in propylene glycol) can be advised.[10]

    4. **Sea bather's eruption**

      a. Severely pruritic papular eruption in areas covered by the swimsuit, seen after swimming in the ocean or salt water.[7] This occurs a few hours after exposure and is primarily seen off the Atlantic or Gulf coasts in March through September.

      b. Recent research has implicated the larvae of the jellyfish *Linuche unguiculata* as the cause.[13]

      c. Disappears completely in one week.

      d. **Prevention:** Showering without swimsuit immediately after getting out of the water. Women should wear two-piece swimsuits and men should not wear t-shirts.[13]

    5. **Swimmer's itch (cutaneous schistosomiasis)**

      a. Pruritic papules in areas uncovered by the swimsuit, seen after swimming in freshwater.[7] Initially, patients will experience a prickly or itchy sensation that lasts a few minutes to an hour (while the cercariae are penetrating the skin). Transient red papules then appear and are replaced by the pruritic papules.

      b. Caused by parasitic cercariae of the family Schistosomatidae that penetrate the epidermis and die.

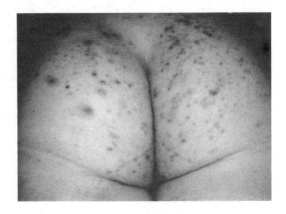

FIGURE 10.   Folliculitis (photograph courtesy of Charles Hammer, MD).

c. Resolves spontaneously in 1 week.

d. **Prevention:** Wash and towel dry promptly after exiting the water.

III. INFECTIONS

A. Bacterial

1. **Impetigo**

   a. Caused by group A β-hemolytic streptococci or *Staphylococcus aureus*. They begin as erythematous papules that rapidly transform into crusted lesions. *S. aureus* may cause bullous lesions.

   b. **Contagious:** Can be rapidly spread in close contact sports.

   c. **Prevention:** Those infected need to avoid close contact until it has resolved.

   d. **Treatment:** Oral antibiotics with coverage for both staphylococci and streptococci, or topical mupirocin.

2. **Folliculitis**

   a. Bacterial infection originating in the hair follicle, usually caused by coagulase-positive staphylococci but may be caused by gram-negative organisms.

   b. Tender follicular papules or pustules may be pruritic and often are exacerbated by occlusive equipment (Fig. 10).

   c. **Prevention:** Wear absorbant clothing next to the skin; avoid occlusive equipment.

   d. **Treatment:** Topical or systemic antibiotics, antibacterial soaps.

3. **Hot tub folliculitis**

   a. Eight hours to 5 days after exposure to contaminated water, an erythematous, macular, papular, papulopustular, or urticarial eruption can occur on any part that had been submerged in the water.[12] They are usually pruritic. Areas of occlusion may have severe involvement.

   b. *Pseudomonas aeruginosa* is the organism that overgrows when the pH and chemical balance are not regulated closely. High water temperature, water turbulence, and high bather load may be factors leading to the rapid dissipation of the chlorine.[12]

   c. Resolves on its own in 7–10 days.

   d. **Prevention:** Close monitoring of pH and chemical balance (maintain free residual chlorine level at 1 ppm and pH 7.2–7.8).[6]

   e. **Treatment:** Self-limited, although topical compresses with 2.5% acetic acid 2–3 times a day may be helpful. In resistant cases, oral antibiotics may be necessary.[6]

4. **Erythrasma**

   a. Well-demarcated reddish-brown patches with fine desquamation occurring in the intertriginous areas (Fig. 11). The area fluoresces orange-red or coral-pink under the Wood's lamp.

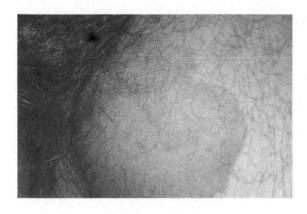

FIGURE 11. Erythrasma (photograph courtesy of Charles Hammer, MD).

    b. Caused by *Corynebacterium minutissimum* which produces a water-soluble porphyrin that fluoresces.

    c. **Prevention:** Wear loose clothing.

    d. **Treatment:** Topical or oral erythromycin, 1 g/day for 5 days.

  5. **Pitted keratolysis**

    a. 1–3 mm discrete craterlike pits on the undersurface of the feet and toes (Fig. 12).

    b. Probably a corynebacterial infection.[6]

    c. **Treatment:** Eliminate local moisture with Drysol (aluminum chloride/anhydrous ethyl alcohol) or Xerac AC (aluminum chloride hexahydrate/anhydrous ethanol). Topical erythromycin and/or benzoyl peroxide may also be applied.[1]

B. **Fungal**

  1. **Tinea cruris, tinea pedis, candidal intertrigo** (Fig. 13)

    a. All are exacerbated by warm, moist environments.

    b. **Prevention:** Wear loose, clean, absorbant clothing. Use of foot and body powder regularly (do not use corn starch since the organisms can use this as a nutrient source). Wear thongs into showers.

    c. **Treatment:** Topical or systemic antifungals. Remember that griseofulvin does not cover candida.

C. **Viral**

  1. **Herpes simplex**

    a. Grouped vesicles on erythematous bases (Fig. 14).

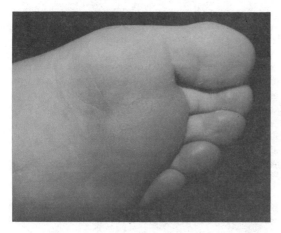

FIGURE 12. Pitted keratolysis.

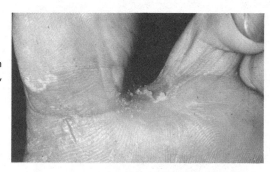

FIGURE 13. Tinea pedis (photograph courtesy of LAC/USC Medical Center, Department of Dermatology).

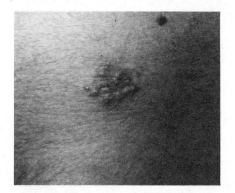

FIGURE 14. Herpes simplex.

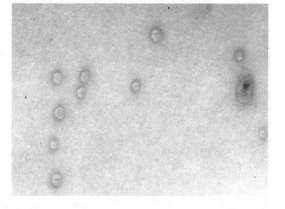

FIGURE 15. Molluscum contagiosum.

      b. Can be readily spread in close contact sports (e.g., "herpes gladiatorum" in wrestling).

      c. Athletes should not be allowed to participate in the contact sport until lesions are healed.

      d. **Treatment:** Acyclovir in recurrent cases.

         i. Initial cases: acyclovir, 200 mg five times a day for 10 days.

         ii. For recurrent cases: acyclovir, 200 mg five times a day for 5 days.

         iii. Suppressive doses range from 200–800 mg/day.

2. **Molluscum contagiosum**

      a. Flesh-colored, dome-shaped papules with central umbilication (Fig. 15).

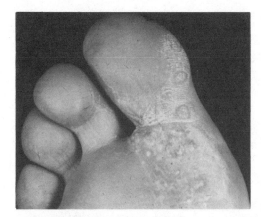

FIGURE 16. Verruca vulgaris: Mosaic wart showing distinctive deviation from skin lines.

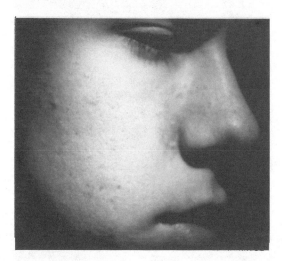

FIGURE 17. Acne.

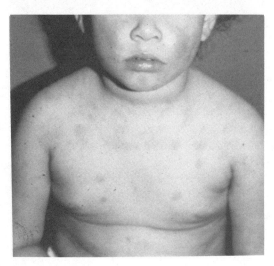

FIGURE 18 Atopic dermatitis (photograph courtesy of LAC/USC Medical Center, Department of Dermatology).

     b. Caused by the pox virus and can be readily transferred by close contact sports.

     c. **Treatment:** Topical therapy with liquid nitrogen, curettage, keratolytics, and canthrone.

   3. **Verruca vulgaris**

     a. Verrucous papules with punctate hemorrhages.

     b. Caused by the human papilloma virus (>40 types) and can be contagious.

     c. They look different from calluses since they deviate the skin lines (Fig. 16).

     d. Plantar warts can cause significant morbidity from pain due to their location.

     e. **Treatment: Do not cause a scar!** Use gentle measures such as keratolytics; other therapies include liquid nitrogen, canthrone, bleomycin, excision, laser, etc.

IV. EXACERBATIONS OF PREEXISTING DISEASE

  A. **Acne vulgaris**

    1. May become pronounced under shoulder pads, head bands, or back packs because of friction, pressure, and occlusion (Fig. 17).

    2. **Treatment:** Use a **benzoyl peroxide** wash in the shower after exercising. Other common therapies include tretinoin (Retin-A); topical antibiotics, including erythromycin and clindamycin; and benzoyl peroxide and oral antibiotics (including tetracycline, erythromycin, and minocycline).

    3. **Prevention:** Washing equipment with soap and water is recommended.

  B. **Atopic dermatitis or xerosis**

    1. Can flare secondarily to sweating, friction, irritation, and drying effects of frequent showering (Fig. 18).

    2. **Treatment:** Use dry-skin precautions, such as short showers or baths (<5 minutes), warm water (not hot), mild soaps, and **moisturizers.**

REFERENCES

1. Basler RSW: Dermatologic aspects of sports participation. Curr Concepts Skin Dis 6:15–19, 1985.
2. Cortese TA, Fukuyama K, Epstein W, et al: Treatment of friction blisters. Arch Dermatol 97:717–721, 1968.
3. Frazier CA: Insect reactions related to sports. Cutis 19:439–444, 1977.
4. Glickman FS: Hiker's hazards. Cutis 19:487–491, 1977.
5. Goldschmidt H: Green hair. Arch Dermatol 15:1288, 1979.
6. Habif TP: Clinical Dermatology, 2nd ed. St. Louis, C.V. Mosby, 1990, pp 105, 205–206.
7. Hicks JH: Swimming and the skin. Cutis 19:448–450, 1977.
8. Houston SD, Knox JM: Skin problems related to sports and recreational activities. Cutis 19:487–491, 1977.
9. Lever WF, Schaumberg-Lever G: Histopathology of the Skin, 7th ed. Philadelphia, J.B. Lippincott, 1990, pp 114, 235.
10. Levine N: Dermatologic aspects of sports medicine. J Am Acad Dermatol 3:415–424, 1980.
11. Pathak MA: Sunscreens: Topical and systemic approaches for protection of human skin against harmful effects of solar radiation. J Am Acad Dermatol 7:285–312, 1982.
12. Silverman AR, Nieland ML: Hot tub dermatitis: A familial outbreak of pseudomonas folliculitis. J Am Acad Dermatol 8:153–156, 1983.
13. Tomchik RS, Russell MT, Szmant AM, Black NA: Clinical perspectives on seabathers eruption, also known as "sea lice." JAMA 269:1669–1672, 1993.

Chapter 30: Rheumatologic Issues

PHILIP MEASE, MD

A rheumatologist's practice is second only to obstetrics/gynecology and perhaps endocrinology in focusing primarily on concerns of women. This is due to the gender-skewed prevalence of rheumatic conditions: rheumatoid arthritis, 2.5:1 female/male ratio; lupus, up to 10:1; fibromyalgia, 4:1; and so on. Only a few rheumatic conditions (e.g., gout and ankylosing spondylosis) are seen predominantly in males. The reason for this imbalance is not entirely clear. Hormonal factors appear to be only a partial explanation.

Many of the problems a rheumatologist focuses on are conditions that have their onset in women in their younger prime, e.g., rheumatoid arthritis, lupus, fibromyalgia, and others. When an active or athletic woman notices persistence of pain or stiffness in joint, tendon, or muscle areas or other more systemic features such as fatigue, it is appropriate to begin investigation for a rheumatologic condition. Unfortunately, it often takes months and sometimes years for a rheumatic condition to be diagnosed, indicating not only that the diagnosis is sometimes hard to make but also that both the treating clinicians and the patients do not include rheumatologic conditions in their differential diagnosis. This chapter is intended as a "sketch" of the field of rheumatology. Its purpose is not to be comprehensive about disease pathogenesis, presentation, and treatment, but rather to trigger one to think about rheumatologic disease while listening to symptoms and to help organize the approach to diagnosis, education, and treatment.

At the start of this chapter are five case examples of patients with common rheumatologic presentations; no diagnosis is given. The cases illustrate certain basic principles about rheumatologic illness which allow us to generate and prioritize the differential diagnosis. The subsequent review of common rheumatologic conditions and treatment approaches should allow us to render a diagnosis and treatment plan in each case, as discussed at the chapter's end.

Case 1: A 34-year-old woman notices pain in the "balls of both feet" upon arising one morning. By the time she is on her way to work, the pain has resolved. This pattern persists, and she attributes it to jogging, which she decides to forgo. However, over the next month, she also notices pain and stiffness, especially in the morning, in her knees, fingers, and wrists. She feels increasingly fatigued and is going to bed soon after returning home from work. Aspirin does not help the pain. On examination she has pain on palpation of the metatarsal joints of both feet and the ulnar aspect of each wrist, with a slightly "doughy" feeling in the wrist. Blood tests reveal a sedimentation rate of 32 mm/hr, hematocrit 33%, rheumatoid factor and antinuclear antibody negative. Radiographs of affected joints are normal.

Case 2: A 40-year-old woman sustains a whiplash injury in a touch football game and develops persistent neck pain. Radiographs of the cervical spine are normal. Appropriate physical therapy and antiinflammatory treatment are prescribed. At her eighth visit in 6 months, she complains of generalized aching and fatigue, fitful sleep, and headaches. A referral to a psychologist is made.

Case 3: A 28-year-old ballet dancer develops low back pain which becomes a persistent problem. The back is stiff in the morning. She works with a physical therapist who specializes in the musculoskeletal problems of dancers and takes ibuprofen, obtaining partial relief of pain. She then develops persistent pain in the back of the heel. On physical examination, she has pain on palpation of an area to the left of L5–S1 and at the insertion of the right Achilles tendon. Radiographs of the spine and pelvis are normal. A bone scan shows light-up in the left sacroiliac joint and right Achilles tendon area. Blood studies (complete blood count, sedimentation rate, rheumatoid factor, and antinuclear antibody) are normal.

Case 4: A 54-year-old woman develops severe pain and swelling of the right great toe at its base. A radiograph of the area is normal. Serum uric acid level is 4.5 mg/dl.

Case 5: A 26-year-old woman presents with chest pain, fever, facial rash, pain and stiffness of her hands and wrists, as well as fatigue. She has had two miscarriages. Examination reveals an erythematous rash on her cheeks. Her white blood count is 3.5×10^3, hematocrit 32%, sedimentation rate 19 mm/hr; urinalysis shows 5–10 red blood cell casts (she is not having a period) and 1+ protein; IgG anticardiolipin level is 54 GPL (normal, 0–23.9 GPL).

I. ELICITING THE SYMPTOM HISTORY

In the following chapter, characteristics such as disease definition, prevalence, pathogenesis, clinical presentation, and treatment approaches are discussed. With each disease process, also consider how the elements of a symptom history would be described by the patient.

A. **Pain** will be the most common presenting symptom.
 1. What are its qualities and characteristics?
 2. Where is the pain located?
    a. Joint (arthritis)?
    b. Tendon (tendinitis)?
    c. Tendon insertion site (enthesium, thus enthesopathy)?
    d. Bursa (bursitis)?
    e. Muscle (myositis, myofascial/fibromyalgia)?
    f. Serosa (serositis)?
    g. Spine (arthritis, discogenic, other)?
    h. Nerve (neuropathy)?
 3. Does it have local or general distribution?
 4. Is the pain persistent, transient, or waxing and waning?
 5. Is the pain sharp, aching, associated with neuropathic qualities?
 6. What relieves and aggravates the pain?
 7. Was the pain associated with trauma or overuse at onset or did it appear "out of the blue"?
B. Is fatigue present? Is it consistently more pervasive and severe than previously experienced? Does it occur continuously or cyclically, worsen with exercise or with any activity?
C. Is **stiffness** present, especially after prolonged lying or sitting?
D. Has abnormal **fatigue** developed?
E. Are there other signs of **inflammation**, such as swelling, warmth, or redness of joints or other connective tissue structures?
F. Are there **other signs of systemic disease**, such as fever, rash, sicca symptoms (dryness), or Raynaud's phenomenon? Any signs of neurologic, pulmonary, renal, or dermatologic disease?
G. Is there a **family history** of rheumatologic disease?

II. RHEUMATOID ARTHRITIS (RA)

A. **Prevalence:** 1–2% of population, with female predominance of 2.5:1.
B. **Age of onset:** 25–55 years; it may also occur in children and the elderly.
C. **Pathology**
 1. Hypertrophy of the synovial membrane of joints with growth of granulation tissue (pannus) over articular surfaces and destruction of cartilage and bone.
 2. Release of proteolytic enzymes and other injurious molecules via cytokine activation.
 3. Humoral, cellular, and nonimmune mechanisms implicated in the process.
D. **Clinical presentation**
 1. Initial presentation is usually polyarticular, of insidious or sudden onset, but it may be oligoarticular and rarely monoarticular.
 2. Initial diagnosis may be difficult, and the patient may need to be observed over time, especially if symptoms are subtle and periodically quiescent.

    3. Distinguishing characteristics from osteoarthritis:
       a. Joints involved in RA but not osteoarthritis include the metacarpophalangeals, wrists, elbows, metatarsophalangeals, and ankles.
       b. Joint warmth, swelling, and erythema are prominent in rheumatoid arthritis. Synovium may feel "doughy" and there may be deforming changes.
       c. Tenosynovitis is more likely in rheumatoid arthritis.
       d. Joint symptoms often are symmetric and wax and wane in concert.
    4. Fatigue and other constitutional symptoms prominent.
    5. Extraarticular features:
       a. Nodules in subcutaneous tissue
       b. Interstitial lung disease
       c. Pulmonary nodules
       d. Pleural effusion
       e. Carpal tunnel syndrome
       f. Fibromyalgia
       g. Sicca syndrome (dry eyes, dry mouth—Sjögren's syndrome)
       h. Vasculitic skin lesions
       i. Neuropathy
       j. Sclerosis
       k. Pericarditis
    6. There may be overlap features with polymyalgia rheumatica, especially in the elderly.
    7. **Severity** ranges from mild joint aching with periods of natural remission and few extraarticular features or laboratory abnormalities, ranging upward to severe multiple joint synovitis with rapid destruction in the articular cartilage and adjacent bone along with troublesome extraarticular features.
    8. Correlations with more severe prognosis:
       a. Rheumatoid factor positive
       b. Elevated sedimentation rate
       c. Extraarticular features, e.g., nodules
       d. Rapidity of erosive changes
E. **Laboratory data**
    1. Anemia, elevation of sedimentation rate, and/or C-reactive protein may be present. White blood cell count may be low in rare Felty's variant.
    2. Radiographic changes (over time) include periarticular demineralization, erosions in periarticular bone, joint space narrowing.
    3. White cells in joint fluid typically number $<50,000$ and $>5,000/\mu L$.
F. **1987 Revised Criteria for Classification of Rheumatoid Arthritis:** At least 4 of the following 7 must be present (items 1–4 must be present for at least 6 weeks):
    1. Morning stiffness
    2. Arthritis of three or more joint areas
    3. Arthritis of hand joints (metacarpophalangeal, proximal interphalangeal, or wrist)
    4. Symmetrical arthritis
    5. Rheumatoid nodule
    6. Serum rheumatoid factor
    7. Radiographic changes (erosions or periarticular osteopenia)

III. TREATMENT CONSIDERATIONS IN RHEUMATOID ARTHRITIS

The following treatment approaches can also be applied to the other arthritides, especially inflammatory ones.
A. **Consider treatment of the whole patient** in the context of family and work life
B. **Educate the patient and family members** about disease pathophysiology, range of natural history, and treatment options.

1. Utilize nurse educators
2. Educational resources
    a. Lay books (e.g., *Arthritis*, by James Fries, MD, and *Arthritis Help Book*, by Kate Lorig and James Fries)
    b. Video tapes
    c. Support groups (if appropriate)
    d. Local chapter of the Arthritis Foundation
3. Consider emotional counseling, especially if social support is inadequate
4. Anticipate future depression and disability, as well as family, vocational, and recreational problems.

C. **Multimodal therapy:** Emphasize a team approach.
1. **Physical therapy**
    a. Strengthening muscle groups adjacent to involved joints as well as stretching and myofascial technique for tight and painful tendon and muscle groups.
    b. Use of heat and cold; typically heat is used for chronically painful joints and muscles, cold for acutely inflamed joints. The key is to do what feels good and helps.
    c. Encourage physical therapist to emphasize education and home treatment as opposed to passive modality.
    d. Consider electrotherapy modalities such as transcutaneous nerve stimulation.
2. **Occupational therapy**
    a. Educate about joint protection for hands.
    b. Use splinting to rest inflamed joints and support optimal hand/wrist functions.
    c. Lifestyle assessment
    d. Job site evaluation and adjustment
    e. Energy conservation
3. **Orthopedic surgery**
    a. Reconstructive and joint replacement surgery with goals of optimized function and decreased pain.
    b. Synovectomy may be useful for severely involved joints not well controlled by medication.
4. **Podiatry:** Orthotics, dealing with painful calluses and structural deformities.
5. **Biofeedback therapy:** Relaxation techniques for pain control.
6. **Vocational counseling**
    a. Desirable to create a flexible work schedule to accommodate variable flares of disease.
    b. Disability process, if necessary, is arduous, and most individuals need assistance.
7. **Aerobic conditioning**
    a. Encourage aerobic conditioning, as it may lead to increased function, decreased overall pain, and improved muscle tone for joint protection.
    b. Swimming is an excellent exercise because it combines stretching, aerobic conditioning, and strengthening of multiple muscle/tendon groups. It also is performed in a relatively weightless state to avoid stress on weight-bearing joints.
    c. Other acceptable modes of exercise include bicycling, exercycle, Nordic track, aerobics, dance, and jogging (if lower extremity joint not significantly involved).
    d. Take care not to aggravate pain in weight-bearing joints. If a joint is excessively inflamed, avoid exercising it aggressively.

D. **Medications**
1. Nonsteroidal antiinflammatory drugs (NSAIDs): The drugs of first choice in treatment.
    a. Inhibit production of inflammatory molecules, e.g., prostaglandins.

    b. Prompt effect. May be used long-term if tolerated and helpful.
    c. Individual responses to drugs vary; if one is not effective after 2–3 weeks, another should be tried.
    d. Side effects include dyspepsia, nausea, platelet inhibition, elevated serum transaminases, and renal toxicity. Periodic monitoring of renal function is advised.
    e. Agents include:
       i. Salicylates
      ii. Indomethacin
     iii. Sulindac
     iv. Meclofenamate
      v. Ibuprofen

2. **Steroids (glucocorticoids):** Appropriate use needs to be individualized.
    a. Prompt anti-inflammatory effect
    b. Occasional corticosteroid joint injections for mono- or oligoarticular flare, or brief tapering use of prednisone for polyarticular flare
    c. Long-term prednisone may occasionally be used at the lowest dose possible, preferably <10 mg/day, in some patients whose symptoms are not controlled on combination therapy.
    d. Adverse effects of prolonged prednisone use include accelerated osteoporosis and atherosclerosis. Employ appropriate antiosteoporosis and cholesterol-lowering measures.
    e. For more severe flares, "pulse" intravenous methylprednisolone (Solu-Medrol), 500–1000 mg/day for 1–3 days, may be used, possibly with fewer side effects than daily moderate to high-dose prednisone.

3. **Disease-modifying drugs** (DMARDs): These so-called "remittive" agents have a more fundamental modifying effect on inappropriate immune cell function. They generally need 1–6 months to take effect and may be added in combination with NSAIDs, steroids, or other DMARDs.
    a. **Hydroxycholoroquine** (Plaquenil): An antimalarial compound which reduces pain and inflammation, occasionally helping with fatigue in patients with mild to moderate rheumatoid arthritis.
       i. Typical dose is 200–400 mg/day.
      ii. Rare adverse effects: Occasional rash, gastrointestinal disturbance, of retinal toxicity.
    b. **Sulfasalazine** (Azulfidine)
       i. Used alone in mild RA or in combination with other DMARDs in more severe RA.
      ii. Rare adverse reactions include leukopenia, anemia, transaminitis, and nausea.
     iii. Typical dosage: 1 g twice daily.
    c. **Methotrexate**
       i. Used since the late 1970s in low-dose form to avoid excessive toxicity.
      ii. May be effective in 80% of patients.
     iii. Adverse effects include potential hepatotoxicity and marrow suppression, gastrointestinal effects such as nausea and diarrhea, and rarely, interstitial lung reaction.
     iv. Typical dosage: 7.5–20 mg/week in oral or injectable form. Injectable liquid may also be ingested.
    d. **Gold**
       i. Most effective form is injectable, 25–50 mg, weekly or every other week. Oral form is not as effective.
      ii. Potential side effects include marrow suppression, proteinuria, rash.
    e. **Other medications,** used less frequently, include ᴅ-penicillamine, azathioprine, cyclophosphamide, and cyclosporine.

4. **Analgesic medications** such as acetominophen can be used; **narcotic analgesics** are to be avoided in chronic illness because of potential habituation.

IV. SPONDYLOARTHROPATHIES

A. **Definition:** A family of chronic inflammatory arthritides affecting both spinal and peripheral joints as well as prominent involvement of tendon insertion sites. Unifying features include:
   1. Sacroiliac and spinal arthritis (sacroiliitis, spondylitis)
   2. Peripheral arthritis usually asymmetric, migratory, or oligoarticular
   3. Involvement of tendon insertion sites (enthesium) with inflammation (enthesopathy)
   4. Male predominance in several subsets
   5. Usually negative for rheumatoid factor
   6. Strong, but not uniform, association with Class I HLA antigen such as HLA-B27
   7. Interaction between genetic proclivity and infectious agents is important in pathogenesis in several subsets.
   8. Extraarticular features are similar, e.g., uveitis, aortitis.
   9. Persistent "sausage digits" are a distinctive trait.

B. **Disease subsets**
   1. **Ankylosing spondylitis**
      a. Predominantly affects the spine, which may fuse over decades (bamboo spine).
      b. Prevalence 0.1%
      c. Male:female ratio 3:1
      d. Rare in blacks
   2. **Reiter's syndrome**
      a. Oligoarticular arthritis
      b. Often associated with nongonococcal urethritis (especially chlamydial)
      c. Conjunctivitis, and mucocutaneous or skin lesions may accompany.
   3. **Reactive arthritis**
      a. Similar to Reiter's syndrome
      b. Accompanies diarrheal infection with *Shigella, Salmonella, Yersinia,* or *Campylobacter.*
      c. Both syndromes are self-limited, lasting 3–12 months in most cases, but chronic symptoms occur in 15–20%.
   4. **Psoriatic arthritis**
      a. Usually peripheral arthritis seen in approximately 7% of patients with cutaneous psoriasis
      b. In patients without active psoriasis, look for nail pitting as a clue.
   5. **Enteropathic arthritis**
      a. Seen in association with inflammatory bowel disease (Crohn's disease, ulcerative colitis) in which arthropathy occurs in 20% and spondylitis in 10%.
      b. Arthropathy symptoms do not necessarily correlate with bowel symptoms temporally or in severity.
   6. **"Undifferentiated spondyloarthropathy"**
      a. Useful categorization of individuals with elements of spondyloarthropathy without historical associations such as infection, or who do not follow characteristic clinical paths such as spine ankylosis.
      b. Actual incidence not well characterized, probably more frequent than recognized.

C. **Pathology**
   1. Mononuclear cell infiltration of synovium, periarticular bone, cartilage, joint capsule.
   2. Increased tendency toward ossification of tendon insertion site.

D. **Laboratory findings**
   1. May be normal, including radiographs and bone scan, especially early in course. Abnormalities may include mild anemia, elevated C-reactive protein, increased sedimentation rate.
   2. Radiographs: Consider a screening radiograph of pelvis to look for sacroiliac narrowing, irregularity, and sclerosis. Lateral view of foot may reveal calcaneal spurs.
   3. Bone scan: Variable light-up in sacroiliac and other symptomatic joints.
   4. Presence of HLA-B27 is not diagnostic.
E. **Treatment considerations:**
   1. Similar to rheumatoid arthritis.
   2. Physical therapy should include spine extensor posturing in patients with spondylitis.
   3. Mild to moderate disease may be managed with NSAIDs alone.
   4. Hydroxychloroquine may rarely lead to flare of psoriasis in psoriatic arthritis. Be cautious of "post-steroid flare" of psoriasis if steroids employed.
   5. In high-risk population, consider screening for HIV (*see* section on HIV/AIDS below) prior to use of steroids, methotrexate, or cytotoxics, which may facilitate the onset of AIDS-related infection.

V. **LUPUS ERYTHEMATOSUS**

A. **Definition:** Lupus is a prototype autoimmune disease with a broad range of presentation from cutaneous to systemic and severity from mild to fatal (rarely).
   1. **Prevalence:** 0.01–0.1% in the general population; higher in black, native American, and certain Asian groups
   2. **Peak age of onset**: 20–50 years
   3. **Female/male ratio:** Up to 10:1, depending on age
   4. **Genetic proclivity:** present
B. **Pathology**
   1. Heterogeneous disorder with a variety of cellular and humoral immunologic abnormalities that vary among patients. Both host and environmental factors influence disease expression. Disease manifestations generated by cellular dysfunction or destruction due to deposition of immune complexes and antibodies, influence of cytokines, or vasculitic-induced ischemia and inflammation.
   2. Lupus may arise from exposure to certain drugs: e.g., procainamide, hydralazine, and isoniazid.
C. **Clinical presentation and diagnosis**
   1. **Diagnosis is based on observation of at least 4 of 11 major criteria** established by the American College of Rheumatology:
      a. Malar rash
      b. Discoid rash
      c. Photosensitivity
      d. Oral/nasopharyngeal ulcers
      e. Nonerosive arthritis
      f. Pleuritis or pericarditis
      g. Proteinuria (>500 mg/24 h) or cylindruria
      h. Psychosis or seizure
      i. Hemolytic anemia, leukopenia (<4,000/mm), lymphopenia (<1,500/mm), or thrombocytopenia (<100,000/mm)
      j. Antinuclear antibody
      k. Anti-dsDNA, anti-Sm, false-positive VDRL, or LE preparation
   2. Many patients will present with fewer than four criteria and possibly other symptoms, such as fatigue and Raynaud's phenomenon, which are not elements of the formal criteria list. These patients cannot be classified as having lupus.
      a. Diagnostic "labels" for these patients include "undifferentiated arthropathy," "undifferentiated autoimmune disease," "lupus-like illness," or "incomplete lupus."

    b. Over time, some of these patients will develop more disease manifestations and can be classified as having lupus or related conditions.

    c. Those who do not may have either intermittent mild symptoms or temporary conditions. Such patients may benefit from a rheumatologic consult, primarily for education and reassurance.

  3. Limited forms of lupus involve just the skin—**subacute cutaneous** or **discoid lupus**.

  4. Because the inflammation in lupus can occur anywhere in the body, disease manifestations can be protean; thus, the clinician should be an open listener and inquisitive, helping to put together pieces of the clinical picture as they emerge over time and helping the patient make treatment choices.

D. **Laboratory findings**

  1. Appropriate screening laboratory studies include:

    a. **Complete blood count** to check for leukopenia, thrombocytopenia, and anemia

    b. **Urinalysis** to check for proteinuria, excess red or white cells, and cellular casts

    c. **Chest radiograph** to assess for pleural effusion or pulmonary infiltrates

    d. **Serum creatinine or creatinine clearance** to assess renal function

  2. **Antinuclear antibody test** is sensitive but not specific. Its presence in high titer, along with other clinical elements, is diagnostically supportive. Low titers with few or "soft" clinical elements must be interpreted cautiously.

  3. **Antibody** to DNA or extractable nuclear antigen (ENA) and its subsets are less frequently positive than ANA in lupus patients, but when positive, are very specific for the diagnosis or its variants.

  4. **Tests correlating with disease severity**

    a. Complement levels: low levels indicate increased disease activity.

    b. DNA antibody: high levels indicate increased disease activity.

    c. Degree of urinary sediment changes or other markers such as chest radiograph changes

    d. These tests need to be correlated with clinical symptomatology before modifying medications.

E. **Treatment approaches**

  1. **Mild disease**

    a. Use NSAIDs for arthralgias, topical steroids for rash, calcium channel blockers for Raynaud's phenomenon.

    b. Consider low doses of selective serotonin reuptake inhibitors for fatigue and depression.

    c. Advise sun avoidance, protective clothing, and sunscreen for those who are photosensitive.

  2. **Moderate/severe disease with internal organ involvement** (e.g., pleuro-pericarditis, ctyopenias, or some renal disease)

    a. Prednisone more likely advised; use with antiosteoporosis measures. Advise about potential side effects, including osteonecrosis.

    b. Hydroxychloroquine is useful as a steroid-sparing agent, particularly for arthritis, skin disease, and fatigue.

  3. **Severe disease** (e.g., with neurologic, renal, or hematologic manifestations)

    a. Addition of "pulse" intravenous steroids, cytotoxic agents, plasmapheresis, or other methods may be advised.

    b. Treatment of specific symptoms (e.g., seizures with antiseizure medications) is individualized.

  4. Lupus is characterized by flares and remissions, often with neurocognitive features, depression, and significant impact on the patient's life within the family and work. Advise living life in balance. Consider the need for psychologic referral.

F. **Pregnancy**
  1. Increased incidence of fetal loss or small-for-date infants. This incidence increases further if antiphospholipid antibodies (anticardiolipin and lupus anticoagulant) are present.
  2. Advise that clinical and laboratory signs of disease should be in remission prior to conception.
  3. Monitor blood pressure, complete blood count, creatinine, urinalysis, and selective autoimmune serology more frequently during pregnancy.
  4. Prednisone may be used during pregnancy, preferably in doses <10 mg, but more if necessary to control disease manifestations.
  5. If antiphospholipid antibodies are positive, consider use of baby aspirin.
  6. Avoid other drugs if possible.
G. **Prognosis** has improved dramatically during the last 25 years.
  1. Current 10-year survival estimate, depending on study population, is 70%.
  2. The major causes of death are infection and renal failure.

VI. SJÖGREN'S SYNDROME

A. **Definition**
  1. Sjögren's syndrome is an autoimmune disease occurring primarily in women, characterized by sicca syndrome (dry eyes, mouth, vagina), and often the presence of antinuclear antibodies, SS-A and/or SS-B.
  2. Its **primary form**, when there is no other autoimmune disease present, may include other clinical symptoms: polyarthritis, fatigue, renal tubular acidosis, and other internal organ involvement. The condition is frequently seen in a **secondary form** accompanying other autoimmune diseases such as lupus or rheumatoid arthritis.
B. **Prevalence:** Uncertain. Estimates range from 1/2,000 individuals upward, depending upon the criteria used and population studied.
C. **Pathology**
  1. Decreased ocular wetting caused by mononuclear cell infiltration of tear glands is measured by **Schirmer's test** or other measures. Salivary gland infiltration with immunologic cells determined by minor **salivary gland biopsy**.
  2. Sjögren's equivalent in AIDS is called **diffuse infiltrative lymphocytosis syndrome** (DILS), in which the salivary glands are infiltrated by CD8 cells.
  3. There is a rare incidence of **late-stage lymphoma**.
D. **Treatment:**
  1. Similar to treatment of lupus or rheumatoid arthritis
  2. Attention is focused on increasing moisture, particulary in the eyes, mouth, and vagina. Numerous artificial tear products are available. Tear duct micro-surgery may be performed. Protective glasses decrease wind-induced tear evaporation.
  3. Artificial saliva and pharmacologic salivary stimulation are not widely accepted so frequent fluid ingestion is still the primary method for treating mouth dryness.
  4. Vaginal lubrication is an important issue in sexually active women.

VII. OSTEOARTHRITIS

Also termed degenerative joint disease and osteoarthrosis
A. **Prevalence**
  1. Increases with age, most frequently beginning in the fifth decade.
  2. Radiographic evidence of hand osteoarthritis is present in >70% of individuals older than 65 and <5% of individuals under 35 years. However, only a certain proportion of those with radiographically evident disease will have symptoms.
  3. There is a a slight female predominance.

B. **Pathogenesis:** multifactorial
  1. Loss of integrity of articular cartilage secondary to either abnormal stresses on normal cartilage or normal stresses on abnormal cartilage.
  2. A genetic component may be present.
C. **Primary (idiopathic) osteoarthritis**
  1. Tendency to be passed through female generations
  2. Joints involved:
     a. Distal interphalangeal joints (Heberden's nodes)
     b. Proximal interphalangeal joints (Bouchard's nodes)
     c. Carpometacarpal joint
     d. First metatarsal phalangeal joint
     e. Spine
     f. Hips
     g. Knees
D. **Secondary osteoarthritis**
  1. Numerous factors may lead to disruption or alteration of normal cartilage; osteoarthritis results from subsequent normal use of abnormal cartilage.
  2. Insults to cartilage include trauma, joint infection, and crystalline or rheumatoid destruction of cartilage.
E. **Clinical presentation**
  1. Pain is the chief symptom, especially with joint use and weight bearing.
  2. Stiffness is typically less than in rheumatoid arthritis.
  3. Signs of inflammation are minimal; systemic features are absent.
F. **Radiographic features:** As disease advances, radiographs show joint space narrowing, subchondral bone sclerosis, periarticular spur formation.
G. **Treatment**
  1. Primarily for symptomatic reduction of pain and restoration of function
  2. NSAIDs or occasional steroid injections
  3. Restorative treatment with surgical approaches, especially joint replacement, may be helpful for severe joint disease.
H. **Prevention**
  1. Appropriate conditioning and stretching prior to sport activities will reduce the incidence of bone fracture and tendon/ligament strain, which in turn can set the stage for secondary osteoarthritis.
  2. Regular and even aggressive exercise performed in the context of normal joints and well-conditioned muscles, tendons, and ligaments does not appear to lead to premature degenerative arthritis.
I. **Prognosis:** Usually slow progression of degenerative changes

VIII. **CRYSTALLINE ARTHRITIS**

A. **Definition:** Formation of crystals in joint fluid may incite an inflammatory cell response and resultant intense pain and swelling.
B. Several forms of crystalline arthritis occur:
  1. **Gout**
     a. When uric acid, a purine metabolite, is overproduced or underexcreted, elevated serum and joint fluid levels occur. Uric acid crystals then may form in supersaturated joint fluid.
     b. **Peak age of onset** is 40–60 years; it occurs more frequently in males.
     c. Approximately 90% of first attacks involve a single joint and are self-limited. Chronic gout may be polyarticular.
     d. **Prevalence** is approximately 0.2%.
     e. **Diagnosis**
        i. Demonstration of uric acid crystals in aspirated joint fluid, or observation of characteristic clinical presentation and elevated serum uric acid level.

    ii. Careful follow-up observation is required to rule out joint infection.

    iii. In chronic forms, deposits of urate can be seen in soft tissues, e.g., the helix of the ear or radiographic evidence of "punched out" erosions of bone adjacent to the involved joints.

2. **Calcium pyrophosphate dihydrate deposition disease (CPPD, pseudogout)**

   a. Results from shedding of crystals of calcium pyrophosphate dihydrate from cartilage.

   b. Occurs in an acute monoarticular form or a more chronic, often polyarticular arthropathy.

   c. Prevalence is about half that of gout, or 0.1%.

   d. Although often occurring on its own, CPPD may sometimes be a clue to an associated disease, such as hemochromatosis or hyperparathyroidism.

   e. **Diagnosis** is made by demonstration of CPPD crystals in joint fluid by polarized microscopy.

3. **Treatment of acute gout or CPPD**

   a. NSAIDs or colchicine (which is more effective in gout). If these are ineffective or not tolerated, injectable or oral steroids may be employed.

   b. If recurrent attacks occur and affect function, add either daily allopurinol to inhibit uric acid formation or a uricosuric agent to increase renal excretion of uric acid. These medicines are not useful in acute attacks, but can help prevent recurrent attacks.

   c. Dietary reduction of purine-rich foods may have a slight effect on uric acid levels.

   d. No medication is available to prevent formation of CPPD crystals. Dietary factors do not play a significant role in CPPD.

IX. INFECTIOUS ARTHRITIS

A. Infection of the joint space represents a **rheumatologic emergency** because of the long-term consequences of untreated infection. Whenever suspected, infection must be ruled out, usually by joint aspiration and culture.

B. **Pathogenesis**

1. In persons aged 15–40 years, 60–90% of cases are caused by *Neisseria gonorrhoeae*.

2. In those over age 40 years, *Staphylococcus aureus* is the predominant organism.

3. In chronically ill patients, those on chronic immune-modifying medications, or those with urinary tract infections, consider gram-negative organisms such as *Escherichia coli* or *Pseudomonas*.

4. The typical mechanism of joint entry is hematogenous spread.

5. Staphylococcus and gram-negative infections usually are monoarticular.

C. **Dissemination** of *N. gonorrhoeae* from the genitourinary tract occurs more commonly in women.

1. The patient presents with polyarthralgias with little or no joint effusion and prominent erythematous macules, papules, or vesicular lesions.

2. Occasionally, gonococci can be seen on gram stain or culture of skin lesions, blood, or joint fluid. Most often, joint fluid is sterile. It is appropriate to culture genitourinary sites.

3. Occasionally, the patient may have a monoarticular presentation with typically positive joint fluid culture.

D. **Treatment**

1. Use an appropriate antibiotic regimen for suspected organisms, usually initially in intravenous form and for a prolonged course.

2. Recurrent joint effusions should be aspirated.

E. **Post-viral arthropathy**, presumably immune-complex mediated, is a common reason for polyarticular inflammation. It typically resolves over several weeks.

F. **Tuberculous arthritis** usually presents in an insidious, monoarticular, and destructive manner.

G. **Lyme disease:** A multisystem illness with skin, joint, neurologic, and cardiac manifestations, caused by a spirochete, *Borrelia burgdorferi*, borne by ticks of the genus *Ixodes*. In the U.S., cases are mainly clustered in the Eastern and Western seaboards and upper midwest.

  1. The disease progresses through stages.

    a. In the first 3 weeks, a key feature is the presence of a rash, erythema chronicum migrans.

    b. The second stage, beginning a few weeks to months later, is characterized by cardiac conduction abnormalities, fatigue, and neurologic abnormalities.

    c. The third stage often entails an oligoarticular migratory arthritis, an array of neurologic signs and symptoms, fatigue, and skin changes.

  2. **Diagnosis** is made by identification of a characteristic clinical syndrome, observation of rash, and positive antibody test. The latter may be negative, especially in early disease. False-positive tests may occur, especially if other disease (e.g., autoimmune) is present.

  3. **Treatment** of early disease is with tetracycline or amoxicillin. In later stages, high-dose penicillin, tetracylcine, or ceftriaxone is used.

  4. If arthritis symptoms persist, symptomatic antiinflammatory treatment may be employed.

  5. Because of frequent media attention, many patients present with concern about Lyme disease, even when there has been little chance of exposure and they are not living in an endemic area. An appropriate level of concern and willingness to educate are important to reassure such patients who may have symptoms of fatigue and arthralgias but are not infected.

H. **Human immunodeficiency virus and acquired immunodeficiency syndrome:** A number of rheumatologic syndromes have arisen in AIDS patients, and these mimic several previously mentioned conditions.

  1. **Spondyloarthropathy**

    a. There is an increased frequency of an inflammatory oligoarticular arthritis, similar to Reiter's syndrome, psoriatic arthritis, and other reactive spondyloarthropathies.

    b. When a patient in a high-risk group presents in this way, HIV status should be tested.

    c. Although immunomodulatory medications are not contraindicated, use them cautiously so as to avoid opportunistic infections.

  2. **Arthropathy:** "Rheumatoid-like" symmetric arthropathy may be present in HIV patients.

  3. **Myopathy:** HIV-associated polymyositis, non-polymyositis myopathy, and azidothymidine-related myopathy may occur.

  4. **Sjögren's syndrome/diffuse infiltrative lymphocytosis syndrome (DILS):** This is a sicca syndrome in which salivary and lacrimal glands are infiltrated with CD8 cells instead of CD4 cells, as seen in standard Sjögren's syndrome.

X. SARCOIDOSIS

A. A multisystem disorder characterized by the presence of noncaseating granulomata infiltrating affected tissues. The cause is unknown.

B. Affects young adults, male and female equally.

C. Often presents with acute polyarthritis, erythema nodosum, and evidence of bilateral hilar adenopathy on chest radiograph.

D. May evolve into chronic arthritis, interstitial lung disease, or other manifestations depending upon which organs are affected.

E. **Treatment:** Steroids or other immunomodulatory medications in more severe disease.

XI. INFLAMMATORY MUSCLE DISEASE (POLYMYOSITIS, DERMATOMYOSITIS)

A. **Incidence**
   1. 5–8 cases/million/year
   2. 2:1 female predominance
B. Characterized by progressive muscle weakness, often with swallowing difficulty, mild myalgias and arthralgias, elevated creatine phosphokinase and aldolase levels, abnormal EMG, and muscle biopsy with lymphocytic infiltrate.
C. **Treatment:** Steroids and/or methotrexate. Intravenous immunoglobulin in certain cases.

XII. RHEUMATOLOGIC MANIFESTATIONS OF ENDOCRINE DISEASE

A. **Hypothyroidism:** Polyarthritis, carpal tunnel syndrome, fibromyalgia, frozen shoulder, myopathy
B. **Hyperthyroidism:** Myopathy, frozen shoulder, fibromyalgia, osteopenia
C. **Diabetes mellitus:** Cheiroarthropathy (fibrosing hand stiffening), Dupuytren's contracture, tenosynovitis, frozen shoulder, carpal tunnel syndrome
D. **Adrenal insufficiency** (and steroid withdrawal): Arthralgia, fibromyalgia
E. **Cushing's syndrome** (and steroid administration): Myopathy, osteopenia, osteonecrosis

XIII. FIBROMYALGIA (FIBROSITIS)

A. **Prevalence**
   1. Present in approximately 2% of the general population, 5% of a general medical clinic population, and up to 20% in a general rheumatology practice
   2. 80–90% female predominance, particularly ages 20–50
B. **Clinical criteria**
   1. History of generalized aching
   2. Presence of at least 11 of 18 specific tender points (Fig. 1).[7]
   3. Associated symptoms
      a. Sleep disturbance
      b. Fatigue
      c. Headaches
      d. Irritable bowel syndrome
      e. Interstitial cystitis (irritable bladder)
      f. Dysmenorrhea
   4. May occur alone or in association with other chronic pain, rheumatologic, or other medical conditions.
C. **Diagnosis:** There are no specific diagnostic tests; diagnosis is based on history and physical examination.
D. **Modulating factors:** Improves with heat, vacation, mild activity; worsens with cold, emotional stress, over- or underexertion.
E. **Pathogenesis:** Several possible mechanisms may be involved simultaneously:
   1. Neurotransmitter imbalance
   2. Muscle biochemical or deconditioning changes
   3. Response to stress, depression, anxiety
   4. Sleep physiology disturbance
F. **Treatment:** Patient education and reassurance. Be willing to spend time with the patient.
   1. Minimize stress
   2. Improve sleep habits and environment
   3. Aerobic exercise
   4. Physical therapy, especially myofascial technique
   5. Acupuncture

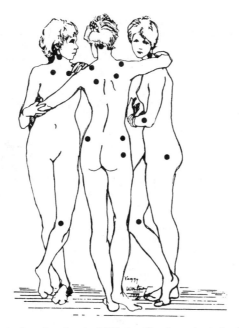

FIGURE 1.   Tender point locations for the 1990 classification criteria for fibromyalgia:
Occiput: bilateral, at the suboccipital muscle insertions
Low cervical: bilateral, at the anterior aspects of the intertransverse spaces at C5–C7
Trapezius: bilateral, at the midpoint of the upper border
Supraspinatus: bilateral, at origins, above the scapula spine near the medial border
Second rib: bilateral, at second costochondral junctions, just lateral to junctions on upper surfaces
Lateral epicondyle: bilateral, 2 cm distal to the epicondyles
Gluteal: bilateral, in upper outer quadrants of buttocks in anterior fold of muscle
Greater trochanter: bilateral, posterior to the trochanteric prominence
Knee: bilateral, at the medial fat pad proximal to the joint line
(*The Three Graces*, after Baron Jean-Baptiste Regnault, 1793, Louvre Museum, Paris. From Wolfe
et al: The American College of Rheumatology 1990 criteria for the classification of fibromyalgia.
Arthritis Rheum 33:169, 1990, with permission.)

      6. Low-dose tricyclic antidepressants, e.g., amitriptyline, 10–50 mg at bedtime, helpful for pain and sleep disturbance, if present.
      7. Selective serotonin reuptake inhibitors useful for fatigue component; may be used in combination with low-dose tricyclics.
      8. NSAIDs, if helpful
    G. **Prognosis:** Chronic waxing and waning symptoms; not commonly seen in elderly women

XIV. CHRONIC FATIGUE SYNDROME

    A. Similar demographics as fibromyalgia
    B. **Clinical findings**
      1. Often history of viral or viral-like illness at onset.
      2. Multisymptom complex of fatigue, neurocognitive symptoms, headache, fibro-myalgia, and multiple other symptoms is frequently observed.
      3. Depression and anxiety frequently coexistent.
      4. Criteria established for purposes of investigation (Table 1); key is to rule out other medical conditions or preexisting major psychiatric illness that could cause similar syndrome.

TABLE 1. Definition of Chronic Fatigue Syndrome

The case definition of chronic fatigue syndrome (CFS) was formally defined by the working group. A case must fulfill both major criteria and selected minor criteria (6 or more of the 11 minor *symptom* criteria and 2 or more of the 3 *physical* criteria *or* 8 or more of the 11 *symptom* criteria):

Major criteria for CFS

1. *Fatigue of at least 6 months' duration:* New onset of persistent or relapsing debilitating fatigue or easy fatigability in a person with no previous history of similar symptoms that does not resolve with bedrest and that is severe enough to reduce or impair average daily activity below 50% of the patient's premorbid activity level for a period of at least 6 months.

2. *Exclusion of other causes of chronic fatigue:* Other clinical conditions that may produce similar symptoms must be excluded by thorough evaluation based on history, physical examination, and appropriate laboratory investigations. These conditions include malignancy, autoimmune disease, infections, chronic psychiatric disease, neuromuscular disease, endocrine disease, drug dependency, or other known or defined chronic pulmonary, cardiac, gastrointestinal, hepatic, renal, or hematologic disease.

Minor criteria for CFS

1. *Symptom criteria:* The symptoms must have begun at or after the onset of increased fatigability and must have persisted over a period of at least 6 months.
   a. Mild fever: oral temperature of 37.5–38.6° C if measured by the patient.
   b. Sore throat
   c. Painful cervical or axillary lymph nodes
   d. Unexplained general muscle weakness
   e. Myalgia
   f. Prolonged (>24 hours) generalized fatigue after levels of exercise that would have been easily tolerated in the patient's premorbid state
   g. Generalized headaches (of a type, severity, or pattern that differs from any premorbid headaches)
   h. Migratory arthralgia, without swelling or erythema
   i. Neuropsychologic complaints (photophobia, transient scotoma, forgetfulness, excessive irritability, confusion, difficulty thinking, inability to concentrate, depression)
   j. Sleep disturbance (hypersomnia or insomnia)
   k. Description of the main symptom complex as initially developing over a few hours to a few days

2. *Physical criteria:* These must be documented by a physician on at least two occasions, at least 1 month apart.
   a. Low-grade fever: oral temperature 37.6–38.6° C
   b. Nonexudative pharyngitis
   c. Palpable or tender cervical or axillary lymph nodes (<2 cm in diameter)

From Holmes GT: Chronic fatigue syndrome—A working case definition. Ann Intern Med 108:387–389, 1988.

    C. **Pathogenesis:** Uncertain, probably heterogeneous; a number of mechanisms are postulated based on various experimental observations, including:
       1. Neurotransmitter imbalance, either biologically or psychologically induced
       2. Cytokine-mediated effects
       3. Allergen-mediated effects
       4. Sleep physiology disturbance
       5. Stress-related mechanisms
       6. Putative viral-mediated mechanisms
    D. **Treatment**
       1. Similar to fibromyalgia
       2. Selective serotonin reuptake inhibitors may be helpful for fatigue and neurocognitive symptoms
       3. Multidisciplinary approach useful
       4. Experimental treatment approaches have been used but are incompletely studied as regards efficacy.
    E. **Prognosis:** Chronic waxing and waning symptoms with a tendency in most to improve gradually over time; some may have persistent symptoms.

XV. MYOFASCIAL AND OVERUSE SYNDROMES

A. Chronic regional pain syndromes, often related to an original tendon, muscle, joint, or nerve trauma or overuse problem
   1. Trigger points and referred pain patterns are common.
   2. Equal incidence in males and females.
   3. Patients usually present without sleep disorder or other systemic symptoms.
B. **Treatment:** Regional physical therapy techniques, stretching, elimination of aggravating factors; occupational therapy modalities, including ergonomic assessment; NSAIDs, if helpful
C. Prognosis is good.

XVI. REFLEX SYMPATHETIC DYSTROPHY SYNDROME

A. Suspect reflex sympathetic dystrophy (RSD) when limb pain is especially distal, persistent, diffuse, and associated with generalized swelling, erythema, and fluctuating temperature and color changes.
B. **Pathogenesis:** Possibly related to dysfunctional neural networks—"spilling over" of signal from afferent pain fibers to efferent sympathetic fibers—setting up a chronic feedback loop even when original pain or other noxious stimulus has resolved.
C. **Treatment:** Sympathetic nerve blocks performed by an anesthesiologist; several-week steroid course; physical therapy
D. **Prognosis:** Good if recognized early and treated promptly; variable to poor if it becomes chronic

XVII. CONCLUSIONS

Although this survey of rheumatology is incomplete, we can now look back on the original case presentations and make the following points and conclusions.

Case 1: A young woman has pain and "gelling" in a polyarticular distribution that persists and is associated with fatigue. The examination reveals evidence of synovitis and symmetric joint distribution consistent with an inflammatory arthritis. Although antibody studies and radiographs are normal, her sedimentation rate is elevated, suggesting inflammation. The diagnostic label that could be applied is **seronegative arthropathy** or **undifferentiated arthropathy**. Given the physical evidence of synovitis, this condition will more likely behave like rheumatoid arthritis than lupus. Her seronegative status suggests a probable milder course. Treatment should include education, family counseling, trials of NSAIDs, referral for physical therapy, and early consideration of second-line remittive medications (DMARDs).

Case 2: This patient will likely have multiple characteristic tender points of fibromyalgia on examination. The theory is that the experience of chronic neck pain has, in some way, upset normal neurotransmitter function, helped engender sleep disturbance, and now, perhaps with other endogenous factors, led to **fibromyalgia**. Psychological referral may be appropriate, but to do so without acknowledging the biophysical aspect of her problem may prove alienating to the patient. A multidisciplinary approach using low-dose tricyclic antidepressants (e.g, 10–30 mg of amitriptyline if tolerated), NSAIDs if helpful, myofascial and physical therapy, and a structured aerobic conditioning program (e.g., swimming) would be worthwhile.

Case 3: Persistent back pain associated with morning stiffness, Achilles tendinitis, and a positive bone scan of the sacroiliac joint suggest a spondyloarthropathy. With no history of urethritis, enteropathic infection, psoriasis, or inflammatory bowel disease, nor evidence of spondylitis on radiograph, this could be labeled **undifferentiated spondyloarthropathy**. Because the patient had only partial improvement with one NSAID, other NSAID trials could be added; if these yield no better results, consider sulfasalazine as well as a physical therapy consult.

Case 4: Sudden-onset monoarthritis of the first metatarsal suggests crystalline arthritis. Given a low normal uric acid level, a likely diagnosis is **calcium pyrophosphate crystal inflammation**. Aspiration of the joint would show characteristic calcium pyrophosphate crystals by polarizing microscopy, and culture would be negative, thus ruling out infection. Some patients with inflammatory or degenerative arthritis will present in a monoarticular fashion, but this would probably be less likely in this case.

Case 5: Pleurisy, rash, arthritis, low white blood cell count, anemia, and the presence of red blood cells and protein in urine fulfill the criteria for **lupus**. The presence of fatigue and fever is supportive. The elevated IgG anticardiolipin antibody level, seen in association with lupus, helps explain her previous miscarriages. NSAIDs may be helpful for arthralgias, but should be used cautiously in the presence of renal disease (check creatinine periodically). A nephrology consult is advisable for better characterization of nephropathy and its optimal management. Prednisone therapy will help ameliorate most symptoms and signs; rheumatology consult to guide therapy and to educate patient and family is recommended. Advise avoidance of excessive exposure to sun. Use of aspirin and/or subcutaneous heparin as well as prednisone therapy may be of benefit in a future pregnancy.

When faced with a woman with musculoskeletal pain, fatigue, or other systemic symptoms that are acutely inflammatory or chronic and without clearcut explanation from a history of trauma, consider the rheumatologic syndromes. The material presented in this chapter should serve as a springboard for further questioning and thought. Sometimes, the clinical picture and diagnostic studies can be unclear, and clarification results from careful observation over time and/or consultation.

REFERENCES

1. Holmes GT: Chronic fatigue syndrome—A working case definition. Ann Intern Med 108:387–389, 1988.
2. Kelley WN, et al (eds): Textbook of Rheumatology. Philadelphia, W.B. Saunders, 1993.
3. Klippel JH, Dieppe PA (eds): Rheumatology. London, Mosby, 1994.
4. McCarty DJ (ed): Arthritis and its Allied Conditions. Malvern, PA, Lea & Febiger, 1989.
5. Schumacher HR, et al (eds): Primer on the Rheumatic Diseases, 9th ed. Atlanta, Arthritis Foundation, 1988.
6. Tan, et al: 1982 revised criteria for the classification of systemic lupus erythematosus. Arthritis Rheum 25:1271–1277, 1982.
7. Wilson JD, et al (eds): Harrison's Principles of Internal Medicine. New York, McGraw-Hill, 1991.
8. Wolfe F, Smyth HA, Yunus HB, et al: The American College of Rheumatology 1990 criteria for the classification of fibromyalgia. Arthritis Rheum 33:160–172, 1990.

Chapter 31: Thyroid Disorders

NORMAN ROSENTHAL, MD

In this chapter, issues related to thyroid disease, the most common endocrinologic abnormality confronting women, are reviewed. Other important problems, such as menstrual disturbances and metabolic bone diseases, are reviewed in other chapters.

I. **CLINICAL APPROACH TO THYROID DISEASE**

With the recent recognition that hyperthyroidism, either overt or subclinical, can result in accelerated bone loss, the assessment of possible osteoporosis in the exercising woman must not only include evaluation of estrogen status but also consideration of unrecognized thyroid disease. This chapter reviews the signs and symptoms of thyroid disorders as well as presents a cost-effective approach to its diagnosis.

A. **Overt hyperthyroidism**
   1. **General manifestations**
      a. **Skin:** The skin is warm and smooth, with increased sweating commonly noted. Softening and loosening of the nails occur rarely.
      b. **Eyes:** Lid lag, retraction, and stare can occur in hyperthyroid patients, but inflammation, swelling, and proptosis are hallmarks of *only* Graves' disease.
      c. **Respiratory system:** Dyspnea on exertion is a common complaint by all who exercise.
      d. **Cardiovascular system:** Tachycardia and palpitations along with a rise in systolic pressure reflect the variety of changes on this system. A notable increased incidence in atrial fibrillation occurs.
      e. **Gastrointestinal system:** Hyperdefecation occurs much more frequently than does malabsorption and steatorrhea. Unexplained diarrhea, especially in the elderly, should be screened with thyroid tests.
      f. **Hematologic system:** A mild normochromic, normocytic anemia will infrequently occur, and rarely, one can see associated idiopathic thrombocytopenic purpura.
      g. **Genitourinary systems:** In the woman, oligo- or amenorrhea can be the initial presenting complaint.
      h. **Bone metabolism:** Stimulation of bone resorption by excessive thyroid hormone results in increased cortical bone turnover as well as permanent reductions in trabecular bone.
      i. **Neuromuscular system:** Tremor, emotional lability, insomnia, and hyperactive deep tendon reflexes are common. Symptoms of proximal muscle weakness may also be present.
      j. **General:** Lethargy and heat intolerance are prominent features.

B. **Subclinical hyperthyroidism:** Defined as a subnormal thyroid-stimulating hormone (TSH) level in the face of a normal serum thyroxine level.
   1. The most common cause of this entity is **overzealous thyroid hormone replacement therapy.** Many physiological abnormalities, such as an increase in nocturnal heat rate, reduced systolic time intervals, and abnormal liver enzymes, have been described in patients taking levothyroxine in doses that result in subclinical hyperthyroidism, but the finding that **bone density** is also reduced has generated the greatest concern. Several studies have shown significant reductions in bone density of 5–12% after 5 years of subclinical disease.
   2. Subclinical hyperthyroidism can also occur in patients with either autonomous nodular thyroid disease or mild Graves' disease.

3. In the absence of classical signs and symptoms, patients who are evaluated for osteopenia, unexplained atrial fibrillation, or unexplained diarrhea should be screened with a serum TSH level.

C. **Laboratory diagnosis**

1. The use of the "sensitive" TSH assay system, now in use by all laboratories, has allowed separation of euthyroid from hyperthyroid individuals with >99% confidence. The degree of hyperthyroidism is best determined by the magnitude of the serum thyroxine level.

2. It is important to remember that a "normal" serum thyroxine level, commonly the only test on chemistry battery panels, does *not* exclude subclinical disease, and serum TSH must be measured.

D. **Differential diagnosis:** Once the biochemical parameters establish the diagnosis of thyroxine excess, the next challenge is to identify the underlying mechanism of disease so as to help guide therapeutic intervention.

1. **Graves' disease:** Accounting for the majority of cases (>70%), this process can be suspected on clinical grounds but *must* be proven with the radioactive iodine uptake study. Findings on examination consistent with this diagnosis include:

   a. **Excessive adrenergic stimulation.** These patients exhibit marked tremulousness and palmar moisture, a rapid heart beat, impressive weight loss, and disrupted sleep patterns as well as heat intolerance.

   b. **Ophthalmopathy:** The presence of periorbital edema, chemosis, restricted extraocular muscle function, and/or proptosis are all specific for autoimmune thyroid disease.

   c. **Thyroid examination:** The gland is typically diffusely enlarged but can be normal in size in 10–15% of cases. A thyroid bruit is rarely present.

2. **Thyroiditis.** This mechanism of disease is caused by inflammatory destruction of thyroid parenchyma with leakage of preformed hormone into the circulation. The process is self-limited and therefore resolves spontaneously. Two forms of this disease exist:

   a. **Painless thyroiditis:** This disease is characterized by lymphocytic infiltration and typically mild symptoms of thyroxine excess. It occurs commonly in the postpartum period. Although the thyroid might be normal in volume, the texture can be lumpy. The clinical picture as well as biochemical abnormalities will resolve in 3–4 months.

   b. **Painful thyroiditis:** Commonly known as **subacute granulomatous thyroiditis,** this disease has a dramatic presentation described as severe anterior neck pain frequently following an upper respiratory tract infection. The thyroid gland is swollen and very tender and associated with fever, malaise, a high sedimentation rate, and signs of mild to moderate thyrotoxicosis. Its clinical course runs similar to the lymphocytic variant.

3. **Autonomous nodular thyroid disease**

   a. This disease process can present either as a solitary nodule, more common in the younger age group, or as multiple nodules such as seen in the elderly. Adenomatous disease is easily palpated but multinodular goiters may be substernal and difficult to feel in the elderly.

   b. Many patients with nodular thyroid disease who are biochemically euthyroid can develop overt hyperthyroidism either with the addition of exogenous thyroid hormone intended for suppression purposes or with exposure to an iodine load, such as with radiocontrast dye, kelp, or amiodarone.

E. **Diagnosis**

1. The two most common forms of hyperthyroidism—Graves' disease and thyroiditis— can be easily distinguished with the use of the radioactive iodine uptake study. Although a 24-hour study is most accurate, a modified 4-hour uptake will suffice in most cases.

a. Patients with **autoimmune disease** will demonstrate *elevated* rates of iodine uptake, reflecting the stimulation of iodine entry into the thyroid by immunoglobulins acting on the TSH receptor.

b. **Thyroiditis** will show a *suppressed* rate of uptake, reflecting reduced iodine uptake into thyroid cells in the absence of TSH.

2. **Nodular thyroid hyperthyroidism** should be considered when a nodular gland is palpated or when evaluating hyperthyroidism in the elderly. As mentioned, substernal glands are common in this age group and imaging studies are necessary. The use of the thyroid scan, preferably with iodine-123, is indicated in this disease category only.

a. Diagnosis of a **toxic solitary nodule** requires the image of a "hot" nodule with suppressed surrounding thyroid tissue.

b. For the **toxic multinodular gland,** heterogeneous activity is described and can be visualized beneath the sternum.

c. In both, the radioactive iodine uptake is commonly normal but can be elevated.

F. **Treatment**

1. **Graves' disease**

a. **Radioactive iodine ablation:** The most common form of therapy, this modality is safe, highly effective, and relatively inexpensive. In the premenopausal woman, concern about adverse effects upon the gonads has not been proven, but this material is *contraindicated in pregnancy* as it is teratogenic to fetal development. The endpoint in therapy is to render the patient hypothyroid and lifetime thyroxine replacement therapy should be expected.

b. **Antithyroid medications:** The thionamides, methimazole, and propylthiouracil are safe and highly effective medications, and comprise the treatment of choice for thyroid storm as well as treatment during pregnancy. Remission rates after 12–24 months are about 10–20%. Medication is well tolerated, but patients must be informed about the 1–2% chance of skin rash and the 0.5% incidence of agranulocytosis.

c. **Surgery:** This option has played an increasingly smaller role in the care of these patients and is best reserved for the rare patient who reacts adversely to drug therapy and/or fails to respond to radioactive iodine therapy.

II. CLINICAL APPROACH TO HYPOTHYROIDISM

This common thyroid abnormality is characterized by an elevated TSH level in the setting of a low serum thyroxine level (overt hypothyroidism) or a normal serum thyroxine level (subclinical hypothyroidism).

A. **General manifestations**

1. **Skin:** Cold, dry, puffy skin can be seen, as can loss of hair in more advanced cases.

2. **ENT:** Hoarseness is uncommon as is tongue enlargement.

3. **Respiratory system:** Exertional dyspnea and sleep apnea may occur.

4. **Cardiovascular system:** Diastolic hypertension and bradycardia can occur, as can pericardial effusions.

5. **Gastrointestinal system:** The hallmark is constipation, but ileus can occur with longstanding unrecognized disease.

6. **Neurologic system:** Prolonged relaxation of reflexes, proximal muscle weakness of lower extremities, and muscle cramping can commonly be elicited.

7. **Genitourinary system:** Metrorrhagia is common, and galactorrhea uncommon.

8. **General:** Decreased energy and cold intolerance are prominent features, as can be depression and apathy.

B. **Clinical syndromes suggesting hypothyroidism**

1. **Pituitary enlargement** in the context of galactorrhea and elevated prolactin levels. An elevated TSH will preclude the misdiagnosis of prolactinoma.

2. **Diastolic hypertension** as a manifestation of acute hypothyroidism.

3. **Sleep apnea**
4. **Intestinal pseudo-obstruction**
5. **SIADH** (syndrome of inappropriate secretion of antidiuretic hormone)
6. **Anemia,** either due to metromenorrhagia or folate and/or vitamin B_{12} deficiency
C. **Etiology**
   1. **Hashimoto's thyroiditis,** the most common cause, is a form of autoimmune thyroiditis and typified by an enlarged gland, firm in texture, with a lumpy contour. The bossellated surface can sometimes be misdiagnosed as nodules. Although commonly positive, *antithyroid antibodies* are rarely needed to make the diagnosis. Other forms of autoimmune diseases, such as pernicious anemia, vitiligo, Addison's disease, or diabetes mellitus, may be present.
   2. Post-radioactive iodine therapy
   3. Post-external radiation therapy for malignancy
   4. Postsurgical intervention
   5. Drug-induced changes, which may be reversible:
      a. Lithium
      b. Iodine
      c. Interleukin or interferon
      d. Propylthiouracil or methimazole
D. **Thyroid hormone therapy**
   1. The goal of replacement therapy is to normalize the serum TSH level.
   2. The mean replacement dosage is 1.6 mcg/kg/day, with about a 10–20% reduction for the elderly.
   3. Initiation of therapy should be gradual if concern for underlying heart disease is present.
   4. An interval of 12 weeks is necessary *before* rechecking a serum TSH level.
   5. Generic thyroxine preparations are unreliable and should be avoided.
   6. Drugs, such as cholestyramine and ferrous sulfate, can markedly diminish absorption.
E. **Subclinical hypothyroidism**
   1. Increasing recognized, especially in women over 65 years of age, this entity is defined as a normal thyroxine level in the setting of an elevated TSH.
   2. For TSH levels >10, all agree that thyroxine should be started expectantly; however, disagreement exists about the need for replacement therapy in patients whose TSH level is 6–10. This mild rise in TSH can regress to the normal range over time. Therapy in this setting would be justified if the endpoint of treatment was correction of an elevated LDL cholesterol, a reversible metabolic abnormality of hypothyroidism.

REFERENCES

Hyperthyroidism

1. Farrar JJ, Taft AD: Iodine-131 treatment of hyperthyroidism: Current issues. Clin Endocrinol 35:207–212, 1991.
2. Roti E, Emerson CH: Postpartum thyroiditis. J Clin Endocrinol Metab 74:3–5, 1992.
3. Spaulding SW, Lippes H: Hyperthyroidism: Causes, clinical features, and diagnosis. Med Clin North Am 69:937, 1985.
4. Solomon B: Current trends in the management of Graves' disease. J Clin Endocrinol Metab 70:1518, 1990.
5. Woeber NA: Thyrotoxicosis and the heart. N Engl J Med 327:44, 1992.

Hypothyroidism

6. Ehrman DA, Sarne DH: Serum TSH and the assessment of thyroid status, Ann Intern Med 110:179, 1989.
7. Fish LH, Schwartz HI, Cavanaugh J, et al: Replacement dose, metabolism and bioavailability of levothyroxine in the treatment of hypothyroidism. N Engl J Med 316:764, 1987.
8. Hall R, Scanlon MF: Hypothyroidism: Clinical features and complications. Clin Endocrinol Metab 8:29, 1979.
9. Staub JJ, Althaus BU, Engler H, et al: Spectrum of subclinical and overt hypothyroidism. Am J Med 92:631, 1992.

Chapter 32: Neurologic Disorders

LYNNE P. TAYLOR, MD

Most neurologic disorders associated with sports are benign and self-limited. Because they can mimic more serious conditions, such as stroke or subarachnoid hemorrhage, however, they can give rise to fear in both patient and health care provider.

Headache, common compression neuropathies, head trauma, vascular and vestibular disorders and diving injuries are the focus of this chapter. Because exercise is not only for the able-bodied, the special role of physical exertion in persons with multiple sclerosis and the wheelchair-bound will be noted at the end.

I. HEADACHE

   A. **Migraine:** A common hemicranial (localized in one side) or holocranial (in both sides) headache associated with various systemic complaints such as nausea, vomiting, and diarrhea as well as mood changes..

      1. **Prevalence:** 30% of women in child-bearing years, decreasing with age and equally distributed across all socioeconomic levels and races.

      2. **Pathophysiology:** Unstable central serotonergic transmission leading to inflammation in the walls of major cranial arteries.

      3. **Helpful historical points**

         a. Family history of migraine, with "sick" or "sinus" headache in 60–90% of first-degree relatives.

         b. 92% of patients have onset of symptoms before age 40.

         c. **Common triggers** include hormonal changes (usually dropping estrogen levels in the few days prior to the onset of the menstrual cycle), weather, stress, caffeine, aged cheeses, alcohol, lack of sleep, and *exercise.*

      4. **Migraine subtypes**

         a. **Common migraine:** Severe, diffuse headache, often with systemic complaints but without neurologic symptoms.

         b. **Classic migraine:** Headache ushered in by scintillating scotomata or visual-field deficits, hemianesthesia, or hemiparesis, followed 10–20 minutes later by headache, often hemicranial.

      5. **Treatment**

         a. **Classic migraine:** Ergots taken immediately at the onset of the aura, usually ergotamine 1 mg plus 100 mg caffeine, oral or rectal; dihydroergotamine 1 mg intravenously; or sumatriptan 6 mg subcutaneous.

         b. **Common migraine:** Aspirin or nonsteroidal antiinflammatory drugs (NSAIDs), particularly indomethacin 50 mg orally three times daily, are often sufficient. For more severe headache, consider isometheptene, once every 30 minutes for a maximum of 8/day. Avoid butalbital combinations and narcotics if possible. Ergots and sumatriptan may also be helpful.

         c. **Prophylactic therapy** is usually initiated for headaches if they occur more frequently than once or twice a week—generally propranolol LA, 80 mg orally in the morning tapering upwards, or verapamil, 80 mg orally three times daily. Nortriptyline or amitriptyline, 10–75 mg each night, are also very often effective.

         d. **Pregnancy:** All drugs noted above (particularly aspirin and ergotamine) are contraindicated in pregnancy. Use acetaminophen or oral meperidine

(Demerol), 50–100 mg, for severe pain during the first trimester. Migraines often abate spontaneously during the second and third trimesters. Prophylactic propranolol, if absolutely necessary, is also safe.

B. **Exertional headache or effort migraine**
   1. Triggered by brief, intense exercise or prolonged athletic activity in deconditioned individuals.
   2. Treat with prophylactic indomethacin, 25–50 mg, before exercise.
   3. Careful graded warm-up has also been successful.

C. **Coital headache**
   1. Sudden, severe, explosive headache peaking in the seconds during or just after orgasm.
   2. Angiogram or a neurologic consult should be performed with the first episode to rule out aneurysm or subarachnoid hemorrhage.
   3. Prophylactic therapy: Indomethacin as for migraine.

D. **Goggle headache**
   1. Throbbing bitemporal headache sometimes associated with sudden, sharp pain in the frontal area, caused by tightly fitting swim goggles and thought to be related to compression of the supraorbital nerve by the rim of the goggle (Fig. 1).
   2. Treated by changing the position of the goggles daily and the use of goggles which do not require a tight headstrap.

E. **Low-pressure headache**
   1. Severe positional headache, worse with standing or sitting and improved with lying supine. It has been described following vigorous exercise (racket sports) and presumably is related to a traumatic tear in the dura and subsequent leakage of spinal fluid.
   2. Generally it spontaneously improves with strict bedrest after 2–3 days.
   3. Patients should be evaluated by a neurologist, as this syndrome is quite rare. Sometimes it is treated, in addition, with epidural blood patching.

II. ARM AND HAND COMPLAINTS

A. **Long thoracic neuropathy**
   1. **Pathophysiology**
      a. Long thoracic nerve derives from the C5, 6, and 7 branches (Fig. 2) and courses downward just behind the midaxillary line to the serratus anterior.

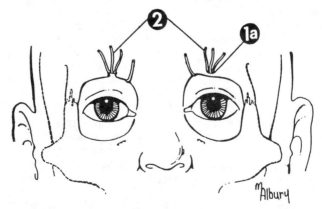

FIGURE 1. The orbital cavity, showing the location of the supraorbital foramen (*1a*) and the supraorbital nerves (*2*). (From Jacobson RI: More "goggle headache": Supraorbital neuralgia [letter]. N Engl J Med 308:1363, 1983; with permission.)

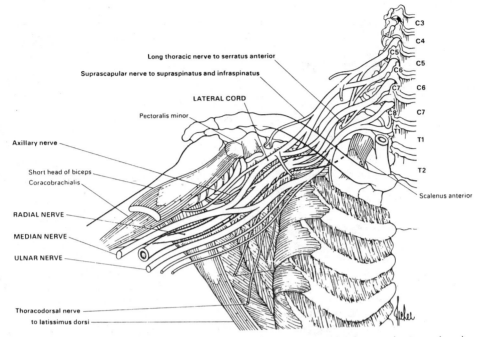

FIGURE 2. Diagram of the brachial plexus, its branches, and the muscles they supply. (Reproduced by permission of Guy's Hospital Medical School and the Guarantors of Brain, London.)

Function of this muscle is to maintain the scapula against the thorax and allow the arm to rotate upward.

b. Generally injured in any movement which requires an overhead serve. It most likely is related to traction forces on the nerve from the belly of the serratus anterior muscle itself. Seen commonly in tennis, golf, baseball, archery, gymnastics, bowling, soccer, ballet, and weight-lifting.

c. Also known as "backpack paralysis," in which the nerve is directly compressed by pressure from a heavy pack.

2. **Clinical presentation**

a. Presents with sharp pain in the shoulder area that radiates into the axilla, though patients occasionally notice prominence of the scapula without shoulder pain.

b. Winging of the lower border of the scapula is found with the patient's arms outstretched (seen best when asking the subject to perform a push-up).

c. Diagnosed by clinical history and examination; sometimes supplemented with electrophysiologic studies (electromyography, or nerve conduction velocity).

3. **Treatment**

a. Initially rest and avoidance of movements where the arm is directly overhead, followed by physical therapy to maintain range of movement and increase strength (exercises should be done supine to allow gravity to fixate the scapula against the body).

b. Prognosis is good, usually with full recovery within 9 months to 2 years.

B. **Suprascapular neuropathy**

1. **Pathophysiology**

a. Stretching of the nerve across the lateral edge of the scapula, likely related to the final phase of the overhead serve in volleyball from contraction of the posterior muscles of the shoulder.

b. Suprascapular nerve is made up of C5 and 6 roots, and the nerve follows a course through the infraspinous process, where the nerve bends around the spine of the scapula.

2. **Clinical presentation**
   a. Poorly localized shoulder pain which increases with shoulder flexion (arm across the chest).
   b. There is weakness in external rotation and abduction of the shoulder, atrophy of the muscles of the upper border of the scapula, and weakness in the supra- and infraspinatus muscles.

3. **Treatment**
   a. Initially rest and avoidance of movements where the arm is directly overhead, followed by physical therapy to maintain range of movement and increase strength (exercises should be done supine to allow gravity to fixate the scapula against the body).
   b. Prognosis is good, usually with full recovery within 9 months to 2 years.

C. **Radial neuropathy**
   1. **Pathophysiology:** Usually direct compression of the nerve in the axilla from improperly fitting crutches or related to humeral fractures.
   2. **Clinical presentation:** As the radial nerve is a predominantly motor nerve, there is usually a painless weakness of the wrist extensors producing a wrist drop. If the wrist is fixated in extension, it is usually possible to demonstrate that the intrinsic hand muscles remain strong.
   3. **Treatment:** Splinting until spontaneous improvement occurs, which might take place over many months.

D. **Ulnar neuropathy**
   1. **Pathophysiology**
      a. The ulnar nerve passes medial to the elbow and is generally damaged by calcification, direct compression, or trauma related to osteoarthritis.
      b. Ulnar nerve compression can occur at the elbow from the pitching motion of tennis, volleyball and baseball; at the wrist from the pressure of hands on poorly padded handle bars (often racing bicycles); or at the palm in cheerleaders or with prolonged clapping.
   2. **Clinical presentation**
      a. Tingling in the fifth digit, which increases with elbow flexion, followed by weakness of grasp and pinch in the affected hand.
      b. Physical examination generally reveals numbness in the distal fingertips of the fourth and fifth fingers as well as intrinsic hand weakness.
   3. **Treatment**
      a. Protection of the ulnar nerve in the ulnar groove at the elbow by a pad.
      b. Avoidance of repetitive motion.
      c. Generally recovery is spontaneous within months.
      d. Occasionally, a nerve transfer is considered, though only if the symptoms persist for more than 1–2 years.

E. **Posterior interosseous neuropathy**
   1. **Pathophysiology:** May be the cause of many cases of "resistant tennis elbow."
   2. **Clinical presentation:** Often presents with lateral elbow pain which increases at night. Physical examination reveals tenderness over the posterior interosseous nerve in the upper forearm and increase in pain with resisted supination of the forearm.
   3. **Treatment:** Rest, though occasionally release of the posterior interosseous nerve surgically is required.

F. **Median neuropathy**
   1. **Pathophysiology:** Classic nocturnal hand pain or "carpal tunnel." Appears to be no more common among athletes than in the general population.

    2. **Clinical presentation:** Compression of the median palmar digital nerve can occur deep in the palm and present with numbness and tingling on the ring and middle fingers. It has been described in a cheerleader doing vigorous cartwheels and clapping.

    3. **Treatment:** Wrist splint, surgical release.

G. **Median digital neuropathy in the thumb**

    1. **Pathophysiology:** Has been seen in bowlers, known as "bowler's thumb."

    2. **Clinical presentation:** Painless thumb numbness.

    3. **Treatment:** Patients do well when treated conservatively with avoidance of trauma.

H. **Brachial plexopathy**

    1. **Pathophysiology:** Obscure, most likely a traction injury.

    2. **Clinical presentation:** Known as "stingers" or "burners." Sharp pain, followed by transient numbness, felt in the shoulder and arm of football players in face-to-face tackling.

    3. **Treatment:** None.

I. **Cervical radiculopathies**

    1. **Pathophysiology:** No more common in athletes than in the general population. Usually related to acute herniated discs, often brought on by rowing machines, Nautilus equipment, and weight-lifting.

    2. Detailed discussion of individual cervical radiculopathies beyond the scope of this chapter.

III. **LEG AND FOOT COMPLAINTS**

A. **Peroneal neuropathy**

    1. **Pathophysiology:** Anatomic course of the common peroneal nerve is between the tendon of the biceps femoris muscle and the lateral head of the gastrocnemius, through the deep fascia of the leg and across the fibular neck (Fig. 3). Can be compressed by myofascial bands or osteophytes.

    2. **Clinical presentation**

        a. Presents with tingling and pain in the lateral aspect of the leg, brought on by running.

        b. Physical examination *after exercise* may demonstrate tingling with percussion of the nerve at the fibular neck (Tinel's sign) and an occasional foot drop.

    3. **Treatment:** Some cases have been successfully treated with tapered shoe inserts and occasional exploration and surgical release of the nerve.

B. **Sciatica**

    1. **Pedal pusher's palsy**

        a. **Pathophysiology:** Produced by compression of the sciatic nerve by direct pressure between the symphysis pubis and the ischial tuberosities from the seat of a racing bicycle, unicycle, or exercise cycle.

        b. **Clinical presentation:** Hip pain with radiation down the posterior aspect of the leg to the foot, tenderness with palpation over the sciatic notch.

        c. **Treatment:** Avoidance of compression.

    2. **Catamenial sciatica**

        a. **Pathophysiology:** Endometrial implants compress the sciatic nerve in the pelvis.

        b. **Clinical presentation:** Cyclical radiating pain timed to the menstrual cycle.

        c. **Treatment:** Suppression of endometriosis.

C. **Tarsal tunnel**

    1. **Pathophysiology:** Compression of the posterior tibial nerve and the tarsal tunnel from forced flexion or eversion of the foot.

    2. **Clinical presentation**

        a. Pain and paresthesias at the medial malleolus radiating into the sole of the foot. Often worsening at night or with exercise.

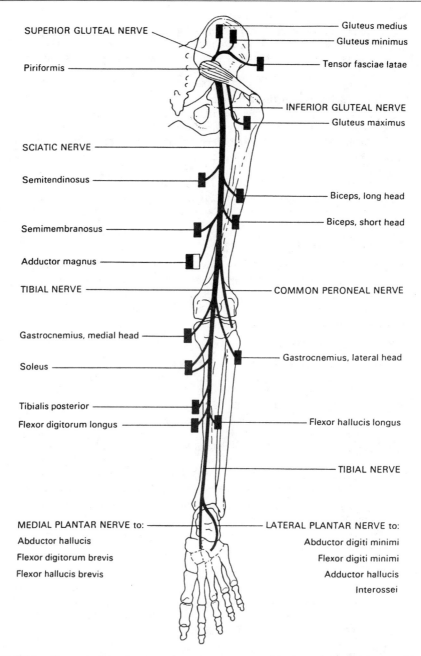

FIGURE 3. Diagram of the nerves on the posterior aspect of the lower limb and the muscles they supply. (Reproduced by permission of Guy's Hospital Medical School and the Guarantors of Brain, London.)

      b. Physical examination may show a positive Tinel's sign with tapping over the nerve and weakness of the intrinsic muscles of the foot.

     • c. Requires EMG testing for diagnosis.

    3. **Treatment:** NSAIDs, local steroid injections, improved foot wear, surgical release.

IV. HEAD INJURY

A. **Concussion**
   1. Sudden rotational force applied to the cranium produces diffuse axonal injury, cerebral edema, and petechial hemorrhage which is clinically expressed as **concussion.**
   2. Common in football, boxing, gymnastics, water sports, and martial arts.

B. **Second concussion**
   1. A player who suffers from a minor head trauma has a **fourfold increased risk of second concussion** over a previously uninjured athlete.
   2. "Second impact syndrome" can occur with reinjury, which can lead to uncontrolled increases in intracranial pressure and herniation leading to sudden death.
   3. Such risks have led to the development of conservative evaluation strategies to protect the head-injured athlete from further neurologic compromise.

C. **Grading system:** A proposed grading system for concussion in sports considers confusion, amnesia, and loss of consciousness and specifies criteria for return to play which are easy to apply (Table 1).

V. VASCULAR DISEASE

A. **Arterial dissection/occlusion:** The vertebral arteries travel through the foramen in the cervical vertebral bodies and can be occluded by any sport which produces **rapid head turning.** Spinal cord infarction (from occlusion of the anterior spinal artery) and brainstem and cerebellar strokes have been reported from gymnastics, swimming, and archery.

VI. VESTIBULAR DISEASE

A. **Benign positional vertigo**
   1. Intense sense of false movement brought on by changes in head position, fatiguing rapidly until the head is turned again.
   2. Caused by dislodgement of a subpopulation of otoliths from directional hairs in the inner ear. Usually degenerative but can be precipitated by vigorous high-impact aerobics, basketball or racket sports.
   3. Spontaneously improves over weeks to months.

VII. DIVING INJURIES (SCUBA)

Decompression sickness and cerebral air embolism are the neurologic manifestations of diving injury. Accidents can occur if divers negligently fail to strictly follow U.S. Navy dive tables but have also been reported in sports divers without clear explanation.

TABLE 1. Grading System for Concussion

Grade	Confusion	Loss of Consciousness	Criteria for Return to Play
1. Mild	Yes (without amnesia)	No	May return to play if asymptomatic at rest and after exertion (with at least 20 min of observation)
2. Mild-moderate	Yes (with post-traumatic amnesia <24 hrs)	No	May return to play after asymptomatic for 1 week.
3. Moderate-severe	Yes (post-traumatic amnesia >24 hrs)	Yes (<2 min)	No play for at least 1 month. May then return after asymptomatic for 1 week.
4. Severe	Yes	Yes (>2 min)	No play for at least 1 month. May then return after asymptomatic for 2 weeks.

A. **Decompression sickness**
   1. Produces paresthesias and sensory loss in the limbs with varying degrees of weakness and paraparesis in more severe cases.
   2. Onset of complaints is sometime after the diver surfaces and usually involves breach of diving tables.
   3. Pathology is of patchy spinal cord infarction thought to be related to changes of protein structure at the interface between blood and air bubbles within the circulation.

B. **Cerebral air embolism**
   1. Associated with breath-holding while ascending. Gas is trapped within the lungs, ruptures into the pulmonary vein, and produces systemic air embolism, often with immediate syncope on surfacing.
   2. Air embolism is often fatal because victims drown.
   3. Survivors may have seizures, cognitive dysfunction, and focal neurologic findings.

C. **Treatment**
   1. Patients with either disorder should be transported immediately to the nearest hyperbaric chamber for recompression therapy (obtained from Divers Alert Network, 919-684-8111).
   2. Breathing 100% oxygen is probably also helpful.

VI. EXERCISE AND THE DISABLED

A. **Multiple sclerosis**
   1. A common neurologic disorder of unknown etiology affecting primarily young to middle-aged women and producing multiple episodes of nervous system dysfunction over months to years.
   2. Inflammatory cells digest the myelin sheath around central nervous system axons (white matter) and create plaques in the cerebral hemispheres, optic nerves, brainstem, and spinal cord.
   3. Most affected women are able to exercise without symptoms, but some patients have recurrence of old deficits with raised body temperatures during vigorous activity.
   4. Swimming in a cold pool allows dissipation of body heat and is the best form of therapy.

B. **Wheelchair athletics**
   1. Because spinal cord injuries affect young people engaged in active sports, it is not surprising that elite ultramarathon wheelchair athletics is becoming more common and competitive.
   2. Knowledge about the exercise physiology of the disabled athlete is just beginning to emerge from studies on this unique population.

REFERENCES

1. Dick APK, Massey EW: Neurologic presentation of decompression sickness and air embolism in sport divers. Neurology 35:667–671, 1985.
2. Ferretti A, Cerullo G, Russo G: Suprascapular neuropathy in volleyball players. J Bone Joint Surg 69A:260–263, 1987.
3. Garcia-Albea E, Cabrera F, Tejeiro J, et al: Delayed postexertional headache, intracranial hypotension and racket sports [letter]. J Neurol Neurosurg Psychiatry 55:975, 1992.
4. Haig AJ: Pedal pusher's palsy [letter]. N Engl J Med 320:63, 1989.
5. Hallet M: Entrapment neuropathies in sports. Presented as a course at the Annual Meeting of the American Academy of Neurology, April 26, 1993, New York. (pages 276-15 through 276-29.)
6. Hankey GJ, Gubbay S: Compressive mononeuropathy of the deep palmar branch of the ulnar nerve in cyclists. J Neurol Neurosurg Psychiatry 51:1588–1590, 1988.
7. Jackson DL, Haglund B: Tarsal tunnel syndrome in athletes: Case reports and literature review. Am J Sports Med 19:61–65, 1991.
8. Jacobson RI: More "goggle headache": Supraorbital neuralgia [letter]. N Engl J Med 308:1363, 1983.

9. Jordan BD: Selected clinical syndromes in sports neurology: Acute brain injury. Presented as a course at the Annual Meeting of the American Academy of Neurology, April 26, 1993, New York. (pages 276-6 through 276-12.)
10. Krejcova H, Krejci L, Jirout J, et al: Vestibular and neurological disorders in diving competitors. Ann NY Acad Sci 374:839–845, 1981.
11. Lambert RW, Burnet DL: Prevention of exercise induced migraine by quantitative warm-up. Headache 25:317–319, 1985.
12. Leach RE, Purnell MB, Saito A: Peroneal nerve entrapment in runners. Am J Sports Med 17:287–291, 1989.
13. Morris AF: A case study of a female ultramarathon wheelchair road user. Paraplegia 24:260–264, 1986.
14. Pestronk A, Pestronk S: Goggle migraine [letter]. N Engl J Med 308:226–227, 1983.
15. Raskin NH: Headache, 2nd ed. New York, Churchill-Livingstone, 1988.
16. Schultz JS, Leonard JA: Long thoracic neuropathy from athletic activity. Arch Phys Med Rehabil 73:87–90, 1992.
17. Shields RW, Jacobs IB: Median palmar digital neuropathy in a cheerleader. Arch Phys Med Rehabil 67:824–826, 1986.
18. Tramo MJ, Hainline B, Petito F, et al: Vertebral artery injury and cerebellar stroke while swimming: Case report. Stroke 16:1039–1042, 1985.

Chapter 33: Respiratory Disorders

ROBERT B. SCHOENE, MD

Few differences are found in ventilation between men and women, especially among exercising athletes. There are some subtle differences in lung and airway growth during the developmental years. The most significant difference, however, is the hyperventilatory influence of female hormonal fluctuation, primarily progesterone and estrogen, both of which play a role in the menstrual cycle and pregnancy. Exercise-induced bronchospasm is found in both men and women; it is an important condition because of its deleterious effects on performance but can be easily treated in most cases. This chapter focuses on these areas of difference between males and females.

I. **VENTILATION**

   A. **The primary purpose of the lungs is to oxygenate the blood** to provide an adequate oxygen supply for tissue metabolism and to eliminate carbon dioxide generated by oxidative metabolism in the tissues. To accomplish these goals, two functions must be intact:
   1. Matching of perfusion of blood to the lung with ventilation of atmospheric air
   2. Lung mechanics which move air in and out of the lung
   B. At rest, these goals are easily met. **With increased metabolism, such as in exercise, come increased demands:**
   1. The heart must be able to generate an adequate cardiac output to increase perfusion.
   2. The respiratory mechanics must be able to increase ventilation to match the greater demand for obtaining oxygen and eliminating CO_2.
   3. In the normal lung, these goals are easily met, and there is little difference between men and women.

II. **LUNG DEVELOPMENT**

   During the developmental years, several differences have been documented between males and females in growth of the lung. These studies have concentrated on changes in growth of the airways and lung parenchyma using cross-sectional and longitudinal study designs in different age groups using tests of lung mechanics.
   A. **Airways**
   1. Function and growth of airways are measured by **tests of airflow.** Variables derived are:
      a. **Spirometry**
         i. Forced expiratory volume in 1 second (FEV_1)
         ii. Peak expiratory flow (PEF)
         iii. Forced expiratory flow at 25–75% of vital capacity (FEF_{25-75})
         iv. FEV_1/FVC (forced vital capacity) ratio
         v. Various fractionations of the flow curve
      b. **Plethysmography**
         i. Measurements of airway resistance and conductance
   2. From a practical standpoint, spirometry is the easier and more useful measurement available to all practitioners.
   3. **The diagnosis of reactive airway or obstructive disease** is made by a decrease in flow rates compared to normals or, more specifically, by an FEV_1/FVC ratio $<75\%$.

B. **Lung parenchyma**
   1. Function and growth of lung parenchyma are inferred from spirometry by vital capacity (VC).
   2. More precise measurements are derived from measurements of lung volume, particularly total lung capacity (TLC), which require helium dilution, nitrogen washout, or body plethysmography.
   3. **Diagnosis of restrictive airway disease** can only be made accurately with TLC <80% predicted.
C. **Differences in growth rates:** Growth of airways and lung parenchyma is at disproportionate rates in males and females. Comparison of growth rates between airways and lung parenchyma can be made during growth periods by analyzing flow/volume ratios, and these techniques have been the primary ones used in large population studies.
   1. **Rates of growth**
      a. **Isoptic:** Airways and lung parenchyma grow together at equal rates.
      b. **Dysanaptic:** Airways and lung parenchyma grow at disproportionate rates.
   2. In normal lung, these growth patterns influence function very little, but **gender differences** in somatic and pulmonary development provide curious findings.
      a. Body height provides the best marker for lung size, but because boys and girls have different growth spurts, there are some differences in lung growth and function during formative years.
      b. At <11 years old, females have more rapid growth, although the chest wall grows more slowly and reaches a smaller volume compared to body size at the end of teenage years. Males continue to expand lung size later in their teen years compared to females.
      c. Peak growth is reached at age 16 years in girls and 18 years in boys.
      d. When lung size is compared to airway size from ages 11–19 years, females have larger airways and exhibit dysanaptic growth patterns—i.e., lung and airspace growth lags behind airway development. Males have isoptic growth patterns—i.e., lower airflow initially but greater flows by the end of somatic development.
   3. **Racial differences:** Blacks have smaller lung volumes than whites, but the gender differences in other parameters of pulmonary function are similar.

III. **CONTROL OF VENTILATION**

   A. Breathing is controlled in humans by a complex interaction of chemical and mechanical events that result in a finely tuned homeostatic balance in which oxygen is perfectly supplied and CO_2 is eliminated and maintained at a precise level in the arterial blood during rest and moderate levels of exercise.
      1. At higher levels of exercise, a **metabolic acidosis** results from an accumulation of lactic acid which plays a partial role in an accelerated burst in ventilation which results in a **respiratory alkalosis** which compensates in part for the metabolic acidosis.
      2. From a mechanical standpoint, an optimal relationship between larger tidal volumes and higher respiratory frequencies is maintained in a biomechanically efficient manner so as to minimize the work of breathing.
      3. Chemically, chemoreceptors in the brainstem and carotid bodies instantaneously sense changes in PO_2, CO_2, and pH and send signals to the spinal cord which activate the muscles of respiration (diaphragm, intercostals, and accessory), which result in higher levels of ventilation.
         a. Carotid bodies or the peripheral chemoreceptors primarily sense changes in PO_2 and pH.
         b. Central chemoreceptors in the brainstem are sensitive to fluctuations in PCO_2 and pH.

4. Mechanically, a number of receptors (primarily stretch, flow, and irritant) are present in the lung parenchyma and help to modulate the pattern (tidal volume and rate) of breathing to achieve metabolic stability in an efficient manner.

B. **Hormone-related hyperventilation:** A number of endogenous and exogenous factors can affect the control of breathing. One important factor which modulates the control of ventilation which differs between men and women is the normal fluctuation of progesterone during the menstrual cycle and pregnancy. The stimulatory effect of progesterone may be potentiated by the presence of estrogen.

1. **Pregnancy**

   a. In the 1950s, hyperventilation was documented during pregnancy. At first, this was attributed to mechanical stimulation from the increasing size of the uterus.

   b. Hyperventilation occurred, however, early in pregnancy long before uterus size could play a role. Later, the progressive increase in progesterone levels was found to be responsible.

   c. Several studies showed similar hyperventilatory effects in men who were given exogenous progesterone, and such therapy is used successfully in patients with chronic alveolar hypoventilation syndrome.

2. **Menstrual cycle**

   a. Hyperventilation occurs in women during the luteal phase of the menstrual cycle, when progesterone levels are high. Hyperventilation occurs both during rest and exercise and results in greater alveolar ventilation, a higher work of breathing, and greater dyspnea during exercise.

   b. In competitive athletes, this modest increase in dyspnea probably does not impair training or competition but may play an inhibitory role in recreationally active women who are not used to intense levels of exercise and subsequent dyspnea. This may be particularly relevant since highly trained aerobic athletes have blunted ventilatory drives and exercise ventilation than normals.

   c. How these factors affect athletic performance is unknown. Studies of exogenous administration of hormones in women, such as in oral contraceptives, have shown conflicting results with respect to ventilation and performance, but the changes are minimal in either direction such that the consequences on these variables are probably minimal.

IV. VENTILATION IN SPORTS-RELATED SITUATIONS

A. **Exercise-induced bronchospasm:** This remains the major sports-related respiratory condition, although no published studies to date show any differences in its occurrence between men and women.

1. Normally, airway conductance improves with exercise. Subjects with exercise-induced bronchospasm, however, have a decrease in airway caliber during or, more commonly, after exercise. During prolonged exercise, bronchospasm may occur and resolve before the exercise session is over.

2. **Incidence**

   a. Probably the same as asthma in the general population (~10%).

   b. Several studies show the incidence may be higher (~15%) in competitive athletes.

   c. Patients with asthma tend to have exercise-induced bronchospasm, although individuals without clinical asthma may get bronchospasm only during or after exercise.

3. **Pathogenesis**

   a. Cause is unknown. Airway narrowing is probably a result of both smooth muscle contraction and edema from inflammation.

   b. A paradoxical response of catecholamines, thermal loss from high volumes of cold, dry air, and inflammatory mediator release have all been implied, and some or all of these factors may play a role and have complex therapeutic implications.

4. **Symptoms:** May be subtle and present for years before a diagnosis is made.
   a. Includes one or more of the following:
      i. Cough during or after exercise
      ii. Inordinate dyspnea
      iii. Overt wheezing
   b. Coaches and team physicians must be aware of such symptoms in athletes, since treatment is safe, easy, and legal at all levels of local, national, and international competition.
5. **Diagnosis:** Once the diagnosis is suspected, there are several means of confirmation:
   a. **Spirometry:** In the clinic, baseline spirometry should be obtained, followed by either a methacholine or exercise challenge.
      i. The exercise test should be on a treadmill or cycle ergometer, and the patient should exercise at a level that induces a heart rate of 80% of predicted maximum for 6–8 minutes.
      ii. Spirometry should be repeated at 5, 15, and 30 minute intervals after the end of exercise.
      iii. A 15–20% drop in FEV_1 confirms the diagnosis.
   b. **Peak flow meter:** As a screening technique at the practice field, a hand-held peak flow meter can be used to measure airflow before, during, and after practices. A diary should be kept to follow symptoms and results of peak flow measurements.
      i. If peak flow drops, a diagnosis is made.
6. **Treatment:** Must be tailored to the individual.
   a. Most athletes respond favorably to inhaled **beta-2 agonists** taken 15 minutes before exercise. These are the mainstay of therapy and most, but not all, are legal in international competition. **Albuterol** is legal and is the primary therapy.
   b. Others may do better with inhaled **steroids or cromolyn** (or any combination thereof). Inhaled steroids are legal, but physicians must notify meet officials ahead of time.

REFERENCES

1. Anderson SD, et al: Sensitivity to heat and water loss at rest and during exercise in asthmatic patients. Eur J Respir Dis 63:459, 1982.
2. Astrand P-O, Rodahl K: The Initial Textbook of Work Physiology, 3rd ed. New York, McGraw-Hill, 1986.
3. Deal EC, Wasserman SI, Sater NA, et al: Evaluation of role played by mediators of immediate hypersensitivities in exercise-induced asthma. J Clin Invest 65:659–665, 1980.
4. Deal EC, McFadden ER Jr, Ingram RH Jr, et al: Role of respiratory heat exchange in exercise-induced asthma. J Appl Physiol 46:467–475, 1979.
5. Hibbert ME, Couriel JM, Landau LI: Changes in lung, airway, and chest wall function in boys and girls between eight and twelve years. J Appl Physiol 57:304–308, 1984.
6. Larsson K, Hjendahl P, Martinsson A: Sympathoadrenal reactivity in exercise-induced asthma. Chest 82:560–567, 1982.
7. Martin BJ, Morgan EJ, Zwillich CW, Weil JD: Control of breathing during prolonged exercise. J Appl Physiol 50:27–31, 1981.
8. Merkus PJFM, Borsboom GJJM, Van Pelt W, et al: Growth of airways and airspaces in teenagers as related to sex but not symptoms. J Appl Physiol 75:2045–2053, 1993.
9. Schoene RB, Pierson DJ, Lakshminarayan S, et al: Effect of medroxyprogesterone acetate on respiratory drives and occlusion pressure. Clin Respir Physiol 16:645–653, 1980.
10. Schoene RB, Robertson HT, Pierson DJ, Peterson AP: Respiratory drives and exercise performance during the menstrual cycle: A study in athletic and non-athletic women. J Appl Physiol 50:1300–1305, 1981.

11. Schwartz JD, Katz SA, Fegley RW, Tockman MS: Analysis of spirometric from a national sample of healthy 6 to 24 year-olds. Am Rev Respir Dis 138:1405–1414, 1988.
12. Schwartz JD, Katz SA, Fegley RW, Tockman MS: Sex and race differences in the development of lung function. Am Rev Respir Dis 138:1415–1421, 1988.
13. Sherrill DL, Camilli A, Lebowitz MD: On the temporal relationships between lung function and somatic growth. Am J Respir Dis 140:638–644, 1989.
14. Sterling DR, Cotton DJ, Graham BL, et al: Characteristics of airway tone during exercise of patients with asthma. J Appl Physiol 54:934–942, 1983.
15. Wasserman K: Breathing during exercise. N Engl J Med 298:780–785, 1978.
16. Wasserman K, Hansen JE, Sue DY, Whipp BJ (eds): Principles of Exercise Testing and Interpretation. Philadelphia, Lea & Febiger, 1987.
17. Weiler JM, Metzger WJ, Donnally AL, et al: Prevalence of bronchial hyperresponsiveness in highly trained athletes. Chest 90:23–28, 1986.

Chapter 34: Cardiovascular Disorders in Women

PAMELA S. DOUGLAS, MD

Many aspects of the female cardiac response to exercise appear similar to the male response. A number of important physiologic and pathologic differences do exist, including aerobic capacity and diagnostic cardiac exercise testing on both treadmill and gated blood pool testing. An appreciation of the normal female response is vital. These differences apply to the female athlete and the sedentary woman. Much research remains to be done before a complete examination can be made of all the unique aspects of cardiovascular problems in the exercising woman.

I. AEROBIC CAPACITY

A. **Maximum aerobic workload is 15–30% lower in the average sedentary woman,** compared to the average sedentary man due to various factors:
   1. Lower total oxygen-carrying capacity of blood in women
      a. Lower blood volume
      b. Fewer red blood cells
      c. Lower hemoglobin content
   2. Smaller hearts in women
      a. Smaller stroke volume
      b. Higher heart rates for a given cardiac output or oxygen uptake
   3. Higher percentage of adipose tissue and lower percentage of working muscle
B. **Men are more active than women and therefore maintain a more trained state,** particularly as women tend to become more sedentary after puberty.
   1. Training programs produce similar increases in aerobic capacity in both sexes, even when older individuals are examined.
   2. Maximal oxygen uptake in individual, highly trained female athletes can approach and equal that of similarly trained males.
   3. No difference in exercise capacity is noted between boys and girls under age 12.
C. **Accurate interpretation of exercise test results** depends on recognition of the normally lower maximal aerobic capacity and higher heart rate in women.
   1. Sex-specific standards have been developed for maximal aerobic capacity.
   2. Sex-specific nomograms for calculation of maximal capacity from submaximal heart rate and oxygen values should be used.
D. **Aging affects aerobic capacity** of healthy individuals of both sexes similarly, causing:
   1. Decline in maximal oxygen uptake
   2. Decreased maximal achievable heart rate
   3. Decreased mechanical performance of the myocardium
   4. Limitations in the functioning of other organ systems

II. CARDIAC FUNCTION IN RESPONSE TO EXERCISE

A. **Normal cardiac response to exercise** in women may differ from that in men.
B. Exercise gated blood pool scanning generally results in an increased **cardiac ejection fraction** in <50% of women as compared to nearly all men.
C. Mechanisms used to increase **cardiac output** during exercise differ in men and women:
   1. In men, end-diastolic left ventricular size does not change with exercise, whereas end-systolic size decreases, leading to increased stroke volume and ejection fraction.

2. Women achieve a similar increase in stroke volume by increasing end-diastolic size, while end-systolic size remains unchanged.
3. Women dilate their left ventricles, or increase preload, whereas men increase ventricular shortening.
4. Physiologic basis for these differences is unknown, as are their significance for preserved health or training.

D. **Clinical implications:** Since good health is defined by the "normal" male pattern of response, the remainder of the population, or women who normally respond differently, may be *falsely diagnosed as unwell.* In a similar manner, a woman with mild cardiac disease may be classified as having more severe impairment than is actually the case.

III. CARDIAC ADAPTATION TO EXERCISE TRAINING

A. Hearts of both men and women appear to adapt similarly to exercise training.
B. Sports studied in women: field hockey, dance, jogging, swimming, triathlon training.
C. In women, weight training or isometric exercise produces cardiovascular effects similar to those of aerobic, dynamic exercise, including:
   1. **Cardiac enlargement and left ventricular hypertrophy** (enlarged heart on chest radiograph, increased left and right ventricular cavity sizes and wall thicknesses on echocardiography, and increased voltage on ECG, all reflecting an increased myocardial mass).
   2. **Cardiac arrhythmias** (unknown if due to increased vagal tone or altered catecholamine metabolism). Although **sinus bradycardia** is most common, low-grade atrioventricular block, premature atrial or ventricular contractions, and repolarization abnormalities are also seen.
   3. **Multivalvular regurgitation,** especially tricuspid, pulmonic, and mitral valves.
   4. **Clinical implications:** *Adaptive changes to exercise may be similar to those signifying the presence of true heart disease.*
      a. Physical training may lead to physiologic structural and electrical changes in the healthy female heart.
      b. These changes must not be confused with similar findings in cardiac disease states (*see* item C under IX. Hypertrophic Cardiomyopathy below on differentiation of pathologic and physiologic hypertrophy).

IV. ELECTROCARDIOGRAPHIC EXERCISE TESTING

A. Monitoring of ECG recordings capable of detecting cardiac ischemia during a controlled exercise protocol is the most widely used diagnostic procedure for detecting coronary disease.
   1. In men, regardless of symptoms, ECG exercise testing is an excellent screening test, with few false-positive results.
   2. **In women, the incidence of false-positive ECG results** (appearance of ECG changes characteristic of myocardial ischemia in its absence) **is quite high,** perhaps as high as two-thirds of all positive tests.
   3. A negative test is quite reliable in excluding the presence of coronary disease in women (as reliable as in men).
   4. Exercise tests are useful in risk stratification of women with known coronary heart disease.
B. Several factors partially explain this gender difference:
   1. Age-related differences in prevalence of heart disease between men and women (Bayes' theorem). Because coronary disease is relatively less likely in younger and middle-aged women, any given positive test result is more likely to be a false rather than a true-positive. Thus, the diagnostic utility of exercise testing for coronary artery disease in women is lower than in men.

2. Higher prevalence in women of other characteristics that are associated with nondiagnostic results, including:
   a. Poor exercise tolerance
   b. Greater age
   c. Atypical chest pain
   d. Resting ECG abnormalities (nonspecific ST- and T-wave changes)
   e. Medications such as digoxin and anxiolytics
C. **Alternative strategies for diagnosis of coronary heart disease in women:**
   1. Pharmacologic stress testing (adenosine, persantine, dobutamine)
   2. Additional imaging
      a. Thallium-201 or sestamibi myocardial scintigraphy
      b. Echocardiography
   3. Both pharmacologic stress testing and imaging in combination
   4. Drawbacks include greater expense, greater expertise, need for special equipment
D. **Clinical implications**
   1. Women with chest pain due to noncardiac causes are more likely to be wrongly diagnosed by conventional exercise testing, leading to unnecessary medications and/or additional testing.
   2. Higher false-positive rate of exercise testing in women makes it a very poor screening test for cardiovascular disease.
   3. Use of additional imaging modalities and/or pharmacologic stress is important, especially in younger women.
   4. Negative test result is good indication of the absence of heart disease, even in women.
   5. Limitations of diagnostic testing for coronary heart disease probably contribute to gender bias in its diagnosis and treatment in women.

V. EXERCISE LIMITATIONS IN HEART DISEASE

A. **Effects of exercise in heart disease patients** appear to be similar in men and women.
B. Because little attention has been focused on potential differences between men and women, it is possible that some differences do exist (as they do in many forms of cardiac disease) but have been overlooked.
C. Longitudinal studies of exercise intervention have shown some benefit in improving cardiac risk factors such as **lipid profiles, blood pressure, obesity, and diabetes mellitus,** although the effect is generally smaller in women than in men. Women with higher fitness levels have longer event-free survival than those with lower exercise capacity.
D. Value of exercise in treatment of established coronary heart disease, or rehabilitation following myocardial infarction or revascularization surgery, is unclear in women. Few women have been studied (too few for gender-specific meta-analysis).
E. In general, as in men, **exercise probably hastens recovery and improved quality of life** in the short-term. Longer-term benefits such as reduction of recurrence of myocardial infarction or improved long-term survival are more difficult to prove.

VI. MITRAL VALVE PROLAPSE

In contrast to most forms of either congenital or acquired heart disease, mitral valve prolapse occurs with greater frequency in women than men.
A. **Signs:** Generally a benign syndrome characterized by a broad variety of cardiac findings:
   1. Mid-systolic nonejection click
   2. Late systolic murmur
   3. Echocardiographic or cineangiographic evidence of systolic billowing of the mitral valve leaflets in the left atrium.
   4. Thickened mitral valve

    5. Atypical chest pain, palpitations, dizziness
    6. Abnormal ECG
    7. Atrial or ventricular arrhythmia
    8. Systemic emboli, mitral regurgitation
    9. Marfan syndrome
    10. Syncope
    11. Sudden death

B. **Possible myocardial involvement in mitral valve prolapse**
    1. Reports of left ventricular segmental contraction abnormalities, chest pain, and ventricular arrhythmias
    2. Failure to increase ejection fraction in response to exercise has been reported. This, however, may represent the normal female response and not a cardiomyopathic process.

C. **Participation in competitive or recreational sports**
    1. Complications have rarely been documented during exercise.
    2. Most patients can exercise without restrictions.
    3. American College of Cardiology[9] recommends limited competitive participation in selected patients, including those with:
        a. History of syncope
        b. Family history of sudden death due to mitral valve prolapse
        c. Chest pain worsened by exercise
        d. Repetitive ventricular ectopy
        e. Sustained supraventricular tachycardia (especially if worsened by exercise)
        f. Moderate or severe mitral regurgitation
        g. Dilation of the ascending aorta (associated with Marfan syndrome)

VII. ANOREXIA NERVOSA

A. **Cardiac changes with starvation** include changes in cardiac architecture, load, and function appropriate to decreased blood pressure. These are:
    1. Decreased heart size
    2. Decreased heart rate
    3. Return to normal with weight gain

B. **Death**
    1. Ipecac-induced cardiomyopathy
    2. Cardiac arrest due to electrolyte abnormalities

VIII. SUDDEN DEATH

A. **Risk factors** predisposing to unexpected sudden death in women are somewhat different from those in men:
    1. Age and, marginally, cholesterol are risk factors in both sexes.
    2. Hematocrit, vital capacity, and glucose were significantly related to the incidence of sudden death in women only.
    3. In men, additional risk factors for sudden death were those associated with coronary disease, including elevated systolic blood pressure, obesity, smoking, and ECG evidence of left ventricular hypertrophy.

B. Women dying suddenly are much less likely than men to have coronary heart disease (about 50%).

IX. HYPERTROPHIC CARDIOMYOPATHY

A. Most common cause of sudden death in young people during exercise.
B. Idiopathic, genetically transmitted syndrome characterized by thickened left ventricle with normal chamber size. There may or may not be an outflow tract gradient.
C. **Differentiating between physiologic and pathologic hypertrophy** may be difficult and rests on identification of other pathologic features, including:

      1. Asymmetric septal hypertrophy

      2. Systolic anterior motion of the mitral valve or chordae

      3. Family history of cardiomyopathy or sudden death

      4. Diastolic filling abnormalities

      5. ECG abnormalities

      6. Lack of regression of hypertrophy with exercise cessation

   D. Any athlete suspected of having hypertrophic cardiomyopathy should be evaluated by a cardiac specialist, with specific recommendations for active sports participation.

   E. **Participation in sports:** In patients with documented hypertrophic cardiomyopathy, the American College of Cardiology[9] recommends:

      1. No participation in high-intensity competitive sports, regardless of disease severity.

      2. Low-intensity sports are allowed (bowling, golf).

      3. Patients with marked hypertrophy, significant left ventricular outflow tract obstruction, arrhythmias, or family history of sudden death or syncope should not participate in any form of athletic endeavors.

X. EXERCISE LIMITATIONS IN OTHER FORMS OF HEART DISEASE

   A. **Best reference:** Task Force on Cardiovascular Abnormalities in the Athlete has published recommendations regarding eligibility for competition.[10] This group was sponsored by the American College of Cadiology and by the National Heart, Lung, and Blood Institute. This includes an up-to-date, comprehensive summary of both resistive and dynamic exercise limitations in all forms of congenital and acquired heart disease.

   B. It must be stressed that any person with known or suspected heart disease, regardless of sex, should undergo a full cardiovascular evaluation before undertaking exercise training or sports competition.

   C. Recommendations and limitations apply equally to male and female athletes.

REFERENCES

1. Astrand I: Aerobic work capacity in men and women with special reference to age. Acta Physiol Scand 49:169, 1960.
2. Astrand PO: Human physical fitness with special reference to age. Physiol Rev 36:307, 1956.
3. Blair SN, Kohl HW, Paffenbarger RS, et al: Physical fitness and all-cause mortality: A prospective study of healthy men and women. JAMA 262:2395, 1989.
4. Douglas PS, O'Toole ML, Hiller WDB, et al: Left ventricular structure and function by echocardiography in ultraendurance athletes. Am J Cardiol 58:805, 1986.
5. Douglas PS, O'Toole ML, Hiller WDB, et al: Electrocardiographic diagnosis of exercise-induced left ventricular hypertrophy. Am Heart J 116:784, 1988.
6. Douglas PS, Berman GO, O'Toole ML, et al: Prevalence of multivalvular regurgitation in athletes. Am J Cardiol 64:209, 1989.
7. Higginbotham MB, Morris KG, Coleman E, et al: Sex-related differences in the normal cardiac response to upright exercise. Circulation 70:357, 1984.
8. Huston TP, Puffer JC, Rodney WM: The athletic heart syndrome. N Engl J Med 313:24, 1985.
9. Maron EJ, Gaffney FA, Jeresaty RM, et al: Task force III: Hypertrophic cardiomyopathy, other myopericardial diseases and mitral valve prolapse. J Am Coll Cardiol 6:1215, 1985.
10. Mitchell JH, Maron BJ, Epstein SE: 16th Bethesda Conference: Cardiovascular abnormalities in the athlete: Recommendations regarding eligibility for competition. J Am Coll Cardiol 6:1186, 1985.
11. Seals DR, Hagberg JM: The effect of exercise training on human hypertension: A review. Med Sci Sports Exerc 16:207, 1984.

Chapter 35: Exercise-Related Anemias

SALLY S. HARRIS, MD, MPH

Anemia is perhaps the most common medical condition encountered in athletes. It is more prevalent in females than males and may be more common in female athletes than nonathletes for a variety of reasons. When unrecognized and untreated, anemia can impair athletic performance and sense of general well-being. It is easily diagnosed and treated; it also is usually preventable and therefore is particularly amenable to screening. Iron deficiency anemia is the most common type of anemia seen in both athletes and nonathletes. However, two types of anemia are unique to athletes: dilutional pseudoanemia and exercise-induced hemolysis. The presence of these conditions raises unique concerns when evaluating anemia in the athletic population.

I. HEMATOLOGIC INDICATORS OF ANEMIA

A. **Normal hemoglobin and hematocrit**
   1. Hemoglobin:
      a. Females   12–16 g/dl
      b. Males   13.4–18 g/dl
   2. Hematocrit:
      a. Females   37–47%
      b. Males   40–54%
B. **Interpretation of hemoglobin and hematocrit**
   1. Normal ranges represent 2 SD from the mean (i.e., 95% of the population will fall into this range).
   2. Values are 0.5 g/dl lower in blacks.
   3. Add 4% to correct values for each 1000 meters of altitude elevation.
C. **Criteria for Anemia**
   1. By strict criteria, anemia is present if hemoglobin or hematocrit values fall outside the normal range. However, significant overlap exists between normal and abnormal values. Therefore, anemia should be defined *relative* to an individual's baseline normal range.
   2. For example, a hemoglobin value of 13 g/dl, although within the normal range, may represent anemia for a woman whose normal baseline level is 13.5 g/dl. Alternatively, a hemoglobin value of 11.5 g/dl, although below the normal range, may not represent anemia for a woman for whom this is her normal baseline level.

II. DILUTIONAL PSEUDOANEMIA ("SPORTS ANEMIA")

A. **Definition:** A natural dilution of hemoglobin that occurs as a result of increased plasma volume associated with regular endurance exercise.
B. **Physiology**
   1. **Acute effects of exercise** are reduction of plasma volume (10–20%) and hemoconcentration due to:
      a. Increased capillary hydrostatic pressure due to increased mean arterial pressure and muscular compression on venules
      b. Increased tissue osmotic pressure due to production of lactic acid and other metabolites
      c. Filtered plasma lost as perspiration

2. **Compensatory rise in baseline plasma volume** occurs due to exercise-induced release of aldosterone, renin, and vasopressin.
3. Increase in plasma volume is proportional to amount and intensity of endurance exercise:
   a. Moderate jogging: 5%
   b. Elite distance running: 20%
4. Increase in plasma volume appears and disappears within a few days of initiation or cessation of training.
5. Although hemoglobin concentration is decreased due to dilutional effect, red blood cell mass is normal or often increased.

C. **May represent favorable adaptive response to training**
   1. Increased plasma volume and less viscous blood allow increased oxygen delivery in tissues during exercise.

D. **Diagnosis:** Distinguishing from iron deficiency anemia (Table 1)
   1. Not hypochromic or microcytic
   2. Not usually severe anemia
   3. Normal iron indices
   4. No response to iron supplementation

III. EXERCISE-INDUCED HEMOLYTIC ANEMIA

A. **Mechanisms**
   1. **Runners' macrocytosis**—foot strike hemolysis
      a. Repetitive hard foot strikes destroy red blood cells.
   2. **Intravascular hemolysis**
      a. Endurance exercise causes increased body temperature, acidosis, or muscular contraction that destroys red blood cells.

B. **Diagnostic triad** (Table 1)
   1. **Macrocytosis:** Older smaller red blood cells are preferentially destroyed.
   2. **Reticulocytosis:** Response to hemolysis
   3. **Low haptoglobin with or without hemoglobinuria**
      a. Destroyed red blood cells release hemoglobin that is then bound by haptoglobin.
      b. Haptoglobin delivers hemoglobin to the liver where the iron can be salvaged.
      c. If plasma concentration of haptoglobin is depleted, free hemoglobin is excreted into the urine, producing hemoglobinuria.

C. **Prevention and treatment in runners**
   1. Lean body composition
   2. Run on soft surfaces
   3. Run "light on feet"
   4. Wear well-cushioned shoes and insoles

D. **Consequences**
   1. Usually negligible source of iron loss
   2. May be of importance for performance of world-class athletes where frequent hemolysis may limit expansion of red blood cell mass

TABLE 1. Laboratory Test Profile of Exercise-Related Anemias

	Hemoglobin/ Hematocrit	Red Blood Cell Size	Serum Ferritin	Reticulocyte Count
Nonanemic iron deficiency	—	—	↓	—
Iron deficiency anemia	↓	↓	↓	—
Dilutional pseudoanemia	↓	—	—	—
Exercise-induced anemia	↓	↑	—	↑

IV. IRON DEFICIENCY ANEMIA

A. **Pathophysiology** (Table 2)
   1. Iron stores are depleted before clinically recognized anemia (characterized by hemoglobin and hematocrit below the normal range) occurs. Ferritin values reflect the status of iron stores.
   2. **Iron stores in the body**
      a. Hemoglobin—64%
      b. Bone marrow iron—27%
      c. Transport protein iron—2%
      d. Enzyme iron—2%
   3. **Ferritin values**
      a. <12 μg/L represents complete depletion of iron stores in the liver.
      b. 12–20 μg/L represents minimal iron stores.
      c. >20 μg/L represents adequate iron stores.
      d. Average ferritin values for young women are 30 μg/L.
      e. Ferritin values are elevated by acute inflammation and liver disease.
B. **Stages of iron deficiency**
   There are three stages of iron deficiency. Stages I and II represent nonanemic iron deficiency. Only the last stage is characterized by reduction of hemoglobin and hematocrit resulting in clinically recognized anemia.
   1. **Stage I—iron depletion**
      a. Characterized by ferritin <12 μg/L indicating depletion of iron stores in the liver
      b. Other indices of iron status remain normal.
      c. Duration of several months
   2. **Stage II—iron deficient erythropoiesis**
      a. Characterized by decreased iron transport marked by low serum iron, increased total iron-binding capacity (TIBC), decreased transferrin saturation (<16%)
      b. Hemoglobin and hematocrit remain normal.
      c. Duration of several weeks
   3. **Stage III—iron deficiency anemia**
      a. Clinically recognized as anemia
      b. Characterized by diminished hemoglobin production
         i. Low hemoglobin and hematocrit
         ii. Decreased mean corpuscular volume
         iii. Hypochromic microcytic red blood cells
C. **Differential diagnosis of hypochromic microcytic anemia**
   1. **Iron deficiency:** Most common, characterized by abnormal iron indices
   2. **Lead toxicity:** Rare outside of childhood
   3. **Thalassemia:** Related to family history, ethnicity
   4. **Chronic disease:** Medical history screening should identify

TABLE 2. Diagnostic Values for Iron Deficiency

Test	Normal Range
Serum ferritin	20–200 μg/L
Transferrin saturation	16–55%
Serum iron	
Females	50–150 μg/dl
Males	80–160 μg/L
Total iron-binding capacity	250–410 μg/dl
Serum erythroprotoporphyrin concentration	<1.24 μmol/L
Mean corpuscular volume (MCV)	81–99 fL
Reticulocyte count	0.5–1.5%
Haptoglobin	100–300 mg/dl

D. **Prevalence of iron deficiency**
   1. Prevalent condition among menstruating women
   2. Higher in females than males except for the 11–14-year-old age group.
   3. It is unclear whether the prevalence is higher among female athletes than non-athletes, although a number of factors related to exercise may contribute to iron deficiency.
   4. Prevalence estimates vary according to the population studied.
   5. High school and college female athletes:
      a. 0–19% for iron deficiency anemia
      b. 20–62% for nonanemic iron deficiency
E. **Effects of training on iron status**
   1. Studies following iron status in runners over a competitive season found that 16% of males and 20% of females with initially normal iron status developed nonanemic iron deficiency while none developed anemia.
   2. Iron status did not change during the season in one study of swimmers.
   3. Development of nonanemic iron deficiency during training among female cross-country runners was found to be preventable by iron supplementation.
F. **Mechanisms of iron deficiency in athletes**
   1. **Gastrointestinal (GI) losses**
      a. Occult GI blood loss is common in runners, probably due to bowel ischemia.
         i. 2% of marathoners and triathletes have visible blood in stools after races.
         ii. 20% of marathoners have occult blood in stools.
         iii. 50% of college and serious recreational runners have occult blood in stools more than once during the competitive season.
      b. Use of aspirin or nonsteroidal antiinflammatory drugs (NSAIDs) may increase GI blood loss.
   2. **Impaired gastrointestinal iron absorption**
      a. Iron-deficient runners absorb 16% of iron from the GI tract compared with 30% absorption in iron-deficient nonathletes.
   3. **Sweat losses**
      a. Up to 0.25–1.0 mg/day
      b. Negligible source of iron loss
   4. **Urinary losses**
      a. Mechanisms
         i. Hematuria due to microtrauma of genitourinary tract
         ii. Hemoglobinuria secondary to hemolysis
      b. Usually negligible source of iron loss
   5. **Menstrual losses**
      a. Most significant source of blood loss in female athletes
      b. Can be affected by stress, level of physical activity, and use of oral contraceptives
      c. Average menstrual loss is 0.6–1.5 mg/day.
   6. **Inadequate dietary intake of iron**
      a. May be preeminent cause of iron deficiency in female athletes
      b. More common among athletes in sports emphasizing lean body physique
      c. Dietary requirements
         i. **RDA:** 15 mg/day for females, 10 mg/day for males
         ii. Average diet contains 5–7 mg of iron/100 kcal. Therefore, women need 3000 kcal/day to get the RDA of 15 mg of iron. Many female athletes consume <2000 kcal/day.
         iii. Modified vegetarian diets pose increased risk due to lower bioavailability and quantities of iron in nonmeat foods.
G. **Effects on performance**
   1. Anemia is clearly associated with adverse effects on physical performance, as shown by **diminished maximum oxygen consumption, decreased physical work**

capacity, lower endurance, and increased fatigue. There is a well-proven correlation between hemoglobin levels and exercise capacity.

    2. It is unclear whether nonanemic iron deficiency impairs performance.

H. **Should nonanemic iron deficiency be treated?**

    1. **Iron should not be administered solely to improve athletic performance,** because it is unclear whether nonanemic iron deficiency impairs performance.

    2. **Iron therapy may be indicated for nonanemic iron-deficient women** to prevent development of anemia and reduce nonhematologic manifestations or iron deficiency, such as susceptibility to infection, impaired attention span, or altered mental function.

    3. From a practical standpoint, **it is often difficult to distinguish nonanemic iron deficiency from mild anemia.** Many women with presumed nonanemic iron deficiency do respond to iron supplementation and will show an increase in hemoglobin values. Therefore, these women are actually mildly anemic, although their hemoglobin falls within the normal range, and will benefit from iron supplementation.

I. **Clinical manifestations**

    1. Clinical manifestations of iron deficiency are rare unless anemia is severe.

    2. Potential signs and symptoms of iron deficiency include:

        a. Exercise fatigue   f. Pica

        b. Muscle burning   g. Pallor

        c. Nausea   h. Koilonychia

        d. Dyspnea   i. Cheilosis

        e. Pagophagia (ice eating)   j. Glossitis

J. **Prevention**

    1. **Increase dietary intake of iron.**

        a. Dietary sources of iron

           i. Lean red meat, dark meat of poultry, leafy green vegetables, grains, nuts, iron-fortified cereals

           ii. Heme sources of iron (red meat) are absorbed better (15–33%) than non-heme iron sources of iron (2–20%).

        b. Cook in iron skillets.

        c. Facilitate iron absorption—animal proteins, vitamin C.

        d. Avoid inhibitors of iron absorption—tea, coffee, milk, eggs.

    2. If unable to meet daily iron needs through diet, a supplement containing the RDA for iron (15 mg) is recommended.

K. **Treatment—iron supplementation**

    1. **Dosage**

        a. For iron deficiency anemia (ferritin <12 μg/L, low hemoglobin)

           i. 50–100 mg elemental iron 3 times per day (e.g., 325 mg ferrous sulfate 3 times daily)

           ii. Confirm response to supplementation by rise of 1 g/dl in hemoglobin after 4–6 weeks. Serum hemoglobin concentration is usually completely corrected within 2 months. Reticulocytosis is seen in 5–10 days.

           iii. Continue treatment for 6–8 months to replenish iron stores and restore normal ferritin level.

        b. For nonanemic iron deficiency (ferritin 12–20 μg/L, normal hemoglobin)

           i. 50–100 mg elemental iron once per day (e.g., 325 mg ferrous sulfate daily)

           ii. Continue supplementation until ferritin >20 μg/L (several months)

    2. **Practical tips**

        a. Iron salts contain varying amounts of elemental iron: sulfate 20%, fumarate 11%, gluconate 33%.

        b. Ferrous sulfate is cheapest.

        c. Avoid sustained-release or enteric-coated products.

    d. Enhance absorption by taking supplements with vitamin C, without other competing supplements, on an empty stomach.

    e. GI side effects are lessened by gradual progression of the dosage from once a day to 3 times a day as tolerance develops.

REFERENCES

1. Balaban EP, et al: The frequency of anemia and iron deficiency in the runner. Med Sci Sports Exerc 21:643–648, 1989.
2. Celsing F, et al: Effects of iron deficiency on endurance and muscle enzyme activity in man. Med Sci Sports Exerc 18:156–161, 1986.
3. Clement DB, et al: Iron status and sports performance. Sports Med 1:65–74, 1984.
4. Dallman PR: Manifestations of iron deficiency. Semin Hematol 19:19–30, 1982.
5. Eichner ER: The anemias of athletes. Phys SportsMed 14:122–130, 1986.
6. Eichner ER: Facts and myths about anemia in active women. Your Patient & Fitness 5(1):12–16, 1991.
7. Falsetti HL, et al: Hematologic variations after endurance running with hard and soft-soled shoes. Phys SportsMed 11:118–127, 1983.
8. Lamanca J, Haymes EL Effects of dietary iron supplementation on endurance [abstract]. Med Sci Sports Exerc 21(Suppl 2):577, 1989.
9. Matter M, et al: The effect of iron and folate therapy on maximal exercise performance in female marathon runners with iron and folate deficiency. Clin Sci 72:415–422, 1987.
10. Miller BJ: Haematologic effects of running. Sports Med 9:1–6, 1990.
11. Newhouse IJ, et al: Iron status in athletes: An update. Sports Med 5:337–352, 1988.
12. Newhouse IJ, et al: The effect of prelatent/latent iron deficiency on physical work capacity. Med Sci Sports Exerc 21:263–268, 1989.
13. Nickerson HJ, et al: Decreased iron stores in high school female runners. Am J Dis Child 139:1115–1119, 1985.
14. Nickerson HJ, et al: Causes of iron deficiency in adolescent athletes. J Pediatr 114:657–663, 1989.
15. Risser WL, et al: Iron deficiency in female athletes: Its prevalence and impact on performance. Med Sci Sports Exerc 20:116–121, 1988.
16. Risser WL, Risser JM: Iron deficiency in adolescents and young adults. Phys SportsMed 18:87–101, 1990.
17. Rowland TW, et al: The effect of iron therapy on the exercise capacity of nonanemic iron-deficient adolescent runners. Am J Dis Child 142:165–169, 1988.
18. Rowland TW, et al: Iron deficiency in athletes: Insights from high school swimmers. Am J Dis Child 143:197–200, 1989.
19. Schoene RBP, et al: Iron repletion decreases maximal exercise lactate concentration in female athletes with minimal iron deficiency anemia. J Lab Clin Med 102:306–312, 1983.

Chapter 36: Infections

ELAINE C. JONG, MD

Common infections in active and exercising women can influence confidence, comfort, and optimal performance. In women, some infectious problems are related to gender and anatomy, such as genitourinary tract infections. Other infections are related to minor trauma associated with exercise and physical activities, particularly skin and soft tissue infections. When sports and recreational activities take place outdoors, in special environments, or at foreign sites, these exposures can present a risk for travel-associated or exotic infections, such as diarrhea and parasitic infections. This outline reviews some of the infectious disease concerns for active and exercising women.

I. **URINARY TRACT INFECTION (UTI)**
   A. **Incidence in the U.S.**
      1. 5 million office visits yearly
      2. 20% of antibiotic prescriptions are written for UTI.
   B. **Risk factors**
      1. **Age:** Incidence of UTI increases with age.
      2. **Gender:** Incidence higher in women than men.
         a. **Anatomical factors**
            i. Proximity of urethra to vagina and rectum in female
            ii. Short urethra, urethral stricture
            iii. Relaxation of the perineum with age leads to urine pooling in the bladder.
         b. **Sexual activity**
            i. Introduction of bacteria into female urethra is common during sexual activity.
            ii. Spermicides may increase colonization with gram-negative rods.
         c. **Mechanical obstruction to urinary flow**
            i. Diaphragms
            ii. Pregnancy
            iii. Neurogenic bladder
      3. **Bacterial virulence and adherence factors**
         a. Some strains of uropathogens are more likely to adhere to uroepithelial cells and cause infection than others.
         b. Certain individuals are genetically predisposed to UTI due to the presence of adherence factors on their uroepithelial cells.
   C. **Uropathogens**
      1. *Escherichia coli* accounts for more than 80–90% of UTI.
      2. **Other gram-negative rods:** *Klebsiella pneumoniae, Proteus mirabilis, Proteus vulgaris, Providencia rettgeri, Morganella morganii, Citrobacter* spp., *Serratia marcescens, Acinetobacter* spp., *Pseudomonas aeruginosa, Enterobacter aerogenes, Enterobacter cloacae*
      3. **Gram-positive cocci:** *Streptococcus faecalis* (enterococcus), *Staphylococcus saprophyticus* (common cause of urethral syndrome), *Staphylococcus epidermidis*
   D. **Clinical diagnosis of UTI**
      1. **Cystitis:** Dysuria, cloudy urine, frequency, suprapubic pain, $\geq 10^5$ CFU/mL urine
      2. **Pyelonephritis:** Fever, chills, flank pain, nausea
      3. **Urethral syndrome:** Dysuria, frequency, pyuria, $< 10^5$ CFU/mL

E. **Antimicrobial treatment**
  1. **Cystitis:** Empiric treatment without culture for infrequent occurrence (<3 times a year)
     a. Trimethoprim/sulfamethoxazole (TMP/SMX) double-strength tablets (180/800 mg); one twice daily for 3–5 days
     b. Norfloxacin, 400 mg orally twice daily for 3–5 days
  2. **Acute pyelonephritis in early mild illness,** able to take oral antibiotics, no underlying systemic illness or urinary obstruction: Start one of the following antibiotics, and change if appropriate after results of pending urine culture and sensitivity testing are known:
     a. TMP/SMX double-strength tablet orally twice daily for 14 days
     b. Norfloxacin, 400 mg orally twice daily for 14 days
     c. Ciprofloxacin, 500 mg orally twice daily for 14 days
     d. Ofloxacin, 300 mg orally twice daily for 14 days
  3. **Acute pyelonephritis with systemic toxicity,** underlying systemic illness or urinary obstruction, unable to take medications by mouth: Start one of the following antibiotics, pending results of urine culture and sensitivity testing:
     a. Ampicillin, 2 g intravenously every 6 hr plus gentamicin, 1.0 μg/kg intravenously every 8 hr
     b. TMP/SMX intravenously
     c. Ceftriaxone, 1 g intravenously or intramuscularly every 24 hr
     d. Ciprofloxacin, 400 mg intravenously every 12 hr
     e. Ofloxacin, 300 mg intravenously every 12 hr
     f. Adjust antibiotic therapy as needed after culture and sensitivity testing results are known. Switch to oral therapy when the patient is able to tolerate oral medication. Complete a 14-day course of treatment.
F. **Prevention**
  1. Drink 8 glasses of water a day (stay well-hydrated).
  2. Urinate shortly after sexual intercourse (urine flow will help to rinse out bacteria contaminating the urethra).
  3. Antimicrobial prophylaxis (for sexually active women reporting frequent UTIs temporally related to intercourse):
     a. TMP/SMX double-strength tablet (160/800 mg), orally twice daily for 3 days after intercourse
     b. TMP/SMX double-strength tablet, ½ tablet orally daily
     c. TMP, 100 mg orally daily
     d. Nitrofurantoin, 50–100 mg orally daily

II. **GENITAL INFECTIONS**
  A. **Vaginal discharge**
    1. *Candida albicans*
       a. Predisposing factors: Antibiotic usage, climate, hormones
       b. Diagnosis
          i. Characteristic white discharge, perineal irritation
          ii. Yeast forms and pseudohyphae on microscopic examination of wet mount of vaginal discharge
       c. Treatment
          i. Stop antibiotics if possible
          ii. Nystatin, miconazole, or clotrimazole vaginal cream for 5–7 days; *or*
          iii. Butoconazole (Femstat) vaginal cream for 3 days; *or*
          iv. Fluconazole, 150–200 mg orally single-dose
       d. Prevention
          i. Wear loose well-ventilated clothing
          ii. Daily ingestion of yogurt containing *Lactobacillus acidophilus*

   2. ***Trichomonas vaginalis***
     a. Predisposing factors: Sexual intercourse with infected partner
     b. Diagnosis:
       i. Foul-smelling greenish discharge, perineal irritation
       ii. Trichomonads on microscopic examination of wet mount of vaginal discharge
     c. Treatment: Metronidazole, 500 mg twice daily for 7 days
   3. **Bacterial vaginosis (nonspecific vaginitis)**
     a. Predisposing factors: unknown, possible altered vaginal flora
     b. Diagnosis
       i. Fishy-smelling, gray, watery vaginal discharge
       ii. "Clue cells" on Gram stain
       iii. Culture of vaginal discharge yields *Gardnerella vaginalis* plus anaerobes, including *Mobiluncus.*
     c. Treatment
       i. Metronidazole, 500 mg twice daily for 7 days (90–95% cure rate; single 2-g dose gives lower cure rate; 70–75%)
       ii. Metronidazole, 0.75% vaginal gel, one applicator full in morning and evening for 5 days
       iii. Amoxicillin/clavulanate (Augmentin), 500 mg three times daily for 7 days
       iv. Clindamycin, 300 mg twice daily for 7 days
       v. Clindamycin, 2.0% topical cream, 5 g/day used vaginally for 5–7 days

B. **Genital skin lesions**
   1. **Herpes simplex II**
     a. Predisposing factors: Sexual intercourse with infected partner
     b. Diagnosis
       i. Perineal irritation and neuralgia, sometimes acute urinary retention
       ii. Shallow 2–3 mm ulcerations on the perineum
       iii. Inguinal lymphadenopathy; herpes simplex virus II (HSV II) on culture of ulcer base or cervical secretions
       iv. Serology positive for HSV II 2–3 weeks after primary infection
     c. Antiviral treatment
       i. Acyclovir, 200-mg tablets, one tablet orally 5 times a day for 7 days; *or*
       ii. Acyclovir, 400 mg (2 tablets) 3 times a day for 7 days; *or*
       iii. Hospitalize severely ill patients to give acyclovir, 5 mg/kg intravenously every 8 hr; switch to oral acyclovir when possible; complete 7 days of treatment
     d. Supportive treatment: Sitz baths; antibiotics as needed for secondary infection of skin lesions and UTI; urinary catheterization for urinary retention
     e. Prophylactic treatment: Acyclovir 400 mg (2 tablets) twice daily, is 75–89% effective in decreasing recurrent HSV II attacks during the year following a primary infection.
   2. **Candida:** Perineal irritation with macular erythematous rash (*see* Candida vaginal discharge above)
   3. **Bartholin gland abscess**
     a. Predisposing factors: Sexual intercourse; dehydration; association with *N. gonorrhoeae* infection
     b. Diagnosis: Tender swelling on labia majorum on either side of vaginal vestibule
     c. Treatment: Sitz baths 4–5 times a day until natural drainage occurs; surgical incision and drainage of fluctuant lesions or recurrent lesions; diagnosis and treatment for gonorrhea and other sexually transmitted diseases.
   4. **Condom dermatitis**
     a. Predisposing factors: Sexual intercourse with partner using a latex condom
       i. 1–2% of the population is allergic to latex rubber.
       ii. High-quality latex condoms can have up to a 5% failure rate during use.

    b. Diagnosis: Historical

        i. Vaginal irritation, erythematous skin rash on external genitalia, thighs, lower abdomen, perianal or anal areas following intercourse

        ii. Skin patch-test for latex rubber allergy

        iii. Potential irritants include latex rubber antioxidants (mercaptobenzothiazaole, tetramethyltiuram, zinc dithiocarbamate), lubricants (paraben or silicone), spermicidal jellies

    c. Prevention: Avoid offending material; consider natural gut condoms (*warning:* these provide effective birth control but do not protect against HIV infection), female condom (polyurethane)

C. **Sexually transmitted diseases in women**

Acute infections with *N. gonorrhoeae* in the female may present as a vaginal discharge. However, infections with *N. gonorrhoeae* and *Chlamydia trachomatis* may be asymptomatic in women. The diagnosis of early (mild) pelvic inflammatory disease (PID) is made on the basis of finding lower abdominal tenderness, cervical motion tenderness, and adnexal tenderness on bimanual pelvic examination.

Because PID leads to serious consequences, and since *N. gonorrhoeae* and *C. trachomatis* are implicated most often as causal agents in PID, empiric treatment of women with a history of high-risk exposure to sexually transmitted diseases or with an abnormal pelvic examination is a combination of sequential antimicrobial coverage to cover both pathogens. (Consequences of PID include infertility, ectopic pregnancy, tubo-ovarian abscess, pyosalpinx, chronic pelvic pain, pelvic adhesive disease.)

  1. *Neisseria gonorrhoeae*

    a. Predisposing factors: Sexual intercourse

    b. Diagnosis

        i. History of high-risk contact

        ii. Pelvic examination

        iii. Gram-negative intracellular diplococci on Gram stain

        iv. Culture positive to confirm *N. gonorrhoeae*

    c. Treatment: Presume penicillinase-positive, tetracycline-resistant strains; use one of the following antibiotics:

        i. Ceftriaxone (Rocephin), 250 mg intramuscularly or intravenously

        ii. Cefixime (Suprax), 400 mg orally once

        iii. Ofloxacin (Floxin), 400 mg orally once

        iv. Follow all with a course of antibiotic treatment for chlamydiae.

  2. *Chlamydia trachomatis*

    a. Predisposing factors: Sexual intercourse; possible contact with contaminated wet surfaces

    b. Diagnosis

        i. Infections may be asymptomatic

        ii. Culture cervical secretions for chlamydiae and/or submit for chlamydia immunofluorescent stain

    c. Treatment: Use one of the following antibiotics:

        i. Doxycyline, 100 mg orally twice daily for 7 days

        ii. Erythromycin, 500 mg orally 4 times daily for 7 days

        iii. Erythromycin, 250 mg orally 4 times daily for 14 days

        iv. Ofloxacin (Floxin), 300 mg orally twice daily for 7 days

        v. Azithromycin (Zithromax) 250 mg, 1 g (4 tablets) orally as a single dose (1 hour before or 2 hours after meals)

  3. **Outpatient treatment of PID:** Use one of the following regimens:

    a. Ceftriaxone, 250 mg IM, *plus* Doxycycline 100 mg orally twice daily for 14 days

    b. Ofloxacin, 400 mg orally twice daily for 14 days, *plus* either clindamycin, 450 mg orally 4 times a day, or metronidazole, 500 mg orally twice daily for 14 days

4. **Human immunodeficiency virus (HIV)**
   a. Predisposing factors: Sexual intercourse with high-risk or infected partners; intravenous illicit drug use; blood transfusion; infant of infected mother; accidental needlestick; organ transplantation
   b. Diagnosis
      i. Asymptomatic or an acute infectious mononucleosis-like syndrome may develop after primary infection.
      ii. HIV serology (ELISA test to screen, Western blot test or other supplemental test to confirm)
   c. Treatment: Asymptomatic adults with $300/mm^3$ CD4+ T-cells/μL, and symptomatic adults with <500 CD4+ T-cells/μL, zidovudine 100 mg every 4 hrs (500–600 mg/day) may help to control infection.
   d. Safe sex precautions: Use a high-quality latex condom for sex with all partners.

III. **INFECTIONS IN RUNNERS**
   A. **Athlete's foot (tinea pedis):** Predisposing factors are moisture, minor foot trauma.
      1. Etiology
         a. *Tinea rubrum*
         b. *Tinea mentagrophytes*
      2. Diagnosis
         a. Location: Interdigital spaces of the foot or undersurfaces of lateral aspects of toes
         b. Clinical presentation: Itching, skin maceration, bullae (*T. mentagrophytes*) or erythema and scales (*T. rubrum*)
         c. 10–20% KOH wet mount
      3. Treatment
         a. Foot hygiene
         b. Topical antifungal cream or powder (chlorphenesin, undecylenate, tolnaftate) for 2–4 weeks
   B. **Cellulitis, and blisters and abrasions with secondary infection:** Predisposing factors are minor foot trauma, athlete's foot
      1. Etiology: Streptococci and staphylococci
      2. Diagnosis: Clinical appearance, culture of exudate
      3. Treatment: Wound care and protective covering, plus antibiotic treatment
         a. Dicloxacillin, 500 mg orally every 6 hr for 5–7 days
         b. Cephalexin (Keflex), 500 mg orally every 6 hr for 5–7 days
         c. Ofloxacin, 400 mg orally twice daily for 5–7 days (for persons allergic to dicloxacillin and cephalexin)
   C. **Puncture wound of foot leading to osteomyelitis:** Caused by stepping on a nail while running in rubber-soled shoes
      1. Etiology
         a. *Pseudomonas aeruginosa* living in the inner soles of athletic shoes is inoculated deep into the foot wound
         b. *Pseudomonas maltophilia*
      2. Diagnosis: Mechanism of injury, increasing pain and drainage following puncture wound, radiograph and/or bone scan, culture of bone biopsy specimen
      3. Treatment
         a. Surgical debridement
         b. Ciprofloxacin intravenously followed by oral ciprofloxacin or other antibiotics with activity against *Pseudomonas*

IV. **HIKING AND TREKKING**
   A. **Traveler's diarrhea**
      1. A common ailment among international travelers, especially in developing countries where **food** (storage, preparation, handling), **water** (supply, treatment, storage), and **sanitation** (disposal of human wastes) are suboptimal.

2. Usually a self-limited illness of 3–6 days characterized by frequent movements of watery diarrhea, which may be accompanied by nausea, vomiting, cramping abdominal pain, low-grade fever, and malaise.
3. **Dysentery** implies the presence of blood and mucus in the stool with pain on defecation. This indicates an invasive process and may be caused by bacterial, cytotoxic, or parasitic destruction.
4. **Definition of acute diarrhea:**
    a. Passage of 4 liquid stools in 24 hours
    b. Three stools in 24 hours and fever, abdominal pain, or nausea/vomiting
    c. Greater than 200 mL of stool per day
    d. Duration of less than 2 weeks
    e. Stools assume the contour of the container
5. **Diagnosis:** Acute diarrhea in travelers is usually treated empirically. If symptoms persist or are accompanied by systemic toxicity (fever, moderate to severe abdominal pain) and blood and mucus in stools, formal medical evaluation and culture of a stool specimen are indicated.
6. **Treatment**
    a. **Oral rehydration** using WHO-ORS (Table 1).
    b. **Empiric self-treatment with antibiotics**
        i. Use of one of the antibiotics (trimethoprim/sulfamethoxazole double-strength, norfloxacin 400 mg, ciprofloxacin 500 mg, or ofloxacin 200 or 300 mg) at a treatment dose of one tablet by mouth twice a day for 3–5 days.
        ii. Furazolidone suspension may be useful in treatment of **cholera** in children <8 years old or in people intolerant of the antibiotics listed above (pediatric dose, 1.25 mg/kg orally 4 times daily for 4 days; adult dose, 100 mg orally 4 times daily for 4 days)
    c. **Antiperistaltic medication—loperamide (Imodium)**
        i. Use concomitantly with antibiotic to shorten duration of symptoms (safe for classic watery diarrhea; do not use in presence of grossly bloody diarrhea or high fever).
        ii. Dose is 4 mg for initial dose, and 2 mg for every loose stool, up to a total dose of 8 mg/day.
B. **Giardiasis**
    1. Pathogen: *Giardia lamblia,* commonly acquired from drinking contaminated surface water. After 7–10 day incubation period, explosive onset of watery diarrhea, "sulfur burps," abdominal cramping and distension, foul-smelling intestinal gas.
    2. Diagnosis: Ova and parasite evaluation (up to 3 specimens collected on different days)
        a. Wet mount
        b. Stains
            i. Trichrome
            ii. (Modified acid-fast bacilli to rule out *Cryptosporidium, Cyclospora*)

TABLE 1. WHO—ORS (World Health Organization Oral Rehydration Solution)*

Mix with 1 L of purified water:

Sodium	90 meq/L	Sodium chloride	3.5 g
Potassium	20 meq/L	Potassium chloride	1.5 g
Chloride	80 meq/L		
Base	30 meq/L	Sodium bicarbonate	2.5 g
(bicarbonate, citrate, or lactate)		*or* trisodium citrate	2.9 g
Glucose	20 g/L	Glucose	20 g

* Commercially available as WHO-ORS from the manufacturer: Jianas Brothers, St Louis, MO.

        c. Purged stool specimen

        d. Giardia-specific antigen test on stool specimen

        e. String test to sample proximal jejunal contents

        f. Jejunal aspirate and biopsy

    3. Treatment

        a. Quinacrine (Atabrine), 100 mg orally 3 times daily for 5 days

        b. Metronidazole (Flagyl), 500 mg orally 3 times daily for 5–10 days

        c. Furazolidone (Furoxone), 100 mg 4 times daily for 7–10 days

        d. Metronidazole (Flagyl), 2.5 g as a single oral dose on 3 consecutive days

        e. Tinidazole (Fasigyn, Tinebah), 2.0 g as a single oral dose

C. **Tropical insect bites**

    1. **Myiasis:** Infestation by larvae of flies. Single or multiple erythematous papules; the patient may have "a sense of movement" within each lesion. Dermal myiasis is a variation of cutaneous larva migrans. Botfly myiasis usually invades the skin via another biting insect (mosquito). Tumbu flies lay their eggs on the ground and laundry spread or hung out to dry; the larvae penetrate the skin when the clothing is worn.

        a. Pathogens

            i. **Dermal myiasis:** Central and South America, screw worm fly or black blowfly larvae

            ii. **Furuncular myiasis:** Central and South America, botfly *(Dermatobia hominis)* larvae; Africa, tumbu *(Cordylobia anthropophaga)* larvae

        b. Diagnosis: Clinical appearance; recovery of a larva from a lesion.

        c. Treatment: Excision; occlusive dressings (petrolatum, adhesive bandage, nailpolish, etc.) to smother the larva so it can be expressed from the pore; raw bacon dressing to induce spontaneous exit of the living larva from the pore; antibiotics effective against *Staphylococcus* and *Streptococcus* in lesions with secondary bacterial infection (common occurrence).

        d. Prevention: Protect exposed skin areas from biting insects (protective clothing and insect repellent [Table 2]); iron all clothing in areas of tumbu fly myiasis.

    2. **Tungiasis:** Pruritic erythematous papules, each with a central black punctum; lesions usually occur on the feet or in areas of skin in contact with infested soil or sand.

        a. Pathogen: *Tunga penetrans* flea (Africa, Central and South America)

        b. Diagnosis: Clinical appearance, recovery of flea from lesion

        c. Treatment: Excision; antibiotics for secondary infection

        d. Wear shoes in tropical areas

D. **Lyme disease**

    1. Caused by bite by an *Ixodes* tick followed by development of a rash, **erythema chronicum migrans** (ECM) which appears several days to a month after the bite. Headache, malaise, fever, chills, stiff neck, arthralgia, and myalgia may accompany the rash and persist for several weeks (Stage 1 disease).

    2. Pathogen: *Borrelia burgdorferi* spirochete

    3. Diagnosis: Clinical; serologic tests include indirect immunofluorescence assay (IFA) and ELISA for detection of total immunoglobins or class-specific IgM and IgG.

    4. Treatment

        a. 2 weeks of oral antibiotic therapy following a tick bite in a highly endemic area

        b. Tetracycline or doxycyline for adults, nonpregnant women, and children 8 years of age or older

        c. Penicillin or amoxicillin for pregnant or lactating women and children under 8 years of age

        d. Erythromycin in patients allergic to tetracycline or penicillin; comparative trials under way with cefuroxime versus doxycycline

TABLE 2.   Insect Repellents and Insecticides*

Insect repellents containing deet (*N,N*-diethyl-*m*-toluamide)

Ultrathon insect repellent: 35% deet in polymer formulation, up to 12 hr protection against mosquitoes; also effective against ticks, biting flies, chiggers, fleas, gnats (3M, Minneapolis, MN)

Deet plus insect repellent: 17.5% deet with 2.5% R 326, apply every 4 hours for mosquitoes, every 8 hours for biting flies (Sawyer Products, Safety Harbor, FL)

Skedaddle insect protection for children: 10% deet using molecular entrapment technology (Little Point Corp., Cambridge, MA)

Permethrin-containing insecticides

Permanone tick repellent: Contains permethrin in a pressurized spray can; repels ticks, chiggers, mosquitoes, and other bugs (Coulston International Corp., Easton, PA)

Duranon tick repellent: Contains permethrin in a formula lasting up to 2 weeks; supplied in a pressurized spray can (Coulston International Corp., Easton, PA)

PermaKill 4-week tick killer: 13.3% permethrin liquid concentrate supplied in 8-oz bottle, can be diluted ($^1/_3$ oz permethrin concentrate in 16 oz water) to be used with a pump spray bottle; or diluted 2 oz in 1.5 cups of water to be used to impregnate outer clothing, bednets, and curtains (Coulston International Corp., Easton, PA)

From Jong EC, McMullen R: The Travel and Tropical Medicine Manual, 2nd ed. Philadelphia, W.B. Saunders, 1994.

  e. Treatment of early infection may blunt the subsequent development of a diagnostic serologic response.
 5. Prevention: Avoid tall grass and wooded areas in endemic areas; if outdoor activities are planned, use a deet-containing insect repellent on exposed skin areas, and spray permethrin- containing insecticide on external clothing (Table 2).

V. SWIMMING, WATER SPORTS, AND THE BEACH

 A. **Skin and soft tissue infection with marine microorganisms:** Resulting from abrasions, lacerations and punctures in the marine environment (coral cuts, sea urchin spines, fishhook injuries)
  1. Pathogens
   a. *Pseudomonas* species
   b. *Vibrio vulnificus, V. parahaemolyticus, V. alginolyticus,* and other *Vibrio* species
  2. Diagnosis: Culture of the wound or exudate
  3. Treatment
   a. Remove foreign bodies
   b. Antibiotics
    i. Ciprofloxacin, 500 mg twice daily
    ii. Ofloxacin, 300 mg orally twice daily for 5–7 days
    iii. Tetracycline, 500 mg 4 times daily
    iv. Doxycycline, 100 mg twice daily
    v. Change treatment as appropriate after results of culture and sensitivity testing are known.
 B. **Swimmer's ear (external otitis):** Inflamed, edematous, itching, or painful ear, often with discharge
  1. Risk factors
   a. Wet or humid conditions, especially frequent swimming
   b. Humid tropical or southern climates
   c. Injury to external auditory canal
  2. Pathogens
   a. *Pseudomonas aeruginosa*
   b. *Staphylococcus aureus*

3. Treatment
  a. Topical antibiotic plus corticosteroid otic solution
  b. Drying agents
  c. 2% acetic acid (to reduce growth of *Pseudomonas*)
  d. Antibiotics active against *P. aeruginosa* and *Staphylococcus* for serious cases
C. **Cutaneous larva migrans:** Itching and papules, then serpiginous lesions in the skin, migrating over days to weeks
  1. Etiology: Skin infection with dog or cat hookworm species *(Ancylostoma)*
  2. Diagnosis: Clinical; history of skin contact, especially walking barefoot, on damp soil or sand where dogs and cats have frequented and have deposited contaminated excretment (although physical signs of the wastes may fade, microscopic larvae remain in the ground).
  3. Treatment: Thiabendazole (Mintezol), 50 mg/kg/day in 2 divided oral doses for 2 days (not to exceed 3 g/day)
  4. Avoid walking barefoot and avoid direct skin contact on damp soil or sand in tropical areas.
D. **Schistosomiasis (swimmer's itch, cercarial dermatitis, bilharzia, snail fever):** Itching macular papular rash on skin following immersion in freshwater contaminated with schistosomal cercariae shed by infected snails
  1. Pathogens
    a. Schistosome species of waterfowl in northern temperate climates (swimmer's itch)
    b. Schistosome species of humans *(Schistosoma mansoni, S. haematobium, S. japonicum, S. mekongi)* in areas of the Caribbean, South America, Africa, and Asia
  2. Diagnosis
    a. History of immersion in water in high-risk areas
    b. Ova and parasite examination of stool specimens 6–8 weeks after exposure
    c. Schistosomiasis serum antibody test in chronic cases
  3. Treatment
    a. Swimmer's itch: Topical 1% hydrocortisone cream for skin and/or oral antihistamines (Benadryl, Chlortrimeton, Seldane, etc.) to decrease itching
    b. Schistosomiasis: praziquantel (Biltricide), 20 mg per kg body weight orally 3 times in 1 day
  4. Prevention: Avoid swimming in contaminated freshwater lakes, rivers, and streams. If accidental immersion occurs, towel off skin moisture as quickly as possible; seek expert medical advice if immersion occurred in high-risk areas of Africa, Asia, or South America, where schistosome species pathogenic to humans are endemic.
E. **Erysipelothrix (seal finger, whale finger):** The most common form of this infection is a local skin lesion, usually on the fingers. It commonly appears as a slowly progressive indurated papular lesion that spreads proximally, accompanied by pain and inflammation in the joints in the pathway of regional lymphatic drainage from the infected site. The lesions do not drain. These characteristics usually differentiate it from pyogenic infections (cellulitis) due to streptococci or staphylococci. The *Erysipelothrix* bacteria causing this infection are found in a variety of animals, including swine, sheep, and fish.
  1. Pathogen: *Erysipelothrix rhusiopathiae* (gram-positive rod)
  2. Diagnosis: History of contact with fish, raw seafood, or meat
  3. Treatment
    a. The localized lesions usually resolve spontaneously over 3 weeks.
    b. About 10% of reported cases in the preantibiotic era were septicemia associated with endocarditis.

   c. Intravenous penicillin (12–20 million units/day in divided doses) or cephalosporins in usual therapeutic doses are recommended for treatment of systemic infections.
F. **"Hot tub" folliculitis**
   1. Etiology:*Pseudomonas aeruginosa* contaminating hot tubs, whirlpools, swimming pools
   2. Clinical presentation: a folliculitis involving submerged areas of skin, with especial involvement of buttocks, hips, and axillae; the lesions are erythematous, papular, and pruritic; occasionally develop into pustules within 48 hours; and resolve spontaneously in 5 days.
   3. Drainage is sometimes indicated for furuncles.
   4. Prevention: Disinfection of hot tub by hyperchlorination; scrupulous maintenance of appropriate chlorine levels during daily use

REFERENCES

1. Baltimore RS, Jenson HB: Puncture wound osteochondritis of the foot caused by *Pseudomonas maltophilia.* Pediatr Infect Dis J 9:143–144, 1990.
2. Centers for Disease Control: Cercarial dermatitis outbreak at a state park—Delaware, 1991. MMWR 40:225–228, 1992.
2a. Centers for Disease Control: 1993 Sexually Transmitted Diseases Treatment Guidelines. MMWR 42(RR-14):1–102, 1993.
3. DuPont HL, Ericsson CD, Mathewson JJ, et al: Five versus three days of ofloxacin therapy for traveler's diarrhea: A placebo-controlled study. Antimicrob Agents Chemother 36:87–91, 1992.
4. Ericsson C, DuPont HL, Mathewson JJ, et al: Treatment of traveler's diarrhea with sulfamethoxazole and trimethoprim and loperamide. JAMA 263:257–261, 1990.
5. Ericsson CD, DuPont HL: Traveler's diarrhea: Approaches to prevention and treatment. Clinical Infectious Diseases 16:616–626, 1993.
6. Hilton E, Isenberg HD, Alperstein P, et al: Ingestion of yogurt containing *Lactobacillus acidophilus* as prophylaxis for candidal vaginitis. Ann Intern Med 116:353–357, 1992.
7. Hooten TM, Hillier S, Johnson C, et al: *Escherichia coli* bactiuria and contraceptive method. JAMA 265:64–69, 1991.
8. Kahn JG, Walker CK, Washington AE, et al: Diagnosing pelvic inflammatory disease: A comprehensive analysis and considerations for developing a new model. JAMA 266:2594–2604, 1991.
9. Kirby P: Ectoparasites, cutaneous parasites, and coelenterate envenomation. In Jong EC (ed): The Travel and Tropical Medicine Manual. Philadelphia, W.B. Saunders, 1987, pp 190–200.
10. Livengood CH III, Thomason JL, Hill GB: Bacterial vaginosis: Treatment with topical intravaginal clindamycin phosphate. Obstet Gynecol 76:118–123, 1990.
11. Lugo-Miro V, Green M, Mazur L: Comparison of different metronidazole therapeutic regimens for bacterial vaginosis: A meta-analysis. JAMA 268:92–95, 1992.
12. Peterson HB, Walker CK, Kahn JG: Pelvic inflammatory disease: Key treatment issues and options. JAMA 266:2605–2611, 1991.
13. Rose S: Giardiasis: Epidemiology, diagnosis and treatment. Intern Med 12:47–54, 1991.
14. Schaaf VM, Perez-Stable EJ, Borchardt K: The limited value of symptoms and signs in the diagnosis of vaginal infections. Arch Intern Med 150:1929–1933, 1990.
15. Stapleton A, Latham RH, Johnson C, Stamm WE: Postcoital antimicrobial prophylaxis for recurrent urinary tract infection: A randomized, double-blind, placebo-controlled trial. JAMA 264:703–706, 1990.
16. Taylor DN, Sanchez JL, Candler W, et al: Treatment of traveler's diarrhea: Ciprofloxacin plus loperamide compared with ciprofloxacin alone. Ann Intern Med 114:731–734, 1991.
17. Volberding PA, Lagokos SW, Koch MA: Zidovudine in asymptomatic human immunodeficiency virus infection: A controlled trial in persons with fewer than 500 CD4-positive cells per cubic millimeter. N Engl J Med 322:941–949, 1990.

Chapter 37: Radiographic Evaluation of Sports-related Injuries

MARIE E. LEE, MD

The radiologic evaluation of sports-related trauma relies initially on standard as well as optimal radiographic projections. Certain injuries are more fully evaluated with tomography, fluoroscopy, arthrography, ultrasound, computed tomography (CT), magnetic resonance imaging (MRI), or nuclear scintigraphy.

The clinical history is critical for tailoring the radiologic examination. Certain injuries, such as femoral shaft fractures, have an association with other injuries, in this case dislocation of the hip. Fractures of the pelvis, tibial plateau, ankle, and sternoclavicular joint are often difficult to define on routine radiographs, and CT may be indicated early in evaluation of these fractures if there is strong clinical indication of injury. Routine radiographs are inadequate for evaluation of tendons, ligaments, or bursa; arthrography, CT, or MRI may be indicated if clinical suspicion for soft-tissue injury is high. Coordination of radiologic examinations with the clinician will optimize diagnosis of bone and soft-tissue injuries by maximizing sensitivity and specificity of the radiologic tests ordered and minimizing cost.

I. **UPPER EXTREMITY**

  A. **Shoulder**

    1. Initial views are the standard anteroposterior (AP) view and views that are perpendicular to the glenohumeral joint.

    2. Lateral views of the shoulder include the scapular Y-view, transthoracic lateral view, and axillary view.

  B. **Humeral fractures**

    1. Fractures of the proximal humerus are classified by the number of fragments and degree of displacement or angular deformity.

      a. Fractures may involve one or more anatomic segments, including the humeral head, greater tuberosity, lesser tuberosity, and shaft.

      b. A fragment is considered displaced if there is at least 1 cm of separation or 45° angulation.

    2. Usually, conventional radiographs demonstrate complex fractures, but occasionally displacement and rotation of fragments is better appreciated on CT. Axial images on CT clearly reveal displacement or angulation of fracture fragments and the status of the articular surface of the humeral head.

  C. **Clavicle**

    1. Fractures of the clavicle involve the middle third in 80% and the distal third in 15%.

    2. Middle clavicular fractures are commonly displaced as the sternocleidomastoid elevates the middle third and the arm depresses the distal third.

    3. Fractures of the distal third of the clavicle may be associated with intact ligaments, disruption of the coracoid ligament, or fracture at the base of the coracoid process.

    4. The distal clavicle may undergo focal osteolysis following acute injury to the shoulder or after repetitive stress with weight-lifting.

  D. **Sternoclavicular joint**

    1. Dislocation and dislocation-fracture of the sternoclavicular joint are commonly overlooked. Most occur from an indirect blow to the sternoclavicular joint in a motor vehicle accident or football injury.

2. Posterior dislocations of the sternoclavicular joint are the most serious and may involve the great vessels, trachea, or esophagus.
3. CT is the best way to evaluate the sternoclavicular joint.

E. **Acromioclavicular joint separation**
1. Separation is classified into 3 grades:
   a. Grade I separation is a ligamentous sprain, and radiographs are negative.
   b. Grade II separation involves rupture of the joint capsule and the acromioclavicular joint space is wide.
   c. Grade III separation occurs when the coracoclavicular ligament is torn and there is an increase in the coracoclavicular distance.
2. Criteria for an increased coracoclavicular distance are values >1.3 cm or 50% asymmetry between the two sides.
3. If the AP view does not show a Grade III separation, then stress views with 10-lb weights may be necessary to define the injury.

F. **Glenohumeral joint**
1. The glenohumeral joint is prone to a high frequency of injury due to a large range of motion.
2. Dislocations of the glenohumeral joint are 95% anterior and 5% posterior.
3. With **anterior dislocation,** a fracture of the posterolateral humeral head may occur as it impacts the anterior rim of the glenoid (Hill-Sachs) or a fracture of the glenoid or glenoid labrum may occur (Bankart lesion).
4. Less than 5% of glenohumeral dislocations are **posterior,** and associated injuries include fracture of the humeral head or posterior glenoid or fracture of the lesser tuberosity of the humerus.
   a. The findings of posterior glenohumeral dislocation on the AP view of the shoulder may be subtle and the scapular Y-view or limited axillary view is most helpful for diagnosis.
5. Damage to the soft-tissue supporting structures of the shoulder, fractures of the humeral head or glenoid, and intra-articular fragments may contribute to an **unstable shoulder.**
   a. There are three types of shoulder instability:
      i. Recurrent dislocation
      ii. Recurrent subluxation
      iii. Functional instability
   b. Double-contrast computed arthrotomography is helpful to evaluate shoulder instability. After the injection of contrast, one should obtain tomograms and CT.
   c. Labral lesions may be detected in up to 90% of patients with shoulder instability.
   d. MRI may also be helpful in the evaluation of shoulder instability. The glenoid labrum is low signal and can be evaluated in axial and coronal planes. A torn labrum on MRI may appear irregular and attenuated and may contain focal or scattered areas of increased signal intensity.

G. **Tendon injury**
1. **Rotator cuff tear**
   a. In rotator cuff injuries, plain films are often negative.
   b. A chronic tear can be associated with secondary radiographic changes including superior displacement of the humeral head with an acromiohumeral interval of 7 mm or less, concave inferior acromial margin, and bony proliferation, sclerosis, or subcortical cysts at the greater tuberosity.
   c. The diagnosis of rotator cuff tear is usually made by arthrography which shows contrast in the subacromial bursa.
   d. Ultrasound evaluation, CT arthrography, or MRI may enhance delineation of rotator cuff tear.

2. **Tendon impingement**
   a. The impingement syndrome with entrapment of the rotator cuff, biceps tendon, and subacromial bursa between the humeral tuberosity and the anterior coraco-acromial region is often secondary to a low-lying acromion or acromial spur.
   b. Radiographs may show a subacromial spur, proliferative and cystic changes at the greater and lesser tuberosity, or acromioclavicular joint degeneration.

H. **Elbow**
   1. **Fractures**
      a. Routine radiographic views of the elbow include AP in extension and lateral with 90° flexion.
      b. The anterior and posterior fat pads are intracapsular and extrasynovial structures that are displaced by fluid or hemarthrosis. Displacement of these fat pads is a valuable clue for intra-articular bone injury (commonly radial head fracture).
      c. In evaluating for elbow fractures, there are two useful tools—the anterior humeral line and the radiocapitellar line.
      d. Incomplete or minimally displaced supracondylar fractures may be difficult to diagnose. A fracture with abnormal alignment is confirmed when, on a true lateral view, a line drawn tangent to the anterior humeral cortex is ventral to or intersects the anterior third of the capitellum.
      e. Avulsion of the medial epicondyle is usually limited to children and adolescents. It is produced by a fall on the outstretched hand or a violent contraction of the flexor pronator muscle group in the act of throwing.
      f. The most common elbow injury in an adult is fracture of the radial head or neck. The fracture is often nondisplaced and difficult to visualize on routine views, although alterations of the anterior and posterior fat pads are typically present.
      g. Osteochondral fractures and associated intra-articular fracture fragments are best seen with CT, CT arthrography, or MRI.
   2. **Dislocations**
      a. Elbow dislocations are usually seen on plain radiographs. The radius and ulna are displaced posterior or posterior-lateral in 90%.
      b. With dislocation of the elbow, there is a high frequency of associated fractures most commonly involving the medial condyle or epicondyle, radial head, and coronoid process. Associated fractures are often better seen on post-reduction views.
      c. Isolated dislocation of the radial head is generally seen in association with a fracture of the proximal or middle third of the ulna (Monteggia's lesion). It should be sought in any patient with an angulated or displaced fracture of the ulna.

II. **WRIST AND HAND**

A. **Wrist**
   1. The standard radiographic views of the wrist are posteroanterior (PA), lateral, and external oblique.
   2. Centering of the x-ray beam on the wrist is critical.
   3. Evaluation of the soft tissues is important as soft-tissue swelling or bowing or obliteration of fat lines may be the only clue that a subtle fracture is present and additional views are needed.
   4. In the normal wrist, a PA view shows three parallel curvilinear arcs:
      a. The first arc traces the proximal articular surface of the scaphoid, lunate, and triquetrum.
      b. The second arc follows the distal articular surfaces of these bones.
      c. The third arc is drawn along the proximal articular surfaces of the hamate and capitate.

5. Disruption of any of these areas signifies dislocation, subluxation, or ligamentous injury.
6. On a true lateral view, the relationship between the radius, carpus, and metacarpals and the alignment of the scaphoid, lunate, and capitate may be determined. The scapholunate angle, formed by the axes of the scaphoid and lunate, normally measures 30–60°. Additional radiographic views and fluoroscopy may help in evaluating wrist alignment.
7. The most common fracture in the wrist involves the distal radius and ulna.
   a. A fracture of the distal radius may occur with dorsal (Colles') or volar (Smith) angulation or displacement.
   b. Subluxation or dislocation of the distal radioulnar joint may occur in association with a distal radial fracture or as an isolated injury.
8. Conventional radiography is limited in evaluating this joint because as little as 10° supination or pronation away from a true lateral projection may mask a subluxation or dislocation.
9. Alignment of the distal radioulnar joint is best evaluated by CT.

B. **Carpal fractures**
   1. The **scaphoid** is the most commonly fractured carpal bone.
      a. A scaphoid series consists of PA, lateral, and external oblique views and a PA view with ulnar deviation.
      b. Nondisplaced fractures may be difficult to detect and usually become apparent 7–10 days later.
      c. Because the principal arterial supply enters at the waist of the scaphoid, the risk for ischemic necrosis and nonunion increases the more proximal the fracture line.
   2. The **triquetrum** is the second most commonly injured carpal bone; the injury is most often a dorsal avulsion fracture.
      a. The triquetral fracture is often only visualized on the lateral view and may be suspected when there is dorsal soft-tissue swelling or a bone fragment at the dorsal-level, proximal carpal row.
   3. **Lunate** fractures are relatively uncommon; pain in the lunate bone should raise the possibility of avascular necrosis of the lunate bone.
   4. A fracture of the body of the **hamate** may occur as an isolated injury or as part of a perilunate-fracture-dislocation.
      a. A fracture of the hook of the hamate often occurs secondary to sports such as golf, racquetball, or baseball.
      b. CT may be helpful in evaluating subtle carpal fractures.
   5. Fractures of the **capitate** usually occur with a fracture of the scaphoid or with perilunate dislocation.

C. **Carpal dislocation and fracture-dislocation**
   1. The classic mechanism of action for fracture-dislocation of the carpus is a fall on the outstretched hand.
   2. Lesser arc injuries are pure dislocations.
   3. Greater arc injuries are fractures or fracture dislocations.
   4. In both injuries, a sequential pattern of fracture or ligament disruption begins at the scaphoid or scapholunate joint and progresses clockwise around the lunate.
   5. Carpal instability increases with each successive stage.
   6. Scapholunate dissociation causes an increase in the scapholunate space by 2–3 mm.
   7. There are five major patterns of carpal instability: dorsal, volar, or ulnar subluxation of the carpus, and dorsiflexion or volarflexion instability.
   8. The two most common carpal instability patterns are dorsiflexion and volarflexion instability.
   9. The radiographic evaluation of a patient with wrist instability begins with an "instability" series, which consists of multiple views in various positions including radial and ulnar deviation, flexion, and extension.

10. A dynamic evaluation under **fluoroscopy** may be the best way to demonstrate certain types of carpal instability.
   a. If a fluoroscopic examination is normal, arthrography may be indicated.
   b. Tears of the interosseous ligaments or triangular fibrocartilage complex are indicated by abnormal intercompartmental communication.
   c. A midcarpal contrast injection is recommended to demonstrate communication between the radiocarpal and midcarpal compartments.
   d. A tear of the triangular cartilage is diagnosed when contrast extends from the radiocarpal joint into the distal radioulnar joint.
11. MRI can show carpal tunnel pathology, post-traumatic ischemic necrosis, and tears of tendons, ligaments, and the triangular fibrocartilage.

D. **Hand**
1. Routine radiographic evaluation of the hand is accomplished with PA, lateral, and oblique views. Radiographs of individual fingers or the thumb and stress views may be helpful.
2. An injury that is often overlooked is dislocation at the carpometacarpal joints.
   a. On a PA view, the carpometacarpal joint spaces should be of uniform width, usually 1–2 mm, and the articular surfaces should be parallel.
   b. With subluxation or dislocation, the articular surfaces overlap.
   c. Oblique or lateral views may be useful to detect soft-tissue swelling and fracture and to determine the direction of dislocation.
3. In the hand, **stress views** are most helpful to rule out ligamentous injury about the first metacarpophalangeal joint.
   a. A collateral ligament injury is often misdiagnosed as a simple sprain, leading to chronic instability and pain.
   b. Routine radiographs are often negative because nearly half of all ligament tears are unaccompanied by fracture.
4. Trauma to the hand may result in a **foreign body** being lodged in the soft tissues.
   a. The most common foreign bodies are pieces of wood, glass, or metal. Metal and glass are almost always visualized on standard radiographs; wood is seen only 15% of the time.
   b. Ultrasound is helpful for detecting nonradiopaque foreign bodies and for preoperative localization of foreign bodies.
   c. CT and MRI may be useful, but are expensive.

III. **LOWER EXTREMITIES**

Adequate evaluation of the skeleton requires a well-performed radiographic examination in two projections that include the articulations proximal and distal to the site of injury. Appropriate interpretation requires a thorough knowledge of common injury problems. Certain activities predispose to predictable injury patterns, and specific skeletal injuries have recognized complications.

A. **Hip dislocation**
1. Dislocation of the femoral head with or without associated acetabular or femoral head fractures occurs from high-energy trauma.
2. Hip dislocations are classified as anterior, posterior, or central depending on the relationship of the femoral head to the acetabulum.
3. **Posterior hip dislocation** is the most common and occurs in 80–85% of cases.
   a. Persistent widening of the joint following reduction suggests osseous or cartilaginous fragments in the joint. CT may be helpful to evaluate these fragments.
   b. Complications of posterior dislocation include secondary degenerative disease, periarticular calcification, or avascular necrosis.
4. **Anterior dislocation** of the hip accounts for 10–15% of dislocations and results from direct or indirect abduction forces. The femoral head may be displaced inferomedial or anterosuperior.

B. **Patellar fractures**
1. Fractures of the patella result from direct trauma or indirect forces from quadriceps contraction.
2. Direct forces may result in comminuted, stellate, or vertical fractures.
3. Indirect forces from the quadriceps may result in transverse or oblique patellar fractures.
4. Injuries to the extensor mechanism, including quadriceps tendon rupture, patellar fracture, patellar tendon rupture, and tibial tubercle avulsion, result from sudden severe quadriceps contraction with knee flexion in weight-bearing.

C. **Patellar dislocation**
1. Acute traumatic dislocation of the patella most commonly occurs in the lateral direction. Lateral dislocation may result from a direct blow or an abrupt change in direction while running.
   a. Powerful quadriceps contraction, a valgus knee force, and external rotation of the leg can drive the patella from the groove.
   b. Dislocation is usually transient.
2. Chondral and osteochondral fractures of the medial facet of the patella or lateral femoral condyle frequently coexist. These injuries result from shearing or impaction forces during dislocation as the patella is driven into the lateral femoral condyle.
   a. Because chondral fractures do not involve the underlying bone, radiographs may show only a joint effusion and arthrography may be necessary.
   b. A caveat is that lipohemarthrosis equals intra-articular fracture.

D. **Recurrent patellar subluxation**
1. The normal relationship between the axis of the quadriceps muscle and the ligamentum patella predisposes to lateral patellar displacement.
2. Similarly, a developmentally deficient lateral femoral condyle, shallow patellofemoral groove, laterally located ligamentum patella, genu valgum, or patella alta may predispose to recurrent dislocation or subluxation. The patient complains of the knee giving out or locking and the findings are confused with a medial meniscal injury.
3. The radiographic examination requires an axial projection in limited flexion (30°) in addition to standard AP and lateral views.

E. **Knee dislocation**
1. Fractures of the patella result from direct or indirect forces from quadriceps contraction.
2. Direct forces may result in a comminuted, stellate, or vertical fracture.
3. Indirect forces from quadriceps may result in transverse or oblique patellar fractures.

F. **Tibial plateau fracture**
1. Tibial plateau fractures occur most commonly in middle-aged patients. They can result from vertical compression, varus or valgus force, or twisting.
2. 80% of tibial plateau fractures involve the lateral tibial plateau. These fractures are often difficult to define and lipohemarthrosis may be the only clue.
3. Coexisting injuries of the medial collateral ligament, anterior cruciate ligament, or lateral collateral ligament are often present.
4. Stress radiography, arthrography, or MRI may be needed to identify injuries to ligamentous structures.

G. **Tibial spine fractures**
1. Fractures of the tibial spine or intercondylar eminence result from avulsion forces at the site of origin of the anterior or posterior cruciates or, rarely, direct impaction of the femoral condyle.
2. Fractures of the anterior tibial spine are most common in children who have a violent hyperextension twisting injury to the knee. A history of a fall from a bicycle is frequently found.

3. In children, this injury is usually isolated, and in adults it may represent a more extensive injury.

4. Tunnel views may help to show avulsion injuries of the anterior or posterior tibial spines.

H. **Proximal fibular fractures**

1. Fractures in this region are uncommon and usually occur in combination with ligamentous injuries of the knee or ankle.

2. Fibular head fractures may result from direct blow, valgus forces, or varus stresses.

I. **Proximal tibiofibular joint dislocation**

1. Dislocation of the proximal tibiofibular joint is uncommon and may result from parachuting, hang-gliding, or horseback riding.

2. **Anterolateral dislocation** occurs from a forced inversion of the ankle with the knee flexed.

3. **Posteromedial dislocations** are often the result of a direct blow and may be associated with peroneal nerve injury.

4. **Superior dislocation** occurs in association with distal tibial fractures.

J. **Tibial and fibular shaft fractures**

1. The tibia is frequently injured in the middle and distal thirds. The degree of comminution and fracture displacement varies with the severity and type of causative force.

2. A compartment syndrome in the leg may result from edema and hemorrhage within the anterior, lateral, or posterior compartments.

3. Radiographic examination should include the entire length of the tibia and fibula on one film to detect fractures remote from the injury site and to enable assessment of rotational deformity.

K. **Stress fractures**

1. Stress fractures have been categorized into two types:

   a. A fatigue fracture resulting from the application of abnormal stress to a bone with normal elastic resistance

   b. An insufficiency fracture occurring when normal stress is placed on a bone with deficient elastic resistance

2. Characteristic locations of fatigue fracture are femoral neck, proximal tibial shaft, mid-shaft of the tibia, and distal fibular shaft in runners, and proximal fibular shaft in individuals in jumping activities.

3. Radiographic findings may lag 2–6 weeks behind the onset of symptoms, and bone scintigraphy may provide early diagnosis of these lesions.

IV. **FOOT AND ANKLE**

A. **Ankle fractures**

1. The major types of injury can be directly related to the patterns of motion of the joint at the time of injury.

2. **Supination–external rotation:** External rotation is the most common injury pattern, resulting in 60% of all ankle injuries.

   a. Initially, rupture of the anteroinferior talofibular ligament results, although alternatively, an avulsion fracture from the anterior tibial tubercle or, rarely, anterior tip of the lateral malleolus may occur.

   b. With further external rotation, the angular forces from the talus against the fibula produce a short oblique spiral fibular fracture.

   c. This may then be followed by an avulsion fracture of the posterior lip of the tibia, fracture of the posterior malleolus, or rupture of the posteroinferior tibiofibular ligament.

   d. Finally, with extreme external rotation, the deltoid ligament becomes stressed with a transverse fracture of the medial malleolus and deltoid ligament rupture.

3. **Supination-adduction:** Approximately 20% of ankle fractures fall into the supination-adduction pattern. With adduction, rupture of the lateral collateral ligaments or a

transverse avulsion fracture of the lateral malleolus results. Further adduction generates a characteristic oblique or nearly vertical fracture of the medial malleolus.

4. **Pronation–external rotation:** External rotation injuries and pronation-abduction injuries include about 20% of ankle fractures.

    a. In pronation-external rotation, one may see a transverse fracture; if more severe injury occurs, a short spiral fracture of the fibula may occur.

    b. Pronation-abduction injuries may mimic the pronation-external rotation injury radiographically.

    c. Pronation-dorsiflexion fractures are rare (<0.5%). They result from axial loading injuries, as a fall from a height.

    d. Initially, a transverse fracture of the medial malleolus is produced.

    e. Other fractures that may occur include fracture of the anterior lip of the tibia, supramalleolar fracture of the fibular shaft, and a transverse fracture of the tibia posteriorly.

B. **Achilles tendon rupture**

1. Rupture of the Achilles tendon usually occurs during exertion with severe contraction of the plantar flexors on the weight-bearing foot.

2. Clinical features usually allow diagnosis. Radiographic examination is performed to rule out associated osseous injury.

3. Lateral radiographs show widening of the tendon, ill-definition of the tendinous margins, and partial or complete obliteration of the pre-Achilles fat pad due to associated hemorrhage.

C. **Fractures and dislocations of the talus**

1. The talus is the second largest tarsal bone (after the calcaneus) and is a vital component of complex ankle motion and axial weight-bearing. It is a frequent site of injury, second only to the calcaneus.

2. Avulsion fractures are the most commonly encountered of talar injuries, generally resulting from combinations of rotational forces with flexion and extension.

    a. Oblique or vertical fractures of the talar neck or body, occurring in the coronal plane, are the next most common fractures of the talus.

    b. Ischemic necrosis of the talus, delayed union or non-union, and secondary degenerative disease of the talar articulations may be complications of these fractures.

    c. Osteochondral fractures of the talar dome are thought to be traumatic in origin, and typical sites include the middle third of the lateral margin or posterior third of the medial margin of the talar dome.

    d. Routine radiography is generally adequate to detect this injury, and evaluation should include AP, lateral, and internal and external oblique views. In some instances, tomography or CT may be required to fully define the injury.

D. **Fractures of the calcaneus**

1. The most frequently injured tarsal bone is the calcaneus.

2. Compressive fractures, generally intra-articular with involvement of the subtalar joint, constitute 75% of calcaneal fractures.

3. They result from axial loading as occurs in a vertical fall.

4. Conventional tomography or CT may be useful in defining the nature of joint involvement and the fractures fragments.

5. Extra-articular fractures constitute 25% of calcaneal fractures and typically are avulsion injuries resulting from twisting injuries. Axial and oblique views are helpful for detection of these fractures.

REFERENCES

1. Dalinka M (ed): Radiographic imaging in orthopedics. Orthop Clin North Am 21(3): 405–624, 1990.
2. Kerr R: Diagnostic imaging of upper extremity trauma. Radiol Clin North Am 27:891–909, 1989.
3. Mitchell M, Ho C, Resnick D, Sartoris D: Diagnostic imaging of lower extremity trauma. Radiol Clin North Am 27:909–929, 1989.

Chapter 38: Upper Extremity Injuries

JO A. HANNAFIN, MD, PhD

The active or athletic woman involved in sports that require the use of the upper extremity may develop traumatic or overuse injuries of the shoulder and forearm. Historically, overuse injuries in the upper and lower extremities were more common in female athletes than their male counterparts. However, with the addition of strength training to upper extremity conditioning programs, the incidence and type of upper extremity injuries sustained by the female athlete are no different than those described for male athletes. The diagnosis and treatment of traumatic and overuse injuries sustained by athletes are described in the following sections.

I. SHOULDER

In evaluation of the active or athletic woman with shoulder pain, a variety of diagnoses must be entertained, including occult cervical spine disease and injuries to the glenohumeral joint, acromioclavicular joint, and scapulothoracic articulation. These injuries may result from repetitive application of intrinsic forces (overuse) or acute application of an extrinsic force (trauma) to the shoulder.

A. **Differential diagnosis of shoulder pain**
   1. Cervical radiculopathy
   2. Clavicular osteolysis
   3. Instability
   4. Primary and secondary impingement
   5. Adhesive capsulitis
   6. Muscle-tendon strain
   7. Suprascapular neuropathy
   8. Fractures
   9. Epiphyseal injuries (in the adolescent athlete)

B. **Shoulder anatomy and biomechanics**
   1. **Ligamentous and muscular anatomy:** The glenohumeral ligament complex provides static restraints to anterior, posterior, and inferior motion of the humeral head on the glenoid. The rotator cuff musculature provides a joint compressive force and functions as a humeral head depressor, preventing superior migration of the humeral head during glenohumeral abduction.[12] These active and static systems attempt to center the humeral head on the glenoid during overhead motion. Injury to either part of this complex may result in transfer of higher forces to the other, with ultimate overload and failure.
   2. **Biomechanics:** Overhead motion, as seen in throwing or serving in tennis, can be broken down into three phases:
      a. **Cocking or windup phase:** The shoulder is positioned in abduction and external rotation by the actions of the deltoid and posterior rotator cuff, while the subscapularis and pectoralis major provide an anterior stabilizing force through eccentric contraction.[12] Cocking results in an anteriorly directed force on the capsule which may be symptomatic in the unstable shoulder. Superior migration of the humeral head may also be seen with resultant impingement.
      b. **Acceleration phase:** During this phase, there is an abrupt reversal of motion. The trunk precedes the body as the arm is maintained in abduction. The subscapularis and pectoralis major are active, resulting in an internal rotation

moment, while the posterior rotator cuff contracts eccentrically to stabilize the humeral head.[12] Stress is focused on the anterior capsule and labrum.

c. **Follow-through:** During this phase, the entire rotator cuff is active. The subscapularis continues internal rotation of the humerus, while eccentric contraction of the posterior cuff and biceps aids in deceleration of the humeral head.[12] Stresses are localized to the capsule, biceps tendon, and anterosuperior labrum secondary to traction during follow-through.

3. **Physical examination**
   a. **Inspection and palpation:** Allows evaluation of the presence of muscular atrophy, asymmetry of scapulothoracic motion, or bony deformity.
      i. Asymmetry of the supraspinatus, infraspinatus and biceps may reflect chronic rotator cuff pathology in the older athlete.
      ii. Isolated infraspinatus atrophy may reflect an injury to the suprascapular nerve.
      iii. Asymmetry or instability of the acromioclavicular joint
   b. **Range of motion:** Evaluation of active and passive range of motion combined with manual motor testing is critical.
      i. Adhesive capsulitis: Early loss of internal rotation, followed by a loss of motion in all planes.
      ii. Discrepancy between active and passive motion or asymmetry of scapulothoracic motion suggests rotator cuff dysfunction.
      iii. Apprehension and loss of external rotation in 90° of abduction is often seen in patients with anterior instability.
   c. **Impingement sign:** May be elicited with forceful abduction of the internally rotated arm against the undersurface of the acromion.
      i. The impingement test as described by Neer[15] may help confirm a diagnosis of impingement but is a nonspecific test.
      ii. Assessment of glenohumeral stability is critical in differentiating primary vs secondary impingement.
   d. **Stability examination:** Estimation of anterior, posterior, and inferior glenohumeral translation in the standing and supine position is important in evaluation of instability.
      i. Must examine the contralateral extremity to assess baseline laxity.
      ii. **Sulcus sign:** Demonstration of inferior translation of the humeral head by application of downward traction on the humerus. Demonstration of a sulcus between the top of the humeral head and the acromion is indicative of capsular laxity.
      iii. **Supine stress test:** Most useful test for glenohumeral instability. Anterior, posterior, and inferior stress is applied to the proximal humerus in neutral rotation and translation of the head on the glenoid is measured (Fig. 1). Anterior or posterior translation of up to 50% is considered normal.
      iv. **Relocation test:** Highly sensitive and specific when evaluated for apprehension; significantly less sensitive when evaluated for pain.
   e. **Evaluation of cervical spine** for degenerative or radicular symptoms is also warranted.
C. **Glenohumeral instability:** Instability of the glenohumeral joint is defined as pathologic laxity that produces symptoms and may result from application of a high extrinsic force in an isolated setting (trauma) or from excessive or repetitive intrinsic force (overuse) resulting in soft tissue laxity.
   1. **Traumatic dislocation**
      a. **Anterior dislocation:** Generally results from forceful abduction and external rotation as a result of a collision or fall.
         i. **Radiographic evaluation** should be performed prior to reduction maneuvers to rule out an associated fracture of the humeral head or neck.

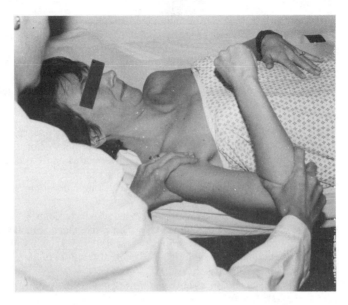

FIGURE 1.   Supine stress test for shoulder instability.

ii. **Treatment:** Reduction under intravenous sedation followed by sling immobilization. Acute operative stabilization has recently been advocated for the elite athlete involved in contact sports because of a significant rate of recurrence.

iii. Evaluation of **axillary nerve function** prior to and following closed reduction.

iv. **Recurrent dislocations** warrant operative intervention for arthroscopic or open anterior stabilization.

b. **Posterior dislocation:** Significantly less common than anterior dislocation of the shoulder. This injury can be seen following a fall on an outstretched adducted arm. Posterior dislocations can also occur as a result of a generalized seizure and are frequently missed in this population.

i. **Radiographic evaluation** is warranted prior to reduction.

ii. **Postreduction immobilization** in neutral glenohumeral rotation.

iii. **Recurrent dislocation** warrants operative open posterior stabilization only after failure of conservative treatment (physical therapy).

2. **Recurrent subluxation:** The most common form of instability related to repetitive intrinsic force.[24]

a. Athletes may complain of **pain in the deceleration phase of sports activity.** This complaint may become more pronounced with rotator cuff fatigue.

b. **Inflammation or degeneration of the rotator cuff may follow** as the rotator cuff attempts to actively resist the anterior or posterior displacement of the humeral head during activity.

c. **Diagnosis** of recurrent subluxation is complex and relies extensively on the history and documentation of the arm position that provokes symptoms.

i. **Anterior instability:** Pain or a sense of abnormal joint movement with arm abduction and external rotation.[18]

ii. **Posterior instability:** Pain with shoulder flexion and adduction in the follow-through phase.[7]

d. **Instability may progress to frank dislocation with activities or during sleep.**

e. **Radiologic evaluation**

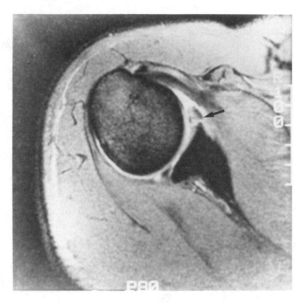

FIGURE 2. Axial MRI of the shoulder demonstrating a complex tear of the anterior labrum (*arrow*).

      i. **Anteroposterior films** in internal and external rotation, West Point, and Stryker notch views to evaluate humeral and glenoid morphology and to determine the presence of Hill-Sachs or Bankart lesions.

      ii. **MRI** may be useful in evaluation of capsular laxity or detachment (Fig. 2), labral injury or detachment, articular surface injuries, loose bodies, and the status of the rotator cuff.

  f. **Treatment:** Based on the results of history, physical findings, and diagnostic procedures in light of subjective complaints and disability.

      i. Most patients will benefit from an aggressive rotator cuff and scapulo-thoracic strengthening program.[4]

      ii. Existence of distinct pathology related to trauma (e.g., Bankart lesion, labral degeneration or stripping, significant capsular laxity, or loose bodies) may warrant earlier surgical exploration and treatment.[10]

      iii. In patients with subluxation and secondary impingement, surgical intervention is reserved for those who fail the rehabilitation program and is designed to address the underlying instability, not the impingement syndrome.

D. **Impingement syndrome:** Defined as injury or inhibition of the rotator cuff, allowing abnormal superior migration of the humeral head with activities involving forward flexion and abduction of the glenohumeral joint. It is commonly seen in two groups of patients: (1) young patients with glenohumeral instability and secondary impingement[23] and (2) older patients with overuse, degenerative rotator cuff disease, and primary impingement syndrome as described by Neer.[15]

  1. **History**

    a. Pain may be poorly localized and may radiate to the mid-humerus.

    b. Patients may also note fatigue, catching, stiffness, or weakness of the shoulder.

    c. Night pain may accompany impingement and is thought to be characteristic of rotator cuff tendinitis or tear.

    d. Important to glean from the history is whether the onset is acute and traumatic or insidious and secondary to progressive rotator cuff dysfunction.

2. **Radiographic evaluation**
  a. **Primary impingement**
    i. Anteroposterior films in internal and external rotation to evaluate the position and morphology of the humeral head.
    ii. Outlet view to evaluate acromial morphology.
    iii. Axillary view to evaluate the width of the glenohumeral space and presence of degenerative changes.
    iv. The presence of sclerosis or cystic changes of the greater tuberosity, acromial osteophyte formation, or proximal migration of the humeral head is indicative of chronic rotator cuff dysfunction.
    v. Arthrography may be useful in documenting the presence and extent of rotator cuff tears.
    vi. MRI is useful to document the presence of rotator cuff tendinitis or impingement, partial and full-thickness rotator cuff tears, and the quality of the cuff musculature in chronic cuff dysfunction (Fig. 3).
3. **Treatment:** The treatment of impingement syndrome or rotator cuff pathology can be broken down into three groups:
  a. **Preventive treatment**
    i. Maintenance of adequate body conditioning, flexibility, and endurance with a rotator cuff and scapulothoracic strengthening program.
    ii. Careful attention to proper shoulder mechanics with overhead activities and sports.
  b. **Nonoperative treatment** for the symptomatic patient with secondary instability as outlined above.
  c. **Nonoperative treatment** for symptomatic primary impingement is similar:
    i. Range of motion, stretching, and strengthening of rotator cuff, scapulo-thoracic and upper extremity musculature.
    ii. Modification of overuse patterns and careful attention to shoulder mechanics are important.

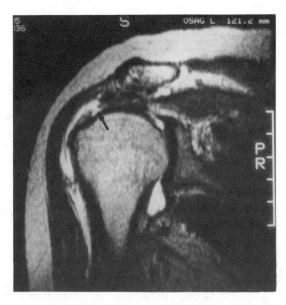

FIGURE 3. Oblique coronal MRI of the shoulder demonstrating a full-thickness tear of the supraspinatus tendon with mild retraction.

     d. **Operative intervention:** Reserved for patients who fail a course of nonoperative treatment.

        i. **Primary impingement:** Arthroscopic or open subacromial decompression, debridement, and repair of the rotator cuff is indicated.

        ii. **Secondary impingement:** Operative treatment of the underlying instability.

E. **Acromioclavicular joint injuries:** These injuries generally result from a fall onto the posterolateral corner of the shoulder with the arm in an adducted position. Application of this acute force may result in dislocation of the acromioclavicular (AC) joint, fracture of the clavicle, or, on rare occasion, dislocation of the sternoclavicular joint.

   1. AC joint injuries may result from acute trauma (AC dislocation) or repetitive overload (clavicular osteolysis).

   2. **Classification and anatomy of AC injuries**

     a. **Type 1:** Minor strain to the fibers of the AC ligament. The ligament remains intact and the AC joint is stable.

     b. **Type 2:** Disruption of the AC joint resulting in widening and mild upward displacement of the distal clavicle. A mild sprain of the coracoclavicular ligaments may be appreciated.

     c. **Type 3:** Disruption of the AC and coracoclavicular ligaments with resultant dislocation of the AC joint and superior migration of the distal clavicle.

     d. **Type 4:** Dislocation of the AC joint with posterior displacement of the distal clavicle into the trapezius muscle.

     e. **Type 5:** Dislocation of the AC joint with gross displacement of the distal clavicle superiorly toward the base of the neck.

     f. **Type 6:** Dislocation of the AC joint with displacement of the clavicle inferior to the acromion or coracoid.

   3. **Diagnosis**

     a. **Inspection and palpation** of the clavicle and AC joint may be diagnostic.

     b. **Radiographic evaluation** (anteroposterior and lateral views of the clavicle) is essential to determine the degree and direction of clavicular displacement.

   4. **Treatment**

     a. **Type 1 and 2:** Treated conservatively with sling or harness immobilization until symptoms subside (generally 7–14 days), followed by controlled remobilization of the shoulder until there is full, painless range of motion.

     b. **Type 3:** There is ongoing controversy over the conservative vs operative treatment of the complete AC dislocation. "Skillful neglect" of these injuries has been advocated with excellent functional outcome in the nonmanual laborer.[16]

     c. **Type 4, 5, and 6:** Require operative treatment because of the significant displacement of the distal clavicle.

   5. **Clavicular osteolysis:** Thought to result from repetitive application of high load to the AC joint.

     a. Presents with pain localized over the AC joint which is more pronounced with weight-bearing activity.

     b. Seen primarily in power lifters and body builders.

     c. **Radiographic evaluation** reveals erosion of the lateral border of the clavicle and widening of the AC joint.

     d. **Treatment:** Rest from inciting activity and use of nonsteroidal antiinflammatory drugs (NSAIDs). Athletes with persistent pain and limitation of function may require operative excision of the distal clavicle (Mumford procedure).

F. **Suprascapular neuropathy:** An uncommon but important cause of shoulder pain in the overhead athlete. Entrapment of the suprascapular nerve may occur as the nerve passes through the suprascapular notch under the transverse scapular ligament or as it passes through the spinoglenoid notch lateral to the border of the scapular spine.

   1. **History and physical examination**
      a. Poorly localized aching or burning pain in the posterolateral shoulder. Pain can often be elicited by direct palpation over the suprascapular notch.
      b. Entrapment in the suprascapular notch will result in weakness or atrophy in the supraspinatus and infraspinatus.
      c. Entrapment in the spinoglenoid notch will result in isolated weakness or atrophy of the infraspinatus.
   2. **Diagnosis**
      a. The diagnosis is dependent upon documentation of abnormal nerve conduction and electromyography studies and concomitant physical findings.
      b. MRI may provide useful information as to the location and type of suprascapular nerve impingement.
   3. **Treatment**
      a. **Initial treatment is conservative** with rest from overhead activity, use of NSAIDs, and physical therapy to maintain strength and range of motion.
      b. **Surgical exploration and decompression** may be indicated for athletes who fail a minimum 6-month course of conservative treatment but remains controversial.
   G. **Injuries in the skeletally immature athlete:** Special attention must be paid to overuse injuries in the skeletally immature athlete. This syndrome is characterized by pain in the shoulder and proximal humerus of a skeletally immature, overhead athlete.
      1. **Diagnosis**
         a. History of repetitive overhead activity
         b. Pain in the shoulder and proximal humerus
         c. Radiographs reveal widening of the physis of the proximal humerus (Fig. 4). It is unclear whether this widening represents a subacute Salter I fracture or the response of the physis to a repetitive traction stress.

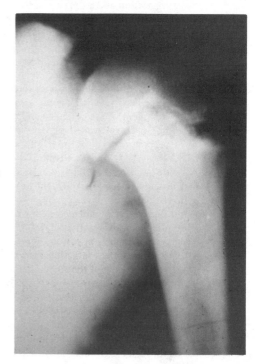

FIGURE 4. Anteroposterior radiograph of the shoulder demonstrating widening of the humeral physis in "little league shoulder."

2. **Treatment:** Cessation of repetitive loading until there is radiologic evidence of healing and full, painless range of motion of the shoulder.

II. ELBOW

Overuse injuries in the elbow may involve muscle, tendon, nerve, ligament, bone or cartilage. Injuries may also involve the physis or epiphysis in the skeletally immature athlete. They are most conveniently grouped by the anatomic area in which they occur.

A. **Lateral elbow pain**

1. **Lateral epicondylitis** ("tennis elbow"): Most common injury involves the extensor musculotendinous unit.

   a. **Anatomy**
      i. Musculotendinous unit spans two joints. Susceptible to injury with repetitive activity as seen in racquet sports.
      ii. Mechanism of injury is most often due to late racquet preparation on the backhand stroke (only 10% people get lateral epicondylitis from playing tennis).
      iii. Most common in older athlete (30–60 years).

   b. **Physical examination:** Pain over the lateral epicondyle and proximal extensor origin which increases with passive volar flexion and resisted wrist dorsiflexion. Both signs are accentuated with elbow extension.

   c. **Treatment**
      i. Judicious rest, use of NSAIDs, and physical therapy to improve flexibility and strength (concentric and eccentric).
      ii. Attention to proper stroke mechanics
      iii. Use of elbow strapping or braces
      iv. Surgical intervention: Local debridement of the focal area of tendon degeneration with primary repair of the tendon defect. Surgical intervention is reserved for cases that fail a minimum of 6-months to 1 year of conservative treatment.[14,20]

   d. **Pathophysiology**
      i. Unclear whether intrinsic injuries result from a single traumatic event or repetitive overuse.
      ii. Tendon injury occurs near insertion to bone.
      iii. Maturation and aging may have a deleterious effect on tendon with alteration in the water content of the tissue and its mechanical properties.
      iv. Regan et al.[20] evaluated microscopic pathology of refractory lateral epicondylitis and described vascular proliferation, focal hyaline degeneration, and no evidence of inflammation. These changes were felt to be more characteristic of a degenerative than an inflammatory process.

2. **Nerve entrapment syndromes**

   a. **Posterior interosseous neuropathy** ("radial tunnel syndrome")
      i. Presents with pain in the proximal extensor mass of the forearm and has been called "resistant tennis elbow."[21]
      ii. **Physical examination**
         (a) Pain over the extensor mass may radiate to the wrist.
         (b) Pain is exacerbated by passive wrist flexion and pronation, and active resisted supination and long finger extension.

   b. **Musculocutaneous neuropathy**
      i. Compression of the lateral cutaneous branch of the musculocutaneous nerve has been described in association with repetitive elbow extension and forearm pronation.[3]
      ii. Results from compression of lateral cutaneous nerve between the biceps tendon and underlying brachialis muscle.

      iii. **History:** Pain, paresthesias, or dysesthesias over the distal dorsal and volar forearm.

      iv. **Physical examination.** Pain on palpation over the anterolateral elbow and lateral epicondyle.

  c. **Initial treatment of nerve impingement syndromes is conservative,** with avoidance or modification of precipitating activity and use of NSAIDs. **Surgical intervention** is reserved for cases refractory to conservative treatment for a minimum of 6 months.

3. **Lateral joint compression with valgus overload:** Involves repetitive injury to the radial head and capitellum with resultant degenerative changes and possible loose body formation.

  a. **Physical examination:**

      i. Localized pain over the radiocapitellar joint.

      ii. History of clicking or locking may be elicited.

      iii. Radiographic examination warranted to rule out loose body formation.

B. **Medial elbow pain:** The medial aspect of the elbow is under significant valgus stress during the tennis serve and the acceleration phase of throwing.

1. **Flexor-pronator injuries ("medial epicondylitis")**

  a. Flexor-pronator group spans the elbow and wrist and is subjected to significant tensile load with valgus stress.

  b. **Physical examination:** Localized pain over the tendinous origin and musculotendinous junction, with increases with passive wrist dorsiflexion or resisted volar flexion. Both signs are accentuated with elbow extension.

  c. **Treatment**

      i. Judicious rest and physical therapy to improve flexibility and strength.

      ii. Attention to proper mechanics of the sport.

      iii. NSAIDs

      iv. Surgical intervention for recalcitrant cases:

        (a) Local debridement of focal area of tendon degeneration

        (b) Primary repair of the tendon defect

  d. **Pathophysiology:** The histopathology of refractory medial epicondylitis is characterized by angiofibroblastic hyperplasia and fibrillary degeneration of collagen without evidence of acute or chronic inflammation (Fig. 5).

2. **Ulnar collateral ligament injuries:** The ulnar collateral ligament (UCL) and medial capsule lie under the flexor-pronator mass. With overload of the musculotendinous supporting structures, stress is transferred to the underlying UCL. Injuries may result from repetitive microtrauma and fiber elongation or from acute failure of the ligament.

  a. **Physical examination**

      i. Patient may provide a history of pain along the medial elbow during the acceleration phase of overhead activity.

      ii. Application of a valgus stress with the elbow in 20–30° of flexion will increase symptoms.

      iii. Symptomatic increase in medial laxity with valgus stress is suggestive of capsuloligamentous injury.

  b. **Radiographic evaluation**

      i. Anteroposterior and lateral views of the elbow may reveal:

        (a) Spur formation in region of the coranoid at the insertion of the UCL.

        (b) Rare ossification of the UCL.

      ii. MRI or arthrography can provide information concerning the integrity of the UCL and the underlying capsule (Fig. 6).

  c. **Treatment**

      i. Initial treatment includes rest, NSAIDs, and physical therapy to improve strength and flexibility.

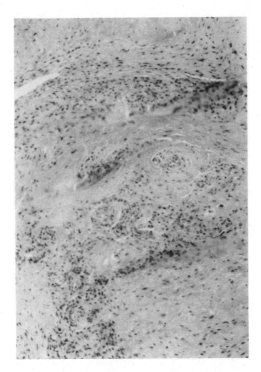

FIGURE 5. Histologic specimen of medial epicondylitis demonstrating angiofibroblastic hyperplasia.

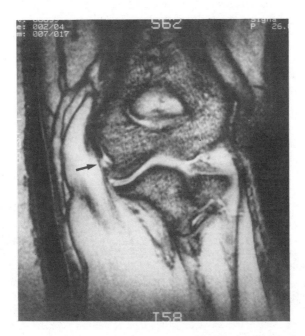

FIGURE 6. Coronal MRI of the elbow demonstrating a partial injury to the ulnar collateral ligament.

ii. Failure of nonoperative treatment in the active athlete may warrant repair or reconstruction of the UCL.[5,11]

d. **Pathophysiology**

i. UCL strain is thought to result from repetitive overload with microscopic fiber failure. An "acute" rupture is thought to represent an endstage of chronic weakening stemming from cumulative overload.

ii. Pathologic changes may alter the material properties of the ligament with subsequent "acute" failure in response to valgus load. •

3. **Nerve entrapment**

a. **Cubital tunnel syndrome, ulnar nerve entrapment:** Well-documented neuropathy in baseball players; thought to result from repetitive valgus stress.[6]

i. **Symptoms** include pain in the medial proximal forearm and paresthesias or dysesthesias in the ring and little finger.

ii. **Physical examination**

(a) Positive Tinel's sign over the cubital tunnel.

(b) Intrinsic muscle atrophy may be present in longstanding cases.

(c) Elbow flexion test: 5 minutes of full elbow flexion may elicit or result in exacerbation of symptoms.

iii. Electrodiagnostic studies are used to confirm the site of ulnar nerve compression.

iv. **Treatment:** Early surgical decompression and submuscular transposition of the ulnar nerve is recommended for symptomatic high-performance athletes.[6]

C. **Posterior elbow pain:** Posterior elbow injuries are also seen in racquet sports and throwing secondary to repetitive elbow extension. Elbow extension and valgus stress combine and result in compression of the olecranon against the medial wall of the trochlea and may result in formation of peripheral osteophytes or loose bodies.

1. **Physical examination**

a. Pain is localized to posterior elbow. In the early stages, pain may be activity-related only; with progression of posterior impingement and onset of degenerative changes, the pain may become more chronic.

b. History of clicking, grinding, or locking.

c. Documentation of active and passive range of motion

i. **Active elbow extension** may be limited by an injury to the triceps.

ii. **Passive range of motion** may be limited by loose bodies or osteophytes in the posterior compartment or by contracture of the anterior capsule of the elbow joint.

d. **Radiologic evaluation**

i. Anteroposterior and lateral views of the elbow may reveal osteophytes or loose bodies.

ii. CT arthrography to evaluate cartilaginous loose bodies and the status of the articular surface.

2. **Treatment**

a. Rest, NSAIDs, and physical therapy to improve flexibility and strength.

b. Arthroscopic intervention is indicated if loose bodies or significant posterior osteophytes are present.

D. **Anterior elbow pain**

1. **Flexion contracture:** Repetitive hyperextension of the elbow may result in traction injuries to the anterior capsule with resultant scar formation.

a. **Treatment**

i. Active and active assisted range of motion exercises.

ii. Cessation of hyperextension loading until resolution of the flexion contracture.

2. **Nerve entrapment**
   a. **Pronator teres syndrome** is uncommon but has been reported in baseball players.[2] The syndrome is defined as compression of the median nerve as it passes between the two heads of the pronator teres. Anterior entrapment can also occur at the ligament of Struthers, lacertus fibrosis, or arch of the flexor digitorum superficialis.
      i. Electrodiagnostic studies are used to confirm the site of median nerve compression.
      ii. Symptoms include pain in the proximal, anterior forearm that increases with activity, and diminished sensation in the volar thumb, index, and middle finger.
      iii. **Symptoms** may be elicited by resisted forearm pronation and wrist flexion, with a positive Tinel's sign over the pronator teres.
      iv. **Treatment**
         (a) Initially conservative with a decrease in repetitive pronation and use of NSAIDs.
         (b) Surgical intervention is indicated if there is no improvement after 6 months of conservative care of if finger flexor weakness develops.
E. **Elbow injuries in the skeletally immature athlete:** Most frequent type of elbow injuries in the adolescent are related to **overuse.** Injury patterns appear to be linked to the stage of development and include abnormalities of ossification, physeal injuries, and osteochondritis dissecans.[19]
   1. **"Little league or gymnast's elbow"**
      a. Athlete may present with medial, lateral, or posterior elbow pain.
      b. Thought to be the result of repetitive overuse.
      c. Radiographs may reveal:
         i. Hypertrophy or fragmentation of the medial epicondyle
         ii. Fragmentation of the trochlea or olecranon
         iii. Ossification abnormalities of the radial head or capitellum
         iv. Osteochondritis dissecans
      d. With the exception of osteochondritis dissecans, these overuse injuries are felt to be self-limited with a benign course.
      e. **Treatment**
         i. Rest from overuse
         ii. Maintenance of strength, range of motion, and conditioning
         iii. Slow, progressive return to sports when no longer symptomatic
         iv. Attention to proper throwing mechanics and avoidance of overload training regimens
   2. **Osteochondritis dissecans** is thought to result from excessive, repetitive compression or shear.
      a. Athletes may present with pain, development of flexion contracture, or symptoms consistent with loose body formation.
      b. Radiographic evaluation
         i. Cystic changes, sclerosis, or loose body formation involving the capitellum
         ii. The radial head is frequently flattened or deformed.
         iii. MRI or CT arthrography may assist in evaluation of the integrity of the overlying cartilage, and extent of injury to the underlying bone.
      c. **Management**
         i. Initially includes rest and maintenance of range of motion, strength, and flexibility.
         ii. Return to sport is strongly contraindicated.
         iii. Loose body formation warrants surgical intervention for debridement, curretage of the donor site, and drilling.[13]

REFERENCES

1. Andrews JR, Carson WG, McLeod WD: Glenoid labral tears related to the long head of the biceps. Am J Sports Med 13:337–341, 1985.
2. Barnes DA, Tullos HS: An analysis of 100 symptomatic baseball players. Am J Sports Med 6:62–67, 1978.
3. Bassett FH, Nunley JA: Compression of the musculocutaneous nerve at the elbow. J Bone Joint Surg 64A:1050–1052, 1982.
4. Burkhead WZ, Rockwood CA: Treatment of instability of the shoulder with an exercise program. J Bone Joint Surg 74A:890–896, 1992.
5. Conway JE, Jobe FW, Glousman RE, Pink M: Medial instability of the elbow in throwing athletes: Treatment by repair or reconstruction of the ulnar collateral ligament. J Bone Joint Surg 74A:67–83, 1992.
6. Del Pizzo W, Jobe FW, Norwood L: Ulnar nerve entrapment syndrome in baseball players. Am J Sports Med 5:182–185, 1977.
7. Fronek J, Warren RF, Bowen M: Posterior subluxation of the shoulder. J Bone Joint Surg 71:205–212, 1989.
8. Garth WP, Allman FL, Armstrong WS: Occult anterior subluxations of the shoulder in noncontact sports. Am J Sports Med 15:579–586, 1987.
9. Hirasawa Y, Sakakida K: Sports and peripheral nerve injury. Am J Sports Med 11:420–426, 1983.
10. Jobe FW, Giangarra CE, Kvitne RS, Glousman RE: Anterior capsulolabral reconstruction of the shoulder in athletes in overhand sports. Am J Sports Med 19:428–434, 1991.
11. Jobe FW, Stark H, Lombardo SJ: Reconstruction of the ulnar collateral ligament in athletes. J Bone Joint Surg 68A:1158–1163, 1986.
12. Jobe FW, Tibone JE, Perry J: An EMG analysis of the shoulder in throwing and pitching. Am J Sports Med 11:3–5, 1983.
13. McNamara GB, Micheli LJ, Berry MV, Sohn RS: The surgical treatment of osteochondritis of the capitellum. Am J Sports Med 13:11–21, 1985.
14. Morrey BF: Reoperation for failed surgical treatment of refractory lateral epicondylitis. J Shoulder Elbow Surg 1:47–55, 1992.
15. Neer CS: Impingement lesions. Clin Orthop 173:70, 1983.
16. Neer Cs, Rockwood CA: Fractures and dislocations of the shoulder. In Rockwood CA, Greene DP (eds): Fractures in Adults, Vol. 1. Philadelphia, J.B. Lippincott, 1984.
17. Nicholas JA, Hershman EB: The Upper Extremity in Sports Medicine. St. Louis, Mosby, 1990.
18. O'Brien SJ, Warren RF, Schwartz E: Anterior shoulder instability. Orthop Clin 18:395–408, 1987.
19. Pappas AM: Elbow problems associated with baseball during childhood and preadolescence. Clin Orthop 164:30–34, 1982.
20. Regan W, Wold LE, Coorad R, Morrey BF: Microscopic histopathology of chronic refractory lateral epicondylitis. Am J Sports Med 20:746–749, 1992.
21. Roles NC, Maudsley RH: Radial tunnel syndrome: Resistant tennis elbow as a nerve entrapment. J Bone Joint Surg 54B:499–508, 1972.
22. Tibone JE, Elrod B, Jobe FW, et al: Surgical treatment of the rotator cuff in athletes. J Bone Joint Surg 68A:887–891, 1986.
23. Tibone JE, Jobe FW, Kerlan RK, et al: Shoulder impingement syndrome treated by anterior acromioplasty. Clin Orthop 198:134–140, 1985.
24. Warren RF: Subluxation of the shoulder in athletes. Clin Sports Med 2:339–354, 1983.

Chapter 39: Knee Injuries

ELIZABETH A. ARENDT, MD

The knee is a complex joint in which the musculoskeletal components are beautifully orchestrated to propel us in upright activity. A well-functioning knee is paramount for activities of daily living as well as sport and exercise. Knowledge of the knee and its injured states is mandatory for health care personnel working with an active population. Both acute and overuse injuries are common in the knee; however, they require different investigative processes to diagnose and treat properly.

I. **FOUNDATION OF INJURY DIAGNOSIS**
   A. **Knowledge of anatomy** (Fig. 1)
      1. **Static structures:** Continuous stabilizers of a joint (always present, do not depend on an active unit)—ligaments, joint surface congruency, menisci
      2. **Dynamic structures:** Intermittent stabilizers of a joint (depend on a motor unit for function)—muscles and their tendinous units
   B. **Clinical correlation**
      1. History
      2. Physical examination
      3. Tests and their interpretation
      4. Treatment

II. **APPROACH TO THE ACUTELY INJURED KNEE**
   A. **History**
      1. **What was the mechanism of injury?:** Helps analyze potential structures that might have been damaged by an application of force or rotatory twist.
      2. **Was a "pop" heard?:** A pop frequently signifies a tearing of a ligament, most commonly, the anterior cruciate ligament (ACL).
      3. **Could one return to play?:** The degree of pain and/or disability cannot be used as a reliable indicator of the seriousness of injury. Pain can be felt at the time of injury and quickly subside. However, continued play with little to no impairment in performance diminishes the likelihood of a serious knee injury.
      4. **Has this joint been previously injured?:** Frequently, this uncovers an acute-on-chronic injury, such as recurrent patella dislocation, or a subluxation event due to chronic ligament injury.
      5. **Was the joint swelling noticed? How soon after the injury?:** Joint swelling within 12 hours of an injury is, by definition, hemorrhage to the joint. Effusion that occurs after 12–24 hours is suggestive of synovial fluid accumulation that can be caused by irritation to an intraarticular structure.
   B. **Physical examination:**
      1. **Inspection**
         a. **Swelling:** The absence of notable intraarticular swelling does not rule out ligament rupture. A severe ligament rupture can have associated large, capsular disruption, and the fluid can escape into the surrounding tissue. The absence of knee swelling may also indicate an extraarticular source of pain.
         b. **Color, deformity, and previous scars:** Localized bruises and abrasions can be useful to identify the point of contact in a contact injury.

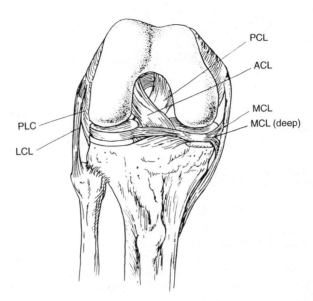

FIGURE 1. Anatomy of the knee. ACL = anterior cruciate ligament; LCL = lateral collateral ligament; MCL = medial collateral ligament; PCL = posterior cruciate ligament. (From Arendt EA: Assessment of the athlete with a painful knee. In Griffin LY (ed): Rehabilitation of the Injured Knee, 2nd ed. St. Louis, Mosby, 1990, with permission.)

    c. **Muscle atrophy**
    d. **Limb alignment**
  2. **Hemarthrosis:** The differential diagnosis of an acute hemarthrosis is:
    a. **Ligament injury:** The cruciate ligaments are intraarticular/extrasynovial structures. Lateral collateral ligament and superficial medial collateral ligaments are extraarticular structures. Deep medial collateral ligament is a thickening of the joint capsule and is intraarticular. The most common ligament torn in acute hemarthrosis is the ACL—70%.
    b. **Peripheral meniscus tear:** The outer or peripheral one-third of the meniscus is vascular. A tear in this region is a source of hemarthrosis. Meniscus tears in this zone have the potential for healing and are repairable.
    c. **Fractures:** In addition to obvious condylar fractures, occult osteochondral fractures can be a cause of hemarthrosis. These include avulsion fractures of ACL and posterior cruciate ligament (PCL) (more common in developing adolescents) and fractures secondary to patella dislocation.
    d. **Synovial/capsular tears:** Patella dislocations, even in the absence of a fracture, are a source of hemarthrosis. This category also includes other disruptions of the extensor mechanism, including quadriceps and infrapatellar tendon ruptures.
  3. **Palpation**
    a. **Direct palpation** of the injured area corresponds to anatomic structures. This is most useful in meniscal, patellofemoral, and collateral ligament injuries.
    b. **The cruciates do not have a palpable attachment to the capsule** and therefore palpation examination is less useful for these structures. However, an ACL injury is associated with anterolateral subluxation of the tibia on the femur (pivot-shift), and therefore anterolateral joint-line tenderness is not uncommon.
    c. **Patella subluxation/dislocation** is associated with medial tenderness along the patella retinaculum. A documented patella dislocation in the absence of

swelling suggests patella laxity due to chronic injuries, hypermobile tissue, and/or a dysplastic patellofemoral joint.

4. **Range of motion**
   a. **Locked knee:** Inability to obtain full passive motion of the joint secondary to a mechanical block. Common causes are displaced meniscus and loose body.
   b. **Pseudolocked knee:** Full range of motion is unable to be obtained secondary to pain (hamstring spasm) or swelling.
   c. **Active range of motion:** Assesses the integrity of motor units surrounding the knee. Frequently missed are disruptions of the extensor mechanism, i.e., quadriceps and patellar tendon injuries.

5. **Stability testing:** The *sine qua non* of a ligament disruption is the presence of pathologic joint motion.
   a. **Straight plane instabilities**
      i. Medial: medial collateral ligament (MCL)
      ii. Lateral: lateral collateral ligament (LCL)
      iii. Anterior: anterior cruciate ligament (ACL)
      iv. Posterior: posterior cruciate ligament (PCL)
   b. **Rotatory instabilities** (i.e., rotation of the tibia around its vertical/longitudinal axis (Fig. 2)
      i. Anterolateral: Associated with ACL injury
      ii. Posterolateral: Associated with structures of the posterolateral corner of the knee (iliotibial band, arcuate complex, popliteus tendon). Frequently associated with PCL and LCL injuries.
      iii. Posteromedial: Rare
      iv. Anteromedial: Associated with ACL/MCL injury

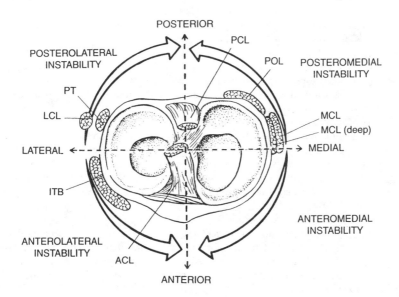

FIGURE 2. Rotatory instability of the knee. PCL = posterior cruciate ligament; POL = posterior oblique ligament; MCL = medial collateral ligament; ACL = anterior cruciate ligament; ITB = iliotibial band; LCL = lateral collateral ligament; PT = popliteal tendon. (From Arendt EA: Assessment of the athlete with a painful knee. In Griffin LY (ed): Rehabilitation of the Injured Knee, 2nd ed. St. Louis, Mosby, 1990, with permission.)

    c. **Extensor mechanism**

        i. Apprehension sign: Passive lateral movement of the patella causing pain and/or apprehension is suggestive of patella subluxation/dislocation.

        ii. Straight leg raising against light resistance establishes the integrity of the extensor mechanism, including quadricep and patella tendons.

C. **Tests and their interpretation**

  1. **Plain radiographs**

    a. **Anteroposterior view**

        i. Primary usefulness is to rule out pertinent negatives and assess overall tibiofemoral alignment.

        ii. Standing views are preferred, but if pain/swelling limit full extension and/or full weight-bearing, supine views are performed.

    b. **Lateral view**

        i. Evaluates position of the knee cap.

        ii. Avulsion fractures, especially PCL, are well seen in this view.

    c. **Axial view**

        i. Evaluates position of patella in the trochlea groove.

        ii. Different views are established (Laurin's, Merchant's). The clinician should become familiar with one technique and utilize that view.

        iii. **Axial views are a must for the complete evaluation of all acute knee injuries.**

    d. **Notch or tunnel view**

        i. Most useful to evaluate avulsion fractures off the tibia, osteochondritis dissecans, and loose bodies.

  2. **Stress radiographs**

    a. Most useful to rule out epiphyseal injuries, especially Salter I growth plate injuries.

  3. **Bone scans**

    a. Most useful in occult infections and to rule out stress fractures.

    b. Usefulness in diagnosing reflex sympathetic dystrophy is variable.

  4. **Computed tomography (CT)**

    a. Has few specific applications for routine imaging of acute knee injuries.

    b. Continues to have application in evaluating complex fractures around the knee, especially those involving cortical surfaces.

    c. When used with contrast, can be useful to evaluate osteochondral defects such as osteochondritis dissecans.

  5. **Magnetic resonance imaging (MRI)**

    a. For the knee, MRI has its largest application in evaluating meniscus and cruciate ligament injuries. Overall accuracy rate for these structures is >90%.

    b. Can diagnose injury to a collateral structure; however, differentiation between grades depends largely on clinical examination. Its ability to "see" cartilage lesions is less accurate.

    c. Can be used to estimate the age of an injury.

    d. Subchondral bone changes, i.e., a bone bruise, have been characterized recently by MRI and are not seen by conventional radiographs or arthroscopy. These MRI changes may lead to cartilage degeneration. Their role in the development of post-traumatic arthritis continues to be investigated.

D. **General treatment**

  1. **Tapping of the knee joint:** Not advised as a routine part of the evaluation of a knee injury. At times can be therapeutic, as in the case of a tense effusion.

  2. **Immobilization/crutches:** Certainly, this is the safest way to protect the injured part until a repeat examination can be performed by the same or referral physician. When feasible, removal of the brace to perform gentle range of motion

exercises is useful to help resolve an effusion. Partial weight-bearing, depending on the patient's comfort level, can also be therapeutic.

3. **Repeat examination:** Very helpful in establishing a more firm diagnosis, especially when pain and/or apprehension is limiting the initial examination. Strategies to reduce swelling, including ice and range of motion, should be utilized. Antiinflammatory medication can be used for pain control if needed. Their role in reduction of acute effusion is debated.

4. **Role of MRI:** MRI should be used as an adjunct in the evaluation of an acutely injured knee only if it will alter the treatment protocol. It should never be used in the absence of a thorough and knowledgeable history and physical examination.

E. **Special considerations:** There is currently an increasing body of epidemiologic data that reveals that injury to the ACL is higher in women, in particular those participating in jumping and pivoting sports. The etiology of the increased ACL injury rate is unclear. Much has been theorized:

1. **Intrinsic factors**
   a. Ligament size or ligament laxity
   b. Intracondylar notch dimensions
   c. Muscular strength and coordination
   d. Limb alignment

2. **Extrinsic factors**
   a. Level of skill or experience
   b. Shoe/floor interface (friction)
   c. Gender-specific avoidance patterns

III. OVERUSE SYNDROMES

A. **Definition:** Repetitive submaximal or subclinical trauma that results in an inflammatory response that causes pain. The injured area has suffered macro- and microscopic damage to its structural unit and/or blood supply. Time is required for healing:

1. **Exogenous:** Identifiable forces being placed on the involved structure from outside—e.g., prepatellar bursitis, supraspinatus/biceps tendinitis.

2. **Endogenous:** Mechanical circumstances in which the musculoskeletal tissue is subjected to greater tensile force or stress than it can effectively absorb. Most overuse syndromes fall into this category.

B. **History:** Overuse injuries are characterized by the absence of an injury, or at least no injury significant enough to explain the current clinical situation. Detailed review of the patient's activities frequently gives insight into a *change* of circumstances. This should be sought in the analysis of all overuse injuries.

1. **Transitional athlete:** At high risk for development of overuse injuries; defined as any athlete with a change in her internal or external environment. This includes:
   a. Change in intensity (distance/time)
   b. Change in frequency or duration
   c. Footwear changes
   d. Surface changes, including material composition and slope
   e. Change in competitive climate
   f. Weather conditions
   g. Life-cycle changes, puberty, aging
   h. Pregnancy and post-partum

2. Location of pain with aggravating or reducing activities, if present

3. Past history of an injury? This frequently uncovers a chronic injury.

4. Recurrent swelling, redness, or warmth

5. Prodromal swelling? Important to establish when dealing with stress fractures.

6. Menstrual history, eating patterns, nutritional intake

C. **Physical examination**
   1. **Inspection**
      a. **Alignment of limb:** A must in evaluating any overuse injury of the lower extremity. A common anatomic complex is **miserable malalignment syndrome** (Fig. 3), which includes femoral anteversion, high Q-angle, tibiofemoral valgus, external tibial torsion, and subtalar pronation. This alignment can cause tissue overload injuries anywhere along the kinetic chain (foot to hip) with lower extremity activities.
      b. **Q-angle:** Indicates potential lateral force for patella subluxation. Not diagnostic.
      c. **Effusion:** Indicates intraarticular pathology. Not common in most overuse injuries around the knee.
      d. **Redness and warmth:** Not common in overuse injuries, but may indicate the presence of an acutely inflamed bursa or tendon region.
   2. **Palpation:** Locate focal areas of tenderness, specifically in the area of the bursa or tendon sheath. Particular attention to the presence of crepitus or fluctuance is helpful.
   3. **Range of motion**
      a. **Patella tracking:** Any abrupt changes should be regarded as abnormal.
      b. **Crepitus of the patellofemoral joint:** Poor correlation with pain, but may be indicative of chondrosis.
      c. **Resisted motion of a joint:** May be indicative of tendinitis of that motor unit.
   4. **Stability (patellofemoral joint)**
      a. **Medial/lateral displacement of the patella:** The patella should not displace more than one-half its width with the knee in full extension. Decrease in medial motion may indicate lateral tightness. Increase in both medial and lateral motion may indicate a hypermobile patella.

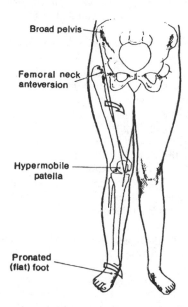

FIGURE 3. Miserable alignment syndrome—femoral neck anteversion, hip varus, knee valgus, and external placement of tibial tubercle with pronation of the heels— is a difference in the athletic female that has been misinterpreted as malalignment. (From Ciullo JV: Lower extremity injuries. In Pearl AJ (ed): The Athletic Female. Champaign, IL, Human Kenetics, 1990, pp 267-298, with permission.)

D. **Investigational tests**
  1. **Strength tests**
     a. Limb to limb variation in strength
     b. Concentric and eccentric strength
     c. Agonist to antagonist strength (quadriceps/hamstring ratio)
     d. Peak torque strength to body weight ratio
  2. **Evaluation of flexibility** (especially in key muscle groups)
     a. Quadriceps
     b. Hamstrings
     c. Achilles tendon
  3. **Radiographs**
     a. **Plain radiographs:** Infrequently necessary for evaluation of overuse injuries. However, radiographic views of the patellofemoral joint, in particular axial views, may be helpful to define patella position.
     b. **Bone scans:** Most useful to assess stress fractures. Its role in diagnosing reflex sympathetic dystrophy is not confirmed.
     c. **MRI:** Main advantage is its ability to view intra- and extraarticular structures. Gold standard for viewing meniscal pathology.
     d. **CT:** Infrequently used to judge patella position in relationship to its femoral groove. Disadvantages of this use of CT include high radiation exposure and poor correlation of current studies to clinical parameters and outcome measures.
  4. **Blood work:** Evaluate for systemic disease (e.g., collagen vascular diseases, Lyme disease)
E. **Treatment**
  1. **Reduce inflammation**
     a. Nonsteroidal antiinflammatory drugs (NSAIDs)
     b. Physical therapy modalities
     c. Relative rest of injured part (reduce activity, substitute activity, protect injured part)
     d. Ice
     e. Compression if swelling is present
  2. **Correct anatomic problems**, when possible (patella sleeves, orthotics to control overpronation, braces, surgery)
  3. **Correct biomechanical errors** when possible (training, sequence, sports style and form, strengthening and stretching of musculoskeletal units)
  4. **Correct environmental concerns**, when possible (new shoes, change to more absorbent running surface, adequate clothing in the cold)
  5. **Sports-specific rehabilitation**
     a. **Recovery of strength**
        i. **Closed chain:** For lower extremity activities, closed chain techniques are more functional. For the patellofemoral joint, closed chain activities for strengthening of the quadriceps complex are more sound biomechanically with less patella femoral contact stresses within the 30–60° arc of motion.
        ii. **Concentric/eccentric**
           (a) Concentric muscle contraction occurs when a muscle shortens as it contracts. In an eccentric contraction, the muscle lengthens as contraction occurs—e.g., as the arm lowers the weight in a biceps curl, the biceps muscle undergoes controlled lengthening as it contracts to properly lower the weight to rest.
           (b) Eccentric strengthening has long been favored for recovery of strength in treatment of tendinitis, though no studies have confirmed this scientifically. For the patellofemoral joint, eccentric muscle activity is an important part of the functional use of the joint. Recovery of

eccentric strength, greater then concentric strength, has been shown to help reduce patellofemoral pain syndrome.

   b. **Maintenance of endurance/aerobic fitness**

   c. **Flexibility** of the kinetic (motion) linkage system

F. **Physician's role**

   1. Diagnose injury

   2. Render appropriate treatment

   3. Educate patient: Patient education is the best treatment for prevention of overuse injuries.

G. **Patient's role**

   1. Understand causative factors in injury

   2. Understand the progression from injury to wellness, including activity modifications

   3. Implement paced return to full activities

IV. SUMMARY

The last quarter century has seen an explosion of knowledge in the biology and biomechanics of knee function, injury, and healing. The challenge of the next quarter century is to use this knowledge to render effective and efficient care, to maximize the health and fitness of the recreational athlete in a manner compatible with individual goals, and to maximize the potential of the elite athlete in a healthful and ethical manner.

REFERENCES

Acute knee inuries

1. Arendt ER, Dick R: Gender specific knee injury pattern in basketball and soccer. Presented at the American Orthopaedic Society of Sports Medicine, Sun Valley, 1993.
2. Daniel D: Assessing the limits of knee motion. Am J SportsMed 19(2):139–147, 1991.
3. DeHaven K: Diagnosis of acute knee injuries with hemarthrosis. Am J Sports Med 8(1):9, 1980.
4. Donaldson W, Warren R, Wickiewicz T: A comparison of acute anterior cruciate ligament examinations. Am J Sports Med 13(1):5–10, 1985.
5. Gray J, Taunton JE, McKenzie DC, et al: A survey of injuries to the anterior cruciate ligament of the knee in female basketball players. Int J Sports Med 6:314–316, 1985.
6. Ireland ML, Wall C: Epidemiology and comparison of knee injuries in elite male and female United States basketball athletes. Med Sci Sports 14:1990.
7. Katz J, Fingeroth R: The diagnostic accuracy of ruptures of the anterior cruciate ligament comparing the Lachman test, the anterior drawer sign, and the pivot shift test in acute and chronic knee injuries. Am J Sports Med 14(1):88–91, 1986.
8. Laurin CA, et al: The tangential x-ray. Clin Orthop 144:16, 1979.
9. Merchant AC, et al: Roentgenographic analysis of PF congruence. J Bone Joint Surg 56A:1391, 1974.
10. Noyes F, Cummings J, Grood E, et al: The diagnosis of knee motion limits, subluxations, and ligament injury. Am J Sports Med 19(2):163–171, 1991.
11. Schutzer, et al: CT classification of PF pain patients. Orthop Clin North Am 17:235, 1986.
12. Vellete AD, Marks P, Fowler P, Mururo T: Occult posttraumatic lesions of the knee: Prevalence, classification, and short-term sequelae evaluated with MR imaging. Radiology 178:271–276, 1991.

Overuse injuries

13. Carson, et al: Patella femoral disorders. Clin Orthop 185:165–184, 1984.
14. DeHaven K, et al: Chondromalacia patella in the athletes: Clinical presentation and conservative management. Am J Sports Med 7:5, 1979.
15. Ericson MO, et al: PF forces during ergometric cycling. Phys Ther 67:1365, 1987.
16. Ficat RP, Hungerford DS: Disorders of the Patello-Femoral Joint. Baltimore, Williams & Wilkins, 1990.
17. Frederick EC: Biomechanical consequences of sports shoe design. Exerc Sport Sci Rev 14:375–400, 1986.
18. Fyfe I, Stanish WD: The use of eccentric training and stretching in the treatment and prevention of tendon injuries. Clin Sports Med 11(3):601–624, 1992.
19. Hungerford DS, Lennox DW: Rehabilitation of the knee in disorders of the patellofemoral joint. Relevant biomechanics. Orthop Clin North Am 14:397, 1983.
20. Hunter L (ed): Overuse injuries. Clin Sports Med 6(2), 1987.

21. Inoue, et al: Subluxation of the patella: CT analysis of PF congruence. J Bone Joint Surg 70A:1331, 1988.
22. McKenzie DC, et al: Running shoes, orthotics, and injuries. Sports Med 2:334–347, 1985.
23. Micheli LJ, Fehlandt AF Jr: Overuse injuries to tendons and apophyses in children and adolescents. Clin Sports Med 11:713–726, 1992.
24. Pavone, et al: Isometric force of the quadriceps muscle after concentric, eccentric and isometric training. Arch Phys Med Rehabil 66:168, 1985.
25. Reilly, et al: Experimental analysis of the quadriceps muscle force and PF joint reaction force for various activities. Acta Orthop Scand 43:126, 1972.

Chapter 40: Physical Therapy Approaches to Patellofemoral Stress Syndrome

CHERYL CLAYPOOLE, PT
SARA AGASSIZ, PT

Pathology related to the patella is a very common source of knee pain. *Patellofemoral stress syndrome* (PFSS) is a term used to describe compression syndromes of the patellofemoral joint. Physical therapy is extremely important in treating this common and aggravating condition. Inherent in this is educating the patient about the problem, addressing flexibility and strength deficits, assessing and correcting biomechanical abnormalities, and modifying the patient's activity profile.

I. **DEFINITION**

   A. Pain, inflammation, imbalance, and/or instability of any component of the extensor mechanism of the knee

   B. **Common diagnoses within this definition**
   1. Anterior knee pain
   2. Patellofemoral malalignment
   3. Extensor mechanism malalignment
   4. Extensor mechanism dysfunction
   5. Patellofemoral pain
   6. "Runner's knee"
   7. Chondromalacia patellae
   8. Patellar subluxation
   9. Patellar dislocation
   10. Plica syndrome
   11. Patellar tendinitis
   12. Quadriceps tendinitis
   13. Osgood-Schlatter disease

   C. **Common symptoms**
   1. Dull aching knee pain
   2. Unable to localize pain—however, most commonly "it hurts somewhere under my kneecap."
   3. Pain with stairs and hills, especially when going down and sometimes up
   4. Pain with prolonged sitting
   5. Pain with squatting or kneeling
   6. Complaint of clicking and popping and/or grinding of knee ("noisy knee")—*not* associated with pain
   7. In severe cases, may have giving way secondary to pain and quadriceps inhibition

   D. **Common causes:** A sound understanding of patellofemoral anatomy and biomechanics is needed for proper diagnosis, treatment, and rehabilitation of patellofemoral disorders.
   1. Direct trauma
   2. Repetitive direct pressure (constant kneeling)
   3. Constant repetitive motion with bent knee against resistance (i.e., crew, cycling)
   4. Malalignment/biomechanic abnormality
   5. Combination of the above

II. ANATOMY

A. **Patella acts as a fulcrum** to increase the extending moment of the quadriceps. The forces transmitted from the patella to the femoral sulcus increase as knee function increases (sitting for long period and/or descending stairs involve high and prolonged patellofemoral compressive loading).

B. **Patellar stabilization is provided by static and dynamic mechanisms.**

   1. **Passive stabilizers**
      a. Femoral sulcus
         i. Depth of patellofemoral groove
         ii. Height of lateral femoral condyle
      b. Configuration of patella
      c. Thickening of capsule
         i. Patellofemoral ligaments; medial patellofemoral ligaments prevent dislocation.
         ii. Lateral patellofemoral ligament—expansion of vastus lateralis and iliotibial band. May be tight and contribute to lateral patellar tilt and malalignment.

   2. **Active stabilizers**
      a. Oblique fibers of vastus medialis obliquus (VMO) keep patella centralized in groove and provides some static stability secondary to insertion.
      b. Pes anserinus group—sartorius, gracilis, and semitendinosus: Internal rotation of proximal tibia helps maintain alignment of the tibial tubercule with the femoral sulcus.

III. EVALUATION

A thorough evaluation can lead to an effective rehabilitation program.

A. **Standing alignment**
   1. Genu valgum or varum
   2. Patellar position—squinting patella or patella alta (high-riding patella)
   3. Tibial or femoral torsion
   4. Subtalar joint pronation

B. **Supine examination**
   1. **Q-angle:** Angle between a line from the midpoint of the patella to the tibial tubercle and midpoint of the patella and the anterior superior iliac spine
      a. Average Q-angle: male = 13°; female = 18°
   2. **Palpation**
      a. Most consistently tender area is the medial facet and medial undersurface of patella.
      b. Tenderness at patellar or quad tendon indicates tendinitis.
      c. Tenderness at tibial tubercle may indicate Osgood-Schlatter's disease.
      d. Medial retinaculum tenderness may indicate subluxing patella.
      e. Tenderness at superior pole of patella or medial femoral condyle may indicate plica syndrome.
   3. **Range of motion** is usually within normal limits for patellofemoral stress syndrome.
   4. **Swelling** may be associated with patellar subluxation and/or dislocation.
   5. **Quadriceps**
      a. Inspect for symmetry, look for atrophy.
      b. Note VMO tone with isometric quadriceps contraction
   6. **Flexibility**
      a. Quadriceps: Athlete should be able to touch heel to buttocks in prone position.
      b. Hamstrings: Straight leg raise should be 90° in supine position.

c. Iliotibial band: Leg should drop to midline in Ober position.

d. Gastric-soleus: Should have 10–20° dorsiflexion.

7. **Patellar mobility:** Normal mobility with knee in extension is lateral or medial motion no more than half the width of the patella; and at 30° of flexion, no patellar movements.

a. May be hypermobile as in subluxing or dislocating patella

b. May be hypomobile usually in the medial direction with tight lateral structures

8. **Patellar tracking:** Contraction of quadriceps should bring the patella in a straight or slightly curved path. Normally the patella should track freely and smoothly.

IV. **REHABILITATION**

A. **Acute pain and inflammation stage:** Goal of physical therapy is to control symptoms and decrease inflammation.

1. **Rest** or a decrease in physical activities, especially those that are stressful on the patellofemoral joint.

2. **Ice** or physical therapy modalities such as electrical stimulation, phonophoresis (especially in the case of tendinitis), etc., to promote resolution of the inflammation.

3. **Pain-free isometric contraction** of the quadriceps, i.e., quad sets, straight leg raises

4. **Stretching** if pain-free

5. **Antiinflammatory medication**

6. **Arch supports** as needed

7. **McConnell strapping** to enhance normal tracking

B. **Subacute stage**

1. **Strengthening of the quadriceps** without increasing the patellofemoral reaction forces. *Pain-free* exercise is key.

a. Quadriceps sets with towel roll

b. Straight leg raise with concurrent quadriceps set

c. Terminal knee extension: Controversy exists on how much range of motion should be used: 10° of motion allows the patella to move outside of the femoral groove.

d. Multiple angle isometrics within the pain-free range of motion

e. Partial arcs of movement from 90–45° when patellofemoral contact is greatest and therefore the force is more dispersed.

2. **Strengthening of the hip adductors:** VMO originates in part from the fascia overlying the adductor magnus. By contracting the adductors, you can facilitate the VMO.

3. **Lower extremity stretching**

a. Quadriceps: If tight, this increases peripatellar soft tissue tension and patello-femoral forces.

b. Hamstrings: If tight, they produce an increase in passive resistance to knee extension, causing increased quadriceps workload.

c. Iliotibial band: Tightness contributes to lateral patellar tracking.

d. Gastroc-soleus: If tight, this causes compensatory foot pronation, tibial rotation, and patellofemoral stress.

e. Patellar mobility: Especially mobilizing medially

4. **External support**

a. A patellar stabilizing brace can help to align the patella, especially with a lateral buttress or pad.

b. Simple knee sleeve or strap has been advocated for patellar or quadriceps tendinitis.

c. Patellar strapping has been advocated by McConnell to correct very specific malalignment of the patella, allow for movement and exercise in a pain-free range, and help to stretch tight lateral structures. With strapping, be sure to check rotation, tilt, and glide of patella and adjust strapping accordingly.

5. **Physical therapy modalities** to help facilitate exercises and strength
   a. **Electrical muscle stimulation** used over the VMO to facilitate strengthening. It has been shown that active contraction is the best way to build strength, but active contraction with concurrent electrical stimulation can help with weak muscles better than active contraction alone.
   b. **Electromyographic (EMG) feedback** can increase VMO output in an exercise or training session and can carry over to functional activities such as stairs, squats, coming to standing from sitting, etc.

C. **Functional or return to activity stage**
   1. **Continue with strengthening**—Incorporate not only quadriceps but entire lower extremity.
   2. **Continue with stretching of entire lower extremity.**
   3. **Incorporate endurance training** that does not increase patellofemoral symptoms.
      a. Swimming (i.e., flutter kick, side stroke)
      b. Bicycling: Start with a seat position that allows for nearly full extension at the bottom of the cycle to minimize knee flexion at the top of the cycle.
      c. Walk-jog regimen that begins with walking and gradually introduces jogging in increasing increments.
      d. Stairclimbing machines can be added as an advanced activity as long as the patient remains asymptomatic.
   4. **Proprioceptive training**, such as balance boards, improves the transition back into activities.
   5. **Strengthening and closed kinetic chain:** Activities that incorporate quadriceps strengthening with the foot on the ground as in partial squats as tolerated, short step-ups and step-downs, terminal knee extension with the foot fixed. It is significant in a closed kinetic chain that the function of one portion of the system (i.e., foot) directly affects the remaining parts (i.e., knee and hip). Forces, if abnormal, are absorbed into other tissues. These forces include:
      a. Abnormal foot function: e.g., increased pronation will cause increased internal tibial rotation, increased Q-angle causing muscles to contract longer and out of phase.
      b. Pelvic involvement with change in leg length will cause change in foot (pronation/supination) or change in total extremity position.
      c. Soft tissue dynamics—strength—flexibility
   6. **Use of EMG in functional activities** helps to increase VMO output and patello-femoral stability.
   7. **Agility drills** as tolerated
   8. **Biomechanical corrections** if needed, such as recommending appropriate shoewear or orthotics for return to sports

V. **SURGERY**

Rarely, a patient does not respond to conservative treatment and may be a surgical candidate. Surgery involves loosening tight lateral retinaculum or reduction of the Q-angle by moving the patellar tendon attachment medially.

VI. **SUMMARY**

One of the main goals in rehabilitation of patients with patellofemoral stress syndrome is to educate them on the problem and rehabilitation and to have them join in setting realistic goals. If they fully understand this, they can move more successfully from a painful state to a pain-free progression of rehabilitation and retraining. It is the judgment of the patient to stop or readjust when symptoms begin, to advance when appropriate, to ice if needed, and to commit to stretching and strengthening exercises.

With the patient being a key player in the rehabilitation., conservative management of patellofemoral stress syndrome has a much better likelihood of succeeding.

Pathology related to the patella is the primary source of knee pain. To minimize compressive loading of the patella, inherent to this syndrome, dynamic stabilization by contraction of the vastus medialis obliquus (VMO) is necessary. During the initial stages of rehabilitation, terminal extension exercises, quadriceps setting and straight leg raises are recommended. As the VMO strengthens and symptoms decrease, closed kinetic chain, multiple angle isometrics, and high-speed isokinetic exercises (submaximally to maximally) can be incorporated.

REFERENCES

1. American Academy of Orthopedic Surgeons: Athletic Training and Sports Medicine. Park Ridge, IL, AAOS, 1984.
2. Antich TJ, Brewster CE: Modifications of quadriceps femoris muscle during knee rehabilitation. Phys Ther 66:1246–1251, 1986.
3. Basmajian J: Muscles Alive: Their Functions, Revised by Electromyography. Baltimore, Williams & Wilkins, 1962.
4. Bentley G, Dowd G: Current concepts of etiology and treatment of chondromalacia patellae. Clin Orthop 189:209–228, 1984.
5. Carson W, James S, Larson R, et al: Patellofemoral disorders: Physical and radiographic evaluation. Clin Orthop 185:165–185, 1984.
6. Gould J, Davies G: Orthopedic and Sports Physical Therapy, vol 2. St. Louis, C.V. Mosby Co., 1985.
7. Hartsell HD: Electrical muscle stimulation and isometric exercise effects on selected quadriceps parameters. J Orthop Sports Phys Ther 8:203–209, 1986.
8. Landry G: Patellofemoral stress syndrome. A common but complex problem. Comprehen Ther 14:21–28, 1988.
9. McConnell J: The management of chrondromalacia patellae: A long-term solution. Aust J Physiother 32:215–223, 1986.
10. Shelton GL, Thiopen LK: Rehabilitation of patellofemoral dysfunction: A review of literature. J Orthop Sports Phys Ther 14:6, 1991.
11. Steadman JR: Nonoperative methods for patellofemoral problems. Am J Sports Med 7:374–375, 1979.
12. Subotnick SL: Biomechanics of the ankle. Presented at the American Physical Therapy Association Annual Meeting, Phoenix, June 1980.

Chapter 41: Back Pain in the Female Athlete

SUZANNE M. TANNER, MD

Lumbar pain is common, accounting for 5–8% of athletic injuries. Women and girls participating in diving, weightlifting, and gymnastics are at the greatest risk for incurring a low back injury. Presented in this chapter are a practical approach to the evaluation of low back pain and a treatment approach to speed an active female's return to sport.

I. PREDISPOSING CONDITIONS

Factors predisposing a female athlete to back injury are both intrinsic and extrinsic:
- A. **Growth spurt:** If the paraspinous tissues do not grow at the same rate as bone, the resultant tight lumbodorsal fascia and hamstrings stress the spine. Emphasis on maintaining flexibility during the adolescent growth phase will mitigate this situation.[2]
- B. **Training errors:** Abrupt increases in training intensity or frequency may precipitate or aggravate low back pain.
- C. **Improper technique:** Excessive lordosis in a dancer performing an arabesque, for example, may precipitate lumbar strain.
- D. **Poor equipment:** Improper bycycle fit, for example, may predispose a cyclist to low back pain.
- E. **Leg length inequality:** A discrepancy in leg length causes an unequal transmission of force across the spine during weight-bearing activities. A 1-cm or greater discrepancy is probably significant.
- F. **Poor fitness:** Strength of both the back extensor muscles and abdominal muscles is important since they support the spine, like guy wires supporting a telephone pole. Inflexibility of the hamstrings increases lumbar strain by accentuating lumbar lordosis. Tight hip flexor muscles limit pelvic movement and strain the lumbar spine.

II. DIAGNOSTIC CATEGORIES

Although a female athlete is exposed to minor trauma more frequently than a nonathlete, an athlete is generally in better physical condition with better development of supporting structures of the spine. Most back injuries in female athletes, therefore, are minor.

Specific entities are listed below, but the diagnosis of low back pain in athletes is complicated by the lack of specificity of pain in many cases.[4] Even if the specific structure injured is unidentifiable, the majority of cases of low back pain in female athletes resolve with conservative therapy.
- A. **Contusion:** Bruise.
- B. **Fracture:** Absence of neurologic deficit does not exclude lumbar spine fractures.
  1. Compression fracture of the vertebral body
  2. Comminuted fracture
  3. Fracture of the growth plate at the vertebral endplate
  4. Lumbar transverse process fracture
  5. Fracture of the spinous process
- C. **Sprain/Strain**
  1. **Sprain** is an injury to ligament; **strain** refers to inflammation, microtears, or tears of muscle or tendon. It is often difficult to differentiate the exact tissue injured.
  2. Mechanisms of sprain/strain:
     a. Acute injury

        b. Chronic or overuse injury
        c. Acute injury imposed on chronic injury[5]
    3. Natural history of these injuries suggests most are caused by lifting or twisting.
    4. Mild to moderate acute low back pain in female athletes usually heals quickly.
 D. **Lumbar facet irritation**
    1. Sports requiring repetitive forceful hyperextension of the lumbar spine place
        individuals at risk of irritating the posterior elements of the spine—e.g., gymnastics,
        diving, power-lifting, golf, tennis.
    2. Characteristic signs are:
        a. Local paralumbar tenderness
        b. Pain with lumbar hyperextension
        c. Buttock or back pain with straight leg raising
        d. Normal neurologic examination
 E. **Spondylolysis/Spondylolisthesis**
    1. **Spondylolysis** indicates fracture; **spondylolisthesis** indicates slippage.
    2. Spondylolysis is a bony defect of the pars interarticularis, usually at L5 verte-
        bra, and may progress to spondylolysis via anterior slippage of the vertebral
        body.
    3. In athletes, the lytic defect is thought to be due to repetitive hyperextension
        maneuvers—e.g., gymnastics, diving, weight-lifting.
    4. In skeletally immature athletes, especially those 9–14 years old, close observation
        for progression to and of spondylolisthesis is advised.[6]
 F. **Sacroiliac disorder**
    1. The sacroiliac joint is one of the largest, yet least mobile, articulations.
    2. Causes of pain include sudden trauma or repetitive microtrauma, such as in a
        runner with leg-length discrepancy.[5]
    3. Localized tenderness over the sacroiliac joint is characteristic.
 G. **Disc herniation**
    1. A focal protrusion of the nucleus pulposus through a defect in the annulus
        fibrosus, usually in the posterolateral portion
    2. Occur in regions of greatest mobility (e.g., L5–S1, L4–L5 levels)
    3. Usually precipitated by trauma, such as lifting a heavy object
    4. Neurologic deficits of lower extremity are usually, not always, found.
 H. **Tumor (spinal disorder simulating athletic injury)**
    1. Primary bone tumors, such as osteoid osteoma and osteoblastoma
    2. Metastatic disease

III. **DIAGNOSTIC TESTS**
    A thorough history and physical examination are usually more productive in determining
    a diagnosis and guiding treatment than are imaging techniques. Often, no specific
    anatomic defect is visible by imaging. The imaging techniques listed below may be
    considered in athletes with severe back pain, acute trauma, or failure to improve after
    several weeks of conservative therapy.
 A. **Radiographs**
    1. In adolescent and young adult females, plain films reveal abnormalities at a low
        rate.
    2. Standard anteroposterior, lateral, and oblique views deliver 11 rad, one of the
        highest doses of radiologic examinations in the gonadal area.[4] Radiation exposure
        during pregnancy is of particular concern.
    3. Oblique films are often necessary to identify a defect in the pars interarticularis
        (i.e., spondylolysis, which presents as a lytic defect, or increased density, in the
        "neck of the Scotty dog") (Fig. 1).
    4. Hyperextension and hyperflexion views may help assess the degree of vertebral
        movement in spondylolisthesis.

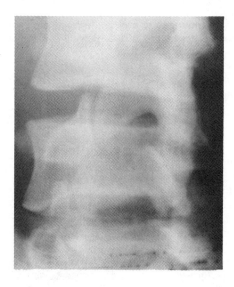 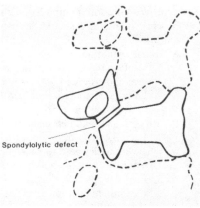

Spondylolytic defect

FIGURE 1.   The spondylolytic defect is seen as a collar on the Scotty dog's neck (pars interarticularis) on an oblique x-ray of lumbar spine. From Wilhite J, Huurman WW: Thoracic and lumbosacral spine. In Mellion MB, Walsh WM, Shelton GL (eds): Team Physician's Handbook. Philadelphia, Hanley & Belfus, 1990; with permission.

   B. **Bone scan** (SPECT scan)
      1. Sensitive modality for detecting spinal infection or malignancy or early spondylolysis.
      2. Although very sensitive, the test is nonspecific.
   C. **Computed tomography (CT)**
      1. Superior to radiographs in defining the extent of spinal fractures
      2. Disadvantages include high radiation dose, poor soft tissue visualization, and limited field of vision[4]
   D. **Magnetic resonance imaging (MRI)**
      1. Provides the most accurate morphologic evaluation of intervertebral discs[4]
      2. No radiation exposure
      3. Abnormalities on MRI must be closely correlated with clinical signs and symptoms, because a high incidence of bulging and degenerated discs is seen in even asymptomatic persons.[1]

IV. INITIAL TREATMENT

   A. **Goals of treatment during the acute phase are to reduce pain and swelling.**
   B. **Avoid strong analgesics,** except to induce sleep. If pain is masked by strong analgesics, the athlete may perform activities that further damage her back.
   C. **Antiinflammatory medications** and **application of ice** reduce swelling and pain. Ice should be applied for about 20 minutes intermittently during the first 48 hours post-injury.
   D. **Other means of pain controls** include microcurrent electrogalvanic nerve stimulation, transcutaneous nerve stimulation, and trigger point injections.
   E. Except for some fractures and severe spondylolisthesis, **complete immobilization is unnecessary.** If bedrest is recommended, it should be limited to 1 day to avoid promoting muscle atrophy and stiffness.

V. REHABILITATION

Goals are to restore motion, strength, and endurance of back and abdominal muscles. General conditioning should be maintained during this period. Rehabilitation should address:

A. Range of motion

1. Gentle passive or active range-of-motion exercises may be started during the first several days after injury, if tolerated.
2. Later, a combination of heat application and stretching may be most beneficial in regaining flexibility.[3]

B. Strength and muscular endurance

1. Exercises may often be started several days after injury. Abdominal as well as back muscles need to be strengthened.
2. Isometric, isotonic, and isokinetic exercises may be used singly or in combination.
3. Pool therapy is less stressful than similar exercises performed on land.
4. Flexion or extension exercises may be recommended first, depending on which is least painful. Flexion exercises may aggravate acute disc herniation, and extension exercises are contraindicated initially in spondylolysis, spondylolisthesis, and facet joint irritation.
5. Later, flexion and extension exercises may be gradually advanced by adding exercises, increasing repetitions performed, and increasing resistance applied to achieve a ratio of 1.3 to 1.0 for back extensor strength to flexor strength.[3]

C. Aerobic capacity

1. Should be performed when resistance exercises are started, to help maintain good cardiorespiratory fitness and improve spinal stabilization.
2. Limit sessions to 20 min/day initially if longer sessions are painful.
3. Walking, pool walking or running, upright cycling on a stationary cycle, and stair-stepping are usually tolerated initially. Add running, swimming, cycling, and cross-country skiing as symptoms subside.
4. Rotatory sports with quick starts and stops (tennis, racquetball) are tolerated last.

VI. PSYCHOLOGIC COUNSELING

Athletes with injuries severe enough to limit sports participation are likely to show shock, disbelief, and denial regarding the extent of their injury. They may have difficulty initially in trusting the physician and may be in a rush to return to sports. The skilled practitioner should help the athlete set and achieve realistic goals.

VII. CONCLUSION

Health care providers of active women and girls have ample opportunity to treat lumbar pain. Although the specific diagnosis of the cause of back pain may be difficult to determine, most back injuries in athletes resolve easily. By eliminating predisposing conditions, starting treatment promptly, and conducting progressive rehabilitation, most female athletes will return to the playing field rapidly.

REFERENCES

1. Boden SD, Davis DO, Dina TS, et al: Abnormal magnetic resonance scans of the lumbar spine in asymptomatic subjects. J Bone Joint Surg 72A(3):1990.
2. Clancy WG: Symposium: Low back pain in athletes. Am J Sports Med 7:361–368, 1979.
3. Maxwell C, Spiegel A: The rehabilitation of athletes following spinal injuries. In Hochschuler SH (ed): The Spine in Sports. Philadelphia, Hanley & Belfus, 1990.
4. Pelz DM: Radiologic investigation of low back pain. Can Med Assoc J 140:289–295, 1989.
5. Triano JJ, Hyde TE: Nonsurgical treatment of sports-related spine injuries: II. Manipulation. In Hochschuler SH (ed): The Spine in Sports. Philadelphia, Hanley & Belfus, 1990.
6. Wiltse LL, Widell EH, Hackson DW: Fatigue fracture: The bone lesion in isthmic spondylolisthesis. J Bone Joint Surg 57:17–22, 1974.

Chapter 42: Stress Fractures in Athletes

CAROL L. OTIS, MD

Stress fractures are a common overuse injury to bone with a complex, multifactorial etiology. Currently accepted concepts about the multiple causes of stress fracture contrast with the previously held notion that stress fractures were simply the result of overtraining. Among the factors that may contribute to stress fractures are bone health, menstrual status, biomechanics, physical and emotional stress, running surface, and an athlete's training program. Collaboration among sports medicine experts is essential to determine the causes and mechanisms of stress fractures, to evaluate an athlete's risk of sustaining such an injury, and to properly direct rehabilitation efforts.

I. **HISTORY**
   A. The first descriptions of probable stress fractures predate radiography. Foot pain and swelling was described in 1855 by Briethaupt in unconditioned Prussian military recruits during basic training.[14] The **"march fracture,"** a stress fracture of the metatarsals, was identified by radiography in the 1890s. They remain a problem in military populations, especially during basic training.
   B. **Athletic stress fractures** are a different syndrome. They were first described in athletes in the 1950s. Etiology is multifactorial and requires assessing the health of the athlete as a whole.

II. **EPIDEMIOLOGY**
   A. Stress fractures are a common injury, representing up to 10% of all sports injuries.[22]
   B. **Runners** are most likely of all athletes to sustain a stress fracture, in whom this accounts for 5–15% of all injuries.[22]
   C. Incidence and location vary according to sport and training. Some stress fractures are felt to be sport-specific, such as a stress fracture of the humerus in a baseball pitcher and multiple stress fractures of the ribs in golfers.[17]

III. **SIGNIFICANCE**
   A. Stress fractures are an aggravating injury occurring in otherwise healthy athletes at their peak of training and conditioning.
   B. Slow onset of pain and disability
   C. Usually there is no significant trauma.
   D. Often, there is a delay in diagnosis:
      1. Plain radiographs are normal initially.
      2. Further tests (bone scan) may be required to make a definitive diagnosis.
      3. Cost and inconvenience may keep an athlete from having a bone scan initially.
   E. They cause the athlete to lose significant time from sports to heal the fracture, then regain training and competitive fitness. Up to a year of rehabilitation and training may be required.
   F. There is no nationwide effort to monitor the incidence of stress fractures among athletes.[14]

IV. **MECHANISM OF INJURY**

   Wolff's Law states that bone constantly remodels to the stress placed on it in predictable patterns.[31]

A. **Force** is transmitted to bone, either compressive or tensile, generating a *stress (force/area)*.

B. **Deformation of bone** is defined by change in length which is defined as *strain* (strain = *deformation*/length).

C. Bone has **elastic properties** that permit it to return to its original configuration after being deformed.

D. A linear relationship exists between stress and strain until **yield strength** is reached (slope of curve = modiolus of elasticity). Beyond this yield strength, bone is irreversibly deformed until breaking point. At **breaking point,** bone is compressed or torn apart in tension,[10] resulting in micro- or macrofractures depending on the amount of stress and strain applied.

E. Repetitive small loads can cause a stress fracture. Repetitive loads that exceed the "critical limit of adaption" result in microfractures. Loads are additive. Estimates of number of cycles or loads required to cause a stress fracture vary depending on the type of bone, maturation of bone, surrounding musculature and other supporting structures, and time between loads (to allow bone repair).

V. TYPES OF FORCE

Multiple dynamic forces are applied to living tissues (compression, tension, rotation) by tendons, ligaments, and muscles. When a long bone is bent, compressive forces are applied on one side and tension forces on the other.

A. **Bone is weaker in tension** (tearing apart). Fractures from *tension* (electropositive force, osteoclastic activity) occur at cement lines of the Haversian system and along osteon.

B. **Compression forces generate greater cellular damage** (electronegative force, osteoblastic activity) and result in diffuse shear microfractures (e.g., calcaneus).

C. **Rotary forces apply tension to all parts** of the bone's column at the surface.

VI. ETIOLOGIC THEORIES

A. **Mechanical theories**

1. Muscle weakness/fatigue may reduce shock absorption potential of bone.[20]

2. Shearing forces from muscles may be transmitted to bone (e.g., humerus of a pitcher).

3. Ground reaction forces—kinetic loads—applied unevenly to bone may overload a specific area of bone, resulting in an inability of that area to adapt.[7]

4. High loading rate due to a high number of repetitions may prevent the bone from daily maintenance and repair.

5. In animal models of stress fracture, the **remodeling** of bone (osteoclasts resorb) predominates over **repair** (osteoblasts reform and construct new bone). The continuum of bone remodeling to bone repair and reformation is interrupted by continued stress/strain. Microstructure of bone is temporarily weakened during initial remodeling, when bone resorption around the Haversian canals is greater than bone formation. Small cracks appear and may propagate. Increased vascularization occurs across the remodeling site. There exists vulnerable area of bone; if stress continues to be applied, then breakdown occurs at this site.

B. **Anthropomorphic theories**

1. Theoretically, although **body dimensions and configuration** could also contribute to stress fracture risk, there are no prospective studies that confirm the potential links between anthropometry and stress fractures. Nevertheless, some proposed factors include:

   a. Shorter individuals may be more prone to stress fractures because their shorter stride length results in more impacts per distance run.

   b. Limited external hip rotation may alter the alignment of the lower extremity, resulting in an inappropriate distribution of forces to bones below the hip.[6]

    c. Foot type (e.g., rigid or pronated foot)[22] or forefoot varus and decreased dorsiflexion[12] may result in an abnormal load distribution.

  2. Despite these numerous hypotheses, the variability and lack of interobserver reliability of these measures limit the usefulness of doing similar prospective anthropomorphic measurements to predict risk.[24] Further research and standardization of methodology are needed.

  3. One **structural factor** that is highly correlated to stress fracture incidence among military recruits is the distribution of bone in the tibia.[23] Measured from tibial radiographs, the tibial area moment of inertia (distribution of bone relative to a bending axis) predicts 92% of stress fractures during the first year of military training in male recruits. This factor has not yet been studied in athletic populations. Preliminary results in a small sample of collegiate women athletes do not support this correlation.[32]

C. **Training theories**

  1. Many experts believe that the repetitive, cyclic loading of bone during heavy training is a major contributor to stress fracture—basically, the notion of "too much, too soon." The nature of the training surface, type of activity, dramatic changes in training intensity, and the speed, distance, and intensity of the training sessions are suspected facets of a training program that place an athlete at risk. Running on concrete surfaces more than two-thirds of the training time, running greater than 32 km/week, and a prior injury history were predictors of lower-extremity injuries in recreational runners in prospective studies.[18,19]

  2. Factors include:

    a. Nature of the training surface

    b. Type of activity

    c. Dramatic changes in training intensity

    d. Speed, distance, intensity of training sessions

    e. Equipment: shoes, devices (orthotics), taping

    f. Level of preseason conditioning may predict stress fracture as it does in other overuse injuries.

  3. Some types of stress fractures appear to be **sport-specific,** caused by the repetitive loads due to type of activity. Fracture is more likely to occur in the part of the body exposed the most to cyclic loads:

    a. Runners—Tibia/fibula/metatarsals

    b. Baseball pitchers—Humerus

    c. Basketball—Os calcis, tarsal navicular

D. **Bone health theories**

  1. The tendency to sustain a stress fracture may be related, at least in part, to an individual's bone mineralization. This bone health theory postulates that osteoporosis (relative lack of bone mineral content due to any cause) may be a cofactor in stress fracture risk.[25]

  2. **Stress fracture** in athletes are thought to be due to abnormal repetitive cyclic loading to a localized area of normal bone beyond its capability to handle these loads.

  3. **Insufficiency fractures** are caused by normal stresses applied to abnormal bone (osteoporosis). In evaluating stress fractures in athletes, factors contributing to osteoporosis may coexist in athletes and should be considered. They include:

    a. Nutrition

      i. Inadequate calcium intake below RDA of 1000 mg/day is common in all women in the U.S.

      ii. Eating disorders have been correlated retrospectively to stress fractures in women athletes in one published study.[1]

    b. Body composition: Low body mass index correlates to low bone density.[3]

    c. Estrogen deficiency at any age lowers bone mass.[3]

      i. Amenorrhea[4]
     ii. Delayed menarche[29]
    iii. Lower rates of oral contraceptive use[25]
    iv. History of irregular menses[3]

  d. Many correlations between amenorrhea or other menstrual irregularities and stress fractures are reported in the literature, but are not conclusive because studies on bone mass and stress fractures have been done retrospectively. Conflicting results from current studies may be due to small sample size, measurement of regional bone mass instead of total bone mass, differences in external loading kinetics, or differences in tibial morphology.[7,21,25]

  e. Delayed puberty in men results in osteopenia.[5] Male runners have been reported with hormone disorders.

  f. Immobilization after prior injury may cause regional bone loss. This is unlikely in athletes unless a severe injury requiring cast or crutches occurs. Could prior fractures predispose?

  g. Metabolic bone disease (increased parathyroid hormone, osteomalacia) may be coexistent in athletes.

  h. Corticosteroid usage

  i. Hyperthyroidism causes loss of bone mineral content.

  4. **More research needed on bone mass and stress fracture risk:**
    a. Is low bone density from any cause a predictor of stress fracture risk?
    b. Should we train individuals with low bone density differently?
    c. Is the euestrogenic state protective?
    d. How and when should bone mass be measured?
    e. Is regional bone mass reliable?
    f. Do athletes have higher bone mass, total vs regional?
    g. Are there differences in bone mass due to training, weight-lifting, genetic, racial, nutritional factors?

VII. PSYCHOLOGIC STRESS AND INJURY

Psychologic factors such as level of perceived stress or life changes[9] and prior incidence of injury[15] may be significant contributors to injury prediction. Emotional stress related to life events may trigger a systemic response, such as an increase in serum glucocorticoids, that influence bone health.[2] Prior injury has been correlated to risk of future injury, via an unknown mechanism.[15]

VIII. DIAGNOSIS

  A. Have a **high index of suspicion** of stress fracture
  B. **History**
    1. Look for an individual doing "too much, too soon," or a recent change in activity such as occurs when an athlete changes schools or coaches or enters intense training.
    2. Any change in speed, distance, surface, intensity, or hills may be a clue.
    3. Shoes (new or old, or design change), increased jumping.
  C. **Symptoms**
    1. Pain of stress fractures generally has a gradual onset with crescendo during activity. Pain is usually localized, rarely diffuse, and resolves with rest or sleep. If there is night pain, rule out osteoid osteoma.
    2. Occasionally pain is described as deep aching (humerus) or foot cramping (tarsal navicular).
    3. Change in gait due to pain may be a clue.
  D. **Differential diagnosis**
    1. Periostitis
    2. Tendinitis

3. Postexertional compartment syndrome
4. Popliteal artery entrapment syndrome
5. True fracture
6. Osteomyelitis
7. Underlying bone cyst or tumor (osteoid osteoma)

E. **Physical examination**
1. Localized pain
2. Pain worse with ultrasound
3. Palpable overlying swelling and edema
4. Bone percussion may lead to transmission of pain to fracture site.
5. Pain elicited when the athlete performs the **hop test** (the athlete jumps up-and-down on the affected limb) is suggestive of a stress fracture.
6. Always have high index of suspicion for upper extremity, pelvic and femoral stress fracture

F. **Radiology**
1. In plain films, detection depends on the continuum of injury in which the x-ray is taken—i.e., the fracture will be visible only in specific positions of the injured part. Plain films are insensitive, but very specific when abnormality is found.
2. The appearance of radiolucency on the bone surface with hazy "cortical crack" may sometimes appear.[14]
3. Periosteal reaction of new bone formation or endosteal thickening occurs at approximately 6 weeks.
4. Callus formation as the bone heals
5. Consider tomograms for bones in which a stress fracture is difficult to detect, i.e., tarsal navicular.

G. **Bone scan**
1. Technetium-99 diphosphonate is incorporated by osteoblast in the physiologic process of new bone formation. There can be positive bone scans in non-stress-fracture cases, as the bone normally remodels as it reacts to the loads, or if another condition is present such as osteomyelitis or bone tumor.
2. Usually the scan is positive within days of onset of pain.
3. There exists a continuum of findings.[14,27] Diffuse uptake indicates stress reaction. Sharp margins to uptake are found in true fractures compared to the diffuse uptake seen in "stress reactions."
4. Linear uptake, in a long pattern, is more likely to be tendinitis.
5. All three phases of triple-phase bone scan[28] are positive in stress fractures. SPECT scanning may increase sensitivity.
6. Differential diagnosis: bone cysts, osteomyelitis, periostitis, tendinitis, "stress reaction."

IX. **TREATMENT**

A. **Phase I:** 2–6 weeks
1. Pain control
   a. Physiotherapy
   b. Nonsteroidal antiinflammatory drugs (NSAIDs)
   c. Ice, massage
   d. Transcutaneous electrical nerve stimulation (TENS)
2. Avoid ultrasound which makes the pain worse.
3. Control activity to allow the bone to heal.
   a. Modified rest
   b. Muscle strengthening
   c. Flexibility
   d. Nonimpact aerobic conditioning (swimming, stationary bicycling); avoid stair-climbing, stepping exercises

B. **Phase II:** 4–8 weeks
    1. After the athlete is pain-free 10–14 days with activities of daily living:
        a. Continue muscle strengthening
        b. Flexibility
        c. Aerobic conditioning
        d. Begin a gradual introduction of sport activities according to pain
        e. Add sports on alternate days—e.g., run 10 minutes on flat grass surface
        f. Correct underlying risk factors, such as surface, shoes, amenorrhea, nutrition
        g. Next, begin a trial of cyclic training, 2 weeks on/1 week off (or less)

C. **Recovery issues**
    1. **Rest** is required for 4–8 weeks as is true for most fractures. Firm-soled shoes for activities of daily living may minimize pain of metatarsal stress fractures.
    2. Longer rest periods may be needed for certain fractures such as tarsal navicular, femur, or pelvis.
    3. **Immobilization (casting)** is not recommended for most.
    4. Avoidance of **weight-bearing** is required for certain fractures, especially those of the femoral neck, as they may progress to a complete fracture and require surgical pins.
    5. Maintain aerobic fitness.
    6. Aircast? One study has found it beneficial.[30]

D. **Evaluate and correct underlying imbalances.**
    1. Consider orthotics
    2. Muscle balance and strengthening
    3. Stretching and flexibility
    4. Limb-length discrepancy
    5. Evaluation of shoes, surface, training

E. **Medical evaluation for bone health** (*see* Chapters 21 and 22)
    1. Amenorrhea: Do full workup for cause.[26] Consider estrogen replacement.
    2. Oligomenorrhea: Do full workup.
    3. Nutrition: Assure adequate calcium, protein, and caloric intake.
    4. Body composition testing may be indicated.
    5. The presence of eating disorders should be assessed (*see* Chapters 13 and 20).
    6. Rule out hyperthyroidism and metabolic bone disease.
    7. Consider bone density evaluation.[13] Know the accuracy of techniques at your institution. Measure trabecular bone (lumbar spine and femoral neck).
        a. Dual photon absorptiometry (DPA)
        b. Quantitative computed tomography (QCT)
        c. Dual-energy x-ray absorptiometry (DEXA)
        d. Total bone mass vs regional bone mass may be the measurement of the future.

F. **Special problem areas**
    1. Tarsal navicular: Hard to diagnose, slow in healing
    2. Femoral neck: May go on to complete fracture
    3. Pubic rami
    4. Anterior tibial: May progress to nonunion
    5. Fifth metatarsal: May not heal
    6. Nonunion stress fractures (anterior tibia, fifth metatarsal) may require surgery, bone grafts, placement of rods, pinning, or prolonged rest.

X. PREVENTION

Begin in preseason to instruct athletes in proper training, proper rehabilitation of prior injuries, and correction of underlying imbalances. Emphasize gradual increase in the "dose" of training.

A. **Training**
    1. "Cyclic"—2 weeks hard, 1 week easy—has been tried in military populations.

    2. Nonimpact alternate training.

    3. Encourage appropriate rest days.

B. **Surface**

    1. Avoid concrete at least two-thirds of the time.[19] Look for grass, sand, bark trails.

    2. Evaluate the floor of gyms and aerobic studios for adequate cushioning.

C. **Shoes:** Footwear should be appropriate for type of activity. Running shoes lose their midsole cushioning after 200 miles.

D. **Strength and flexibility:** A balance of strength and flexibility is important, especially in athletes returning from injury.

    1. Do eccentric and concentric training of lower extremity.

    2. Emphasize anterior tibial muscles, which are usually neglected.

E. Consider correcting underlying **biomechanical factors** if an individual has had prior injuries.

F. **Menstrual status:** Athlete should be euestrogenic. Consider hormone replacement for amenorrheic athletes.

G. **Maximize nutritional status:** Calcium 1000–1500 mg/day.

H. **Watch for early warning signs.** Advise athletes to report and treat overuse injuries early. Use ice whirlpool after the hardest training.

I. **Educate about risks** of eating disorders, amenorrhea and their link to osteoporosis (female athlete triad).

REFERENCES

1. Barrow GW, Saha S: Menstrual irregularity and stress fracture in collegiate female distance runners. Am J Sports Med 16:209–215, 1988.
2. Ding JH, Sheckter CB, Drinkwater BL, et al: High serum cortisol levels in exercise-associated amenorrhea. Ann Intern Med 108:530–534, 1988.
3. Drinkwater BL, Bruemner B, Chestnut CH: Menstrual history as a determinant of current bone density in young athletes. JAMA 263:545–548, 1990.
4. Drinkwater BL, Nilson K, Chestnut CH, et al: Bone mineral content of amenorrheic and eumenorrheic athletes. N Engl J Med 311:277–281, 1984.
5. Finkelstein JS, et al: Osteopenia in men with a history of delayed puberty. N Engl J Med 326:600–604, 1992.
6. Giladi M, et al: External rotation of hip: A predictor of risk for stress fractures. Clin Orthop 218:131–134, 1987.
7. Grimston SK, et al: Bone mass, external loads, and stress fractures in female runners. Int J Sport Biomech 7:293–302, 1991.
8. Grimston SK, Engsberg JR, Kloiber R, Hanley DA: Menstrual, calcium and training history: Relationship to bone health in female runners. Clin Sports Med 2:199–228, 1990.
9. Hardy C: An examination of life stress-injury relationship. Behav Med (Fall):113–118, 1988.
10. Hershman EB, Mailly T: Stress fractures. Clin Sports Med 9:183–214, 1990.
11. Holmes TH, Rahe RH: The social readjustment scale. J Psychosom Res 2:213–218, 1967.
12. Hughes L: Biomechanical analysis of the foot and ankle for predisposition to developing stress fractures. J Orthop Sports Phys Ther 7:96–101, 1985.
13. Johnston CC Jr, et al: Clinical use of bone densitometry. N Engl J Med 324:1105–1109, 1991.
14. Jones BH, Harris JM, Vinh TN, Rubin C: Exercise-induced stress fractures and stress reactions of bone: Epidemiology, etiology and classification. Exerc Sports Sci Rev 17:379–422, 1989.
15. Kraus J, Conroy C: Mortality and morbidity from injuries in sport. Annu Rev Public Health 5:3–92, 1984.
16. Lloyd T, Myers C, Buchanan JR, Demers LM: Collegiate women athletes with irregular menses during adolescence have decreased bone density. Obstet Gynecol 72:639–642, 1988.
17. Lord MJ, Carson W: Multiple rib stress fractures. Phys Sports Med 21(5):81–91, 1993.
18. Macera CA: Lower extremity injuries in runners: Advances in prediction. Sports Med 13:50–57, 1992.
19. Macera CA, Pare RR, Powell KE, et al: Predicting lower extremity injuries among habitual runners. Arch Intern Med 149:2565–2568, 1989.
20. Markey KL: Stress fractures. Clin Sports Med 6:405–425, 1987.
21. Martin AD, Bailey DA: Review: Skeletal integrity in amenorrheic athletes. Aust J Sci Med Sports 19:3–7, 1987.

22. Matheson GO, Clement DB, McKenzie DC, et al: Stress fractures in athletes: A study of 320 cases. Am J Sports Med 15:46–58, 1987.
23. Milgrom C, Giladi M, Simkin A, et al: The area moment of inertia of the tibia: A risk factor for stress fractures. J Biomech 22:1243–1248, 1989.
24. Montgomery LC, Nelson FR, Norton JP, Deuster PA: Orthopedic history and examination in the etiology of overuse injuries. Med Sci Sports Exerc 21:237–243, 1989.
25. Myburgh KH, Hutchins J, Fataar AB, et al: Low bone density is an etiologic factor for stress fractures in athletes. Ann Intern Med 113:754–759, 1990.
26. Otis CL: Exercise-associated amenorrhea. Clin Sports Med 11:351–362, 1992.
27. Roub LW, Rupani HD: Bone stress. Radiology 132:431–438, 1979.
28. Rupani, et al: Three phases of radionuclide bone imaging in sports medicine. Radiology 156:187–196, 1985.
29. Warren MP, Brooks-Gunn J, Hamilton LH, et al: Scoliosis and fractures in young ballet dancers: Relation to delayed menarche and secondary amenorrhea. N Engl J Med 314:1348–1353, 1986.
30. Whitelaw GP, et al: A pneumatic brace for treatment of tibial stress fractures. Clin Orthop 270:301–305, 1991.
31. Woo SL, Kuei SC, Amiel D, et al: The effect of prolonged physical training on the properties of long bone: A study of Wolff's law. J Bone Joint Surg 63A:780–786, 1981.
32. Zernicke RF, McNitt-Gray J, Otis C, et al: Stress fracture risk assessment among elite collegiate women runners [abstract]. Presented at the International Society of Biomechanics Meeting, July 1993.

Chapter 43: Heat and Cold

PAMELA FOYSTER, RN

I. HEAT ILLNESS

Heat illness is a potentially life-threatening spectrum of physiologic responses to hot environments. Heat stroke is the third most common cause of death in athletes.[2a]

A. Physiology

1. **Methods of gaining body heat**
   a. Radiant heat from sun
   b. Dehydration
   c. Exertion
   d. Increased metabolism in cooling process
   e. Humid climates reduce the effectiveness of the body's cooling mechanism.

2. **Methods for losing body heat**
   a. Radiation, as long as ambient air temperature is lower than skin temperature
   b. Evaporation is the body's best heat loss mechanism when air temperature approaches 95° F.
   c. Convective heat dissipation improves with mild wind, but ceases when air temperature exceeds skin temperature. Greater ambient temperature negates the temperature gradient from core to skin to air.
   d. Air conduction is a weak cooling mechanism, as air is a good insulator. Water is highly conductive and a rapid cooling tool.

3. **Physiologic responses to heat**
   a. Peripheral cutaneous vasodilation increases surface area to promote cooling. It is compensated for by intense splanchnic vessel vasoconstriction to maintain blood pressure. However, cutaneous dilatation will exceed the available compensation, promoting hypotension.
   b. Increased sweating: As much as 1–2 L/hr with exertion. Dripping sweat is not effective toward lowering body temperature.
   c. Increased cardiac output. Stroke volume decreases and heart rate increases.
   d. Thermoregulatory control is believed to be contained in the anterior hypothalamus. It is the core temperature rather than skin temperature which denotes the severity of heat illness.

4. **Acclimatization response**
   a. Acclimatization to exercise in heat
      i. Can take up to 14 days
      ii. Requires increased fluid intake to promote plasma volume expansion and increased sweat rate of acclimatization[1]
      iii. Rate of acclimatization is related to VO_2max and previous training in a cool environment prior to heat exposure
   b. Acclimatization involves the cardiovascular, renal, endocrine, and exocrine systems.
   c. Although men have a higher metabolic rate and sweat twice as much as women before and after acclimatization, heat tolerance is similar for given performance level, equal physical condition, lean body mass, body surface area, and weight.[1,5]

B. **Minor heat-related illnesses**
  1. **Heat cramps**
     a. Can occur in heat-acclimatized individuals.
     b. Usually occurs in large muscle groups, such as legs, but abdominal muscles also commonly affected.
     c. Usually occurs after heavy exertion, when muscles are cooling.
     d. Persons have usually rehydrated with water only, and thus are hyponatremic in addition to being dehydrated.
     e. Treat slowly with water and electrolyte replacement based on body water deficit and electrolyte values. Salt tablets are not recommended.
  2. **Heat edema**
     a. Most common in nonacclimatized individuals
     b. More common in women and the elderly
     c. Usually limited to legs and feet
     d. Self-resolving with acclimatization
  3. **Heat syncope**
     a. Lightheadedness related to heat-induced hypovolemia, secondary to vasodilation
     b. Athlete should lie down in a cool place, legs slightly elevated. Give cold water.
     c. Educate on prevention: Adequate hydration, support hose if necessary, and avoiding long periods of standing.
C. **Heat exhaustion**
  1. **Types of heat exhaustion:** Both forms can be serious and usually present together.
     a. Sodium depletion, secondary to large amounts of plain water ingestion
     b. Water depletion, which can lead to heat stroke
  2. **Risk factors**
     a. Not acclimatized to heat
     b. Dehydration
     c. Fluid replacement does not include sodium.
  3. **Signs and symptoms**
     a. Flu-like symptoms: Weakness, malaise, poor appetite
     b. Temperature $<40°C$
     c. **No central nervous system disturbances**
     d. Patient is able to sweat.
     e. May be orthostatic due to dehydration, vasodilation
  4. **Treatment**
     a. Move patient to cool, shaded area.
     b. Perform a neurologic examination to differentiate from heat stroke.
     c. Rehydrate with oral and/or intravenous water, sodium, and glucose. Contents will depend on electrolytes and energy needs.
     d. Most nonelderly individuals will not require hospitalization. Elderly need to be monitored carefully for complications. Treat cautiously. They may require hospitalization.
  5. **Prevention**
     a. Wear light, loose clothing.
     b. Maintain adequate hydration with water and sodium.
     c. Avoid heavy exertion if not acclimatized.
D. **Heat stroke**
  1. **Pathophysiology**
     a. **Body unable to lose heat through two primary mechanisms of cooling: evaporation and radiation.**
     b. **Functional hypovolemia** due to failure of peripheral and splanchnic vessels to constrict and support blood pressure.

TABLE 1.   Severe Complications of Heat Stroke

Cardiovascular	Arrhythmias
	Myocardial infarction
	Pulmonary edema
Central nervous system	Cerebral and spinal infarction
	Coma
	Seizures
Gastrointestinal	Hepatocellular necrosis
	Upper gastrointestinal bleeding
Hematologic	Disseminated intravascular coagulation
	Metabolic lactic acidosis
Musculoskeletal	Rhabdomyolysis
	Myoglobinemia
Pulmonary	Adult respiratory distress syndrome
	Pulmonary infarction
Renal	Acute renal failure

From Mellion MB, Shelton GL: Safe exercise in the heat and heat injuries. In Mellion MB, Walsh WM, Shelton GL (eds): The Team Physician's Handbook. Philadelphia, Hanley & Belfus, 1990, with permission.

    c. **Hypoglycemia** occurs as a result of the body's attempt at cooling, as well as core temperature increase. The increased activity leading to exertional heat stroke will have also consumed a large amount of glucose.

    d. Heat, increased metabolism, and cellular changes decrease pH.

    e. **Complications** (Table 1)

        i. As organ dysfunction progresses, electrolyte imbalances occur.

        ii. Hepatic injury is a consistent component of heat stroke.

        iii. Renal failure is more common with exertional heat stroke, secondary to glomerular injury and acute tubular necrosis.

        iv. Coagulopathies and disseminated intravascular coagulation are most notable in severe heat stroke and are a poor prognostic indicator.

2. **Risk factors**

    a. Age extremes (children, the elderly)

    b. Skin disorders, including disease and burns, skin grafts

    c. Medical history, including cardiovascular disease, central nervous system disturbances, endocrine disorders, alcohol abuse

    d. Medications, including anticholinergics, diuretics, antihypertensives, antipsychotics, antidepressants, salicylates

    e. Athletes, nonacclimatized persons (Heat stroke is the third leading cause of death in athletes, after spinal cord injury and heart failure.[2])

3. **Presentation**

    a. **General**

        i. Most significant observable difference between heat exhaustion and heat stroke is **central nervous system changes:** disorientation, vomiting, coma, convulsion, agitation, ataxia.

        ii. **Febrile.** Rectal temperature $>40°$ C (tympanic readings are more indicative of true core temperature if taken accurately). If the temperature is $<40^0$C, the body may still be trying to cool, but clinical presentation will define heat stroke.

        iii. Tachycardia, tachypnea, hypotension

        iv. Any heat stroke can be life-threatening.

        v. Skin can be moist or dry.

b. **Classic heat stroke**
   i. **Sweating may be present or absent.**
   ii. Multiple system involvements are absent to mild.
   iii. No physcial exertion required.
c. **Exertional heat stroke**
   i. Occurs in young, healthy, active individuals. Common among athletes, men more often than women.
   ii. Results from strenuous exercise in persons not acclimatized to hot environment.
   iii. Sweating can be present or absent.
   iv. Multiple system involvement

4. **Treatment**
   a. **Heat stroke is a medical emergency and is not spontaneously reversible.** It progresses to cardiovascular and nervous system collapse without proper intervention.
   b. **Field**
      i. **Move to cool, shaded area.**
      ii. Remove clothing.
      iii. **Warm or cool water mist** to promote evaporative heat loss, which is the body's most effective cooling method. **Gentle breeze or fan** if possible.
      iv. Nothing by mouth
      v. Cold packs to groin and axilla (but evaporative cooling more important)
      vi. Avoid causing shivering (it raises body temperature and consumes glucose).
      vii. **Evacuate to medical facility as soon as possible.**
   c. **Hospital**
      i. **Rapid cooling takes priority over all other interventions.** Damage is a consequence of the level of core temperature elevation and length of hyperthermia. Rapid cooling reduces complications and promotes optimal outcome.
      ii. Most effective are noninvasive cooling methods such as mists with gentle fanning breeze. Cool water immersion can reduce core temperature to 40°C. Avoid rebound hypothermia.
      iii. Treat shivering and convulsions which may be brought on by treatment modalities.
      iv. Monitor electrolytes, liver function tests, coagulation values, electrocardiogram, arterial blood gases, hemodynamics, ethanol level, fluid balance.
      v. Aspirin and acetaminophen are not effective and may exacerbate existing coagulopathies. Aspirin may paradoxically raise body temperature.

5. **Prevention**
   a. Medical history and evaluation to identify those at risk
   b. Risk factor correction (acclimatization, conditioning)
   c. Weather conditions: High heat and humidity limit the body's ability to dissipate heat.
   d. Reschedule workouts to avoid heat stress, or alter workout to decrease intensity and duration and to add more frequent breaks (Fig. 1).
   e. Wear cool, loose clothing.
   f. Change in body weight of 3–5% from pre-exercise levels suggests caution. Weight loss may indicate dehydration.
   g. Maintain adequate hydration as well as electrolyte intake via food (not just water).

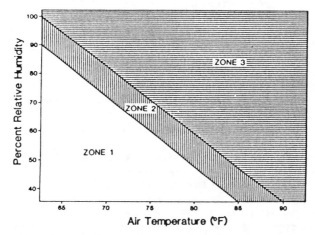

FIGURE 1. Heat Stress Danger Chart. Environmental conditions in **zone 1** are fairly safe for participation. Normal heat stress precautions should be taken. In **zone 2**, moderate heat stress precautions should be taken. Workouts should be less intense, shorter, and with more frequent fluid breaks. In **zone 3**, heat stress danger is at its greatest. Workouts should be rescheduled to a cooler part of the day. Workouts should be relatively easy. Light clothing should be worn. Extra fluids for everyone and close observation for early heat injury symptoms are essential. (Adapted from Fox EL, Mathews DK: The Physiological Basis of Physical Education and Athletics, 3rd ed. Philadelphia, Saunders College Publishing, 1981.)

II. HYPOTHERMIA

Although not often documented as a primary diagnosis, accidental hypothermia is believed to be more common than statistics illustrate, with the highest rates being in inner cities. This condition can also occur among athletes who are exposed to cold for long periods of time, such as skiers, runners, hikers, or long-distance swimmers, or climbers.

A. **Definition:** Hypothermia is an acute or chronic cooling of the body's core temperature to <35°C. Factors such as environment, caloric intake, clothing, fitness, and rest all contribute to the level of impairment. Hypothermia is both a symptom and clinical diagnosis.[15] Unlike heat acclimatization, the human body has no true adaptive ability for cold other than mental tolerance. There are always physiologic responses and consequences when core temperature is threatened.

B. **Types of heat loss**[15]
  1. **Radiant:** Accounts for 65% of heat loss. Can be inhibited with appropriate clothing.
  2. **Evaporative:** In a mild environment, it accounts for 20–30% of heat loss. Can be increased by wet clothing, dry cold air, and wind on exposed skin. High-altitude environments combine all elements.
  3. **Convection:** Can account for 15% of heat loss. Greatest losses occur in moving air and water.
  4. **Conduction:** Possible for 15% of heat loss. Water is a strong conductor, as are ice, snow, rock, and wet clothing.

C. **Risk factors**
  1. Large body-surface-to-mass ratio, as found in women, children, and tall thin adults
  2. Medical conditions, such as endocrine disorders, dermatologic dysfunction, and others
  3. Alcohol use
  4. Poor nutrition and dehydration
  5. Individuals with low body fat percentage

    D. **Gender differences:** Studies of men's and women's cooling rates, metabolic responses, and thermoregulatory responses to cold environments (air or water) show a variety of responses.

        1. Although women have a lower resting metabolic rate, less muscle mass (to generate heat), and greater body-surface-area-to-mass ratio, no gender-specific absolutes exist to compare cooling rates.

        2. In the prevention and treatment of hypothermia, the same general rules apply to all. Basal metabolism and metabolic response to cold are individual and of greater importance in cold injury and illness than gender.[13,23,24]

    E. **Pathophysiology** (Table 2)

        1. **Initially, skin cools and peripheral vessels constrict to limit heat loss.** Cooled blood remains in the periphery to protect core temperature.

        2. **Shivering will initially increase metabolic rate** 5–10 times (10-fold increase with exercise), thereby increasing metabolic heat production. This also increases oxygen demand and convective heat loss. The severely hypothermic patient does not have the glucose available to generate heat or to drive other metabolic processes.

        3. Initial **cold-induced diuresis** will create hypovolemia.

        4. Initially, there is a catecholamine response that shuts off at 29°C, followed by steady decline in all functions: heart rate, respiratory rate, muscle strength and coordination, reflexes.

        5. Other physiologic attempts at heat production include the release of adrenocorticoids, insulin (ineffective in severe hypothermia), and thyrotropin (which leads to an increase in thyroxine release).

        6. **Oxygen utilization**

           a. Decreased oxygen demand with progressive cooling

           b. Initially there is respiratory alkalosis, due to hyperventilation. This progresses to respiratory and metabolic acidosis, as hypoxic tissues convert to anaerobic metabolism.

TABLE 2. Abbreviated Stages of Hypothermia

Stage	Core Temperature °C	°F	Signs and Symptoms
Mild	36	96.8	Shivering, decreased fine motor skills, sensation of being cold, increased metabolism
	34	93.2	Amnesia, dysarthria, maximum respiratory rate, apathy, normotension
Moderate	32	89.6	Irrational behavior, more grossly uncoordinated, paradoxical undressing, shivering stops at 31°C/87.8°F
	30	86	Atrial fibrillation, poikilothermia, insulin ineffective, cardiac output $2/3$ normal
	28	82.4	Ventricular fibrillation threshold decreased
Severe	26	78.8	Loss of reflexes, major acid-base disturbances, no pain response
	25	77	Cerebral blood flow 33% normal; spontaneous atrioventricular fibrillation, pulmonary edema may develop.
	24	75.2	Significant hypotension
	22	71.6	Maximum potential for ventricular fibrillation
	18	64.4	Asystole
	16	60.8	Lowest adult accidental hypothermia survival
	15.2	59.4	Lowest infant accidental hypothermia survival

Adapted from Auerbach, Geehr,[12] and Wilkerson.[32]

7. **Cardiovascular function**
   a. Bradycardia secondary to cold-sensitive pacemaker cells that can delay conduction due to prolonged action potential.
   b. Progressively decreasing mean arterial blood pressure, cardiac index, and subsequent renal blood flow. Hepatic metabolism and lactic acid excretion are also reduced.
   c. Atrial dysrhythmias are common. Ventricular dysrhythmias are more likely at very cold temperatures. Debate continues as to whether ventricular fibrillation or asystole is the more common lethal rhythm.
8. Blood viscosity increases 2% per °C drop in temperature.

F. **Signs and symptoms**
   1. **Field diagnosis**
      a. Victim will be chilled during activity, cold when stopped. Deteriorating level of consciousness and judgment. Apathetic, listless. Decreasing coordination, ataxia. Paradoxical undressing is a sign of severe hypothermia.
      b. Initial shivering but later stops as cooling progresses.
      c. Diagnose by signs and symptoms; do not worry about actual temperature.
   2. **In-hospital diagnosis**
      a. Examine events leading to condition, underlying, contributing, or differentiating factors, temperature.
      b. Diagnose severity by signs and symptoms, not temperature alone.
      c. Expect ongoing fluid shifts as body temperature changes.
      d. Laboratory findings
         i. Increased hematocrit, decreased white blood cells, electrolyte imbalances
         ii. Prolonged clotting times, leukopenia, thrombocytopenia, significant at $<20°C$.
      e. Cardiac instability reflects inadequate fluid volume.
      f. Hyperreflexive between 35–32.2°C, then hyporeflexive. Areflexive at 26°C. Knee jerk last to go, first to return.
      g. Rule out other diagnoses, such as primary alcohol intoxication, hypoglycemia, and narcotic overdose.

G. **Treatment**
   1. **Field**
      a. **Get the patient quickly to shelter, out of cold and wind.**
      b. For **mild hypothermia**, supply food, warm fluids, shelter, and **dry** warm clothes.
      c. Never rub extremities. Focus on warming core.
      d. **Rough handling risks ventricular fibrillation.**
      e. Passive external rewarming to trunk only (i.e., with blankets). Warm humidified oxygen if available. (This is the only active external rewarming technique considered safe in the field.)
      f. If **severe hypothermia**, victim is unable to generate own heat. Treatment is more complex, the condition life-threatening. **Careful evacuation is required.**
      g. Prevent burns during heat application.
   2. **Hospital**
      a. Hypothermia patients are at risk for compartment syndrome and rhabdomyolysis.
      b. As patient is warmed, oxygen demands increase as well as fluid needs. Use warm intravenous fluids, 40–42°C. Each 10° rise in core temperature increases oxygen consumption 2–3 times.
      c. Hypothermia causes protein binding of medications. Expect altered and unpredictable metabolism and excretion secondary to hepatic and renal dysfunction. Use any medication very cautiously.

    d. Electrolyte levels will fluctuate with fluid shifts, as does membrane permeability and sodium-potassium pump function.

    e. Do not correct pH, as it can lead to decreased cardiac output, increased lactic acidosis, and risks ventricular fibrillation.

    f. Coagulopathies are common.

    g. Insulin is ineffective at temperatures $<30°C$.

    h. Watch for fluid shifts and signs and symptoms of fluid overload as patient is rewarmed.

    i. Handle patients gently to reduce risks of dysrhythmias.

    j. Suspect sepsis if patient fails to warm or has signs and symptoms of aspiration infiltrates on chest radiograph or bacteremia.

    k. Rule out other diagnoses such as primary alcohol intoxication, hypoglycemia, and drug overdose.

    l. Atrial dysrhythmias are benign and usually self-resolve with continued warming.

    m. Treatment of ventricular dysrhythmias is controversial. Chemical prophylaxis is not warranted.[14]

H. Prevention

1. **Decrease heat loss:** Dress accordingly for environment, weather, and activity. Avoid sweating by dressing properly for activity, bring change of clothes; avoid wet clothing, wind chill on exposed skin.

    a. Avoid getting insulating layers wet.

2. **Avoid exhaustion:** Allow enough rest and adequate pacing to avoid exhaustion.

3. **Increase heat production:** Encourage adequate caloric intake to provide carbohydrates for activity plus heat production in environment.

4. **Promote positive fluid balance:** Use hydration to counter effects of evaporative heat losses and environment factors (cold, dry air and altitude).

I. Immersion hypothermia

1. Subcutaneous body fat is most significant variable of cooling rate, as is body surface area.

2. Critical factors in cold-water immersion cooling rates:

    a. Water temperature, weather conditions

    b. Victim's body fat

    c. Clothing

    d. Victim's behavior

    e. Amount of body immersed

3. Exercise or movement in cold water increases cooling rate by 35–50% by increasing blood flow to peripheral tissues and by increasing water flow around body surface area (i.e., convection).

4. Important survival factor is to get as much of body out of the water, even if weather is cold and windy.

5. The most significant lifesaving measure is a personal flotation device.

III. OTHER COLD INJURIES

A. Frostbite

1. **Definition:** Frostbite is the **actual freezing of tissues, superficial or deep**. While other cold-related injuries may appear to be frostbite, the differentiating factor is irreversible damage and loss of tissue. It can occur in skiers, skaters, sledders, bicyclists, and runners, as well as hikers and climbers.

2. **Risk factors**

    a. **Predisposing**

        i. History of previous cold injuries

        ii. Smoking (diminishes microcirculation where frostbite occurs)

       iii. Vascular disease

       iv. Age

   b. **Current**

       i. Constricting clothing, poor-fitting boots

       ii. Hypothermia

       iii. Exhaustion

       iv. Dehydration

       v. Sweating (keeps skin wet, expends energy)

       vi. Clothing: Adding warmer clothes is a conscious decision, not a reflex, and cannot be made if mental ability is impaired by cold.

       vii. Skin temperature as determined by blood flow

   c. **Environmental**

       i. Wind chill (only to exposed skin)

       ii. Water is 25 times more conductive than air.

       iii. Snow, especially if deep, cold, and/or wet

       iv. Weather, sudden storms

       v. Accidents producing additional trauma

       vi. Altitude has no direct causal effects, but hypoxia impairs decision-making. Altitude also affects shivering capabilities, resulting in greater energy expenditure and promoting exhaustion and dehydration.

   d. **Gender is not a predisposing factor.**

       i. In studies of men and women's responses to cold, some have shown a strong relationship due to women's higher body fat content, but others have not.[23]

       ii. No difference in peripheral skin temperature in men vs women.[23]

3. **Types of frostbite**[28]

   a. True frostbite (superficial or deep)

   b. Mixed injury: cold-water immersion followed by freezing (very poor prognosis)

   c. Freeze-thaw-refreeze (very poor prognosis)

   d. Hypoxia

   e. Extremity compartment compression, followed by freezing

   f. Extremity fracture and dislocation, followed by freezing

   g. Hypothermia associated with freezing injury

   h. Freezing superimposed on small vessel disease

   i. Freezing in children, with epiphyseal necrosis

   j. Congenital deformity with superimposed freezing

   k. Frostbite with superimposed burns or burn injury with superimposed frostbite

4. **Progressive pathology**

   a. Fingertips, toes, nose tip, ear lobes, and exposed skin are areas most commonly affected.

   b. Pain and discomfort initially (also prickly or itchy), proceeding to numbness

   c. Local vasoconstriction/dilatation occurs in 5–10 min cycles. This is a temporary compensation, which ultimately ceases, to prevent further core cooling.

   d. Once blood flow ceases, local cooling can progress rapidly, at 0.5°C/min or more.

   e. **Four pathologic phases:**[25]

       i. **Prefreeze:** Secondary to chilling. Includes vasospasticity and plasma leakage; tissue temperature is 3–10°C (cutaneous sensation stops at 10°C).

       ii. **Freeze-thaw:** Ice crystals form. Ambient temperature is –15 to –6°C; skin temperature is –4°C. Skin becomes poikilothermic. Most sensitive are endothelium, bone marrow, and nerve cells; less sensitive are muscle, bone, and cartilage tissues.

       iii. **Vascular stasis:** Vascular spasticity and dilatation, capillary leakage, shunting, stasis coagulation

      iv. **Late ischemic phase:** Secondary to thrombosis and arteriole/venule shunting; ischemia, gangrene, autonomic dysfunction

    f. Ice crystal formation

      i. **Intracellular:** mechanically destroys cell

      ii. **Interstitial:** altered intracellular electrolyte concentration, chemically destroys cell

      iii. Denaturation of lipid proteins

      iv. Overlap occurs between phases.

  5. **Clinical presentation**

    a. Frostbite is not numbness followed by tingling with rewarming. This is called frosting and is a warning sign. **True frostbite damages tissue.**

    b. Assessment classification describes the appearance of increasingly severe stages:

      i. **Superficial:** Involves surface tissue only. Skin is waxy and white, edematous, but no blisters. Area is numb, but underlying tissues are soft and pliable. Thawing increases erythema and edema. Superficial blisters appear, filled with clear or milky fluid. Skin is red and edematous, which increases on thawing.

      ii. **Deep:** Full-thickness injury. Deep purple blisters appear, indicating deep structural damage and poor prognosis. Underlying tissue is hard and frozen. Black hard eschar forms in 9–15 days.

      iii. **Full-thickness:** Necrosis and mummification. Skin is purple and burgundy colored; it may take weeks for complete demarcation between viable and nonviable tissue. Body part may be amputated; bone also frozen.

    c. Vesicles and bullae appear within 1–48 hours of rewarming (longer times for high altitude); may continue for weeks.

  6. **Treatment**

    a. **Field**

      i. Assess and treat other injuries, most importantly hypothermia. Keep patient warm and dry. Keep body part frozen and dry.

      ii. Avoid thaw and refreeze. If a frozen body part thaws and then refreezes, further damage **will** result; it is better to leave the part frozen until reaching shelter.

      iii. If hospital is >2 hours away, initiate rapid rewarming. Keep blisters intact. Protect body part by keeping it warm, dry, clean, softly padded and splinted, if necessary.

      iv. Never rub. Do not warm by stove, fire, or heater. Damaged sensory function can allow thermal burn to occur, which will result in poor outcome.

      v. No alcohol or smoking

    b. **Hospital**

      i. Do **not** make a definitive diagnosis as to the extent of damage and possible recovery on initial examination. It can take **weeks** to appreciate the extent of tissues regeneration.

      ii. Frostbitten tissue or body parts will occasionally present still frozen.

      iii. Identify associated traumatic or medical injuries, especially hypothermia. Correct core temperature to at least 34°C *before* rewarming frostbite.

      iv. **Rapid, controlled rewarming** in a warm-water bath, 37°–41°C (104°–108°F). The water should be circulated by whirlpool or manual stirring and water temperature maintained constant. Remove frozen clothing and boots with hot water. Rewarming should be complete in 30–45 minutes. The thawing process may be painful.

      v. **Prognostic signs** (after rewarming)

(a) Favorable
    (i) Pinprick sensation
    (ii) Normal color, warmth, large clear blebs appearing early, edema, erythema. Blebs should develop to distal tips of fingers and toes.
(b) Unfavorable
    (i) Small dark blebs appearing later or not developing to distal ends of fingers and toes.
    (ii) No edema
    (iii) Cyanosis which does not blanch with pressure

  vi. **Post-warming progression**
    (a) Edema: Appears 3 hr after rewarming, lasts 5 days or more
    (b) Blisters or bullae: Appear 1–48 hr after rewarming
    (c) Eschar: Dark, hard, dry; usually appears in 9–15 days
    (d) Mummification: Takes 22–45 days for completion; delay amputation until clear demarcation.

  vii. **Provide supportive care through demarcation period** (22–45 days). Freeze-thaw-refreeze injuries will complete the demarcation process (sometimes to spontaneous amputation) within 7–9 days.

  viii. **Update tetanus toxoid immunization** if not current.
    (a) Intravenous penicillin through edema phase
    (b) Ibuprofen to inhibit arachidonic acid cascade (encourages fibrinolysis)[25,28]
    (c) Topical agents, such as aloe vera or thromboxane[25,28]

  ix. Protect skin with fluffy sterile dressings, bed cradle, no pressure.

  x. **Sensation and pain:** The severity of injury will determine neurologic damage. Tingling or electric-like sensations and burning are caused by ischemic neuritis and are exacerbated with warmth.

  xi. If there is no tissue loss, symptoms are usually gone in 1 month. If tissue is lost, symptoms can last to 6 months.

  xii. Promote physical therapy, especially for joint range of motion, as soon as thawing is complete. Best time is during and after hydrotherapy.

7. **Prevention**
  a. Exercise and train appropriately for event, activity, or expedition.
  b. Wear adequate clothing, especially good-fitting footwear.
  c. Use careful judgment in appropriate pacing, rest, knowing when to stop, knowing when to turn around, based on group ability and weather.
  d. Maintain proper nutrition and hydration to keep up with increased energy expenditure outdoors, especially at high altitudes.

B. **Frostnip**
  1. Reversible ice crystal formation involving skin surface only; no actual freezing of tissue. Also called frosting.
  2. Symptoms: Numbness, frosted appearance
  3. Take as a serious warning.

C. **Chilblains**
  1. Itchy, painful erythema of the skin of the extremities (ears, fingers, tip of nose, lower legs)

D. **Raynaud's phenomenon**
  1. A collection of signs and symptoms representing an underlying vasospastic condition. Although not an environmental injury per se, it is frequently triggered by cold. It occurs in women five times more frequently than men.
  2. **Risk factors**
    a. Female gender
    b. Smoking (nicotine)
    c. Underlying vascular disease

    d. Occupation: Mechanical tasks involving vibration, such as chainsaw or jackhammer operation, farming, typing, piano playing, climbing

3. **Pathophysiology**

    a. **Raynaud's phenomenon** is the clinical presentation of signs and symptoms. **Raynaud's disease** is a primary event, not secondary to other vascular disease, and is an idiopathic, vasospastic condition.

    b. **Vasospasm** is the result of an overreactive sympathetic alpha-adrenergic response from cutaneous perception of cold, either local or systemic. The stimulus must be removed to halt the sympathetic activity.[22] Can also be triggered by stress.

    c. Women have more **sympathetic tone** than men.

    d. Persons with Raynaud's phenomenon have documented lower digital systolic blood pressure (controversial).

    e. More common in hands than in feet

    f. Triggers include cold, stress, nicotine, caffeine.

    g. **Diagnosis, signs, and symptoms**

        i. One or all phases of vasospasm and recovery may be present:

            (a) First phase: Ischemia secondary to vasospasm

            (b) Second phase: Cyanosis after vessels have dilated but carry deoxygenated blood

            (c) Third phase: Red, hyperemic, as blood flow returns to normal bringing oxygenated blood

        ii. Patient may complain of numbness and pain.

        iii. Unlike frostbite, ischemia is irregular between digits and extremities. Also different, warmth, red color, blood flow, and sensation return within minutes after rewarming.

        iv. Severity ranges widely between patients, frequency of attacks, and environments.

        v. **Diagnosis is based on history.** Ischemic attacks may not be reproducible in clinic. Underlying vascular disease must be ruled out to determine Raynaud's phenomenon vs disease.

    h. **Treatment**

        i. Noninvasive

            (a) Apply warm clothing. Keep whole body warm, as well as extremities.

            (b) No smoking

            (c) Discontinue potentially triggering medications.

            (d) Biofeedback

            (e) Hot-cold hydrotherapy

        ii. Pharmacologic

            (a) Sympathetic inhibitors

            (b) Calcium channel blockers

        iii. Surgical

            (a) Sympathectomy: Rarely. Results are variable, but better in lower extremities than in upper.[13,22]

INFORMATION

The **Wilderness Medical Society** is a 3000-member organization of medical and related professionals from all aspects of wilderness care. Their journal, *Journal of Wilderness Medicine*, is published quarterly. They provide a current list of recommended publications as well as offer speakers for various topics and educational slide presentations. They can be reached at PO Box 2463, Indianapolis, IN 46206 (telephone 317-631-1745).

REFERENCES

Heat illness

1. Armstrong, Moresh: The induction and decay of heat acclimatization in trained athletes. Sports Med 12:302–312, 1991.
2. Auerbach PS, Geehr EC: Management of Wilderness and Environmental Emergencies, 2nd ed. St. Louis, Mosby, 1989.
2a. Backer HD, Shopes E, Collins SL: Hyponatremia in recreational hikers in Grand Canyon National Park. J Wilderness Med 4:391–406, 1993.
3. Bracker MD: Environmental and thermal injury. Clin Sports Med 11:419–431, 1992.
4. Haynes EM: Physiological responses of female athletes to heat stress: A review. Phys SportsMed 12(3):45–55, 1984.
5. Knochel JP: Heat stroke and related heat stress disorders. DM 35:301–377, 1989.
6. Travis SPL: Management of heat stroke. J R Naval Med Serv 74:39–43, 1988.
7. Tek D, Olshaker JS: Heat illness. Emerg Med Clin North Am 10:299–310, 1992.
8. Weiss E: Heat illness. Presented at the Wilderness Medicine Conference. Whistler, BC, Canada, July 1991.
9. Wells CL: Sexual differences in heat stress response. Phys SportsMed 5(9):79–90, 1977.
10. Yarbrough BE, Hubbard RW: Heat-related illnesses. In Auerbach PS (ed): Management of Wilderness and Environmental Emergencies, 2nd ed. St. Louis, Mosby, 1989.

Hypothermia and cold injury

11. Auerbach PS: Medicine for Outdoors. Boston, Little, Brown, 1986.
12. Auerbach PS, Geehr EC: Management of Wilderness and Environmental Emergencies, 2nd ed. St. Louis, Mosby, 1989.
13. Bracker MD: Environmental and thermal injury. Clin Sports Med 11:419–436, 1992.
14. Danzl DF: Accidental Hypothermia. Wilderness Medical Society, 1992.
15. Danzl DF, Pozos RS, Hamlet MP: Accidental Hypothermia. In Auerbach PS (ed): Management of Wilderness and Environmental Emergencies, 2nd ed. St. Louis, Mosby, 1989.
16. Danzl DF, Sowers MB, Vicaro SJ, et al: Chemical defibrillation in severe accidental hypothermia. Ann Emerg Med 11:698–699, 1982.
17. Forgey WW: Traveler's Medical Resource. Merriville, IN, ICS Books, 1990.
18. Grahm TE: Thermal, metabolic, and cardiovascular changes in men and women during cold stress. Med Sci Sports Exerc (Suppl 20):S185–S192, 1988.
19. Hayward JS, Eckerson JD, Collis ML: Thermal balance and survival time prediction of man in cold water. Can J Physiol Pharmacol 53:21–32, 1975.
20. Kayser B, Binzoni T, Hoppeler H, et al: A case of severe frostbite on Mt Blanc: A multitechnique approach. J Wilderness Med 4:167–174, 1993.
21. Kocher G, Kahn SE, Kotler MN: Bretylium tosylate and ventricular fibrillation in hypothermia [letter]. Ann Intern Med 105:624, 1986.
22. Loscalzo, Creager, Dzau V (eds): Vascular Medicine. Boston, Little, Brown, 1992.
23. McArdle, Magel, Gergley, Spina: Thermal adjustment to cold water exposure in resting men and women. J Appl Physiol Respir Environ Exerc Physiol 56:1565–1571, 1984.
24. McArdle, Magle, Spina, et al: Thermal adjustment to cold water exposure in exercising men and women. J Appl Physiol Respir Environ Exerc Physiol 56:1572–1577, 1984.
25. Mills WJ: Comment and recapitulation [on frostbite]. Alaska Med 135:70–87, 1993.
26. Mills WJ: Field care of the hypothermic patient. Inter J Sports Med Oct 1992, pp 199–202.
27. Mills WJ, Mills WJ: Peripheral nonfreezing cold injury: Immersion injury. Alaska Med 35:118–128, 1993.
28. Mills WJ, O'Malley J, Kappes B: Cold and refreezing: A historical chronology of laboratory investigation and clinical experience. Alaska Med 35:89–116, 1993.
29. Smith DJ, Robson MC, Heggers JP: Frostbite and other cold-induced injuries. In Auerbach PS (ed): Management of Wilderness and Environmental Emergencies, 2nd edition. St. Louis, Mosby, 1989.

30. Stevens, Grahm, Wilson: Gender differences in cardiovascular responses to cold and exercise. Can J Physiol Pharmacol 65:165–171, 1987.
31. Wagner, Horvath: Influences of age and gender on human thermoregulatory responses to cold exposure. J Appl Physiol 58:180–186, 1985.
32. Wilkerson JA: Medicine for Mountaineering, 3rd ed. Seattle, The Mountaineers, 1985.

PART IV
SPECIFIC SPORTS

Chapter 44: Skiing

PATRICIA GIBBS, MD

There has been relatively little study of the sport of skiing beyond research on epidemiology and risk factors for injury. This chapter presents that information and the small amount of data specifically pertaining to women in skiing.

I. **GENERAL INTRODUCTION**

    A. The history of women in skiing has not been well documented. For centuries, skis were used as a means of military transportation, and as such, participation was, in all likelihood, a male-dominated endeavor.

    B. The first mention of a woman's involvement in ski competition was in 1893. Later, 13 women competed in the first winter Olympics in 1924 at Chamonix, France.

    C. Currently, women participate in all Alpine (downhill) and Nordic (cross-country) events (Fig. 1).

    D. Epidemiologic studies estimate the number of skiers worldwide to be 25–30 million, and possibly as high as 200 million.

II. **WHAT IS SKIING?**

    A. The term *skiing* actually encompasses a variety of diverse events.

       1. **Alpine (downhill) skiing** is the most popular form of the sport in the U. S. Participants wear semirigid ski boots that span the foot and ankle. These attach to the ski through releasable bindings. Mechanical ski lifts carry the skiers to the top of the hill and the skiers then make their way to the bottom.

         a. Competitive events include:

           i. Slalom—competitors navigate closely set plastic gates, making a series of rapid turns in succession.

           ii. Giant slalom—gates are more widely set, allowing slightly greater speed and more fluid progression from gate to gate.

           iii. Super giant slalom—distances between gates are increased even more, necessitating rapid, high-speed turns.

           iv. Downhill—the event with greatest distance between gates; speeds of up to 80 mph are reached by women competitors.

       2. **Freestyle skiing** is a form of downhill skiing that has recently been added to the roster of winter Olympic eventes.

         a. Freestyle events include:

           i. Mogul skiing—competitors must combine "stunts" and fluidity while skiing steep, bumpy terrain.

           ii. Aerials—individuals perform flips, twists, and other acrobatics after launching themselves from the end of a ski jump.

           iii. Ballet—classical ballet moves such as arabesque and tour en l'air are combined with other dancelike movements while skiing down a short, smooth slope.

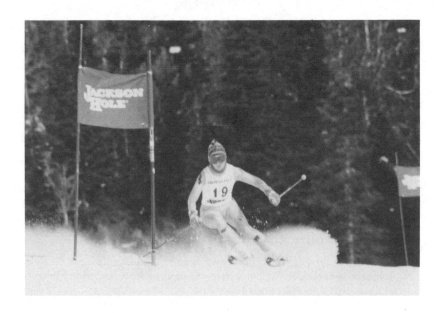

FIGURE 1. Women of all ages now participate in Alpine skiing competition. Shown here, a woman competing in the U.S. Alpine Masters Championships at 60 years of age. (Photo courtesy of Chris Hellman, Powder Shots Action Photographers, Jackson Hole, WY.)

3. In **Nordic (cross-country) skiing**, the ski boots more closely resemble running shoes. They attach to thin, flexible skis at the toe only.
   a. Nordic skiers travel long distances through a combination of diagonal strides, skating motions, and downhill gliding.
   b. The sport requires both endurance and balance.
4. **Other skiing events** include:
   a. Ski jumping
   b. Biathlon: A skiing/shooting event
   c. Telemark skiing: A technique of downhill skiing on sturdy cross-country equipment
   d. Snowboarding: A new discipline in which both boots attach to a single double-wide ski
   e. Speed skiing: Speeds of up to 133 mph have been reached by female speed skiers.

III. INCIDENCE OF INJURY

A. Injury incidence varies with type of skiing. Alpine skiing is the best studied.
B. Most authorities cite the **overall incidence of injury** in downhill skiing at 2–4 injuries/1000 skier days—i.e., of 1000 skiers active on a given day, 2–4 become injured.
   1. Any skier has a 14% chance of injury over a ski season consisting of 14 days skied (the number of days skied per year by the average skier).
   2. Most injuries are caused by falls (70–90%), with the remainder (11–20%) attributed to collision.
C. **There has been an overall trend toward fewer skiing injuries through the past 20 years.** This may be due to improved binding technology and fewer lower extremity equipment-related (LEER) injuries. It has been estimated that LEER injuries decreased by 43% over the years 1972–1978.
   1. **Lower extremity sprains and fractures** have decreased, while the incidence of knee injury has remained constant.

2. Several studies have noted a worrisome increase in the proportion of **knee sprains** which are categorized as severe (3rd degree).

3. Modern binding technology has not yet incorporated features that protect the knee from **rotational injury**.

D. **Upper and lower body injuries** now occur in approximately equal proportions.

1. One study of 1850 skiing injuries found 50% of all injuries were caused by 9 types of injury:

   a. Sprain of the medial collateral ligament (13%)

   b. Facial laceration (10%)

   c. Disruption of the ulnar collateral ligament of the thumb (6%)

   d. Tibial fracture (3%)

   e. Shoulder dislocation (3%)

   f. Lower leg laceration (3%)

   g. Ankle sprain (3%)

   h. Soft-tissue injury of the shoulder (3%)

   i. Tear of the medial meniscus (3%)

E. **Mortality rates** for skiing-related injury/illness range from 0.5–0.87 deaths/million skier days.

1. Of 8 **trauma-related deaths** at an Australian ski area between 1984 and 1987, 7 occurred in men. Most deaths due to trauma were caused by collision with fixed objects.

2. **Cardiovascular deaths** in skiers occurred at a rate of 0.45/million skier days; 14 of 15 such deaths occurred in men.

3. Unclear from these data is the number of men vs women who were participating in skiing over this time span. Thus, the **gender-specific risk of ski-related death is unknown.**

4. These rates compare with an incidence of 2 deaths/100,000 player years in football.

F. **Alpine ski racers** have a high prevalence of injury: Of 150 top competitors surveyed, 83% report injuries which disabled them for 20 or more days.

G. The incidence of **injury in Nordic skiing** appears to be lower than that for Alpine skiing, with a rate of 0.47 injuries/1000 skier days.

1. Nordic skiing involves sustained and repetitive use of upper and lower extremities, so an increased proportion of overuse injury versus trauma might be expected. Studies reporting trauma incidence might overlook overuse injury for which patients may not seek medical attention from an on-site trauma facility.

2. Despite the lower frequency of injury in cross-country skiing, there appears to be a **greater proportion of severe injury** when compared with downhill skiing. This is of concern, given the remote nature of cross-country skiing and the difficulty involved in attaining timely evacuation.

H. **Ski jumping:** A sport involving jumping into the air and soaring hundreds of meters above the ground should carry an excess risk.

1. Incidence studies reveal similar injury rates in ski jumpers as alpine skiers, i.e., 1.2 injuries/1000 skier days in world cup jumpers and 4.3 injuries/1000 skier days in regional jumpers.

IV. PREVENTION OF SKIING INJURY

A. **Risk factors for skiing injury:** Several studies have sought to determine behaviors or conditions predisposing to injury in downhill skiing.

1. Risk factors may be categorized according to the following variables:

   a. **Personal characteristics**

      i. **Age**: Children have similar injury rates as adults, but their injuries appear to be more severe, with a greater proportion of fractures and greater numbers of head and neck injuries.

      ii. **Gender:** Several studies show higher injury rates in women than in men, but others do not support this pattern. Studies may be confounded by the fact that women are more likely to report their injuries to local health care facilities than men.

   (a) Women seem more prone to knee ligament injuries than men, which indicates a problem with binding adjustment or design.

b. **Skill level**
   i. Self-reported "beginners" have a 2- to 3-fold increased risk of injury versus advanced skiers.
   ii. Experience also represents an independent risk factor; a preventive effect remains after adjusting for skill level.
   iii. Ski lessons may help in reducing risk, at least during the first one to two seasons of participation.

c. **Physical conditioning**
   i. Though better physical conditioning would be expected to lower injury risk, this has not been supported with empirical evidence. One study actually indicates an increased risk of accident in skiers reporting better physical conditioning.
   ii. The lack of clear-cut benefit to good physical conditioning may be due to confounding with other risk factors, such as risk-taking behavior.

d. **Behavior**
   i. Skiers who report fearing an accident while skiing have a lower injury rate.
   ii. Paradoxically, "sensation-seeking" skiers appear to sustain fewer injuries than those with lower scores on a questionnaire of behavioral traits.
   iii. Alcohol consumption has been suspected as a significant cause of skiing accidents, but a random testing of injured skiers for alcohol levels identified only 1 of 39 injured skiers with any alcohol at all on blood analysis.
   iv. Glycogen depletion occurs in muscle fibers after a day of skiing. The additive effects of several days of glycogen depletion might predispose to fatigue and injury which could be corrected by carbohydrate loading, but this question has not been studied in clinical trials.

e. **Equipment**
   i. Most skiers adjust their **bindings** at least 50% higher than the recommended release setting. Those with LEER injuries show an even larger increase over recommended settings: The average deviation in binding adjustment in knee injuries is 85%, and that for tibial fractures 150%.
   ii. The reason for this choice of binding settings, skiers report, is a fear of premature binding release.
   iii. A recent randomized study indicated that proper binding adjustment reduced injury risk 3-fold.
   iv. Because **children** <15 years old have an increased risk of lower extremity fracture, an equipment-related problem might exist caused by improperly fitted or outdated boots or inappropriately adjusted bindings.
   v. Children appear to be at increased risk of head injury and thus use of **protective headgear** may be advisable.
   vi. **Thumb injury** is often caused by falling onto a hand that is gripping a pole handle. Special handles have been designed to promote complete pole release when falling; with the standard pole grip, the best policy may be to **avoid using the pole strap** or, if using the strap, to insert the hand from the bottom of the loop upwards, such that the pole will fall away from the hand when dropped.

f. **Environment**
   i. Icy or hard-packed snow leads to more overall injuries and a greater proportion of upper extremity and head injuries.
   ii. Wet snow and powder are associated with more lower extremity injuries.
   iii. A greater number of injuries occur on cloudless than cloudy days.

2. While much can be said about factors associated with increased injury rates, the best method of promoting injury prevention is not yet determined.
   a. The optimal way of determining effective injury prevention strategies would be to do prospective, randomized, controlled studies introducing a variable such as physical conditioning and measuring injury outcomes.
   b. Thus far, this has only been done with binding adjustment, and a significant effect was found with this intervention, as discussed above.

V. PHYSIOLOGY

A. Few physiologic studies have been done on skiers, even fewer focusing on gender-specific physiology.
   1. Studies on **body fat composition of female skiers** reveal an average body fat content of 16% in female Nordic skiers and 20% in female Alpine skiers. These percentages compare with an average value of 21–29% in populations of nonathletic women.
   2. A study comparing female versus male Alpine and cross-country skiers on measures of **power, strength, agility, and aerobic quality** revealed:
      a. **Maximal oxygen uptake** adjusted for lean body weight: male Nordic skiers > male Alpine skiers > female Nordic skiers > female Alpine skiers (though the difference between male Alpine and female Nordic skiers was only 2%).
      b. **Power:** Male Alpine skiers > male Nordic skiers > female Alpine skiers > female Nordic skiers.
      c. **Agility:** Male Alpine skiers > female Alpine skiers > male cross-country skiers > female cross-country skiers.
      d. **Strength** adjusted for weight: Male Alpine skiers > female Alpine skiers = male cross-country skiers = female cross-country skiers.
      e. Investigators found a positive correlation between ability in the slalom event and muscular endurance; this was measured by number of quadriceps extensions on Cybex testing attained before 50% reduction in peak torque. No difference was found between men and women on this measure. Percentage decline in peak torque may correlate positively with the number of fast-twitch muscle fibers, and thus slalom skiers with greater expertise may have a greater percentage of slow-twitch fibers than do less accomplished skiers.

VI. MEDICAL ISSUES IN THE WOMAN SKIER

A. **Iron**
   1. Studies on Olympic athletes revealed a 50% incidence of prelatent iron deficiency and a 7% incidence of anemia in female Nordic skiers. Alpine women have a 20% incidence of both overt anemia and iron deficiency.
   2. These data indicate that screening for ferritin levels may be prudent in competitive skiers.
   3. Proper dietary counseling for these athletes is of importance.

B. **Amenorrhea**
   1. Though incidence and prevalence of amenorrhea in other sports have been well studied and documented, only one report included skiers among its subjects, and this study grouped Nordic women with distance runners. It indicated a frequency of 43% menstrual disturbance and 11.5% secondary amenorrhea in a group of runners and cross-country skiers during a period of intensive training.
   2. No studies as yet have measured rates of menstrual disturbances in Alpine skiers.

C. **Pregnancy**
   1. The effect of pregnancy on skiing has had no systematic study. This places the practitioner in a difficult position: We are asked to provide recommendations to the pregnant skier on the advisability of continuing the sport, but yet we have no firm data to support these recommendations.

a. It is unclear how many women are skiing when pregnant. Some do ski pregnant, and one manufacturer makes special "expanding" ski pants designed for expectant mothers.

b. An Austrian ski team member, Ulrike Maier, won the 1989 world championship Super G while entering her second trimester of pregnancy.*

2. At this point, it is prudent to advise that **pregnant women follow usual guidelines for exercise during pregnancy**, such as those of the American College of Obstetrics and Gynecology (*see* Chapter 21). However, skiing involves additional risks not covered by these recommendations:

a. **Increased risk of trauma**

   i. Abdominal/thoracic trauma comprised 8% of all skiing injuries in one large study.

   ii. Due to a 14% risk of injury over a 14-day season, 1 in 100 average skiers might be expected to sustain significant abdominal/thoracic trauma.

   iii. By comparison, statistics indicate that physical trauma complicates 1 in every 12 pregnancies.

   iv. The risk of first-trimester pregnancy loss following abdominal trauma of any type is not known, though most practitioners feel the relationship is minimal.

      (a) In a study of 1000 cases of spontaneous first-trimester abortion, only 1 case could be linked with trauma. First-trimester spontaneous abortion has not as yet been linked with trauma caused by motor vehicle accident.

      (b) Recreational skiing in the first trimester would not seem to pose any additional risk beyond that imposed by other forms of exercise or travel.

   v. Once the uterus has risen above the pelvic brim, i.e., in the early second trimester, it becomes at risk for direct abdominal injury.

      (a) **Skiing after the first trimester could be discouraged by the practitioner.**

      (b) However, it is important to remember the level of expertise of the pregnant skier. The practitioner should present the known data on risk during skiing and provide information on ways of reducing these risks.

   vi. Pregnancy complicated by maternal cardiac or pulmonary disease, pregnancy-induced hypertension, multiple gestation, fetal-growth retardation, diabetes, premature labor, or other chronic illness should be an absolute contraindication to skiing.

b. **Travel**

   i. Skiing requires the presence of snow and usually mountains, so most skiers must travel to participate in the sport.

   ii. Regarding travel during pregnancy, it is generally agreed that, barring the complications noted above, it is safe to continue air travel up until the 34th week of gestation.

   iii. Travel may be of above-average hazard levels, given the often difficult driving conditions imposed by mountains and snowy roads.

   iv. Travel to the ski area probably imposes greater hazards than skiing itself.

c. **Cold**

   i. Though most research has been done on the effects of increased core temperature on pregnancy outcome, there are no studies designed to answer the opposite question, i.e., the influence of cold exposure on human pregnancy.

---

* Since the writing of this chapter, Ulrike Maier was tragically killed in a skiing accident while competing in a downhill race in January 1994.

    ii. Incidence of death caused by hypothermia in skiers was found to be 0.18/ million skier-days. However, it is uncertain what effect nonfatal episodes of hypothermia would have on placental blood flow and pregnancy outcome.

    iii. Controlled studies on sheep exposed to low ambient temperatures throughout their gestation indicate that fetal birthweight actually increases in cold-exposed animals.

    iv. This question must remain an unknown until appropriate human studies are conducted.

  d. **Altitude**

    i. Studies on populations living at high altitude indicate a negative correlation between fetal birthweight and increasing altitude at altitudes >7000 ft.

    ii. The effect of transient exposure to increased elevation is unknown. Given that physiologic adaptations have not had a chance to compensate for lower oxygen levels at high altitude in travelers, one might expect more acute adverse effects on the average skier than on those accustomed to these levels.

    ii. Again, lack of empiric evidence on this topic compels the practitioner to advise against skiing at altitudes >7000 ft in pregnant women, especially in those accustomed to life at lower altitude.

  e. **Remote access**

    i. Many ski areas are accessible by difficult and tortuous roads. These roads may close due to excessive snowfall, thereby closing off emergency transport to a medical facility.

    ii. After the fetus attains potential viability, access to timely care for premature labor is imperative. Thus, pregnant women should not travel to remote ski areas after 23 weeks' gestation, even if they do not ski.

  f. **Balance**

    i. There is a theoretic risk that alterations in the center of gravity produced by the enlarged uterus could predispose the pregnant woman to falling.

    ii. There is one case report in the literature of a woman in her first trimester who lost her coordination and was unable to ski. Other than this report, the scientific literature is devoid of information regarding the effect of pregnancy on balance in skiing.

VII. SUMMARY

A. Much remains to be learned about medical issues related to skiing.

  1. Future studies should further document risk factors for injury in subgroups of skiers, such as competitive athletes and pregnant women.

  2. Prospective studies on pregnant skiers to determine pregnancy outcomes would greatly aid the clinician in making recommendations.

B. **Current recommendations for injury prevention** include:

  1. **Bindings** should be properly adjusted by trained technicians prior to each ski season and periodically checked throughout the season.

  2. All skiers should use **built-in ski-retaining devices** (i.e., ski brakes) rather than straps to arrest ski descent following binding release.

  3. Individuals should **ski with caution** and within their ability level. Ski lessons are advisable.

  4. Skiers should **maintain awareness of snow and weather conditions**. Pregnant women should not ski if conditions are crowded or icy.

  5. **Alcohol and drug use must be avoided** while skiing.

  6. **Children** should have modern, properly fitted equipment and should optimally wear protective headgear.

  7. **Pregnant women** should not travel to remote ski areas after 23 weeks' gestation and should avoid elevations >7000 ft. Though physicians should advise against skiing after the first trimester, the final decision remains with the pregnant

woman. They should be informed of the hazards and advised of ways to minimize risks if they do decide to ski.

8. **Proper preseason conditioning** seems prudent, despite an absence of empirical evidence on the subject.

ACKNOWLEDGMENT

Much helpful information was obtained from Peggy Chapman at the U.S. National Ski Hall of Fame and Ski Museum., PO Box 191, Ishpeming, MI 49849-0191; telephone 906-485-6323.

REFERENCES

1. Barry M, Bia F: Pregnancy and travel. JAMA 261:728–731, 1989.
2. Bouter LM, Knipschild PG: Causes and prevention of injury in downhill skiing. Phys SportsMed 17(2):80–94, 1989.
3. Clement DB, Lloyd-Smith DR, Macintyre GO, et al: Iron status in winter Olympic sports. J Sports Sci 5:261–271, 1987.
4. Ekeland A, Holtmoen A, Lystad H: Lower extremity equipment-related injuries in Alpine recreational skiers. Am J Sports Med 21(2):201–205, 1993.
5. Ellison AE: Skiing injuries. Clin Symp 29:1–40, 1977.
6. Fiore DC: Death on a ski slope: Response and prevention. Phys Sportsmed 22(2):46–55, 1994.
7. Haymes EM, Dickinson AL: Characteristics of elite male and female ski racers. Med Sci Sports Exerc 12:153–158, 1980.
8. Ronkainen H, Pakarinen A, Kauppila A: Pubertal and menstrual disorders of female runners, skiers and volleyball players. Gynecol Obstet Invest 18:183–189, 1984.
9. Scharplatz D, Thurleman K, Enderlin F: Thoracoabdominal trauma in ski accidents. Injury 10:86–91, 1978.
10. Sherry E: Pregnancy as a risk factor for injury in downhill skiing [letter]. Med J Aust 143:633, 1985.
11. Sherry E, Asquith J: Nordic (cross-country) skiing injuries in Australia. Med J Aust 146:245–246, 1987.
12. Thompson GE, Bassett JM, Samson DE, Slee J: The effects of cold exposure of pregnant sheep on foetal plasma nutrients, hormones and birth weight. Br J Nutr 48:59–64, 1982.
13. Tough SC, Butt JC: A review of fatal injuries associated with downhill skiing. Am J Forensic Med Pathol 14(1):12–16, 1993.
14. Tough SC, Butt JC: A reivew of 19 fatal injuries associated with backcountry skiing. Am J Forensic Med Pathol 14(1):17–21, 1993.
15. Unger C, Weiser JK, McCullough RE, Keefer S: Altitude, low birth weight, and infant mortality in Colorado. JAMA 259:3427–3432, 1988.
16. Wright JR: Nordic ski jumping injuries: A survey of active American jumpers. Am J Sports Med 19:615–619, 1991.

Chapter 45: Scuba Diving and the Marine Environment

GARY BEERMAN, ARNP/PA-C

I. SCUBA

Among the best known examples of diving women are the diving Ama of Japan and Korea, who began as early as 268 BC. There are currently an estimated 3 million active recreational scuba divers in the U.S. More than 300,000 new sport divers are trained each year with approximately 27% being women.

Dysbaric diving problems can result from the mechanical effects of pressure (e.g., barotrauma) and problems caused by breathing air or other gas mixtures in higher-than-normal partial pressures. Examples are decompression sickness and arterial gas embolism. These problems are well described elsewhere, and discussion here will be limited to those areas that pertain to women.

A. **Pregnancy:** The current advice is **do not dive when pregnant**. The physiology of the nitrogen compartments is barely understood in the mother, much less the fetus. Studies are small and conflicting but significant enough to assume:
   1. Diving can increase the incidence of birth defects.
   2. Fetal resistance to bubble formation is offset by the negative consequences of bubble formation that occurs for any reason.
   3. Maternal decompression sickness late in pregnancy entails a high risk of stillbirth. This risk may increase with decompression.
   4. *Any* bubble in the fetus is more ominous than *many* bubbles in the mother.
B. **Menstruation and decompression sickness:** The data are sparse and conflicting, and there are no well-done prospective studies with controls in large enough numbers to be significant.
   1. Patterns of decompression sickness
      a. Several altitude studies have found that women form more nitrogen bubbles than men for a given exposure, but they seem to have a higher incidence of decompression sickness, more delayed onset of symptoms, and more likelihood to suffer more serious Type II bends.
      b. A retrospective questionnaire study by Bangasser of 649 female divers showed a 3.3-fold increase in decompression sickness among women divers. All conditions were not known. Cases with insufficient data were not scrutinized, and no controlled decompression sickness criteria used to determine if decompression sickness occurred.
      c. The incidence of decompression sickness in women is no different from that in men as documented by Divers Alert Network in the U.S. and the equivalent agencies in England and Australia (Table 1).
      d. Hyperbaric chamber studies involve a warm environment with air, and probably do not predict water pressure effects.
   2. In the Hyperbaric Department at Virginia Mason Clinic, Seattle, a slight increase in decompression sickness has been noticed in menstruating employees who work in the chamber. A look at actual diver patients showed in the cold Pacific Northwest waters, there is no increase in decompression sickness (numbers were small).

This chapter is printed with permission of Divers Alert Network.

TABLE 1. Cases of Decompression Syndrome in Males vs Females, 1987–1991

Sex	1991	1990	1989	1988	1987
Female	25.2% (n = 110)	26.4%	26.1%	21.6%	24.1%
Male	74.8% (n = 327)	73.6%	73.9%	78.4%	75.9%
Total number	437	459	391	268	270

The percentage of females in the scuba diving population (approx 27%) is about the same as the percentage of femals in the injury statistics, supporting the notion that females are neither more nor less likely than males to experience decompression illness. Data from Divers Alert Network 1991 Report.[4]

    3. Some experts suggest that the Divers Alert Network data may be skewed because women do not dive as frequently during their menses. The Virginia Mason Clinic hyperbaric data show that they do.

    4. Current advice is that menstruation probably does not increase a woman's risk for decompression sickness. Following dive tables, staying less time than indicated, and taking a 3-minute safety stop at 15 feet after a no-decompression dive will be sound advice for all divers.

  C. **Hormonal contraceptives:** Microsludging from the pill had occurred in earlier formulations that contained 100–400% higher doses than current formulations. There is no increased risk to women divers using any current form of hormonal contraception.

  D. **Intrauterine devices:** Studies show there is movement of water into the uterine cavity during diving, with a theoretical increased risk for infection. Data show no increased risk.

  E. **Breast implants:** One study shows implants do form bubbles under pressure, but these have no significance.

II. ULTRAVIOLET RADIATION EXPOSURE

One of the pleasures of the active and athletic woman in the marine environment is the sun. However, acute effects are sunburn and conjunctivitis. Years later, these effects may manifest as actinic keratoses, basal cell carcinoma, squamous cell carcinoma, malignant melanoma, and cataracts.

  A. The sun's radiation ranges from short-wavelength, high-energy waves such as x-rays, ultraviolet (UV), visible light, and infrared (IR), through lower-energy TV and radio waves. Most high-energy radiation is blocked by the earth's atmosphere.

    1. **UV radiation**

      a. **UVC:** Blocked by the ozone layer; cytotoxic. Present in electric arcs (welding, search lights, germicidal lamps).

      b. **UVB:** Causes most burning, tanning, skin aging, and skin cancers. Partially blocked by the ozone layer. Some exposure is necessary for vitamin D. UVB causes conjunctivitis and contributes to the formation of cataracts and pterygia, reduces cellular immunity, and reactivates herpes simplex virus. Some evidence suggests that latent HIV may be activated by UV.

      c. **UVA:** Originally thought to be less dangerous, it penetrates deeper than UVB. Used in tanning beds; may still cause skin and eye damage; destroys folic acid. It can cause severe reactions when skin is photosensitized by drugs or chemicals such as cosmetics.

    2. **UV facts**

      a. UV radiation is more intense in summer, tropical latitudes, high altitude (increase of 4% per 1000 feet), and mid-day.

      b. Half of UVB arrives scattered from the sky; 80% may pass through overcast sky; reflections from water, snow, or sand can add 85%.

    3. Window glass blocks UVB and half of UVA, but both penetrate several feet into clear water.

B. **Significance to women**
1. **Melasma** (racoon mask, or mask of pregnancy) may be accentuated or initiated due to photosensitizing drugs for urinary tract infection or acne (doxycycline, sulfa, Retin-A, thiazide diuretics, etc.) or cosmetics.
2. Increased risk of skin cancer in women using Retin-A for acne or wrinkles.
3. Older women who use sunscreen regularly may develop vitamin D deficiency and osteoporosis and will benefit from supplementation of vitamin D.

C. **Appropriate protection**
1. Zinc oxide
2. Start with some SPF-15 sunscreen that is broad-spectrum (UVA/UVB), especially those containing Parsol 1789.
3. Apply liberally at least 20 minutes before exposure. Two applications necessary to achieve rated SPF protection.
4. Wide-brimmed hat and eye protection that blocks at least 90% of UVA, IR, and visible light. Contact lenses block approximately 90% UV light. Lateral shields for very bright conditions.

III. **HAZARDOUS MARINE LIFE**

Eventually, every woman who is active in the marine environment, no matter how careful, will be bitten, stung, abraded, or punctured by a hazardous marine animal or plant.

A. **General care (infection control and prevention)**
1. Wounds acquired in the marine environment are often contaminated with seawater, sand, bacteria from the marine animal, venom, and other organic matter. To minimize the infection risk, all wounds should be cleaned as best possible.
2. **Irrigate the wound** with at least 1 L of sterile saline or the cleanest disinfected freshwater available. An alternate choice is to use tap water or disinfected drinking water. The addition of povidone-iodine in a solution not to exceed 10% may help kill bacteria. Never add solvents. Ocean water should be used only as a last resort because it is laden with marine bacteria. Fire coral, anemone, hydroid, and jellyfish sting should be detoxified with vinegar before application of freshwater.
3. **Scrub the wound vigorously** with soap and the irrigating solution, and remove all obvious fragments such as coral, seaweed, and fish spines. Do not pour alcohol, full-strength antiseptics, or hydrogen peroxide directly into the wound.
4. Wounds acquired in the marine environment frequently become infected. Marine bacteria are often different from land or freshwater and can cause serious illness.
   a. **Antibiotics:** Trimethoprim-sulfamethoxazole, adult dose of one double-strength tablet every 12 hr, or doxycycline, 100 mg twice daily, are the antibiotics of choice. A back-up antibiotic is ciprofloxacin, 500 mg every 12 hr, or ofloxacin, 400 mg every 12 hr.

B. **Sharks**
1. Shark attacks occur in the summer and fall seasons:
   a. Tropical zone, 20° North–20° South: All months of the year.
   b. Latitudes 20° N–40° N, May through November.
   c. 20° S–40° S, November to April
2. Until last year, textbooks advised women not to dive during menstruation. The current advice is that the data are inconclusive.
   a. An Australian study showed no difference in the number of shark attacks on men and women. On further examination of the data, however, <50% of the divers were women, and they tended to stay in shallower water.
   b. The Diver Alert Network 1991 data show no difference in number of shark attacks on men and women. The data may be skewed because females may dive less frequently during menses.

    c. Women lose an average of 30 ml of blood/menses, and a 1-hour dive would average 0.25 ml of blood loss. A certain percentage of this blood is hemolyzed, and one Australian study suggested that hemolyzed blood may actually repel sharks.

    d. The conclusion is that more specific studies need to be done, and there may actually be an increased risk of shark attack to women during menstruation.

C. **Human parasitic catfish** (candiru, *Urinophilus erythrurus*)

    1. Located in Amazonia, the fish can penetrate the urethra, vagina, and rectum of humans and animals.

    2. Usually juvenile specimens are involved. They are eel-like, slimy, and elongated and have fang-like erectile teeth in front of mouth.

    3. Natives wear a variety of protective devices.

    4. Once it invades the urethra or vagina, it needs to be sugically removed.

D. **Schistosome dermatitis** (swimmer's itch) and **Bilharzia** (snail fever)

    1. A papular, pruritic dermatitis following freshwater immersion due to penetration of the skin by the cercarial larvae of various flukes (members of the phylum Platyhelminthes). Marine host is a marine bird or other marine vertebrae, and snails shed the cercaria.

    2. First symptoms are prickling sensation of the skin, small papules, and intense itching. Some people are hypersensitive and develop severe reactions.

    3. **Treatment**

        a. Antihistamines

        b. Topical steroid creams

        c. Antibiotics for secondary infections due to intense scratching

        d. Praziquantel, 20 mg orally three times daily in 1 day, for serious systemic infection called **Katayma fever**. This may occur within 6–8 weeks after exposure, especially in tropical areas. Diagnosis is made by examining the stool for ovum and parasites.

    4. **Prevention**

        a. Protective clothing, heavy nylon or rubber dive suit

        b. Dimethyl phthallate solution, 25% in cream base, rubbed on skin before swimming

        c. Medical or industrial-grade protective hand creams applied to the body prior to swimming may help.

        d. Brisk scrubbing with a rough towel immediately after leaving the water is helpful.

IV. HYPOTHERMIA

Thermal stress, especially cold, is a common problem in the marine environment. Temperatures must be in the mid-80° F range to achieve thermal balance. Significant heat loss occurs if the woman is exposed without thermal protection for even brief periods of time. This is especially true in temperate or northern waters for acute hypothermia, and also true in the tropics for chronic hypothermia. This may occur after repetitive dives over days (*see* also Chapter 43).

A. **Mild hypothermia:** Rectal temperature 90° F or above

    1. Signs and symptoms: Shivering, minimal or no alteration of mental status, normal or slightly impaired coordination

    2. Treatment

        a. Field rewarming with external heat source

        b. Remove wet clothes.

        c. Protect head and neck from further heat loss.

        d. Insulate from ground.

        e. Oral hydration and glucose (not orally if altered mental status)

B. **Profound hypothermia:** Rectal temperature <90° F
   1. Signs and symptoms: Altered mental status not attributable to other causes, decreased coordination, lassitude, and apathetic and uncooperative attitude
   2. Treatment
      a. Handle with care. Sudden movements may risk ventricular fibrillation.
      b. Evacuate as soon as possible. Try to reverse heat loss while waiting.
      c. Place in sleeping bag with two normothermic persons.
      d. If available, a portable rewarming suit, with heated humidified air, warmed intravenous hydration, and glucose.
C. Early studies showed women have less thermoregulatory capability than men. The subjects were "matched" college students; in fact, they had no disease, but the men were fit and active, whereas the women were sedentary.
   1. A recent study showed no difference in cold. With all variables equal, women may have a slight theoretical advantage due to subcutaneous fat.
   2. Women sweat less, and because of increased subcutaneous fat have a theoretical decreased heat thermoregulatory mechanism. With fit subjects, women acclimate to heat equal to men in recent studies.
   3. Small individuals of either sex may be at a slight disadvantage in extremely hot or cold environments due to body-surface-to-mass ratio. The male-female difference is very small.
   4. Small muscle mass is a disadvantage in cold because it generates less heat through exercise or shivering.
      a. Women, if equally fit, neutralize this difference with increased subcutaneous fat.
      b. Upper body weight training and aerobic fitness will prevent hypothermia, especially in professional women divers.

V. IMMUNIZATIONS

Often the woman who is working or playing in the marine environment will need to travel. This often involves tropical climates in third-world countries.
A. Immunizations for the marine traveler should include malaria prophylaxis and prevention and treatment of food- and water-borne diseases.
B. The only difference in requirements between men and women concerns the woman anticipating pregnancy (Table 2).
   1. Best to give necessary vaccinations during the last two trimesters of pregnancy for travel in endemic areas. In general, avoid live vaccines in the pregnant traveler (MMR, OPV, and oral typhoid). MMR is absolutely contraindicated in pregnancy.
   2. Yellow fever immunization is given only if travel is necessary and risk of disease substantial.
   3. CDC recommends oral polio vaccine (OPV) to nonimmunized pregnant women only if a strong need for immediate protection exits. Inactivated polio vaccine is preferred.
   4. If risk justifies typhoid immunization, injection is preferred.

VI. MARINE FIRST AID KIT

A. This is a suggested list of supplies to treat a wide variety of medical situations related to marine activity. It may not address every situation and should be modified to meet the needs of the individual and the location.
   1. Medical guidebook (e.g., Clark's *Dangerous Marine Organisms in Hawaii* and Auerbach's *A Medical Guide to Hazardous Marine Life*)
   2. Elastic cloth bandages (Band-Aids), assorted sizes, butterfly bandages or Steri-Strips, assorted sizes
   3. 2 × 2-inch sterile gauze pads
   4. 4 × 4-inch sterile gauze pads

TABLE 2.	Vaccination during Pregnancy

Vaccine		Indications for Vaccination during Pregnancy
Live virus vaccines		
Measles	Live-attenuated	Contraindicated
Mumps		
Rubella		
Yellow fever	Live-attenuated	Contraindicated except if exposure is unavoidable
Poliomyelitis	Trivalent live-attentuated (OPV)	Persons at substantial risk of exposure may receive live-attenuated virus vaccine
Inactivated virus vaccines		
Hepatitis B	Recombinant produced, purified hepatitis B surface antigen	Pregnancy is not a contraindication.
Influenza	Inactivated type A and B virus vaccines	Usually recommended only for patients with serious underlying disease. It is prudent to avoid vaccination during the first trimester. Consult health authorities for current recommendations.
Poliomyelitis	Killed virus (IPV)	OPV, not IPV, is indicated for immediate protection of pregnant females
Rabies	Killed virus Rabies IG	Substantial risk of exposure
Live bacterial vaccines		
Typhoid (Ty21a)	Live bacterial	Should reflect actual risks of disease and probable benefits of vaccine
Inactivated bacterial vaccines		
Cholera	Killed bacterial	Should reflect actual risks of disease and probable benefits of vaccine
Typhoid		
Plague	Killed bacterial	Selective vaccination of exposed persons
Meningococcal	Polysaccharide	Only in unusual outbreak situations
Pneumococcal	Polysaccharide	Only for high-risk persons
Haemophilus b conjugate	Polysaccharide-protein	Only for high-risk persons
Toxoids		
Tetanus-diphtheria (Td)	Combined tetanus-diphtheria toxoids, adult formulation	Lack of primary series, or no booster within 10 years. It is prudent to avoid vaccination during first trimester.
Immune globulins, pooled or hyperimmune	Immune globulin or specific globulin preparations	Exposure or anticipated unavoidable exposure to measles, hepatitis A, hepatitis B, rabies, or tetanus

5. 8 × 12-inch sterile gauze pads
6. 2-inch rolled gauze
7. 4-inch rolled gauze
8. 2-inch elastic wrap or conforming roll bandage (Coban)
9. 4-inch elastic wrap or conforming roll bandage (Coban)
10. 1-inch rolled adhesive tape
11. Scissors
12. Forceps (splinter)
13. Thermometer (hypothermic)
14. Soap (Phresh, pHisoHex, or pHisoDerm)
15. Cotton swabs
16. 3–12-oz sterile eye wash (aerosol)
17. Tincture of benzoin (bandage adhesive)

18. Bacitracin ointment or Mupirocin ointment
19. Hydrocortisone cream 1% and a mid-potency steroid cream
20. Analgesics (acetaminophen, 325 mg, with codeine, 30 mg tablets, or other combination of narcotic and acetaminophen)
21. Prednisone, 10-mg tablets
22. Doxycycline, 100 mg
23. Trimethoprim-sulfamethoxazole
24. Ciprofloxacin, 500-mg tablets
25. Clarithromycin, 500-mg tablets, third-generation cephalosporin, or azithromycin, 250-mg capsules
26. Pen-Vee K, 250-mg tablets
27. Broad-spectrum sunscreen (SPF 15 or greater)
28. Allergy kit: Epinephrine with needle/syringe; diphenhydramine, 25-mg capsules; or nonsedating alternative such as terfenadine or loratadine
29. Providone-iodine, 10% solution
30. Acetic acid, 5% (vinegar)
31. Isopropyl alcohol, 40%–70%
32. Hydrogen peroxide
33. Instant heat pack
34. Snake bite suction device
35. Motion sickness drugs (perchlorparyzine, hydroxyzine, dimenhydrinate, scopolamine patch—injectable, rectal, and oral)
36. Anesthetic eye drops (proparacaine or tetracaine)
37. Cycloplegic, 0.25% scopolamine or Cyclogyl
38. Ophthalmic antibiotic (gentamicin, tobramycin)
39. 18-gauge and 27-gauge sterile needles (helpful for removal of foreign bodies)
40. Allergic conjunctivitis drugs (Ketorolac, ophthalmic, or nedocromil sodium)
41. Airway and breather mask

ACKNOWLEDGMENTS

Direct financial support for this report was provided by the National Oceanic and Atmospheric Administration (NOAA) and the Dive Equipment Manufacturers Association (DEMA). Divers Alert Network also recognizes the dive clubs, stores, instructors, and many individual members who support the organization and diving safety. (Divers Alert Network, Box 3823, Duke University Medical Center, Durham, NC 27710)

REFERENCES

1. Auerbach PS: A Medical Guide to Hazardous Marine Life. St. Louis, Mosby, 1991, pp 1–52.
2. Barry M, Bia F: Pregnancy and travel. JAMA 261:728–731, 1989.
3. Bassett B: Twelve year survey of the susceptibility of women to altitude decompression sickness. Presented at the Aerospace Medical Association Scientific meeting, 1978, pp 31–40.
4. Bennett P, Moon R, Mebane G, et al: 1991 Report on Diving Accidents and Fatalities. Durham, NC, Divers Alert Network, 1992.
5. Centers for Disease Control and Prevention: Health Information for International Travel. Atlanta, CDC, 1993 (published yearly, $4.75).
6. Clark AM, Sims JK: Dangerous Marine Organisms of Hawaii. NOAA Office of Sea Grant, Department of Commerce, Fifth Printing, September 1989.
7. Cresswell J, Ste Leger-Dowse M: Women and scuba diving. BMJ 302:1590–1591, 1991.
8. Fife W: Women in Diving: 35th Undersea and Hyperbaric Medical Society Workshop [UHMS publ no. 71 (WS-WD)]. Undersea and Hyperbaric Medical Society, 1987, pp 1–162.
9. Halstead KW: Dangerous Marine Animals. St. Louis, Mosby, 1993.
10. Kizer KW: Meeting the challenge of scuba diving emergencies: Recognition, resuscitation, and recompression. Emerg Med 12(17):151–159, 1991.
11. Rudge S: Relationship of menstrual history to altitude chamber decompression sickness. Aviat Space Environ Med (July):657–659, 1990.
12. Schirmer JU, Workman WT: Menstrual history and altitude chamber trainees. Aviat Space Environ Med (July):616–618, 1992.

13. Summary of Health Information for International Travel. Washington, DC, U.S. Government Printing Office.

14. Thompson RF: Travel and Routine Immunizations: A Practical Guide for the Medical Office. Milwaukee, WI, Shoreland Medical Marketing.

15. Vorosmarti J: Fitness to Dive: 34th Undersea and Hyperbaric Medical Society Workshop [UHMS publ no. 70 (WS-FD)]. Undersea and Hyperbaric Medical Society, 1987, pp 12–116.

16. WHO: Vaccination Certificate Requirements and Health Advice for International Travelers. Geneva, World Health Organization, 1993 (published yearly).

17. Wilderness Medical Society: Marine and Tropical Medicine Syllabus, February 1993. Indianapolis, IN, Wilderness Medical Society, 1993.

18. Zwingelberg KM, Knight MA, Biles JB: Decompression sickness in women divers. Undersea Biomed Res 14(4):311–317, 1987.

Chapter 46: Swimming and Water Polo

KATHERINE KENAL, MD, MA

Swimming is the most popular recreational activity in the U.S., enjoyed by more than 120 million people. Its popularity lies in its excellent potential for building cardiovascular and musculoskeletal fitness with less risk for injury as compared to other sports. Participants span all age groups, from water babies to Masters swimmers. Over 171,000 (55.5% women) are registered with U.S. Swimming and involved in year-round competitive swimming programs. An additional 33,000 compete on a seasonal basis. Still more compete in colleges and universities. Masters Swimming organized its first national championship in 1972 and now includes incremental age groups from 19 years old up to its oldest member who is 100. Of its 27,500 members, 42% are women, the largest female age group is 30–34 years old, and the oldest female swimmer is in her late 80s.

Distance ocean swimming and open-water swimming have enjoyed increased popularity. A popular competitive ocean swim is the La Jolla Rough Water Swim in California, which attracts several thousand swimmers every summer. The limits have been tested, most notably by Lynne Cox, former English Channel record holder, whose accomplishments include a swim across the Bering Strait from the U.S. to Russia in a water temperature of 39° F (normal pool temperature is 78–82° F).

As a sport, water polo has been around for a century. Long popular on the east and west coasts, there has been a recent surge in growth over the last 5 years, much of it occurring in the midwest. Since the 1970s, the number of registered female players has grown to over 2200 (with estimates of *unregistered* players more than double that number). Women's teams at the community, high school and university level have provided players for the U.S. National Women's Team, which competes internationally at the World Championships.

Even though swimming and its associated sports are considered relatively injury-free, there are common injuries and other medical concerns which are specific to pool swimmers, ocean swimmers, and water polo players.

I. BIOMECHANICS

Water is a highly resistant medium through which a swimmer must propel herself. **Proper stroke biomechanics** is of utmost importance to ensure energy-efficient movement through water as well as reduction of injuries.

A. **Overview**
   1. Serious competitors can swim up to 10,000–14,000 m/day (6–8 miles) 6–7 days/week.
   2. They perform over 1 million arm cycles annually and a greater number of leg kicks.
   3. Four strokes are used:
      a. Freestyle (most efficient stroke)
      b. Backstroke
      c. Butterfly
      d. Breaststroke

B. **Upper extremity:** Greater than 75% of the forward propulsion comes from the arms (except in breaststroke where it is more evenly divided between arm stroke and kick).
   1. **Arm stroke:** 3 out of 4 strokes use the same shoulder motion. The arm stroke is divided into two phases:
      a. **Pull-through:** Arm generates progressive acceleration through this underwater portion.
         i. Hand entry and stroke initiation
         ii. Mid-pull-through

        iii. End push-through

        iv. Lead stroke with hand, keeping hand flat for greatest surface area with fingers in comfortable position.

    b. **Recovery:** Arm is out of water with elbow in horizontal plane above hand (in breaststroke the recovery is underwater).

        i. Elbow lift

        ii. Mid-recovery

        iii. Hand entry leads elbow into water.

  2. **Body position:** Minimize surface area exposure to enhance hydroplaning.

  3. **Body roll:** At its maximum (70–100°) in mid-pull-through, body roll decreases the horizontal arm extension required during recovery to clear the hand above the water and decreases the amount of head rotation required for each breath.

    a. Body roll is minimized in water polo during head-up swimming and when driving with the ball.

    b. In ocean swimming, the swimmer may be forced to single-sided breathing when waves approach from one direction and to a more head-up position in choppy water, both of which tend to limit symmetric roll.

C. **Lower extremity**

  1. **Knee**

    a. In 3 of 4 strokes, the kick is primarily a stabilizing force (with increasing propulsion as the distance shortens).

    b. Stress is in the flexion-extension plane from 0–90°.

    c. The breaststroke gains substantial propulsion from its kick. The knees flex to 130° with thighs abducted, feet dorsiflexed and everted.

        i. This motion places excessive valgus and external rotational stress on the medial supporting structures of the knees as the thighs adduct and extend during the propulsion phase.

    d. The "eggbeater" kick used by water polo players imposes similar stresses to the medial knee, particularly for the goalie and 2-m guard, whose kick provides substantial propulsion for vertical, lateral, and forward motion.

  2. **Ankle**

    a. Flutter and butterfly kicks move the foot in the flexion-extension plane.

    b. In breaststroke, active dorsiflexion and eversion are needed in the propulsion phase. These movements can place considerable stress on the anterior and lateral compartments.

II. ORTHOPEDIC INJURIES

A. **Swimmer's shoulder**

  1. **Generally related to overuse.** It is the most common musculoskeletal injury in swimmers. In a recent survey, 73% of elite swimmers had a history of interfering shoulder complaints at some point in their racing careers.

  2. **Most commonly affects:**

    a. Shoulder on the breathing side

    b. Swimmers involved in sprinting events

    c. Occurs during early to mid season upon rapid increase in workload

  3. **Mechanism**

    a. The shoulder cycles through extremes of abduction and adduction with internal rotation.

    b. At hand entry, the soft tissue structures of the shoulder are impinged underneath the coracoacromial arch. This impingement has also been described in various throwing sports including water polo.

    c. At the end of push-through, decreased blood supply is observed in the area of the supraspinatus and biceps tendon insertions, further fueling inflammatory and degenerative changes.

    d. Glenohumeral instability with resultant abnormal anterior and superior migration of the humeral head has been cited as a major, if not primary, cause for swimmer's shoulder. May involve bony abnormality.

4. **Other injuries:**
   a. Arthritic changes or adhesive capsulitis may be found more commonly in the Masters swimmer.
   b. In water polo, a shot block during the acceleration phase of a throw can cause acute microtrauma to the rotator cuff.

5. **Anatomy:** Structures at risk for impingement:
   a. Rotator cuff muscles: supraspinatus (acute: tendinitis; chronic: tendinosis)
   b. Subacromial bursa (bursitis)
   c. Coracoacromial ligament (inflammation)
   d. Biceps tendon (tendinitis)

6. **Symptoms** described in four stages:
   a. Stage 1: Pain after activity only
   b. Stage 2: Pain during activity, but does not restrict activity
   c. Stage 3: Pain during activity that restricts performance
   d. Stage 4: Chronic, unremitting pain, which prevents competitive swimming

7. **Diagnosis**
   a. **Impingement syndrome**
      i. Pain while swimming, particularly at hand entry/stroke initiation and during end of push-through
      ii. Limited range of motion with pain in extreme arm positions
      iii. Tenderness along coracoacromial ligament
      iv. Tenderness at insertion of supraspinatus tendon on humerus
      v. Impingement sign: anterior and/or overhead
      vi. Instability or anatomic abnormality
   b. **Biceps tendinitis**
      i. Tenderness to palpation of bicipital groove
      ii. Pain at bicipital groove with resisted forearm supination and elbow flexion (Yergason's maneuver) or with resisted forward flexion
   c. **Rotator cuff tear**
      i. History of chronic impingement or acute trauma
      ii. Drop arm test
   d. **Glenohumeral instability**
      i. Backstroke flipturn—apprehension
      ii. Apprehension sign
      iii. Sulcus sign
      iv. Clunck sign for glenoid labral tear
   e. **Posterior shoulder strain**
      i. Follow-through in water polo throw involves deceleration. Posterior shoulder pain during this phase of the throw is due to glenohumeral instability and/or eccentric load placed on weak posterior structures of shoulder, including the posterior rotator cuff muscles and shoulder stabilizers (rhomboid, levator scapulae, and inferior trapezius muscles).
   f. **Adhesive capsulitis**
      i. Decreased range of motion, particularly internal and external rotation and abduction
      ii. Palpable mechanical block to motion that is not necessarily pain-related
   g. **Acromioclavicular arthritis**
      i. Pain at AC joint with extreme horizontal adduction at 90° flexion
      ii. Cross arm test

8. **Other diagnostic tests**
   a. Radiographs

b. CT scan
c. MRI
d. Arthrogram
e. Steroid injection

9. **Treatment**
   a. Most importantly, keep the athlete involved in the sport with an active rehabilitation program.
   b. Ice: 15–20 minutes, 3–5 times a day
   c. Nonsteroidal antiinflammatory drugs (NSAIDs)
   d. Physical therapy modalities (i.e., phonophoresis/iontophoresis, cross-friction massage, ultrasound)
   e. Corticosteroid injection in recalcitrant cases of impingement syndrome
   f. Blatz proximal arm band for biceps tendinitis: Similar to tennis elbow strap, it is purported to work by restoring excursion of the biceps and deltoid muscles.
   g. Coach should assess the stroke for any biomechanical errors, as improper stroke mechanics is a major cause of swimming-related injuries.
   h. Reduce workout intensity and distance covered.
   i. Eliminate butterfly stroke, throwing in water polo, and use of swim paddles, drag suits, and pull buoys during treatment and rehabilitation phase
   j. Continue strength workouts for rotator cuff muscles and scapulae stabilizers, but eliminate other upper body exercises
   k. Continue to kick with skulling at side, but eliminate use of kick board, as it can irritate shoulders when arms are holding board in full extension.
   l. Surgical treatment is rarely needed.

10. **Prevention**
   a. Fundamentals of good stroke biomechanics should be emphasized throughout the season. The coach must be particularly attuned to this when the swimmer becomes fatigued, a time when she is more likely to exercise poor biomechanics.
   b. The coach must provide a proper progression in intensity and duration of swimming and strength training.
   c. Stretching should be an integral part of the warm-up phase; however, partner-stretching for the shoulders should be eliminated because it promotes extremes in range of motion which can stretch the anterior capsule and predispose an athlete to unwanted instability.
   d. Strength training should promote balance in the musculature about the shoulder.
      i. Swimmers tend to have strong **internal rotators,** and therefore work with elastic bands (surgical tubing) should emphasize concentric as well as eccentric load on the **external rotators**.
      ii. Bands can be used to simulate resisted throwing motion for the water polo player.
      iii. Scapulae stabilizers (rhomboids, levator scapula, serratus anterior, and trapezius) are strengthened by the sitted dip exercise, seated rowing and pull-down exercises.
   e. Because hand paddles place extra stress on the shoulder, prudent usage is warranted.

B. **Back and neck**
   1. **Most injuries occur in the lower back.** Strains of lumbar myofacial tissue can occur from the repeated pounding and twisting during flip turns or torsional strain when the body does not roll as a whole unit during the stroke.
   2. **Scheuermann's disease** (butterflier's back)
      a. Uncommon. Most typically presents in swimmers with backache and thoracic kyphosis.

      b. The original lesion is a growth disturbance of the epiphyseal plates of the anterior vertebral body. The cause may be developmental, traumatic, or both.

      c. Progression of the disease appears to be due to repetitive flexion loading of the spine.

  3. **Spondylolysis:** Can occur with or without spondylolisthesis.

      a. Hyperextension motions of the lumbar spine during strenuous training, as seen with the newer style of breaststroke and with the butterfly stroke, places the swimmer at risk for developing or exacerbating this condition. Starts and turns also aggravate it.

      b. Probably caused by repetitive stress in a genetically predisposed athlete rather than by an acute injury.

      c. Radiographically, it presents as a defect in the pars interarticularis (usually unilateral—L5 vertebra, "Scotty dog with collar"). If plain films are unremarkable bone scan should be used to confirm the suspected diagnosis (stress response of bone that has not proceeded to fracture).

      d. It may be asymptomatic; however, if symptomatic and acute or chronic, one can elicit a positive one-leg hyperextension test.

  4. **Disc syndrome and degenerative joint disease of the cervical spine:** Can present in the Masters swimmer with the typical radiculopathy.

  5. **Atlanto-occipital instability:** Of particular concern for the Down's syndrome athlete. These swimmers should avoid diving by starting races in the water. Water polo should be avoided as well.

  6. **Treatment**

      a. **Myofascial strains** can be treated with ice, massage therapy, NSAIDs, rest, and appropriate stretching and strengthening.

      b. In **Scheuermann's disease,** avoid aggravating activities (butterfly, bench press, dumbbell flies).

        i. Treat with extension exercises, rest and a Warm "N" Form brace. Athlete may resume activities (except as noted) when pain-free.

        ii. If 3 or more vertebrae are involved, with kyphosis exceeding 40°, a hyperlordotic Boston-type brace may be required. Swimmers should be followed radiographically until vertebral growth is completed.

      c. Acute lesion of **spondylolysis** requires restricting aggravating activities, starting hamstring flexibility, abdominal strengthening, and gentle extension exercises to strengthen the paraspinous muscles.

        i. Use of an antilordotic brace may allow the swimmer to return to the water.

        ii. Radiographically, a pars defect may persist without symptoms if there is a fibrous union; therefore, resolution of symptoms with a normal bone scan may establish an end point of treatment.

C. **Elbow**

  1. In backstroke and the water polo throw, **medial epicondylitis** is caused by repetitive tension overloading of the wrist flexors, leading to microtears in the tendinous insertion at the epicondyle. The athlete will have tenderness over the medial epicondyle and increased pain with resisted wrist (or middle finger) flexion and forearm pronation.

  2. **Treatment**

      a. RICE (rest, ice, compression, elevation)

      b. Physical therapy

      c. Splint (with wrist in neutral)

      d. NSAIDs

      e. Steroid injections (limit to 3)

      f. If after prolonged time (6–12 months) with failure of conservative treatment, the rare athlete may require surgery involving recession of the flexor tendon at its medial epicondyle origin.

D. **Fingers**
 1. **Interphalangeal joint (IP) injuries**
    a. **"Jammed finger"** commonly occurs in water polo when the outstretched finger is jammed backward by a direct blow to the fingertip, leading to a sprain of the ligaments surrounding the IP joint.
    b. Two specific injuries can result:
       i. **Mallet finger,** caused by hyperflexion of the distal interphalangeal (DIP) joint disrupting the extensor mechanism. This can result in avulsion fracture of the dorsal aspect of the base of the distal phalanx. There will be pain over the dorsal DIP and the athlete will be unable to fully extend the distal phalanx.
       ii. **Hyperextension** of the proximal interphalangeal (PIP) joint, which can lead to avulsion fracture of the volar aspect of the more distal bone.
       iii. Both injuries can be confirmed by a lateral radiographic view.
 2. **Treatment**
    a. RICE
    b. Often, adequate immobilization is provided by buddy taping the injured finger to the adjacent finger, allowing the player to return quickly to the game (within the 3-min time limit for injury treatment).
    c. The PIP joint with volar plate injuries should be immobilized in about 30° flexion for 2–3 weeks. If fracture is displaced or joint is unstable, it may require extended splinting or surgical referral.
    d. An acute mallet finger requires immobilization of DIP in full extension, for 6–8 weeks.
E. **Knees**
 1. **Medial knee pain:** Breaststrokers report an incidence of **medial knee pain** of 73%. Water polo players, particularly goalies and 2-m guards, also report medial knee pain. Applied forces to the knee include increased valgus and rotatory stress with initiation of the kick and subsequent external tibial rotation, circumduction, and knee extension.
 2. Clinically, one finds tenderness over the medial collateral ligament, inferomedial patellar border, medial retinaculum, and medial plica.
    a. **Medial collateral ligament:** Pain can be reproduced with valgus stress at 30° flexion.
    b. **Medial synovitis** with or without medial plica: Localized inflammation secondary to entrapment of peripatellar synovium. May have swollen tender plica.
    c. **Patellofemoral pain syndrome:** Due to malalignment (tilt, rotation, lateral placement) with increased Q-angle, weak vastus medialis obliquus function, imbalance of gluteal muscle strength, overpronation, hamstring/quadriceps inflexibility. Pain with palpation of the patellar facets and adjacent femoral condyles, and positive patellar compression test. May have patellar instability or patella alta.
 3. **Treatment**
    a. RICE
    b. Physical therapy
    c. Corticosteroid injection to plica (not intraarticular)
    d. Change to other strokes in training during acute phase
 4. **Prevention:** This is usually an overuse injury, so stress:
    a. Adequate warm-up with gradual increase in breaststroke distance and intensity
    b. Proper kick biomechanics assessed by coach
    c. Appropriate strengthening and stretching (eliminate partner-stretching of knees)
F. **Ankles**
 1. The repetitive nature of the flutter and dolphin kick can lead to **tendinitis** of the extensor tendons of the foot and ankle where they cross under the extensor retinaculum.

2. **Treatment**
    a. RICE
    b. NSAIDs
    c. Eliminate use of flippers during acute phase
    d. Appropriate stretching with gradual return
G. **Muscle cramps**
    1. Involuntary muscle contraction, particularly of the calves. The cause is uncertain, but several factors are associated:
        a. Dehydration
        b. Fatigue
        c. Electrolyte deficiencies/imbalances (due to prolonged illness with vomiting/diarrhea, bulemia, inadequate electrolyte replacement with prolonged exercise)
        d. Acute cold exposure (ocean swimming)
    2. **Treatment**
        a. Stretch affected muscle
        b. Massage
        c. Ice
        d. Fluid and electrolyte replacement (1 lb of lost weight = 1 pt of fluid)
        e. Regularly occurring cramps require further work-up to rule out diabetes, or neurovascular problems.
    3. **Prevention**
        a. Hydration and electrolyte replacement
        b. Appropriate training to avoid extreme fatigue
        c. Stretching
        d. Allow adequate time to acclimatize to cold water

III. **MEDICAL ISSUES**

A. **Swimmer's ear**
    1. **Diffuse external otitis** is commonly caused by bacteria or fungal infection of the external auditory meatus. Infection is introduced to a hyperhydrated and macerated ear canal. Itching is commonly the first symptom. Pain can be severe and is caused by inflammation.
    2. **Exostoses** (bony growths) in the ear canals may occur in ocean swimmers from prolonged exposure to cold water and wind. The epithelium can become thin and irritated in these areas. Debris, such as sand and seaweed can get trapped behind the exostosis.
    3. **Treatment**
        a. **Irrigation:** Use a 20-mL syringe with high-velocity stream of water and hydrogen peroxide (1:1) to flush debris.
        b. **Mild inflammation** is treated by reacidifying the canal with 2% acetic acid or 2% boric acid otic solution (assuming tympanic membrane is not perforated). **Severe edema** is treated by inserting cotton wick in the canal and adding drops of high-potency steroids, Burrow's solution, or 2% acetic acid.
        c. **Bacterial infections** respond to antibiotic/steroid drops (e.g., Coly-Mycin S Otic, Cortisporin Otic suspension). Treat with 3–4 drops in affected ear 3–4 times daily; may require oral antibiotics or local/oral analgesics. Mild cases may be treated with a 1:1 solution of isopropyl alcohol and vinegar.
        d. **Fungal infections** can be treated with cresylate or thimerosal; tolnaftate after canal is cleared of debris. Eight drops per ear 3 times/day for 7 days.
        e. Remain out of water until acute infection is treated, usually 7–10 days. Athletes may return to water, if absolutely necessary 2–3 days after initiating therapy if painfree and without redness, drainage, or hot burning sensation. *However, this may delay healing.*

4. **Prevention**
   a. Drain water from ears after swimming, by tilting head and jumping vigorously or by drying with a towel. Avoid scratching. Put dropperful of drying agent in each ear. Use newer silicon ear plugs. Protect ears from cold and wind with swim cap.
   b. The addition of ear guards to the water polo cap has drastically reduced the incidence of ruptured tympanic membranes from thrown-ball contact with the ear.

B. **Chlorine-related irritant dermatitis and conjunctivitis**
   1. **Irritant dermatitis** presents with allergic-type symptoms. Swimmers who have preexisting allergies may have heightened adverse reactions such as rhinitis, itchy eyes, and itchy/dry skin.
   2. **Conjunctivitis** should be treated appropriately if infectious. If due to irritation, treat with over-the-counter artificial tears and/or antihistamines. Judicious use of steroid ophthalmic preparations may be tried after viral infection is ruled out.
   3. **Swollen corneas** can result from the freshwater component of pool water. Swimmers may experience haloes, blurriness, and scratchy sensation. Corneas usually repair themselves in a few hours, and the damage is not accumulative.
   4. **Prevention**
      a. Remain in pool no longer than necessary
      b. After leaving the pool, cleanse body thoroughly with soap and water, flushing eyes, nose, and ears.
      c. Use goggles to avoid eye irritation.
      d. Apply moisturizing lotion to skin immediately after showering.
      e. To protect hair, apply conditioner on dry hair before swimming and cover with a cap. Then, use any over-the-counter swim shampoo after swimming.

C. **Contact lenses**
   1. Avoid wearing soft contact lenses, even with goggles. A naturally occurring protozoan, *Acanthamoeba,* has been responsible for more than 100 cases of **acanthamoeba kerititis,** which can lead to blindness.
      a. Recommend goggles with prescription lenses.

D. **Hypothermia**
   1. Open-water swimmers can succumb to hypothermia, which is defined as a generalized physiologic state in which the core temperature is below 95°F.
   2. **Early warning signs** are uncomfortable cold with numbness during the swim. Race officials and crew members should be alert for swimmers with discolored faces, unfocused eyes, and labored/erratic strokes. Sure signs are confusion, lethargy, incoordination, and speech difficulties.
   3. **Treatment**
      a. Removal from water and removal of wet swimming suit; provide warm wool blankets, warm fluids, and slow rewarming in hot bath.
      b. Be aware of the afterdrop phenomenon (continued temperature fall during rewarming—use continual temperature monitoring).
      c. Severe cases (core temperature <85°F) will need hospitalization.
   4. **Prevention**
      a. Key in avoiding hypothermia.
      b. Training should allow for adaptation to cold water by gradual progression of swimming in lower temperatures and lengthening times of exposure.
      c. The greater the percent of body fat, the better the degree of insulation (Lynne Cox swam for 2 hours across the Bering Strait in 39°F water—her body fat was 35%).
      d. National and world federations of long-distance swimming prohibit the use of wet suits. However, unsanctioned races will allow them, offering the added advantage of bouyancy.
      e. Liberal application of anhydrous lanolin to the axilla, inner thigh, neck, back, and chest may help (this may make emergency removal from water difficult).

5. **Heed the warning signs.** Appropriate monitoring by verbal communication is absolutely necessary between swimmer and crew members (touching will automatically disqualify them). Boats for crew and race officials must be adequately equipped to provide immediate treatment of hypothermia.

E. **Exercise-induced asthma**
  1. Warm humid conditions associated with swimming provide a favorable environment for exercise-induced asthma.
  2. Some swimmers may need preexercise medication, 15 minutes before activity, with inhaled beta-agonist or cromolyn sodium. May try nonpharmacologic measures.
  3. Be aware of NCAA- and IOC-banned drugs.

F. **Headache**
  1. **Exertional headache** can come from dynamic or static efforts.
     a. Considered benign; the cause is not known but is probably vascular in origin with certain activities as triggers.
     b. Acute onset, short duration (4–6 min), brought on by exertion, generalized, may recur with gradual resolution over weeks to months. Often positive family history for migraines. Physical examination, CT of head, cervical and skull radiographs, lumbar puncture have normal findings.
     c. **Treatment** is avoiding aggravating activities and/or using NSAIDs. With failure of conservative treatment, antimigraine medications may be helpful.
  2. **Cold-induced headache** possible in distance ocean swimmers. Preventive measures with acclimatization are the best treatment. It is advisable to wear a swim cap.
  3. **Goggle headache** presents with pain in the facial and temporal areas. It occurs from excessively tight-fitting goggles. Thought to be caused by pressure on the superficial cutaneous nerves in the orbital regions. Treat by loosening straps, avoid pressing goggles into occular orbit.
  4. **Headache in the Masters swimmer** may signal onset of **stroke** or may be a "walk headache," which occurs as manifestation of **ischemic heart disease.** Get appropriate history, physical examination, and diagnostic tests as indicated.

G. **Pregnancy**
  1. **Swimming can be safely initiated during pregnancy.** Avoid extremes of cold or hot water to minimize potential effects of hypo- or hyperthermic stress on the fetus. Nutritional intake must equal the caloric demands for both training and pregnancy. Replenish fluids to avoid dehydration.
  2. May continue swimming at same perceived level of exertion during first half of pregnancy. Avoid excessive exercise late in pregnancy. Observe recommendations of maximum heart rate: 220—age × 70%; maximum core temperature: 101°F. Close monitoring by physician is recommended.
  3. **Avoid water polo** due to the contact in the game and potential trauma to abdomen and fetus. The same considerations need to be taken into account for mass starts at open-water swims.
  4. **Swimming is a great postpartum activity,** particularly when joint laxity is prevalent. Resume swimming only after bleeding has stopped.

H. **Coronary heart disease (sudden death)**
  1. Two cardiac-related **deaths** have been reported in Masters swimmers during U.S. National Championships within the last 7 years.
  2. The **benefit/risk ratio favors exercise for the elderly;** however, a preparticipation history, physical examination, and indicated tests which are age-appropriate are imperative. Absolute contraindications for exercise must be understood.

I. **Overtraining**
  1. Excessive training that is nonspecific can lead to a state of overtraining. Inadequate recovery time uncouples the two-part process of training—tissue breakdown and recovery. Swimmers are left unable to match their adaptation response to the training load.

2. Signals of overtraining include problems in training, lifestyle, and health.
3. Research on competitive swimmers has shown no significant difference in performance between one group swimming one-half the distance of a control group over a 4-year period. Therefore, training should be specific to the competitive distance without detrimental overload.
4. Overtraining is important not only as it directly relates to decreased performance, but also for implications in athletic amenorrhea, disordered eating, and decreased function of the immune system.

J. **Other medical concerns**
1. Amenorrhea
2. Eating disorders/disordered eating
3. Hyperventilation training: Underwater lengths can be deadly
4. Skin problems: Sunburn, precancerous and cancerous lesions (particularly in Masters swimmers with accumulation of sun exposure), chafing, athlete's foot, cold-induced urticaria
5. Ocean creature envenomations
6. Psychology: Clinical and performance enhancement
7. Nutrition and dehydration

REFERENCES

1. Ciullo JV, Stevens GG: The prevention and treatment of injuries to the shoulder in swimming. Sports Med 7:182–204, 1989.
2. Dimeff RJ: Headaches in the athlete. Clin Sports Med 11:339–349, 1992.
3. Gambaccini P: Are you allergic to the pool? Fitness Swim 2(3):40–42, 1993.
4. Heinz Schelkun P: Swimmer's ear—getting patients back in the water. Phys SportsMed 19(7):85–90, 1991.
5. Johnson D: In swimming, shoulder the burden. Sportscare Fitness (May/June):1988, pp 24–30.
6. Johnson JE, Sim FH, Scott SG: Musculoskeletal injuries in competitive swimmers. Mayo Clin Proc 62:289–304, 1987.
7. Joy EA, Belgrade MJ: Exertional headache. Phys SportsMed 21(6):94–100, 1993.
8. Knuttgen HG: Training. Penn State Sports Med News 1(8):1–2, 1993.
9. Knuttgen HG: Swimmer's shoulder. Penn State Sports Med News 1(9):2–3, 1993.
10. Knuttgen HG: Swimming and soft contact lenses. Penn State Sports Med News 1(9):7, 1993.
11. McMaster WC, Long SC, Caiozzo VJ: Isokinetic torque imbalances in the rotator cuff of the elite water polo player. Am J Sports Med 19:72–75, 1991.
12. Pacelli LC: Water polo's benefits surface. Phys SportsMed 19(4):118–123, 1991.
13. Vizsolyi P, Taunton J, Robertson G, et al: Breaststroker's knee—An analysis of epidemiological and biomechanical factors. Am J Sports Med 15:63–71, 1987.

Chapter 47: Rowing

DAVID J. MUSNICK, MD

Rowing began in the U.S. as an intercollegiate athletic sport for women in the 1960s and 1970s. It was introduced as an Olympic sport for women in 1976. Women participate in crew in high school, college, club, and masters levels. Overuse injuries are common as these athletes are involved in rigorous training and racing schedules.

I. **OVERVIEW**

  A. **Injury incidence**
   1. **Overuse injuries** occur as listed regionally from most frequent in decreasing order[1]:
      a. Knee
      b. Low back
      c. Upper extremity
      d. Foot
      e. Ankle
      f. Rib cage/thoracic spine
      g. Other
   2. Injury incidence is maximum in the late winter and spring, corresponding to peak training and racing seasons, respectively.

  B. **Terminology**
   1. **Sculling** is rowing with two oars per oarswoman.
   2. **Sweep rowing** is done with one oar kept on only one side of the boat (port or starboard).

  C. **Boat information**
   1. Events are classified as:
      a. **Heavyweight:** Shells with a rower weighing >130 lb
      b. **Lightweight:** All rowers weighing <130 lb
   2. Boat seats move fore and aft.

  D. **Rowing strokes and biomechanics**
   1. **Catch** is when the oar is placed in the water. The knees, hips, and back are flexed and the elbows are extended.
   2. **Drive** is the propulsion phase. The rower begins in catch position with the subsequent rapid extension of knees, hips, and back. The scapula retracts, the shoulders extend, and the elbows flex.

II. **CREW INJURIES**

  A. **Medical history:** Any crew athlete presenting with injury symptoms should have a comprehensive history including:
   1. Description of training
   2. Sculling vs sweep rowing
   3. On-water training schedule
   4. Rowing ergometer training
   5. Weight training program
   6. Other aerobic muscular-toning exercise
   7. History of eating disorders
   8. Symptom in relation to phase of the stroke

9. History of spine symptoms
    a. A facet or disc syndrome can lead to a prolonged extremity overuse syndrome in some cases.
    b. Subtle spine problems can also lead to spine weakness and altered biomechanics resulting in overuse syndromes.

B. **Physical examination**
    1. Should be focused on regional problems
    2. The proximal joint should be examined (in extremity syndromes) along with required spine examination if there are spine symptoms or a prolonged extremity syndrome.
    3. Patterns of joint and muscle restriction should be assessed.
    4. A simulation of rowing technique should be done on an ergometer, if possible.
    5. The athlete should have a technique evaluation in the boat by the coach and trainer or physician.

C. **Injury prevention**
    1. Adequate stretching of Achilles, quadriceps, hamstrings, hip flexors, spine, and shoulder girdle should be done before on-water and conditioning activities.
    2. Strengthening programs of the spine, scapular stabilizers, rotator cuff, and anterior chest are important.
    3. Avoid overuse with rowing ergometer and weight-lifting programs.

III. INJURY TREATMENT

A. In treatment of overuse injuries caused by the rowing stroke, consider:
    1. Discontinue or decrease intensity of rowing ergometer workouts and substitute aerobic activities that will not exacerbate the overuse syndrome.
    2. Discontinue a selective part of the weight-lifting program that may be exacerbating the syndrome.
    3. Use antiinflammatories, physical therapy, and rowing technique analysis early.
    4. Decrease or discontinue on-water rowing if there is a moderately severe condition such as lumbar radiculopathy or a rib stress fracture.
    5. Alter equipment to diminish the load to the athlete (shorten oars, increase inboard length of oar, increase flex of oar).[2]
    6. Discontinue on-water rowing temporarily if the above measures fail and the syndrome continues to be aggravated and significantly affects performance or appears to be developing into a chronic syndrome.
    7. During racing season, temporizing measures may need to be taken to keep a high-level athlete rowing during critical races.

IV. SPECIFIC INJURIES

A. **Spine injuries**
    1. **Lumbar spine syndromes**
        a. **Sport-specific causes:**
            i. Large forces are transmitted through the spine, shoulders, and arms to the oar.
            ii. Sweep rowing can load the disc and facet joints disproportionately with torsional forces.
            iii. Significant forces occur in the discs during sitting and possibly in the rowing stroke.
            iv. Over-reaching at the catch can strain the spine.
        b. **Most back syndromes are "mechanical," "facet syndromes," central disc protrusions, annular disc tears, or a combination.**
            i. A comprehensive spine, sacroiliac joint, hip, neurologic, and biomechanical evaluation is important.
            ii. Plain films are often *not* useful on the initial visit.
            iii. Treatment

(a) Modify or discontinue ergometer and specific weight-training involving significant flexion, extension, or rotation of the spine.
(b) Lumbar support during non-rowing sitting (lumbar roll, etc.)
(c) Consider a swimming program if pain is reduced by swimming. (No diving.)
(d) Assessment of hip flexor and quadriceps/hamstring tightness should be done.
(e) Referral to a therapist with manual spine training should be done early. Include functional assessment of spine strength.
(f) A stabilization set of exercises should begin with emphasis on spine, abdominal, and hip region muscles.

c. **Lumbar disc syndromes**
   i. **Central disc syndromes** without radiculopathy may benefit from the above lumbar program plus an epidural cortisone injection.
      (a) May require stopping all rowing activities for 4–6 weeks if other interventions fail.
   ii. **Herniated discs with motor loss** should be followed very closely after rowing activities have stopped. They may benefit from epidural cortisone and manual therapy but may need surgical intervention if profound or progressive motor loss. Surgical consult is advisable early.
   iii. **Herniated discs with only sensory radiculopathy** may worsen with continued rowing. These patients may be able to participate in very important races if their physical findings are stable and they are informed of the risks.
      (a) Tricyclic antidepressants (nonsedating) may decrease the sensory radiculopathy symptoms.
      (b) MRI is more helpful than CT in localizing the lesions and degree of degenerative changes.
      (c) Patients with sensory radiculopathy with normal MRI may have **radiculitis** and may benefit from manual therapy, tricyclic antidepressants, and nerve sheath injection.
      (d) **Spondylolisthesis** and **spondylosis** should be suspected when there is localized low back pain off the midline made worse by extension.
         (i) Oblique and lateral lumbar films will confirm.
         (ii) Bone scan will confirm a stress fracture of the pars interarticularis.
         (iii) Neurologic symptoms are an indication for MRI.
         (iv) Patients with pars stress fractures should stop all rowing activities and be placed in a brace and started on appropriate physical therapy.

2. **Thoracic spine disorders**
   a. Most thoracic disorders are **strains, mechanical joint syndromes**, or **rib stress fractures**.
      i. Strains and mechanical syndromes are treated with manual physical therapy, technique evaluation and modification, and an upper-body strengthening program.
   b. **Persistent thoracic pain** may be secondary to costovertebral joint dysfunction/sprains, costochondritis (anterior chest), intrathoracic mass, or rib stress fractures.
   c. **Thoracic spine disc herniations** are very uncommon in crew athletes.
      i. Any patient with thoracic pain should have a neurologic examination and tests for upper motor neuron involvement.
   d. **Rib stress fractures**
      i. Suspect if localized and prolonged palpable pain along a particular rib.
         (a) Common locations are posterolateral and periscapula.
         (b) Radiographs may be negative for 3 or more weeks.

(c) Bone scan may be necessary to confirm.

(d) Palpate individual ribs for spring and point tenderness. Other symptoms include pain with deep breathing, rowing, and thoracic motion.

ii. Posterolateral ribs most commonly affected by repetitive motion, by a pull of the serratus anterior and rhomboids, as well as excessive scapular protraction.

iii. Sweep rowers appear to have a greater likelihood of stress fracture than scullers.

iv. The stress fracture often occurs during periods of intense training and racing.

v. Women develop stress fractures more commonly than men, likely secondary to a difference in upper body strength.[3]

vi. Treatment of a confirmed stress fracture involves:

(a) Discontinue rowing, ergometer, and selected weight-lifting for 4–6 weeks.

(b) Begin aerobic cross-training activities such as cycling, stair climbing, etc.

(c) Upper body and spine strengthening

(d) Gradually return the athlete to rowing activities and weight-lifting.

(e) Rowing technique or equipment evaluation and modification. Consider change from sweep to sculler.

(f) Begin physical therapy.

3. **Cervical spine disorders** are unusual and are usually facet syndromes or strains. They are often technique-related and related to posture as well as thoracic spine problems.

B. **Thoracic outlet syndrome**

1. Suspect in an athlete with **sensory radiculopathy primarily involving the lateral hand**. (Although the thumb and first finger may also be involved.)

a. Nighttime paresthesias are early symptoms.

b. Rule out vascular syndromes

c. Check patient in cervical rotation, abduction of arms, and military position.

2. Treatment consists of manual therapy, soft-tissue work, and joint mobilization.

3. If vascular symptoms develop, pursue vascular studies.

C. **Shoulder disorders**

1. **Impingement problems** are most common and often related to inadequate scapular stabilization and rotator cuff muscle strength as well as postural errors.

2. Treatment is standard with correction of the above muscle imbalances, technique modification, and avoidance of impingement position in weight-lifting. Physical therapy should be begun early.

a. Subacromial injection may be tried if conservative program is inadequate.

b. In persistent cuff tendinitis syndromes, the cervical spine should be thoroughly evaluated to rule out a cervical radiculopathy or a corresponding facet syndrome.

c. Surgical opinion should be sought if there is no improvement after rowing has been stopped, cervical spine problems have been treated, and subacromial injection and physical therapy have failed.

D. **Wrist syndromes**

1. **Extensor tenosynovitis** in the first, second, or "intersection" area of the dorsal compartment is more common.

a. Crepitus and swelling indicate moderate to severe involvement.

b. Treatment

i. Technique modification in the stroke finish and catch

ii. Splinting

iii. Nonsteroidal antiinflammatory drugs (NSAIDs)

iv. Cortisone injection into compartments
v. Decreasing ergometer workouts
vi. The rower does not usually need to be removed from water race activities.

E. **Knee disorders**
1. **Patellofemoral arthralgia** and **iliotibial band syndrome** (ITB) are common in rowers due to repetitive knee flexion and extension.
   a. Genu valgum, femoral anteversion, external tibial rotation, and tight hip flexors and quadriceps may predispose to patellofemoral arthralgia.
   b. Genu varum, and tight iliotibial bands may contribute to iliotibial band syndrome.
      i. Knee motion may be from 110° of flexion to full extension in rowing.
   c. Treatment
      i. Early therapy program to reverse patterns of muscle tightness
      ii. Decreasing squatting and knee extension weight-lifting
      iii. Decrease hill running, rowing ergometer, and stair-climbing.
      iv. Patella taping or bracing may be useful.
      v. Quadriceps/vastus medialis obliquus strengthening

F. **Exercise-induced allergic syndromes**
1. **Exercise-induced asthma** is common because of training in cold weather.
   a. Treat with bronchodilators with or without cromolyn sodium.
2. **Exercise-induced angioedema**
   a. Severe angioedema of the tongue with airway compromise is a **medical emergency** and requires epinephrine and usually cortisone treatment.
   b. If a rower has had one episode, she should always have a Medic-Alert bracelet and an epinephrine pen or anaphylaxis kit.
   c. If there are repeated episodes, the team physician should consider taking the athlete off the team because of the danger to the athlete.
3. **Exercise-induced anaphylaxis**
   a. Signs are hypotension, nausea, abdominal pain, anxiety, possible bronchospasm, possible angioedema.
   b. Because this is an unpredictable and **life-threatening problem** and impossible to treat on the water, the team physician should consider making this a medical contraindication for crew participation.

REFERENCES

1. Hosea, Timothy, Boland A, et al: Rowing injuries. In Postgraduate Advances in Sports Medicine, Forum Medicum. Philadelphia, University of Pennsylvania, 1989.
2. Nelson D: Personal communication, September 1993.
3. Holden D, Jackson D: Stress fractures of the ribs in female rowers. Am J Sports Med 13(5):342–348, 1985.

Chapter 48: Gymnastics

AURELIA NATTIV, MD
BARRI KATZ STRYER, MD
BERT R. MANDELBAUM, MD

Physicians who treat young gymnasts face a great challenge. Gymnasts often begin intensive training between 5 and 7 years of age. During their training they undergo immense physical and psychological growth. Peak participation occurs during a very vulnerable stage of physical and psychological development, and sport demands may be developmentally precocious. Gymnasts may sustain serious medical, orthopedic, and/or psychiatric problems which can have potentially permanent sequelae. Therefore, prevention, early detection, and intervention are of utmost importance. Physicians who treat gymnasts—from recreational to elite—must be aware of the various problems and developmental limitations unique to the sport. This knowledge will allow them to provide early intervention and to educate athletes, coaches, and parents regarding prevention and treatment of sports-specific injuries and associated diseases.

I. **MEDICAL CONCERNS**

Nutritional, endocrine, and psychological problems are common for gymnasts and, unfortunately, at least partially promoted by the sport. Education must be provided to increase awareness of these potentially devastating problems and to understand the role the sport plays in their development.[8,29]

A. **Nutritional concerns**
1. **Low-calorie diets and poor nutritional habits**
   a. **Low body weight and lean physique are promoted in the female gymnast.** Judging is quite subjective and is influenced by appearance. A thinner physique is more desirable. However, the sport of gymnastics requires only moderate calorie expenditure, making the maintenance of a thin physique more difficult in comparison to endurance sports, such as distance running.[4,8,29]
   b. **Calorie restrictions** are often the means that gymnasts use to attain these ideals, which often result in deficient nutrition, decreased metabolic rate, and disordered eating.[4,8]
2. **Disordered eating** (*see also* I.C.2)
   a. There is a spectrum of disorders from mild idiosyncrasies and preoccupations to anorexia nervosa and bulimia at the extreme.[28,50]
   b. Many individuals fall somewhere on the continuum, and early recognition is critical to prevention, education, and treatment.
   c. Disordered eating patterns are reported to be more prevalent in sports that emphasize appearance, such as female gymnastics.[28,38,39,50]
   d. Education, as to the prevention of disordered eating, should occur early in sport training, because disordered eating patterns often develop at this time.
   e. May contribute to menstrual dysfunction (*see* I.B.1.).[22,28,30,50]
   f. Anorexia and bulimia may cause serious electrolyte disturbances with subsequent multiorgan pathology and premature death.[31,34]
3. **Calcium**
   a. Requirements for female athletes are greater than for males and ideally met through dietary sources. If not met through diet, calcium supplements are recommended.[29,40]

b. Daily requirement for hypoestrogenic amenorrheic or oligomenorrheic athletes is 1500 mg.

c. Daily requirement for euestrogenic athlete is 1200 mg.

4. **Iron**

a. Requirements for female athletes are greater than for males. Female gymnasts often have inadequate stores due to deficient caloric intake and nutrition.[35,40]

b. Nutritional deficiencies in combination with iron loss through menstruation place the female gymnast at risk for iron deficiency anemia.[4,8,35]

c. Physicians should be astute to this problem and institute prevention, workup, and treatment when clinically indicated.

B. **Endocrine concerns**

1. **Menstrual dysfunction**

a. A spectrum of menstrual irregularities can be seen in the female gymnast, with hypoestrogenic amenorrhea at the extreme and periods of oligomenorrhea at an intermediate point.[22,28,30]

b. **Delayed menarche and secondary amenorrhea** are more common in certain groups of athletes, including gymnasts, than in nonathletes.[22,28,30]

c. The **prevalence of secondary amenorrhea** in gymnasts has not been determined. In female athletes it varies from 3.4% to 66% compared with 2% to 5% in the general population.[22,28,30]

d. **Secondary amenorrhea** in the female gymnast most likely has a multifactorial etiology including: abrupt changes in body composition, inadequate caloric intake, poor nutrition, disordered eating patterns, stress, high intensity and frequency of exercise as well as other variables.[22,28,29,30]

e. **Potential complications** of menstrual dysfunction include:

i. Infertility: Reversible if exercise-related

ii. Premature osteoporosis and an increased risk of fractures[11,12,22,28,30]

iii. An increased risk of scoliosis has been associated with delayed menarche in ballet dancers.[48]

iv. Theoretical problems include possible increased risk of uterine cancer (with unopposed estrogen state) and heart disease (with hypoestrogenic amenorrhea).[40]

f. **Clinical evaluation of amenorrhea:** refer to chapter 21.

g. **Intervention**

i. Early detection and intervention are crucial.

ii. For individuals 16 or older with exercise-induced menstrual dysfunction, hormone therapy may be indicated.[1,22,28,30,40]

iii. Other variables contributing to menstrual dysfunction must be addressed, such as life stressors, exercise intensity, and diet.

iv. Treatment is indicated and important especially if the gymnast has had amenorrhea for 6 or more months and other medical causes have been ruled out.[22,28,30]

v. When hormonal therapy is indicated, low-dose birth control pills or cyclic estrogen and progesterone therapy is recommended (conjugated estrogens 0.625 mg and medroxyprogesterone acetate 10 mg for days 15–25).[30,40,41]

2. **Premature osteoporosis**

a. Premature osteoporosis in the young female athlete refers to bone loss and inadequate bone formation, resulting in low bone mass, microarchitectural deterioration, increased skeletal fragility, and increased risk of fracture.[28]

b. The years of gymnastic participation are during preadolescence, adolescence, and young adulthood. These are the years of most rapid skeleton growth and development, with 60–70% of peak bone mass attained during the adolescent growth spurt.[29]

c. Prevalence of osteoporosis in young female athletes is unknown.[28]

d. Bone loss may be *irreversible* even with treatment including calcium supplementation, resumption of menses, and estrogen replacement therapy.[9,14]

3. **Female athlete triad** *(see also* Chapter 23)
   a. Refers to the **inter-relatedness of disordered eating, amenorrhea, and osteo-porosis.**[28,50]
      i. Each disorder alone is of serious medical concern, but when all three components of the triad are present, there is significant morbidity and risk of mortality.
      ii. Disordered eating may lead to menstrual dysfunction and subsequent premature osteoporosis.
   b. **Risks and contributing factors**
      i. Same as those of disordered eating
      ii. Sport-athlete mismatch: Genetically some athletes may not be able to attain "ideal" body type for their sport.
      iii. Adolescence and young adulthood appear to be periods of increased risk (window of vulnerability). Psychological, societal, and biological factors may contribute to this being a sensitive period.
      iv. Disorders of eating and menses may go undetected for significant time periods.
   c. **Diagnosis, prevention, and treatment**
      i. **Education** is the key to prevention, which is the key to treatment. A high index of suspicion in all female athletes needs to be maintained, as well as an increased awareness of the severity of the problem.
      ii. The **preparticipation examination** represents an opportunity for screening and education. Athletes at risk require follow-up with team or individual primary care physician.[20,28,29]
      iii. **Follow-up examination** for at-risk athletes should include a thorough history, physical, and diagnostic work-up when indicated. A multidisciplinary health care team, including a psychologist and nutritionist, is recommended. Education of the athlete about the short- and long-term sequelae is important.
4. **Growth problems**
   a. Evidence exists that heavy gymnastics training ($>$18 hr/week), starting prior to puberty and maintained throughout puberty, can alter growth rate so that full adult height is not attained.[10,47]
   b. Elite female gymnasts have been found to be considerably lighter and shorter, with narrower hips and shoulders, compared with nonathlete adolescent girls.[10,47]
   c. Mechanisms are unknown, but prolonged inhibiton of the hypothalamic-pituitary-gonadal axis, along with the metabolic effects of inadequate nutrition, may contribute.
   d. Such data emphasize the importance of the "dose-response" relationship and the concept of a threshold of training below which growth potential may not suffer.[23,29]
   e. Intervention may be time-sensitive and most critical prior to and during puberty.
   f. **Recommendations to prevent growth alterations**[10,29,47]
      i. Train $<$18 hours/week.
      ii. Increased calories, iron, and calcium for female gymnasts with skeletal ages 11–13.
      iii. Screen for overuse epiphyseal injuries in lower extremities.
      iv. Continuous psychological support promoting appropriate body image.
5. **Site-specific increase in bone mineral density**[28,37]
   a. May occur with high-intensity exercise in skeletal sites that are maximally stressed and may be related to the mechanical loading regimen.
   b. Bone mineral density has been found to be greater at upper and lower extremity skeletal sites in female collegiate gymnasts with and without menstrual irregularities compared to nonathletes, as well as athletes in other sports in preliminary research data.

    c. High mechanical loads at specific skeletal sites *may* partially offset the adverse effects of amenorrhea on bone density. However,

        i. It is premature to conclude that amenorrheic female gymnasts do not develop premature osteoporosis.

        ii. It is recommended that preventative strategies and treatments be continued in female gymnasts with disordered eating and menstrual dysfunction until further research is available.

C. **Psychological concerns**

  1. **Body image**

    a. The image of Olga Korbut, Nadia Comaneci, and Mary Lou Retton as prototypical gymnasts still generally holds true.

    b. The pressure from coaches, parents, society, and media to fit the prototypical profile is enormous.[5,28,29]

    c. Judging can be subjective, influenced by esthetics, height, weight, age, and physique.

    d. Low percent body fat or weight is often perceived to be associated with improved performance by the gymnast, distance runner, and other athletes, *despite little data to support this belief.*[28,29,50]

    e. This obsession with thinness—"lighter is better"—is often the initial impetus for disordered eating.[28,50]

  2. **Disordered eating**

    a. Disordered eating refers to a spectrum of abnormal eating patterns including: binging, purging, food restriction, prolonged fasting, use of diet pills, diuretics, laxatives, and intrusive thought patterns (preoccupation with food, distorted body image, fear of becoming fat, and dissatisfaction with one's body).[28,50]

    b. Anorexia nervosa and bulimia nervosa represent the extreme of this spectrum.[3,28,50]

    c. Many athletes, although they do not meet DSM-IV criteria for anorexia or bulimia, exhibit many of the behaviors and thought patterns of these illnesses.[3]

    d. Disordered eating patterns place victims at significant risk for the development of serious metabolic, endocrine, skeletal, and psychiatric disorders.[31,34]

    e. **Prevalence**

        i. In young female athletes, 15–62%[13,28,38,39]

        ii. True data difficult to obtain because of the secretive nature of disorder and the denial and minimizing of symptoms. May be an underestimation of risk.

        iii. 1–3% in the general population for bulimia nervosa[3,6,28]

        iv. 1% in the general population for anorexia nervosa[3,6,28]

        v. The prevalence of both anorexia and bulimia in the general population has been reported to be higher in adolescent and young adult women, in those with a higher socioeconomic class, and in those with a family history of eating disorders.[28]

    f. **Contributing factors to disordered eating**

        i. Emphasis on thinness and appearance[28,50]

        ii. Tight uniforms, leotards, revealing clothing[28]

        iii. Pressure to excel[28,50]

        iv. Need to please salient adults: coaches, parents[28,50]

        v. Coaches who use daily or frequent weigh-ins with negative reinforcement, including unsolicited comments and sarcasm for weight gain and in reference to appearance.[7,50]

        vi. Need for control: An athlete feeling out of control, due to parental or coach demands, may feel the need to control her food intake to decrease her anxiety, thereby leading to increasingly regimented diets.[7,28,50]

        vii. Social isolation and lack of support system[7,50]

        viii. Narrow perspective on life—success in sports is their only purpose[28]

       ix. Importance of individual success to notoriety and financial compensation to institution[28,50]

       x. Emphasis by society on athletic excellence and image[28]

       xi. Personality make-up of each individual athlete; psychological importance/significance of contributing factors to the individual.[28,50]

   g. Risk factors to disordered eating

       i. Family history of eating disorders[3]

       ii. Athletes in individual sports, like gymnasts, appear to be at greater risk than athletes in team sports.[28]

       iii. Significance and intensity of contributing factors[28,50]

3. **Psychosocial development**

   a. The peak years for gymnastics training typically coincide with critical developmental years.

   b. During these years gymnastics should allow for *pleasure*, development of discipline and physical fitness, and socialization.[2,42,43,45]

   c. Gymnastics involves competition which needs to be placed in a healthy perspective, to avoid pathologic anxiety and fear of failure, and to promote enjoyment.[42,43,45]

   d. Children need short-term realistic goals, reasonable expectations, and positive reinforcement.[42]

   e. Motivation and improvement are best promoted by supportive and sound technical instruction.[42,45]

   f. Children define themselves, and their self-concept is continually influenced by the feedback they receive from their environment.[42,44]

   g. Prior to 10 years of age, children depend significantly on adult feedback and reinforcement. This progressively shifts to peer comparison with increasing age and, in adolescence, toward adult role models other than parents.[49]

   h. In adolescence, there is an increased desire for autonomy and a struggle between independence and dependence and increased responsibilities and interests.[49]

4. **Coaches**

   a. Most coaches have little knowledge of child development; yet gymnasts may spend more or essentially equal amounts of quality time with their coach as with their parents, during critical developmental years.[5,43,44]

   b. Most coaches have little awareness of the great influence they have on their gymnasts.[44,45]

   c. Coaches' demands may be unrealistic for the gymnast, especially considering all areas of the child's life and not just athletic capability.[5,43,44,45]

   d. Coaches are important role models for these developing athletes,[15,45] especially gymnasts who are typically young and at a vulnerable/impressionable stage when they start with a coach.

   e. Gymnasts frequently have a strong desire or need to please their coach. They will do things which they feel will please their coach which may not be advantageous to their health and well-being.[44,45]

   f. A gymnast's self-esteem is significantly affected by her coach's feelings, attitudes, and behavior toward her and her teammates.[5,44,45]

   g. Unrealistic body fat and weight goals may be promoted by coaches using daily or frequent weigh-ins with punitive measures.[28,50]

   h. Unfortunately, an athlete may have lifelong problems from the harmful training techniques promoted by the coach.[28,50]

II. ORTHOPEDIC CONCERNS

The young female gymnast incurs significant risk of acute traumatic as well as chronic musculoskeletal injury. Her growing and developing body is exposed to constant and repetitive stresses. This repetitive jarring at a vulnerable period of development may have cumulative effects on bone.[23,29]

A. **Epidemiology of gymnastic injuries**
1. Incidence of injury is greatest in the lower extremity, followed by the upper extremity and then trunk.[15,25,46] Ankle sprains are the most common of all traumatic or overuse injuries.
2. Incidence increases dramatically as skill level increases.[15,23,29]
   a. Increased difficulty of tricks
   b. Increased practice and thus exposure time
3. Reported injury rates are highest for floor exercise, followed by the balance beam, uneven parallel bars, and vault.[15,25,29,46]

B. **Spine injuries**
1. **Acute traumatic injuries to cervical, thoracic, lumbar spine**[16,17,19,29]
   a. True emergencies
   b. Neurologic compromise may have catastrophic consequences with the potential for high morbidity and mortality.
   c. **Prevention:** All attempts to maintain safety must be made:
      i. Appropriate level of participation
      ii. Skill
      iii. Fitness
      iv. Adequate spotting
      v. Adequate coaching
2. **Chronic overuse injuries**[17,19]
   a. Significant problem for the young gymnast
   b. Caused by repetitive flexion, rotation, and extension of the spine.
   c. Common problems
      i. Discogenic pathology
      ii. Vertebral endplate abnormalities
      iii. Pars interarticularis damage with resultant spondylolysis and spondylolisthesis
   d. Spondylolysis[17]
      i. Reported incidence in female gymnasts of pars interarticularis defects is 4 times higher than in general white females.
      ii. Predilection in young gymnasts in the 9–13 year age group
      iii. Result of repetitive forces of hyperextension, hyperflexion, torque, and compression of the lumbar spine
      iv. Potential progression to spondylolisthesis
      v. Radiographs of the lumbar spine should include oblique views.
      vi. Bone scan should be obtained if radiographs normal but diagnosis is suspected.
      vii. Rest and possible bracing are usually indicated to ensure adequate healing.
      viii. The length of time for rest and immobilization varies.
   e. Spondylolisthesis[17]
      i. Higher morbidity and less potential for full recovery than spondylolysis
      ii. With persistent pain, surgical intervention may be indicated.
3. **Segmented spinal fragmentation**[16,17]
   a. Occurs at the thoracolumbar junction
   b. Consequence of axial compressive trauma, such as upon dismount, and repetitive flexion and flexion rotation forces
   c. Chronic degenerative changes and localized back pain may result.

C. **Lower extremity injuries**[15,16,25,46]
1. **Ankle**
   a. Gymnasts often land with the foot not flat, subjecting knees and ankles to torsional loads and predisposing them to ligament injuries.
   b. **Recurrent ankle sprains**
      i. Characterized by pain, functional instability, and weakness
      ii. Common

       iii. Typically cause painful dorsiflexion that may lead to anterolateral or anteromedial impingement syndrome

       iv. Pathogenesis: combination of laxity and hypertrophic scar causing impingement of soft tissue, cartilage, or bone

       v. Prevention

          (a) Use of thick floor mats for dismounts

          (b) Spotters assisting at dismounts

          (c) Appropriate conditioning and warm-ups

       vi. Treatment

          (a) Initially rest, nonsteroidal antiinflammatory drugs (NSAIDs), physical therapy

          (b) With 2 months of persistent pain may need imaging study, such as MRI, to rule out avascular necrosis and osteochondritis dissecans.

          (c) Persistent pain may be treated with arthroscopic surgery.

  2. **Knee**[15,18,25,46]

    a. Significant problem with dismounts and floor exercise.

    b. Ligament injuries, meniscal tears, and fractures may result from high-energy trauma.

    c. Anterior cruciate injuries

      i. If the physis is open, repair is often delayed until it closes.

      ii. Knee braces have been effective nonoperative treatment but are generally not liked by gymnasts.

      iii. Postoperative return to the gym within days is recommended for psychological and physical conditioning.

      iv. Activity should be gradually increased.

      v. Full return to gymnastics in about a year

    d. Patellofemoral syndrome

    e. Patellar tendon problems

    f. Common etiologies of knee injury in gymnastics

      i. Premature attempts at new skills

      ii. Poor mental conditioning

      iii. Poor physical conditioning

      iv. Increasing activity too quickly

      v. Overuse

    g. Prevention through education, preparation, and methodical coaching progressions is critical.

D. **Upper extremity injuries**

  1. **Wrist pain**[23,29]

    a. Common (33% prevalence in female gymnasts in one study)

    b. Appears to be correlated with gymnast's age and total hours of gymnastics—"dose"

    c. "Positive ulnar variance" may be present—an increased length of the ulna relative to the radius

      i. Hypothesized etiologies

         (a) Repetitive distal radial physis injury inhibiting radial growth

         (b) Ulna becomes hypertrophic due to repetitive stress ("quadriped theory")

      ii. Possible sequelae

         (a) Triangular fibrocartilage tears

         (b) Chondromalacia

         (c) Ganglion cysts of tendon sheaths or wrist capsule

    d. Treatment goals

      i. Prevention and early treatment

      ii. Minimize morbidity.

      iii. Maximize performance.

    e. Prevention
       i. History and physical
      ii. Consider anteroposterior wrist radiographs to define abnormalities in those gymnasts with wrist pain.
     iii. Avoid overloading wrists early—progressive weight-bearing over several years.
     iv. High-repetition, low-weight flexibility and strength exercises
      v. Cyclically progressive training—each escalation followed by decrease in total load for 1 week then next increase to allow for autorepair of connective tissues
     vi. Alternate swinging and support events.
    vii. Do not participate with pain—cross train.
  2. **Elbow**
    a. **Elbow dislocation** is most likely to occur on the uneven bars.[33]
       i. May have associated fracture (such as of medial epicondyle)
      ii. Result of acute traumatic injury
     iii. Avoid outstretched arm position when falling.
    b. **Hyperextension**
       i. Causes injury to capsule and posterior and medial ligamentous structures
      ii. Treatment includes early mobilization, range-of-motion exercises, and conditioning.
     iii. Adherence to treatment may allow full gymnastic function within 3 months.
    c. **Medial epicondylitis/tendinitis** of the common flexor tendon origin
       i. Secondary to repetitive upper extremity weight-bearing
      ii. Treatment includes restricting activity, strengthening involved muscle groups and NSAIDs.
  3. **Shoulder**
    a. **Instability disorders**[15,16,29]
       i. Gymnasts tend to have increased ligament laxity (hyperlaxity)
         (a) Results in a spectrum of glenohumeral instability disorders
         (b) Makes diagnosis and treatment of subluxations, dislocations, and labrum abnormalities difficult
      ii. MRI may be helpful for diagnosis of glenohumeral and rotator cuff pathology.
     iii. Treatment
        (a) Strengthening and physical therapy
        (b) Surgical repair can be used if physical therapy is unsuccessful.
    b. **Impingement syndromes**
       i. Common
      ii. May be secondary to
        (a) supraspinatus tendinitis (most common)
        (b) Bicipital tendinitis
        (c) Both
     iii. Treatment
        (a) Initially NSAIDs, icing, and rest
        (b) Strengthening and conditioning
        (c) Arthroscopy has been effective in decreasing pain.

III. CONCLUSION

Gymnastics is a tremendously demanding sport. Young gymnasts train and perform at levels of physical and psychological stress that can potentially result in various detrimental disorders. Further compounding the severity of this stress is that intensive gymnastic training is coincident with critical developmental years. At times, physical and psychological demands may exceed the developmental capacity of the gymnast.

A. **Preparticipation screening**
   1. A place to screen for medical and psychological problems and to educate, prevent, and intervene in areas of concern.
   2. Specific questions must be asked, and a comfortable private setting is ideal to facilitate the physician–athlete interaction.
   3. Age of initiation, sport selectivity, progression of advancement, and technique should be individualized and periodically reevaluated by physician and multidisciplinary health care team.
   4. Age, developmental level, physical and psychological factors, as well as individual environmental factors must be considered.
   5. Titrating the "dose" of the gymnastic stress to the "response" of the gymnast's body and emotional capacity should be understood by all.
   6. Adherence to specific recommendations is essential to ensure safe, enjoyable, and successful participation.

B. **Team approach to medical care**
   1. When problems arise, it is critical that a multidisciplinary team approach is utilized for treatment.
   2. This team may include a primary care physician, orthopedist, nutritionist, psychologist and/or psychiatrist, athletic trainer, and physical therapist.
   3. Communication with the gymnast's coach and parents, when indicated, is important.
   4. The team approach is paramount to ensure optimal health throughout a young gymnast's years of participation.

C. **Maintenance of psychological well-being**[29]
   1. Gymnastic participation is coincident with critical years for psychosocial development, during which children are very impressionable.
   2. It is essential that coaches and parents are aware of the psychological needs and capacity of each individual and tailor programs, interactions, and expectations accordingly.
   3. A psychologist and/or psychiatrist with knowledge of athletics and child development should be available to gymnasts, coaches, and parents.

REFERENCES

1. American Academy of Pediatrics, Committee on Sports Medicine: Amenorrhea in adolescent athletes. Pediatrics 84:394–395, 1989.
2. American Academy of Pediatrics, Committees on Sports Medicine and School Health: Organized athletics for preadolescent children. Pediatrics 84:583–584, 1989.
3. American Psychiatric Association: Diagnostic and Statistical Manual of Mental Disorders—IV (4th ed rev). Washington, DC, American Psychiatric Press, 1994.
4. Benardot D, Schwarz M, Heller DW: Nutrient intake in young highly competitive gymnasts. J Am Diet Assoc 89:401–403, 1989.
5. Brown BR, Butterfield SA: Coaches: A missing link in the health care system. Br J Med 146:211–217, 1992.
6. Brownell KD, Nelson Steen S, Wilmore JH: Weight regulation practices in athletes: Analysis of metabolic and health effects. Med Sci Sports Exerc 19(6):546, 1987
7. Brownell KD, Rodin J, Wilmore JH (eds): Eating, Body Weight and Performance in Athletes. Philadelphia, Lea & Febiger, 1992.
8. Calabrese LH: Nutritional and medical aspects of gymnastics. Clin Sports Med 4:23–30, 1985.
9. Cann CE, Cavanaugh DJ, Schnurpfiel K, et al: Menstrual history is the primary determinant of trabecular bone density in women runners [abstract]. Med Sci Sports Exerc 20(suppl 2):S59, 1988.
10. Claessens AL, Malina RM, Lefevre J, et al: Growth and menarchial status of elite female gymnasts. Med Sci Sports Exerc 24:755–763, 1992.
11. Drinkwater BL, Bruemmer B, Chestnut III CH: Menstrual history as a determinant of current bone density in young athletes. JAMA 263:545, 1990.
12. Drinkwater BI, Nilson K, Chesnut CH III, et al: Bone mineral content of amenorrheic and eumenorrheic athletes. N Engl J Med 311:277–281, 1984.
13. Dummer GM, Rosen W, Heusner WW: Pathogenic weight-control behavior of young competitive swimmers. Phys SportsMed 15(5):75, 1987.
14. Emans SJ, et al: Estrogen deficiency in adolescents and young adults: Impact on bone mineral content and effects of estrogen replacement therapy. Obstet Gynecol 76:585, 1990.

15. Garrick JG, Requa RK: Epidemiology of women's gymnastics injuries. Am J Sports Med 8:261–264, 1980.
16. Goldberg MJ: Gymnastics injuries. Orthop Clin North Am 11:717–726, 1980.
17. Hall SJ: Mechanical contribution to lumbar stress injuries in female gymnasts. Med Sci Sports Exerc 18:599–602, 1986.
18. Hunter LY, Torgan C: Dismounts in gymnastics: Should scoring be reevaluated? Am J Sports Med 11:208–210, 1983.
19. Jackson DW, Wiltse LL, Cirinccoine RJ: Spondylolysis in the female gymnast. Clin Orthop 117:63–73, 1976.
20. Johnson MD: Tailoring the preparticipation exam to female athletes. Phys SportsMed 20(7):61, 1992.
21. Lloyd T, Triantafyllou SJ, et al: Women athletes with menstrual irregularity have increased musculoskeletal injuries. Med Sci Sports Exerc 18:374, 1986.
22. Loucks AB, Horvath SM: Athletic amenorrhea: A review. Med Sci Sports Exerc 17(1):56–72, 1985.
23. Mandelbaum BR, Bartolozzi AR, Davis CA, et al: Wrist pain syndrome in the gymnast: Pathogenic, diagnostic, and therapeutic considerations. Am J Sports Med 17(3):305–317, 1989.
24. Marcus R, Drinkwater B, Dalsky G, et al: Osteoporosis and exercise in women. Med Sci Sports Exerc 24(suppl 6):S301, 1992.
25. McAuley E, Hudash G, Shields K, et al: Injuries in women's gymnastics: The state of the art. Am J Sports Med 15:558–565, 1987.
26. Moffatt RJ: Dietary status of elite female high school gymnasts: Inadequacy of vitamin and mineral intake. J Am Diet Assoc 84:1361–1363, 1984.
27. Myburgh K, Hutchins J, Fataar AB, et al: Low bone density is an etiologic factor for stress fractures in athletes. Ann Intern Med 113:754, 1990.
28. Nattiv A, Agostini R, Drinkwater B, et al: The female athlete triad: The inter-relatedness of disordered eating, amenorrhea and osteoporosis. Clin Sports Med 1994 (in press).
29. Nattiv A, Mandelbaum BR: Injuries and special concerns in female gymnasts: Detecting, treating and preventing common problems. Phys SportsMed 21(7):66, 1993.
30. Otis CL: Exercise-associated amenorrhea. Clin Sports Med 11:351, 1992.
31. Palla B, Litt H: Medical complications of eating disorders in adolescents. Pediatrics 81:613–623, 1988.
32. Pettrone FA, Ricciardelli E: Gymnastics injuries: The Virginia experience, 1982–1983. Am J Sports Med 15:58–62, 1987.
33. Priest JB, Weise DJ: Elbow injury in women's gymnastics. Am J Sports Med 9:288–295, 1981.
34. Ratnasuriya RH, Eisler I, Szmukler GI, et al: Anorexia nervosa: Outcome and prognostic factors after 20 years. Br J Psychiatry 158:495, 1991.
35. Risser WL, Lee EJ, Poindexter HB, et al: Iron deficiency in female athletes: Its prevalence and impact on performance. Med Sci Sports Exerc 20(20):116–121, 1988.
36. Rigotti NA, Neer RM, Skates SJ, et al: The clinical course of osteoporosis in women with anorexia nervosa: A longitudinal study of cortical bone mass. JAMA 265:1133, 1991.
37. Robinson T, Snow-Harter C, Gillis D, et al: Bone and mineral density and menstrual cycle status in competitive female runners and gymnasts [abstract]. Med Sci Sports Exerc (suppl 25)S49, 1993.
38. Rosen LW, Hough DO: Pathogenic weight control behaviors of female college gymnasts. Phys SportsMed 16(9):14, 1988.
39. Rosen LW, McKeag DB, Hough DO, et al: Pathogenic weight control behaviors of female college athletes. Phys SportsMed 14(1):79, 1986.
40. Shangold MM, Mirkin G: Women and Exercise: Physiology and Sports Medicine, 2nd ed. Philadelphia, FA Davis Co., 1994.
41. Shangold M, Rebar RW, Wentz AC, et al: Evaluation and management of menstrual dysfunction in athletes. JAMA 263:1665–1669, 1990.
42. Smith RE: A positive approach to enhancing sport performance: Principles of positive reinforcement and performance feedback. In Williams JM (ed): Applied Sport Psychology: Personal Growth to Peak Performance. Mountain View, CA, Mayfield Publishing Co., 1993.
43. Smoll FL: Enhancing coach-parent relationships in youth sports. In Williams JM (ed): Applied Sport Psychology: Personal Growth to Peak Performance. Mountain View, CA, Mayfield Publishing Co., 1993.
44. Smoll FL, Smith RE: Educating youth sports coaches: An applied sport psychology perspective. In Williams JM (ed): Applied Sport Psychology: Personal Growth to Peak Performance. Mountain View, CA, Mayfield Publishing Co., 1993.
45. Smoll FL, Smith RE: Psychology of the young athlete: Stress-related maladies and remedial approaches. Ped Clin North Am 37:1021–1046, 1990.
46. Snook GA: Injuries in women's gymnastics: A 5-year study. Am J Sports Med 7:242–244, 1979.
47. Theintz GE, Howald H, Weiss U, et al: Evidence for a reduction of growth potential in adolescent female gymnasts. J Pediatr 122:306–313, 1993.
48. Warren MP, Brooks-Gunn J, Hamilton LH, et al: Scoliosis and fractures in young ballet dancers: Relation to delayed menarche and secondary amenorhhea. N Engl J Med 314:1348–1353, 1986.
49. Weiss MR, Bredemeier, BJL: Moral development in sport. Exerc Sport Sci Rev 18:331–377 1990.
50. Yeager KK, Agostini R, Nattiv A, Drinkwater B: The female athlete triad: disordered eating, amenorrhea, osteoporosis [commentary]. Med Sci Sports Exerc 25(7):755, 1993.

Chapter 49: Figure Skating

ANGELA D. SMITH, MD

Figure skating continues to grow in popularity at both the recreational and competitive levels. Like gymnasts and dancers, female figure skaters must meet not only athletic but esthetic standards. The combination of the requirements for both long hours of training and weight control may lead to inadequate nutrition and injury. In many areas of medical concern, figure skating does not differ from almost all other sports. This chapter provides the background knowledge needed to understand the training regimen of a competitive figure skater and to care for the most common physical problems resulting from the sport.

I. **DEFINITIONS**

    A. **Edges:** The two sides of the concavely ground figure-skate blade; skaters should always skate on only one edge at a time, except during brief changes of edge; inside edge is medial, outside edge is lateral.

    B. **Stroking:** Forward or backward skating, includes straight steps and crossovers.

    C. **Footwork:** Usually rapid steps including turns, hops, and arm movements.

    D. **Spins:** If rotating to the left (the easiest direction for most skaters), a forward spin is on the left foot, a backward spin on the right; upright or scratch spin; sit spin; camel spin (in arabesque or spiral position); change foot spins involve step-over change; flying spins have a jump for the change of foot.

    E. **Jumps:** All take off from skating backward except axel; named by take-off position and number of revolutions; e.g., double loop takes off right foot and rotates through two revolutions, double toe loop takes off from left toe pick and rotates through two revolutions; axel has one half more revolution, e.g., single axel is $1\frac{1}{2}$ revolution, etc.

    F. **Lifts:** One skater lifts another by the waist, both hands or one hand; ice dancers have limitations on the height and types of lifts.

    G. **Throw jumps:** The female jumps using her own power as she is also lifted into the air by her partner—the additional force from her partner markedly increases the height and distance of the jump, as well as the force absorbed on landing the jump.

II. **TYPES OF EVENTS**

Organized by discipline and by test level. Some competitive events have age criteria in addition to the test level. Some tests have special versions for adults.

    A. **Singles**

        1. **Figures**

            a. Few skaters do figures competitively now, and they are not done in international competition. Judged by carriage, flow, and tracings viewed on the ice.

            b. Aerobic and anaerobic fitness requirements: None. (Some participants hold their breath during certain figures, however.)

            c. Flexibility required: None

            d. Injuries: Rare, of overuse type

            e. Somatotype: Any

            f. Requires good vision, mental discipline

        2. **Free skating**

            a. Jumps, spins, connecting moves, and footwork

            b. Aerobic and anaerobic fitness requirement: Relatively high anaerobic, moderately high aerobic; while doing difficult jumps within a competitive program, heart rates reach supramaximal levels.

  c. Flexibility required: Extremely good in lower extremities

  d. Injuries: Repetitive overuse problems and acute injuries

  e. Somatotype: All body types, but somatotypes more pleasing to judge's eye may be scored more highly.

B. **Pair skating**

 1. Aerobic and anaerobic fitness requirement: Relatively high anaerobic, moderately high aerobic

 2. Flexibility required: Extremely good in trunk and upper and lower extremities

 3. Injuries: Repetitive overuse problems and acute injuries in equal percentages, but acute injuries in pairs are often the more severe because of the additional force behind them; concussions are not unusual.

 4. Somatotype: Large size difference needed between the partners to make lifts and throws successful; few elite female pair skaters are much over 5 ft 1 in and 100 lb.

 5. Very athletic and acrobatic; greater risk-taking behavior required than in other skating disciplines

C. **Ice dancing**

 1. Judged on carriage, flow, style, speed, interpretation, difficulty

 2. Aerobic and anaerobic fitness requirement: Relatively high anaerobic, moderately high aerobic

 3. Flexibility required: Extremely good in trunk and upper and lower extremities

 4. Injuries: Might suspect more overuse, but the only comparative study showed overuse and acute injuries equal in incidence and severity (judged by training time lost).[5]

 5. Somatotype: More classical line required, so very slender somatotype required at the elite level. Even at less advanced levels, esthetic component is present.

 6. Overuse problems occur related to the extreme and constant knee flexion and ankle dorsiflexion required.

D. **Precision team skating**

 1. Usually 16 or more skaters, all doing the same moves. In the last decade, this has become a competitive sport, with international contests.

 2. Aerobic and anaerobic fitness requirement: Less than for singles, pairs, or ice dancing. Except at highest levels, skating speeds tend to be much slower; no jumps, which are the element that increases the singles skater's heart rate the most.

 3. Flexibility required: Depends on the team's choreography

 4. Injuries: No reports in the literature; author's experience suggests primarily overuse and boot-related injuries among younger precision skaters, but fractures have occurred among older adult team members.

 5. Somatotype: All but the markedly obese

 6. A rapidly evolving sport that will probably become even more athletic as rules modifications continue.

III. TRAINING

A. **Figures:** 2–4 hr/day

B. **Free skating:** 2–3 hr/day on-ice free skating practice; may include 3–5 hr/week of ice dancing to improve line and depth of edges, and 3–10 hr/week total of strength training, ballet or other dance, and aerobic training.

C. **Ice dancing:** 2–3 hr/day on-ice and 3–10 hr/week ballet, ballroom dance, or other choreography off-ice.

D. **Precision team skating:** 1–5 hr/week practicing precision team skating, but most also skate an additional 2–10 hr/week.

IV. EMOTIONAL STRESSES OF COMPETITIVE SKATERS

A. **Coach/athlete interactions**

B. **Parent/athlete/sibling** interactions and expectations: Related to the understanding that all family members often sacrifice financially for the skater and unequal attention often is paid to the skater. The skater may feel intense pressure to perform at or above level of realistic expectations.

  C. **Atypical social life:** Few competitive skaters beyond intermediate level attend typical schools for the usual school hours; many young grade-schoolers already do home tutoring or professional school correspondence curricula. Even those who attend day school rarely are present for lunch, recess, gym, and before- or after-school activities. For most, social life revolves around skating friends.

V. EPIDEMIOLOGY

  A. **Limitations of existing studies**
    1. No published long-term prospective studies with accurately recorded denominators of all actual activity found in MEDLINE and SIRC computer searches.
    2. Most studies are retrospective, based on questionnaire, which is often given during a stressful time, as during the National Championships.

  B. **Cross-sectional studies**
    1. By questionnaire, combined with gathering of physiologic data in some small studies: None of these provides data on more than 100 athletes, male and female combined. They show that approximately half of injuries of national championship-level competitors are from overuse and half are acute; lower extremities most frequently involved.[1,2]
    2. Accident reports from emergency rooms from cities with recently opened ice rinks: Incidence of injury that requires emergency room care is 1/10,000 for the first few months of operation of a new rink when no previous one was in the region. Most injuries occur among skaters who have skated fewer than 10 times and include fractures, lacerations, and contusions, of both upper and lower extremities.

  C. **Longitudinal studies**
    1. Only 1 published article[5] and 1 abstract[7] of prospective longitudinal study that continued for longer than 1 year. These followed elite and junior elite pair skaters and ice dancers and found that instituting required ballet class for flexibility training in year 2 and a strength training class in year 3 was associated with decreased incidence of both acute and overuse injuries over a 4-year period. Most injuries involved the lower extremities, even among pair skaters.

VI. INJURIES BY CAUSE

  A. **Repetitive microtrauma:** Mainly lower extremities
  B. **Acute macrotrauma:** In 4-year longitudinal study, after both flexibility and strength training programs were required, lift-related injuries decreased markedly. Two concussions occurred in each of the first 2 years of study (3 in females), but no concussions in the last 2 years of study.[7]
  C. **Boots:** In 4-year longitudinal study, boot-related injuries were eliminated in years 3 and 4, apparently because skaters requested assistance as soon as they thought there might be a problem.
    1. Tendinitis from pressure of boot top and laces[8]
    2. Pressure over malleoli
    3. Problems with flexion creases over ankle and sinus tarsi

VII. INJURIES BY LOCATION

  A. **Foot and ankle**
    1. Boot-related problems predominate.
    2. Also injuries off ice
    3. In the 4-year study, there was only 1 acute severe peroneal muscle strain/ankle sprain, but no other significant on-ice ankle injuries.

  B. **Knee**
    1. Primarily overuse

2. Anterior cruciate ligament tear from figure skating training has not been reported; isolated medial collateral ligament injury does occur.

C. **Hip and thigh**
   1. Groin muscle strain, mainly hip flexors and adductors
   2. Hamstring strain rare; quadriceps strain very rare
D. **Trunk:** Mainly lumbar strains.
E. **Shoulder:** Strains, mostly in male pair skaters and ice dancers; rare among females.
F. **Arm and elbow:** Rare
G. **Hand and wrist**
   1. Ganglions
   2. Hand fractures; most in the author's series occurred off-ice.
H. **Head and neck**
   1. Concussions from falls, usually from an overhead lift
   2. Cervical strain

VIII. **INJURY PREVENTION**

A. **Preparticipation history**
   1. **Training history**
      a. Type of event (singles, pairs, etc.)
      b. Level of recreation or competition (beginner, novice elite, etc.)
      c. Hours per week of on-ice training
      d. Hours per week of off-ice training
      e. Recent changes
         i. Coach
         ii. Competitive program, technical changes in a move, making many consecutive attempts to complete a new maneuver
         iii. Training program, off-ice and on-ice
         iv. Boots: brand, style, or new pair
         v. Change in ice surface (e.g., larger area to cover)
   2. **Injury history**
      a. Remote injury, whether seems related or not
      b. Recent injury
   3. **Growth status:** If skeletally immature, current and recent rate of growth; rapid growth may contribute to injuries related to lack of muscle flexibility or boot fit.
   4. **Menstrual history**
   5. **Nutrition diary**
      a. Total calories per day
      b. Percentage of carbohydrates in diet
      c. Calcium-containing foods
   6. **Emotional stresses**
      a. Support system: Many young skaters live away from home and often lack readily available affection, personal attention, positive statements, and finances.
      b. Conflicts among competitors: Significant conflicts are rare, but some may compete for attention from coach in some settings.
      c. Coach/athlete conflict
      d. Internal concerns about performance
B. **Preparticipation examination**
   1. **Lean body mass**
   2. **Muscle flexibility**
   3. **Muscle strength**, especially rehabilitation of previous injuries
   4. **Feet/ankles and boots**[8]
      a. Malleolar bursas and oddly shaped toes usual, even with most flexible boots
      b. Boggy tenosynovitis is not unusual over the anterior tendons at the ankle, especially with stiffer boots that do not flex with ankle dorsiflexion.

    c. Note blade placement: generally it is just medial to the center seam at toes and center of heel; if blade is more than a few millimeters away from this alignment, check for significant angular or torsional malalignment of the skater's lower extremities.

IX. MEDICAL PROBLEMS

A. Disordered eating

1. One study of 23 female junior and senior competitors showed consumption of 55 ± 22% of RDA for calories, and diets were deficient in iron, calcium, vitamin D, niacin, and vitamin B6.[3]
2. On Eating Attitudes Test (EAT), these skaters indicated:[3]
   a. 87% exercise strenuously to burn off calories.
   b. 78% terrified of becoming overweight.
   c. 65% have desire to be even thinner.
   d. 48% scored within the anorexic range on EAT.
   e. 10 competitors had menstrual cycle irregularity.
3. Most elite skaters, especially if their primary event is pair skating or ice dancing, listen to nutritional advice whole-heartedly but avoid dairy foods ("too fattening") and do not take in sufficient carbohydrates ("too many calories").
4. Incidence of bulimia nervosa and anorexia nervosa still appears to be low.

B. Menstrual irregularity and contraception

1. Small numbers, 10 of 23 in the above study,[3] reported irregularity; of 20 post-pubertal skaters in another study,[4] 4 reported amenorrhea and 4 reported oligomenorrhea. Both have similar results—approximately 40% of competitive skaters have irregular menses.
2. No information on incidence of oral contraceptive use; some skaters hesitate to use oral contraceptives because of feared or real bloating and weight gain.
3. Menarche usually delayed in elite skaters.
4. Pregnancy may not be recognized; in the author's experience, both an atypically poor championship performance and a case of presumed prolonged postconcussion nausea in extremely lean athletes eventually were found to be related to pregnancy.

C. Osteoporosis

1. Study of 22 skaters, 11–23 years old, using dual-energy x-ray absorptiometry for measurement, found bone mineral density (BMD) of legs and pelvis higher in skaters than in sedentary controls.
2. For those with abnormal menses, BMD was 2% lower than in other skaters, but the difference was not significant.
3. No difference between skaters and sedentary females in BMD of spine or upper extremities.[4]
4. Study of 5 elite skaters, using quantitative CT scan of lumbar spine, found 3 competitors had BMD more than 2 SD below mean for age and gender.[2a]
5. May need to consider hormone replacement if indicated.

X. TREATMENT OF PROBLEMS SPECIFIC TO FIGURE SKATERS

A. Acute injuries

1. **Ankle sprains**
   a. RICE (rest, ice, compression, elevation), early motion (protected if necessary)
   b. May begin basic skating, such as stroking, as soon as foot can fit into boot reasonably comfortably, if skater wishes to tolerate it.
   c. Progress activity as healing proceeds; no double or triple jumps until normal peroneal strength.
2. **Wrist and hand fractures**
   a. Consider allowing full skating activity, as long as immobilizing devices provide sufficient protection.

      b. No limitations necessary for figures.

      c. May not be able to achieve firm handgrips required for precision team skating

  3. **Groin muscle strains**

      a. Relative rest, ice, compression; other physical therapy modalities may be appropriate.

      b. Strengthen adjacent muscle groups to compensate.

      c. Flexibility training

      d. Avoid injurious activities (usually spins, multirevolution jumps) until healing is sufficient.

  4. **Concussions**

      a. Generally do not allow multirevolution jumps and any lifts until postconcussive symptoms have cleared; however, competitive skaters rarely listen to this advice because of their concerns about loss of training time.

B. **Repetitive overuse injuries**

  1. **Anterior knee pain syndromes:** Related to lack of quadriceps flexibilty in study of junior elite figure skaters[6]

  2. **Shoulder strains**: Along with impingement and subluxation; treat with strengthening and symptomatically. Rare, even among female pair skaters.

  3. **Wrist ganglions**

      a. Very common among pair skaters; caused by weight-bearing/lifting with forcibly dorsiflexed wrists.

      b. Skaters function well with these injuries—not one in the author's practice has ever requested injection or excision, and even mild temporary pain is rare.

  4. **Exertional compartment syndromes of the leg**

      a. Occur especially among ice dancers, who must maintain position of ankle dorsiflexion

      b. No specific treatment has proved useful except stopping ice dancing or surgical release of the affected compartments.

  5. **Lower-leg posteromedial tibial stress syndrome**

      a. May respond to strengthening of posterior tibial muscle or padding of medial boot top.

      b. Orthotics possibly helpful on rare occasions, but orthotics in skates cause many problems due to lack of space and rigidity of boot.

      c. Look at blade placement and balance of skater standing in skate (without skate guards on—they may have terrycloth blade-protectors on).

  6. **Low back pain**

      a. Endemic among competitive skaters and coaches

      b. Most frequent among female pair skaters, who are at greater risk for spondylolysis, probably due to the need for holding the free leg very high in the air at all times.

C. **Boot-related injuries**

  1. **Malleolar bursitis**

      a. Push out boot over malleolus to relieve pressure.

      b. Fabricate a doughnut-shaped pad of dense foam; two pieces of adhesive-backed foam, stick adhesive sides together, with the cut-out over the prominence of the malleolus; usually works well.

      c. Aspiration, with or without corticosteroid injection, is generally not useful as fluid almost always reaccumulates rapidly.

      d. Surgical excision has never been necessary in this author's practice; the enlarged bursa may remain, but pain has always been relieved by boot or padding modifications.

      e. Surgical excision, if performed, generally ablates the mass but does not always relieve the pain, since the boot pressure remains.

2. **"Pump bumps"** (Haglund's deformity of the calcaneal tuberosity)
   a. Caused by excessive motion of the heel within the boot
   b. Change fit of boot by narrowing heel, if possible, or change to another boot with a narrower heel.
3. **Tenosynovitis anterior to the ankle**
   a. Usually caused by the upper two crossing laces in boots that are very stiff.
   b. Treatment options
      i. More flexible boots
      ii. More dense or thicker padding of tongue of boot
      iii. Partially detach the tongue padding in the area of the tenosynovitis, cut to size a piece of heat-moldable plastic (available from orthopedic bracemakers or from occupational therapists), heat the plastic, and place it between the leather and the padding of the tongue (with the boot already on the skater, untied). Then, have the skater lace up the boot slightly more loosely than usual to make only small grooves in the plastic as it hardens. Finally, reglue the padding to the plastic and to the exposed portion of the tongue. The plastic now distributes the force of the laces over a larger area.
4. **Achilles tendinitis**
   a. May be caused by jumping, usually repetitive double or triple toe jumps, with the athlete plantarflexing as much as the boot allows in order to plant the toepick. If this is the cause, pad the proximal rim of the boot and decrease the frequency of practicing the harmful jumps until symptoms abate.
   b. May be caused by pressure from the excessive padding that is immediately adjacent to both sides of the tendon in many current, expensive styles of boots. If this is the cause, the boot-fitter in the local skate shop or orthopedic brace shop may be able to compress the excessive padding sufficiently; otherwise, the boot manufacturer can remove the extra padding.
   c. May be caused by off-ice activities (the boots of competitive skaters rarely allow any dorsiflexion of the ankle beyond neutral, so repetitive tension stress is relatively unlikely from on-ice activities); treat as usual for the off-ice activity.
5. **Callosities over toes or bony prominences**, such as accessory naviculars
   a. Toes may look bad, but they have never been painful in the author's experience, unless the boots are too small.
   b. Pad or relieve (by punching out overlying boot) painful foot prominences.

REFERENCES

1. Brock RM, Striowski CC: Injuries in elite figure skating. Phys SportsMed 14(1):111–115, 1986.
2. Garrick JG: Figure skating injuries. Med Sci Sports Exerc 14:141, 1982.
2a. Provost-Craig M, personal communication, 1993.
3. Rucinski A: Masters thesis. Quoted in Provost-Craig M: Too thin to win. Syllabus material for conference on Medical and Orthopedic Issues of Active and Athletic Women, Pennsylvania State University, State College, PA, April 1993.
4. Slemenda CW, Johnston CC: High intensity activities in young women: Site specific bone mass effects among female figure skaters. Bone Miner 20:125–132, 1993.
5. Smith AD, Ludington R: Injuries in elite pair skaters and ice dancers. Am J Sports Med 17:482–488, 1989.
6. Smith AD, Stroud L, McQueen C: Flexibility and anterior knee pain in adolescent elite figure skaters. J Pediatr Orthop 11:77–82, 1991.
7. Smith AD: Reduction of injuries among elite figure skaters: A 4-year longitudinal study. Med Sci Sports Exerc 23(Suppl 4):1991.
8. Smith AD: Foot and ankle injuries in figure skaters. Phys SportsMed 18(3):73, 1990.

Chapter 50: The Child Dancer

MARIE D. SCHAFLE, MD

In the present economic climate, primary care providers are called upon with increasing frequency to provide care for special populations who previously sought care in sports and dance medicine centers. Many of these patients are children and adolescents. Some of the most frequent questions and concerns of ballet dancers and their parents are addressed here.

I. POPULATION

    A. Fifteen to twenty thousand audition for professional schools each year.

    B. Approximately one percent of these are admitted.

    C. One or two of these will go on to professional careers.

    D. Average training is ten years to reach the level expected to apprentice to a company.

II. TRAINING

    A. **Beginning levels**
1. Vast majority of ballet participants
2. 1 or 2 hours of class per week
3. Soft shoes or slippers with suede soles
4. Basic foot and arm positions, torso control, and proper turnout are emphasized.
5. Strength, coordination, and grace as well as concentration skills are developed.
6. Common injuries are associated with forcing turnout and other technique errors.
7. Utilize the expertise of the instructor in ferreting out errors in technique.

    B. **Intermediate levels**
1. Fewer participants
2. Time and intensity are increased. Commitment to dance is greater.
   a. 3–5 classes/week
   b. Pointe work for girls, increased height and complexity of jumps, and more advanced *attitudes* for both sexes
   c. Summer workshops greatly increase the time spent dancing per week and also may cause an abrupt change in technique.
   d. Slight increase in lumbar lordosis and flexion at the hip is the most common technique error and is an attempt to increase turnout.

    C. **Advanced levels**
1. Serious pointe work separates the serious from the recreational dancers.
2. Strength and technique are the criteria for determining readiness for pointe.
   a. Solid "passe" is a good indicator of sufficient strength and technique.
3. First two metatarsals bear most of the weight en pointe.
   a. Second metatarsal is at risk for **stress fracture**, manifested as gradual onset of soreness at the base of the second metatarsal, increased with pointe work at first and gradually becoming painful most of the time.
      i. Rule out dietary deficiencies and eating disorders.
      ii. Check for menstrual irregularities or delayed onset of menarche.
      iii. Treatment is rest from painful activities and physical therapy.
      iv. Definitive treatment can be delayed if professional demands are great.
4. **Overuse injuries** associated with pointe work
   a. **Lumbar facet joint stress and pars stress fractures:** Due to increased lumbar lordosis with forced turnout.

       b. **Hip flexor tendinitis:** Due to increased flexion at the hip secondary to increased lumbar lordosis.

       c. **Patellofemoral problems,** patellar subluxation, and overuse tendinitis of the hip adductors, and the patellar tendon
   - i. Insufficient strength to maintain turnout at the hip in stiffer pointe shoes.
   - ii. Medial drift of the knee on landing jumps due to lack of external rotator strength.

       d. Lack of foot and ankle strength
   - i. Acute ankle sprains
   - ii. Peroneal tendinitis, Achilles tendinitis, flexor hallucis longus tendinitis

5. **Partnering**
   a. Males are often far less advanced in technique than females.
   b. Men are not specifically prepared for the work of partnering.
   c. Combined inexperience of the partners increases the chance of injury.
      - i. Acute injuries from being dropped
      - ii. Low back strain and stress fractures in men due to lack of strength for stabilization

6. **Leaping**
   a. Men begin to learn the grand leaps. Multiple repetitions may lead to tibial and fibular stress fractures.
   b. Women begin to learn more advanced leaps with the same risks.

D. **Preprofessional and professional levels**

1. **Career-related problems**
   a. Increased anxiety concerning weight and fitness for company
   b. Increased physical stress due to greater time commitment and greater intensity of training
   c. Greater difficulty in resting any injury due to real fear of harming career chances

2. **Choreography**
   a. Classical ballet barre is ill suited to preparing the dancer for many modern choreographies.
   b. Choreography selection is not the option of the dancer but of the artistic director

III. **ETIOLOGY OF INJURY**

A. **Forcing turnout**
1. Increased lumbar lordosis
2. Flexion at the hip
3. Rolling in or pronation of the foot
4. Gripping the floor with the toes
5. Turning the feet out with knees and hips flexed; then extending the knees

B. **Measuring turnout**
1. The dancer should be supine, hips at 0° flexion and 0° abduction.
2. Externally rotate each hip to maximum degree without changing the alignment above.
3. Have dancer hold the hip in external rotation against resistance to check symmetry of strength.

C. **Effects of growth**
1. Epiphysitis at the calcaneus, tibial tubercle, iliac crest
2. Tendinitis associated with rapid bone growth
3. Worsening of scoliosis associated with delay of menarche

D. **Eating disorders and drug abuse**
1. Ignorance about nutrition and health
2. True psychological disturbances requiring expert help

3. Abuse of laxatives and purgatives
4. Other drug abuse not specifically related to dance but common in the adolescent population

IV. CONCLUSION

Like any other physical pursuit, ballet has its own unique set of related injuries. Because ballet class is so structured and the movement so deliberate, it is relatively easy for the dancer to discover and correct technique errors, and to modify class until injuries have improved. Injuries to young dancers are usually minor and usually self-induced, with the single-minded pursuit of 180 degrees of turnout being the most likely culprit. The free exchange of information between physician and instructor is extremely important in the treatment of a dancer since it provides both with information which each would otherwise not be able to gleam from his or her own perspective. In the event that either physician or instructor feels unable to interact with or trust his or her opposite number, the nearest professional dance school can be contacted for referrals to more experienced professionals. Thorough evaluation and explanation of physical complaints and technique errors will allow the young dancer to improve technique and strength over time, and will reinforce in the dancer's mind that ballet is a long-term pursuit. A time of injury is often a good one to counsel overeager parents. Not every talented young dancer achieves the goal of membership in a professional company. It is important for the parents to realize that the discipline and grace acquired by every ballet student are important assets for the future, regardless of the eventual choice of career.

REFERENCES

1. Braisted JR, Mellin L, Gong EJ, et al: The adolescent ballet dancer: Nutritional practices associated with anorexia nervosa. J Adolesc Health Care 5:365–371, 1985.
2. Contompasis J: Common adolescent dance injuries. Clin Podiatry 1:631–644, 1984.
3. Hammond SN: Ballet Basics. Mayfield Publishing Co., 1984.
4. Hardaker WT Jr: Medical considerations in dance training for children. Am Fam Physician 35(5):93–99, 1987.
5. Klemp P, Chalton D: Articular mobility in ballet dancers: A follow-up study after 4 years. Am J Sports Med 17(1):72–75, 1989.
6. McLain D: Artistic development in the dancer. Clin Sports Med 2(3):563–570, 1983.
7. Sammarco GJ, Miller EH: Forefoot conditions in dancers. Part I. Foot Ankle 3(2):85–92, 1982.
8. Teitz CC: Sports medicine concerns in dance and gymnastics. Clin Sports Med 2:571–593, 1983.
9. Warren MP, Brooks-Gunn J, Hamilton LH, et al: Scoliosis and fractures in young ballet dancers: Relation to delayed menarche and secondary amenorrhea. N Engl J Med 314:1348–1353, 1986.
10. Whiteside PL: The teacher's role in treating dance injuries. Dance Teacher Now (April):32–34, 1986.

Chapter 51: Dance

JAMES G. GARRICK, MD

I. GENERAL CONSIDERATIONS

A. Ballet

  1. **Training**

     a. **The successful begin young.**

        i. **Novices in late teens prone to more problems.**

           (a) Unique problems among college dance students

        ii. Training may begin as early as age 5 (weekly).

        iii. Serious training (daily) begins early teens.

        iv. Generally professional status must be attained by late teens.

        v. Professionals may dance into 40s and 50s.

           (a) Ballet activities often continue into adulthood for the "recreational" dancer.

     b. **Training highly structured**

        i. **Practitioner <u>MUST</u> know what goes on in classes.**

        ii. Classes are precisely structured around a gradual warm-up (at the barre) with increasing speed and range of motion, concluding with actual "steps" and jumps carried out around and across the classroom.

        iii. Classes are taken daily, even during the performing season.

           (a) Performance season days include classes, rehearsals, and performances.

     c. Year-round

        i. May perform only a few months.

        ii. Classes continue virtually every day, throughout the entire year.

  2. **Sex differences**

     a. **The majority of dancers are female.**

        i. Professional companies have nearly equal numbers of males and females.

     b. Male dancers often begin later (teens)

        i. Many with previous athletic experience (and injuries)

     c. Male/female differences

        i. Female dancers dance en pointe (on their toes).

           (a) Usually begin pointe work at age 12.

           (b) Going en pointe depends on training and strength, not musculoskeletal maturity.

        ii. Males dance on metatarsal heads (MTP joint dorsiflexion 90°).

        iii. Males responsible for lifting (partnering).

           (a) Lifting begins mid to late teens.

           (b) Boys frequently ill-prepared with respect to upper body strength, which can pose a risk to females during lifts.

  3. **Psychology**

     a. **Pyramid system**

        i. Hundreds of thousands of little girls take ballet lessons.

        ii. Only hundreds achieve professional status.

        iii. Competition continues within professional companies.

           (a) Corps de ballet

           (b) Soloist

           (c) Principal dancer

    b. **Advancement based on subjective judgments.**
       i. Students must audition (compete) for entry into professional schools.
       ii. Body type (dancer unable to alter)
       iii. Weight
          (a) Among the most weight-conscious of all athletes
          (b) Anorexia nervosa and bulimia nervosa more common than in perhaps any other activity.
    c. **Teenage dancers often separated from parents.**
       i. Live where training is appropriate.
       ii. Only adult input/supervision may come from teachers.
    d. **Education usually ceases with high school.**
       i. Some do not complete high school.
    e. **Experience with medical care often bad.**
       i. Practitioners do not understand demands of continuous training.
       ii. Treatment of injuries often superficial and expedient.
          (a) Most injuries are of overuse variety, and cause must be found to prevent recurrence.

B. **Modern**
  1. From the artistic standpoint, modern dance differs appreciably from ballet. From a medical standpoint, the differences seem largely related to the factors presented below.
  2. Generally, modern dance is:
    a. Performed barefoot.
    b. Does not emphasize external rotation of the hips.
    c. Involves more movements requiring hyperflexion of the knees.
    d. Involves more abrupt movements.
  3. There are greater differences among the characteristics and demands of the various forms of modern dance than in ballet.
  4. Most modern dancers (like all dancers) have some background in ballet.
  5. Modern dance training usually begins later than ballet, often in the late teens and 20s.
  6. Modern dance companies are usually smaller than ballet companies and thus are less likely to have structured medical care systems.

C. **Jazz**
  1. Among teenagers, jazz may be the most popular form.
  2. Weight restrictions are not as demanding as in ballet.
  3. Choreography does not demand external rotation of the hips as in ballet but generally requires better than average hip motion (splits and high kicks).

II. MEDICAL PROBLEMS

A. **Menstrual abnormalities**
  1. Both primary and secondary amenorrhea are common.
  2. Delayed onset of menses is the rule rather than the exception in the serious dance student.
B. **Contagious diseases** spread rapidly within a dance company or school because of daily, close contact of participants.
C. **Smoking** appears to be more common in the dance (ballet) community than in the general population.
D. **Nutritional disorders are common in the dance community.**
  1. Bulimia and anorexia nervosa occur more frequently in the dance community than in the general population.
  2. Found mainly in teenagers but can occur at any age.
  3. May enhance the problems associated with injuries (demineralization, slowed healing, worsened side effects with medications).

III. INJURIES

While virtually any acute or overuse injury can be seen among dancers, **some injuries are so closely related to the specific demands of dance** (ballet in most instances) that their diagnosis and treatment merit special consideration.

A. **Types**
   1. **Acute: Few are unique to ballet.**
      a. Generally same as seen with any running/jumping sport.
      b. Occasional "environmental" injuries are seen.
         i. Falls from sets
         ii. Objects falling on dancers
   2. **Overuse: Cause of vast majority of injuries**
      a. **Frequently related to turnout (external rotation of hips) or lack thereof.**
      c. Related to activity variances:
         i. Following layoffs
         ii. New demands from new choreography
         iii. Increased activity during performance season
      d. Most difficult to treat
         i. Not totally disabling
         ii. Gradual onset and thus presented for treatment late in course

B. **Diagnosis**
   1. **Must be precise.**
      a. Often related to the very specific demands of dance technique (knowing the demands makes treatment easier).
      b. If vague, cause will not be found and reinjury will occur.
   2. **Must be immediate.**
      a. Little time available for reflection (dancer is de-training while waiting).
   3. **Must be explained to dancer** (and often teacher or artistic director).

C. **Treatment**
   1. **Maintenance of conditioning (strength, flexibility, and endurance) is of paramount importance.**
   2. Programs must allow continuation of as much training as possible.
      a. Must understand classwork and training in order to manipulate activities during treatment.
   3. Dancer must understand goals and rationale of treatment.
      a. Must actively participate in program.
      b. Muscular rehabilitation (strength, endurance, and flexibility) is involved in the management of *every* injury.
   4. Program must be taught so dancer can carry it out on her own (away from medical facility).
   5. Frequent demands for expedient treatment (i.e., corticosteroid injection, etc.) must be tempered with long-term goals.
   6. Side effects of medications must be considered.
      a. Muscle relaxants—loss of timing and coordination
      b. Nonsteroidal antiinflammatory drugs (NSAIDs)—food intake is irregular.

D. **Trunk and thoracic spine**
   1. **Parathoracic strains—often actually involve the scapular stabilizing muscles** (rhomboids, trapezius, and levator).
      a. Seen in males, with cause often related to lifting partner.
   2. **Scoliosis** has been reported to be more common in female ballet dancers than in the general population.
      a. May be related to a combination of two common problems
         i. Delayed onset of menses
         ii. Dietary anomalies

E. **Lumbar spine**
  1. **Spondylolysis**
     a. **Cause**
        i. May be prompted by lordosis secondary to inadequate external rotation of hips.
           (a) External rotation of the hips is increased by slight hip flexion.
           (b) In order to maintain an upright posture, increased lordosis is used to compensate for hip flexion.
        ii. Condition may be more common in dancers than in general population.
     b. **Diagnosis**
        i. Midline pain with hyperextension
           (a) Arabesque position in ballet
        ii. Oblique x-rays to reveal defect
        iii. Bone scan to reveal maturity of lesion
     c. **Treatment**
        i. Pain-free activity is the keystone for management.
        ii. Brace is necessary for pain-free activities of daily living.
        iii. Abdominal strengthening exercises are helpful.
        iv. Gradual resumption of dance activities
           (a) Jumping and partnering resumed last.
F. **Hips**
  1. **Overuse**
     a. **Piriformis syndrome**
        i. Cause: Inadequate external rotation of hips or weak external rotators
        ii. Diagnosis
           (a) Deep posterior hip (gluteal) pain
           (b) Pain when arising from a deep chair or car seat
           (c) May be sciatic radiation
           (d) Pain on exam with increased internal rotation or external rotation against resistance
        iii. Treatment
           (a) Stretching and strengthening of external rotators of hips
     b. **Degenerative joint disease**
        i. Cause: Possibly long-term dance activities with repetitive microtrauma
        ii. Diagnosis
           (a) May be seen in younger age groups than generally expected
           (b) Anterior hip pain: activity-related
           (c) Limitation of motion: Rotation, pure flexion, and abduction
           (d) Weakness of musculature
        iii. Treatment
           (a) Strengthen hip musculature
           (b) Surgical treatment usually means an end to dancing.
G. **Thigh**
  1. **Overuse**
     a. **Sartorius tendinitis**
        i. Cause: Overuse as an external rotator of hip (weight-bearing or nonweight-bearing leg)
        ii. Diagnosis
           (a) Tenderness at origin
           (b) Pain with resisted hip flexion, external rotation, and abduction
        iii. Treatment
           (a) NSAIDs
           (b) Physical therapy local modalities for symptoms
           (c) Stretching and strengthening exercises

H. **Knee**
1. **Acute**
   a. **Sprains**
      i. **ACL injuries** do occur in ballet.
         (a) Treatment: Surgical management is not necessarily indicated, as a substantial number of dancers are known to perform with an absent ACL and no appreciable disability. Any surgical complication, even in small limitation of knee extension, is career-halting for a ballet dancer.
   b. **Meniscal injuries**
      i. Definitive diagnosis should be established early, as prolonged, watchful waiting results in deterioration of conditioning. Early use of MRI or arthroscopy is often indicated. Meniscus repairs should not be mindlessly performed, because the period of immobilization may in itself be career-threatening.
2. **Overuse**
   a. **Patellofemoral dysfunction is very common.**
      i. Cause
         (a) Inadequate quadriceps (vastus medialis) strength for demands of dancing
         (b) External rotation of leg to compensate for inadequate hip external rotation (increase of Q-angle)
         (c) Inadequate rehabilitation of prior knee injury
      ii. Diagnosis
         (a) Activity-related, retro- or peripatellar pain
            (i) More often in region of medial retinaculum
         (b) Occasional effusion if seen late in course
         (c) Decreased tone or bulk of vastus medialis
         (d) Radiographic changes and crepitation are usually of confirmatory value only.
      iii. Treatment
         (a) Relative rest
         (b) Avoidance of deep squats (grand plié)
         (c) Physical therapy modalities if effusion present
         (d) NSAIDs
         (e) Quadriceps isometrics (full extension)
         (f) Electrical muscular stimulation for vastus medialis if exercises are painful or ineffective
         (g) Neoprene sleeve with lateral pad
         (h) Surgical intervention should be considered only as a last resort and then only if the alternative is to stop dancing.
   b. **Patellar tendinitis**
      i. Cause: May be repetitive jumping; relative quadriceps inflexibility (tight quadriceps not uncommon in ballet dancers)
      ii. Diagnosis
         (a) Activity-related infrapatellar pain
         (b) Focal tenderness at origin of tendon fibers at inferior pole of patella
         (c) Rarely swelling or radiographic changes
      iii. Treatment
         (a) Relative rest (jumping)
         (b) NSAIDs
         (c) Ice
         (d) Quadriceps stretching and strengthening
         (e) Neoprene sleeve with lateral pad
         (f) Steroid injections not indicated

I. **Leg**
  1. **Acute**
     a. **Achilles tendon rupture**
        i. Cause often previous episode(s) of Achilles tendinitis.
        ii. Males predominate.
        iii. Diagnosis
           (a) Sudden, often loud, snap in distal calf
           (b) Dancer describes being struck in calf
           (c) Defect in tendon
           (d) Positive Thompson test
        iv. Treatment
           (a) Surgical treatment favored by most, but closed management has been effective in dancers.
  2. **Overuse**
     a. **Achilles tendinitis**
        i. Cause
           (a) Usually overuse but may be minor sprain
           (b) May be mechanical from pressure
              (i) Ribbons on toe shoes tied too tightly
              (ii) Footwear used with character roles (e.g., cowboy boots)
        ii. Diagnosis
           (a) Achilles tendon pain with activities
           (b) Pain with passive dorsiflexion
           (c) Pain with (or inability to) arise on toes (relevé)
           (d) Swelling
           (e) Crepitation (uncommon)
        iii. Treatment
           (a) Physical therapy modalities
           (b) Relative rest (may have to avoid all dancing temporarily and use heel lift in shoes for daily activities)
           (c) Stretching and strengthening are helpful.
           (d) Gradual return to dancing with avoidance of all pain
           (e) Steroid injections not appropriate
        iv. **Cautions**
           (a) Posterior ankle impingement often misdiagnosed as Achilles tendinitis
           (b) May enhance likelihood of rupture of Achilles tendon
     b. **Stress fractures:** May involve distal tibia or fibula or (more uncommon) anterior border of mid-shaft of tibia with transverse fracture line through anterior cortex on radiograph (the "dreaded black line" of Hamilton).
        i. Cause: Usually change in activity
        ii. Diagnosis
           (a) Activity-related, localized pain at site of fracture
           (b) Focal tenderness
           (c) Radiograph may not reveal if seen early in course
           (d) Bone scan
        iii. Treatment
           (a) Rest to the point of **pain-free activities of daily living** for 7–10 consecutive days
           (b) Gradual resumption of dancing activities—must remain pain-free
           (c) Stress fracture of anterior border of mid-tibia must be treated with extreme caution, as this lesion has a propensity to go on to overt fracture. Surgical drilling of the fracture site hastens safe return to dancing activities.

J. **Ankle**
 1. **Acute**
  a. **Sprains—usually lateral (inversion)**
   i. Treatment
    (a) With grade III sprains, some advocate surgical repair because instability in plantarflexed position (de riguer in ballet) is so disabling.
    (b) We prefer active, aggressive rehabilitation.
    (c) Cast immobilization results in needless time loss.
   ii. **Cautions**
    (a) **Peroneal tendon dislocations often mistaken for lateral ankle sprains.**
     (i) Tenderness localized to posterior distal fibula
     (ii) Ecchymosis may be extensive along course of peroneal tendons.
     (iii) Flake of bone off lateral malleolus (radiograph)
     (iv) Should be managed surgically when acute
    (b) **Avulsion fracture of base of the fifth metatarsal styloid**
     (i) Similar mechanism of injury
     (ii) Pain and tenderness at base of fifth metatarsal
     (iii) May usually be treated as ankle sprain
  b. **Ankle impingement**
   i. **Posterior**
    (a) Cause: Impingement of posterior process of talus or os trigonum
    (b) Diagnosis
     (i) Posterior ankle pain with plantar flexion
     (ii) Pain reproduced with active or passive plantar flexion
     (iii) Presence of large posterior process of talus or os trigonum on radiograph
    (c) Treatment: First (few) episodes
     (i) NSAIDs
     (ii) Physical therapy modalities for swelling
     (iii) Contrast baths
     (iv) Ankle strengthening (invertors and evertors)
    (d) Treatment: Recurrent episodes
     (i) Surgical removal of posterior process of talus or os trigonum
   ii. **Anterior**
    (a) Cause: Usually osteophytes of anterior tibia and/or anterior articular margin of dome of talus
    (b) Diagnosis
     (i) Anterior ankle pain with extreme of dorsiflexion
     (ii) Radiographs reveal impingement of osteophytes.
    (c) Treatment
     (i) First episode: as above
     (ii) Recurrent episodes—surgical excison of osteophytes
K. **Foot**
 1. **Acute**
  a. **Spiral fracture of shaft of fifth metatarsal (dancer's fracture)**
   i. Cause: Inversion injury while on toes
   ii. Diagnosis by radiography
   iii. Treatment: Short period of immobilization followed by protection with taping and attenuated dance activities
 2. **Overuse**
  a. **Stress fractures**
   i. Cause: Usually activity changes
    (a) May involve **metatarsal shaft** (metatarsals 2–4)
    (b) May involve base of second metatarsal

        (i) A "ballet-specific" injury often resulting in long-term disability
        (ii) Usually requires bone scan for diagnosis
        (iii) Uncommon
    (c) **Sesamoids**
        (i) Utilize bone scan to assist in differentiating from bipartite sesamoid or sesamoiditis
  ii. Diagnosis
    (a) Activity-related pain, often well-localized
    (b) Tenderness (focal) at fracture site
    (c) Radiographs (may not reveal if seen early)
    (d) Bone scan
  iii. Treatment
    (a) Activity attenuation until activities of daily living are pain-free for at least 7 consecutive days (longer for base of second metatarsal)
    (b) Gradual resumption of dance activities—must remain pain-free

b. **Degenerative joint disease of first MTP joint**
  i. Cause: More often seen in male dancers, because their positions require more frequent dorsiflexion of this joint.
  ii. Diagnosis
    (a) Pain at dorsum of MTP joint with hyperdorsiflexion (worsened with weight-bearing in this position)
    (b) Loss of dorsiflexion at MTP joint
    (c) Tenderness at dorsum of joint
    (d) Radiographs reveal osteophyte at articular margin of dorsum of metatarsal head.
  iii. Treatment
    (a) Early: NSAIDs, contrast baths, taping to restrict motion of toe (which also compromises dancing)
    (b) Late: Surgical excision of osteophytes

c. **Morton's neuroma**
  i. Cause
    (a) May be related to constrictive footwear
    (b) Usually at 3–4 interspace
  ii. Diagnosis
    (a) Weight-bearing, activity-related pain
    (b) Often "shock-like" sensation in involved toes
    (c) Usually relief with removal of footwear
        (i) Can be seen with barefoot dancing (rare)
  iii. Treatment
    (a) Metatarsal pad placed just proximal to metatarsal heads
    (b) Local injections of corticosteroid (3 or fewer)
    (c) Surgical excision (probably successful in no more than 80% of cases)

ACKNOWLEDGMENT

This chapter appeared previously in Mellion MB, Walsh WM, Shelton GL (eds): The Team Physician's Handbook. Philadelphia, Hanley & Belfus, 1990, with permission.

Chapter 52: Running

JULIE WENTWORTH COLLITON, MD

Women have become increasingly active in all aspects of society. Running is one activity that has proved appealing to women for many reasons. It is an efficient way to maintain a general level of fitness, relieve stress, maintain weight, boost self-esteem, socialize with friends, or engage in healthy competition. Running, however, can also be taken to extremes and lead to self-destructive consequences, such as overuse injuries and eating disorders. This chapter reviews the issues pertinent to women runners and helps physicians guide these women toward safe and reasonable running goals.

I. WOMEN AND RUNNING—A HISTORICAL PERSPECTIVE

1891—First recorded woman's running event, near Dublin, Ireland. It was approximately 100 yards and was won by Eva Francisco in 13.0 s.

1896—First modern Olympic marathon. A woman with the pseudonym Melpomene competed unofficially and completed the race in 4 hr, 30 min.

1913—L. Aaltonen ran 1,500 m in 5 min, 44 s.

1918—Marie Ledru complete the French Marathon.

1919—Alice Milliat was unsuccessful in petitioning the International Olympic Committee (IOC) to add women's athletics to the 1920 Games (women had been competing in more "feminine" sports, such as figure skating, tennis, and swimming, since 1900).

1924—Women's athletics were rejected again by the IOC.

1926—Violet Piercy of Great Britain ran a 3 hr, 40 min, 22 s marathon.

1928—Majority vote overrode IOC president and women's athletics were added. Included were the 100 m, 800 m, 4 × 100-m relay, high jump, and discus. Many of the women were not properly conditioned to compete in longer distances; because of this, women were not allowed to compete in distances longer than 200 m until 1960.

1965—The first U.S. nationally recognized cross-country race of 1.5 miles was run around Seattle's Green Lake and was won by Marie Mulder.

1967—Katherine Switzer was the first woman to officially run the Boston Marathon. When race director Jock Semple discovered a woman in the race, he attempted to physically remove her from the field. She eventually completed the race in 4 hr, 20 min. Another woman in the race that year, Roberta Gibb Bingay, ran unofficially and crossed the finish line at 3 hr, 40 min.

1971—A woman's time for 3 miles on the track of 17 min, 7 s, run by Cheryl Bridges, was officially recorded.

1972—Title IX of the U.S. Education Amendments was passed, making sex discrimination illegal in institutions using federal funds; therefore, women's sports had to be provided in schools.

1973—A Connecticut judge ruled against a girl who wanted to run on her school's cross-country team. He stated, "Athletic competition builds character in our boys. We do not need that kind of character in our girls."

1975—Liane Winter set a women's world record at the Boston Marathon with a time of 2 hr, 42 min, 42 s. A second woman, Katherine Switzer, finished at 2 hr 51 min.

1978—Grete Waitz ran her first New York Marathon with a time of 2 hr, 32 min, 30 s.

1979—International Runner's Committee (IRC) was formed to lobby for women's runner-related issues.

1980—U.S. Olympic Track and Field Trials held women's exhibition events in 5,000 and 10,000 m.

1981/82—National Collegiate Athletic Association took over women's collegiate sports and held coed championships for the first time in cross-country and track.

1982—International Amateur Athletic Federation (IAAF) recognized world records for women at 5,000 and 10,000 m.

1984—Addition of the 3,000 m and marathon to the women's events at the Olympics.

1988—The 10,000 m was added to the Olympics.

1991—The New York City Marathon became known as the "marathon of the moms," as the top three contenders, Liz McColgan, Lisa Ondicki, and Joan Benoit Samuelson, were all mothers.

II. PHYSIOLOGY IN FEMALE VS. MALE RUNNERS

The basic physiology and components of performance do not differ between women and men, but there is a difference in the size of the physiologic response to various stimuli.

A. Body composition

1. **Body fat**

   a. Trained male runners have 4–10% body fat, compared to approximately 16% in elite female runners (although some have less). The average untrained female has approximately 25%.

   b. The higher percent body fat in women yields an extra 9–12 lbs that they transport when compared with men, requiring additional energy expenditure during running and placing a greater demand on the oxygen transport system.

   c. **Women must not attempt to lower their body fat to unnaturally low levels through energy restriction and excessive training.** Although many top female distance runners have body fat levels <10%, many record holders have body fat values >14% (e.g., Joan Benoit Samuelson and Lynn Jennings).

   d. The reduction in the runner's body fat value is primarily due to training and a diet high in complex carbohydrate and low in total fat, not because of caloric restriction.

2. **Muscle composition**

   a. Muscle fiber composition is similar between men and women, comprising approximately 52% slow-twitch and 48% fast-twitch. In both male and female elite distance runners, the percentage of slow-twitch fibers is higher, ranging from 60–98%, in the leg muscles.

   b. Untrained adult men have substantially thicker muscle fibers than untrained females. In equally trained men and women distance runners, the difference in muscle fiber thickness was 8%. Female runners have an average fiber area that is 79% larger than that of untrained women and approximately the same size as untrained men.

   c. Muscle mass is one component to strength and speed, so the size of muscle fiber is clearly a determinant of performance where men have an advantage over women. However, there is no evidence to suggest that men have a greater number of muscle fibers than women.

B. Muscle metabolism

1. **Circulation**

   a. Capillaries surrounding the muscle fibers deliver fuels to and remove wastes from muscles. Female runners have approximately 4.9 capillaries around each muscle fiber, and male runners have about 5.6 capillaries/fiber.

   b. Females do not receive less circulation per fiber, but rather the volume of muscle served by each capillary is less and fewer capillaries are needed.

   c. Running can increase the number of capillaries around each leg muscle in both sexes. Training level is more significant than gender in determining the capillary density in the muscle.

2. **Fuel preference**
    a. The greater degree of fat stores, which would spare the use of glycogen as fuel, has been suggested to make women better suited to longer-distance endurance events, like the marathon, than men. However, men have a greater fat-burning capacity.
    b. In men and women running at marathon pace for 1 hour, both derived about 50% of energy from fat. Thus, there is no significance different in performance based on fat utilization between men and women.

3. **Energy production**
    a. In a study comparing concentrations of the mitochondrial enzymes succinate dehydrogenase, malate dehydrogenase, and carnitine palmityl transferase from leg muscles of men and women, the only significant difference was found to be a higher concentration of **succinate dehydrogenase** in men.
    b. This enzyme difference did not afford a greater endurance capacity, as men and women were equally good at distances of 10 km and the marathon.

4. **Oxygen transport**
    a. **VO_2max:** Values in elite female athletes are 20–25% lower than in elite males. If corrected for lean body mass, this difference becomes 8–9%.
    b. **Cardiac output:** In men and women elite runners, heart volume differs by 33%, giving men an aerobic advantage by allowing them to pump a greater volume of blood per minute. No data are available on men and women who have performed equally in distance events.
    c. **Hemoglobin:** In men and women with equivalent VO_2max values, women have lower hemoglobin levels. To compensate, one proposed mechanism is that 2,3-diphosphoglyceric acid, which facilitates the unloading of O_2 at the muscle, is higher in female than male distance runners.

C. **Conditioning response**
  1. **Trainability**
      a. Men and women who train together have almost equal adaptative responses: VO_2max increased by 15% and 14.2%, respectively; heart rate and blood lactate changes did not vary between the sexes.
      b. Therefore, although men and women demonstrate differences in aerobic endurance and muscle strength, they adapt to and benefit from training in a similar manner.
  2. **Strength and speed**
      a. The **strength** of a single muscle fiber is determined by the size of the muscle fiber, not by the individual's sex. The larger the muscle, the more contractile filaments and the greater potential for generating a force when activated, hence **speed.**
      b. In strength training, men respond with a greater degree of hypertrophy than do women. Hypertrophy in muscle is regulated primarily by testosterone, which is approximately 10 times higher in men than women.
      c. In comparison of strength per kilogram of lean body weight in men and women runners, women had equal leg-extension strength compared with men. However, men had significantly greater **upper-extremity strength** than women. This disparity in strength is most apparent in 100- and 200-m sprints, which require maximal force development in both upper and lower extremities and where men have a 9–10% performance advantage.

III. ENDOCRINOLOGIC FACTORS

A. **Menstruation**
  1. **Normal cycle**
      a. Research has shown that the menstrual cycle has **no significant physiologic effect** on performance, and women in all stages of the menstrual cycle have won Olympic medals.

b. In actual races, some women show better performance times during the follicular phase (prior to ovulation); other women *perceive* that they perform better at this phase.

c. The reason for these results may relate to **premenstrual syndrome** (PMS), which is the constellation of symptoms related to the menstrual cycle, including water retention, irritability, increased appetite, mood swings, anxiety, headaches, depression, and heavy and tender breasts. These symptoms may be related to hormonal levels or changes at the time of menstruation.

d. The impact of PMS on performance for many athletes may be psychological. But water-weight gain may be as much as 5 lb and can affect performance.

e. Women should be encouraged to continue their running programs, as exercise alleviates the symptoms.

2. **Amenorrhea and oligomenorrhea**

   a. **Prevalence**

      i. As many as 50% of competitive athletes may be amenorrheic.

      ii. Both amenorrhea and oligomenorrhea are more prevalent among athletes, with the overall incidence being 10–20% compared with 5% for the general population.

      iii. In runners, there is no correlation with menstrual dysfunction and average weekly mileage, running pace, or number of years training. There is a correlation with menstrual irregularities prior to beginning a running program.

   b. **Effects of menstrual irregularities**

      i. Decreased bone density and osteoporosis, which can lead to an increased risk of fractures and stress fractures, both at a young age and later.

      ii. Alterations in blood lipid profiles and increased risk of coronary artery disease

      iii. Athletes in training who have lost their menses should be concerned that they may be consuming too few calories or exhibiting symptoms of an eating disorder.

   c. **Treatment approach**

      i. First, determine the cause of the menstrual dysfunction, to rule out problems unrelated to running or exercise.

      ii. Treatment of choice is a reduction in mileage, small weight gain, or increase in calorie intake. Usually a 10% reduction in mileage and a 4–5 lb weight gain are enough to allow normal menstruation to resume.

      iii. If the patient is not willing to comply, **patient reluctance** may be due to training and competition goals or related to an eating disorder. Appropriately trained professionals must be called for assistance in guiding the athlete to appropriate treatment.

      iv. Hormonal therapy may be administered during this time to protect from the deleterious effects of menstrual irregularity.

B. **Fertility**

1. **Infertility** is increased among elite runners, probably due to the menstrual dysfunction common in this population.

2. As athletes decrease running intensity, menstrual dysfunction usually resolves enabling successful pregnancies.

3. In less competitive runners, there is no increased incidence of infertility.

C. **Contraception**

1. **Amenorrhea/dysmenorrhea**

   a. Menstrual dysfunction is *not* a reliable means of contraception.

   b. For many runners who have gone without their periods for some time, pregnancy is the first indication that they are once again ovulating.

2. **Rhythm**
   a. The rhythm method is unreliable.
   b. Many runners have shortened luteal phase in their menstrual cycle during times of intense training, reducing the time from ovulation to onset of bleeding from the usual 12 days to about 8 days and allowing fewer days for safe unprotected intercourse.
3. **Oral contraceptives**
   a. Oral contraceptive pills are used less often among elite runners.
   b. Water-weight gain, nausea, severe cramping, and heavy bleeding are side effects unacceptable to the runner.
   c. These symptoms are less common with the lower-dose pills now available.
4. **Mechanical/barrier**
   a. Mechanical methods (sponge, foam, diaphragm, condoms) tend to be popular among runners, probably because they cause no side effects related to running.
   b. The diaphragm must be left in place for at least 6 hours after intercourse, at times during training or competing, and may be uncomfortable for some women. If this is the case, a smaller size may be tried, or an alternative method should be sought.
   c. All mechanical methods require motivation and planning on the part of the partners; this should be considered when advising a runner.

D. **Pregnancy**
   1. **Potential contraindications to running while pregnant**
      a. Past miscarriages
      b. History of placenta previa
      c. Incompetent cervix
      d. Vaginal bleeding
      e. Anemia, moderate to severe
      f. Renal disease
      g. Hypertension, uncontrolled
      h. Diabetes, poorly controlled
      i. Thyroid disease
      j. Coronary artery disease
      k. Cardiac disease, especially mitral or aortic valve disease
   2. **Potential benefits of running while pregnant**
      a. Improved muscle tone
      b. Improved fitness
      c. Enhanced self-esteem
      d. Fewer varicose veins
      e. Decreased backache
      f. Improved sleep
      g. Sense of control
      h. Possibly easier pregnancy, labor, delivery, and recovery (related to fitness and muscle tone)
      i. Improved ability to dissipate heat
      j. Improved blood glucose homeostasis
   3. **Guidelines for pregnant runners**
      a. Intensity of running should be reduced; never run to exhaustion.
      b. Maximal benefits are gained by running at least 3 times weekly for 20–30 minute durations.
      c. Heart rate should be kept between 120–140 beats/min or 25–30% below normal training heart rate. Heart rate should return to resting within 10 minutes following exercise (a patient's resting heart rate will rise during pregnancy, and this should be determined before running).

d. If strenuous exercise is done, it should not exceed 15 minutes in duration. A pregnant runner should be able to talk while running.

e. Remain adequately hydrated. Dehydration will alter circulation, which may trigger premature labor.

f. Avoid getting overheated; maternal core temperature should not exceed 38°C. Avoid exercising in hot humid weather.

g. Be sure to account for increased nutritional/caloric demands of both pregnancy and running.

h. Warm-up and cool-down are crucial. It should include slow prolonged stretching as well as gradual change in heart rate.

i. A light-weight maternity girdle may offer support for low back discomfort.

E. **Postpartum:** After delivery, there are numerous changes in the new mother's body and lifestyle. Many factors—personal, psychologic, and physiologic—must be considered when advising a woman about resuming running and to what intensity, duration and frequency.

1. **General guidelines for postpartum running**

a. If an episiotomy was performed, wait until soreness has resolved before beginning a vigorous running program.

b. Vaginal bleeding associated with running that is heavy or bright red is a contraindication to running.

c. Fatigue will be more common shortly after giving birth, due to many factors: e.g., anemia, sleep deprivation, inadequate calories (especially if breast feeding), infant care, and household maintenance. Running should be tapered accordingly.

d. Incontinence is not uncommon after giving birth and may last several months. Kegel exercises may help alleviate some of this, as will the normalization of hormone levels.

e. Additional breast support is indicated, especially if the mother is breast feeding. An elastic wrap over a running or nursing bra may be helpful.

f. Regular exercise at least 3 times a week is preferable to intermittent exercise.

g. Vigorous exercise in hot humid weather or during febrile illness should be avoided.

h. Postpartum joint and soft tissue laxity may predispose to injury. Extremes of motion that put added stress on joints and soft tissues should be avoided: e.g., stretching to the point of maximum resistance, running stairs, and hill training.

i. Warm-up and cool-down periods that include stretching and a gradual change in heart rate are crucial.

j. Hydration is very important; advise on the importance of fluids before, after, and, when appropriate, during exercise.

k. A postpartum exercise program should begin and increase very gradually.

IV. COMMON INJURIES

The overall incidence of injuries in female runners is no greater than it is for male runners. The greatest difference between female and male injury patterns relates to biomechanics. Women tend to have a greater degree of femoral anteversion as well as a wider pelvis and greater Q-angle. This tends to put greater stress on the medial compartment of the knee, patellofemoral complex, and medial aspect of the ankle.

A. **Stress fractures** (*see* Chapter 42)

1. **Mechanism:** Repeated microtrauma to the bone to where osteoblasts cannot lay down new bone fast enough to meet demand.

2. **Risk factors**

a. Menstrual dysfunction

b. Eating disorders

c. Change in running intensity, duration, or frequency

    d. Change in running surface
    e. Running in inappropriate or overly-worn shoes
  3. **Common sites**
    a. Femoral neck
    b. Pubis
    c. Tibia
    d. Fibula
    e. Metatarsals
  4. **Symptoms:** Pain during a run that decreases or stops after the run
  5. **Signs**
    a. Local tenderness
    b. Pain may be made worse with ultrasound over the fracture.
  6. **Diagnosis**
    a. Bone scan most sensitive
    b. Radiographs may not become positive until after many weeks and callus formation is seen.
    c. Clinical suspicion often adequate to make diagnosis.
  7. **Treatment**
    a. Relative rest until pain subsides
    b. Cross-training while injured to maintain strength and flexibility
    c. When pain-free, begin gradual return to running.
  8. **Prevention**
    a. Avoid abrupt changes in training schedule.
    b. Avoid frequent changes in training surfaces.
    c. Replace running shoes after every 300 miles of use.
B. **Patellofemoral stress syndrome** (*see* Chapter 40)
  1. **Description:** Retropatellar pain resulting from patellofemoral malalignment. There may also be patellar instability, which can result from overuse injury with extreme and/or repetitive loading of the patellofemoral joint.
  2. **Symptoms**
    a. Anterior knee pain, often made worse when sitting in tight places with knee flexed
    b. Pain worse when descending stairs or hills
    c. Mild swelling
    d. May have the sensation of snapping or popping around the patella
  3. **Signs**
    a. Increased Q-angle
    b. Femoral anteversion, squinting patella
    c. Genu valgum
    d. Painful patellofemoral compression test
    e. Crepitation around the patella when knee is flexed or extended
    f. Mild effusion possible
    g. Tenderness to palpation around the patella
    h. Excessive pronation/supination or leg-length discrepancy
    i. Vastus medialis obliquus (VMO) hypoplasia
  4. **Radiographs**
    a. May be normal
    b. Infrapatellar views may show lateral tilt and/or lateral subluxation.
  5. **Treatment**
    a. Ultrasound, phonophoresis, iontophoresis
    b. Flexibility training
    c. Nonsteroidal antiinflammatory drugs (NSAIDs)
    d. Strengthening
    e. Orthotics or lifts, where appropriate
    f. Progressive return to running

C. **Achilles tendinitis**
1. **Symptoms:** While running, there is a gradual onset of pain 1–3 inches proximal to the insertion site of the Achilles tendon into os calcis. More common in runners older than 35.
2. **Signs**
   a. Rigid pes cavus
   b. Pes planus
   c. Local tenderness or swelling
   d. Tight gastrocsoleus complex
3. **Treatment**
   a. Relative rest
   b. Modalities: Ice when acutely inflamed and following a stretching session. Heat may be helpful prior to stretching program. A trial of ultrasound prior to stretching may be helpful.
   c. NSAIDs
   d. Heel lifts, arch supports, and orthotics, when appropriate
   e. Stretching of the Achilles tendon and plantar fascia
4. **Prevention**
   a. Flexibility to gastrocsoleus complex with the knee in both flexed and extended positions
   b. Balancing of strength between the foot plantar and dorsiflexors
   c. Running shoes should have a slightly elevated heel and well-supported longitudinal arch.
D. **Retrocalcaneal bursitis**
1. **Description:** Bursal inflammation immediately anterior to the insertion of the Achilles tendon
2. **Symptoms:** Aching pain with exercise. The runner's heel-counter may be too constrictive, causing friction in this area.
3. **Signs:** Tenderness and swelling are localized anterior to the insertion of the Achilles tendon.
4. **Radiographs** may demonstrate a prominent superior projection of the calcaneus or obliteration of the normal radio-opaque space anterior to the tendon.
5. **Treatment**
   a. Nonsurgial treatment is similar to Achilles tendinitis.
   b. Failed nonoperative therapy may require debridement of the bursa and excision of the superior projection of the calcaneus.
E. **Posterior tibialis tendinitis**
1. **Symptoms:** Gradual onset of pain posterior and inferior to the medial malleolus, present in foot-flat and toe-off phase of running
2. **Signs**
   a. Tenderness localized over the course of the posterior tibialis tendon around malleolus
   b. Mild swelling over course of tendon
   c. Pain with resisted inversion/plantar flexion or attempt at single-limb heel rise
3. **Treatment**
   a. Modalities: as for Achilles tendinitis
   b. NSAIDs
   c. Running shoe or orthotic designed to prevent overpronation
F. **Iliotibial band friction syndrome**
1. **Symptoms:** Pain localized to the lateral aspect of the knee and is worse with running down hills or on banked surfaces
2. **Signs**
   a. Tenderness over the lateral epicondyle of tibia/femur
   b. Pain localized at lateral epicondyle as flexed knee is extended top 30°

     c. Pain at lateral epicondyle as the runner supports all of her body weight with her knee flexed at 30°.

     d. Genus varus may be seen.

     e. Hyperpronated foot causing excessive internal tibial rotation may be present.

  3. **Treatment**

     a. Relative rest; avoid running downhill and on banked surfaces.

     b. Modalities: as for Achilles tendinitis

     c. NSAIDs

     d. Iliotibial band stretching

     e. Correct foot malalignment with appropriate shoes or orthotics, if indicated.

G. **Shin splints**

  1. **Symptoms**

     a. **Anterior:** Pain or tenderness along the medial or lateral anterior border of the tibia associated with running

     b. **Posterior:** Posteromedial leg pain in women who run on crowned roads, banked track, or uneven terrain

  2. **Signs**

     a. **Anterior**

       i. Pain with resisted dorsiflexion or passive plantar flexion of the foot

       ii. Diffuse tenderness over anterior tibial border

     b. **Posterior**

       i. Tenderness along posteromedial border of the tibia

       ii. Foot pronation

  3. **Treatment**

     a. NSAIDs

     b. Modalities: ice following activity

     c. Relative rest

     d. Correct foot biomechanics with appropriate shoes or orthotics, if indicated.

     e. Improve strength and flexibility of ankle plantar and dorsiflexors.

H. **Plantar fasciitis**

  1. **Symptoms:** Pain acutely or subacutely localized to the plantar surface of os calcis. Pain is usually worse when the athlete first arises after having been non–weight-bearing for a time.

  2. **Signs**

     a. Pain and tenderness over plantar-most aspect of os calcis or slightly distal and medial to that point

     b. Pain may be reproduced with stretch of plantar fascis.

     c. Tightness in Achilles tendon

  3. **Treatment**

     a. Modalities: ultrasound combined with deep friction massage

     b. NSAIDs

     c. Stretching of plantar fascia and gastrocsoleus complex

     d. Orthotics to support longitudinal arch

I. **Metatarsalgia**

  1. **Symptoms:** Pain under metatarsal heads due to repetitive impact from running

  2. **Signs**

     a. Tenderness localized to metatarsal heads

     b. Callus formation present over prominent metatarsal heads

  3. **Treatment**

     a. Orthotics for cushioning of metatarsal heads

     b. Rocker-bottom sole for refractory cases

J. **Morton's neuroma**

  1. **Symptoms:** Pain in the foot localized to the third, or less commonly the second, interspace (Fig. 1). Paresthesias or numbness may be present along the involved

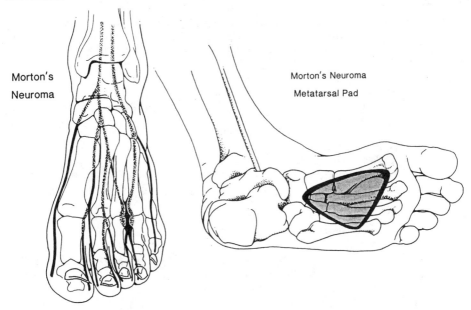

Morton's
Neuroma

Morton's Neuroma

Metatarsal Pad

FIGURE 1. Morton's neuroma. (From Hunter SC, Cappielo WL, Hess GP, Joyce D: Foot problems. In Mellion MB, Walsh WM, Shelton GL (eds): The Team Physician's Handbook. Philadelphia, Hanley & Belfus, 1990, with permission.)

digital nerves. There may be a history of wearing shoes with a narrow toe box (i.e., pumps).

2. **Signs**
   a. Tenderness in involved interspace
   b. Reproduction of symptoms by side-to-side compression of the foot.

3. **Treatment**
   a. Properly fitting shoes
   b. NSAIDs
   c. Orthotics with metatarsal pads to relieve pressure on metatarsal heads
   d. Surgery to alleviate compression on the digital nerve when nonoperative treatment fails

K. **Tarsal tunnel syndrome**
   1. **Symptoms:** Numbness and paresthesias on the plantar aspect of the foot
   2. **Signs:**
      a. Positive Tinel's sign
      b. Tenderness to palpation in the tarsal canal
      c. Electrodiagnostic evidence of slowing in the distal motor latencies of the medial and lateral plantar nerves
   3. **Treatment**
      a. Modalities: ultrasound combined with deep friction massage in the region of the tarsal tunnel
      b. NSAIDs
      c. Properly fitting shoes with adequate shock absorption
      d. Surgical release of compression within the tunnel when indicated.

V. OVERUSE SYNDROMES IN RUNNERS

Overuse syndromes can affect any part of the lower extremity and the list of potential injuries is almost limitless. These syndromes are chronic musculoskeletal problems resulting from microtraumatic stress to localized tissues, which leads to inflammation.

Usually caused by excess mileage in training, the inflammation develops faster than the body's ability to repair, and eventuates in macroscopic irritation and tissue disruption. These syndromes often affect tissues that are biomechanically critical to running.

A. **History of injury**
 1. **Nature of the present injury**
    a. When the injury was noticed
    b. Part injured
    c. Treatment in progress
    d. Recent foot or leg injuries that may have changed gait pattern
    e. Past medical or orthopedic problems
    f. Past use of orthotics or other pedal modifications (e.g., for leg-length discrepancy)
 2. **General training practices of the individual**
    a. Weekly mileage
       i. Changes in mileage
          (a) Rate of advancement should not be $\geq$10% per week.
       ii. Changes in intensity or pattern of running
       iii. Excessive mileage: Injury rises over the 30-mile/week training threshold.
          (a) $\geq$15% per year for males
          (b) $\geq$20% per year for females
    b. Surface
       i. Type of surface (grass, asphalt, clay, etc.) and recent changes from one to another
       ii. Surface grade
          (a) Uphill stresses gastroc-Achilles tendon system.
          (b) Downhill stresses tibial stabilizers or anterior tibialis muscle group.
       iii. Bank of roadway or track
          (a) Pronation of upper foot
          (b) Supination of lower foot
    c. Nature and extent of running in leisure activities.
    d. Use of lower extremities in activities of daily living.
 3. **Nature of specific training practices**
    a. Interval training—sprints can increase biomechanical strain.
    b. Footwear use
       i. Training footwear
          (a) How often changed? Shoes lose 50% of shock absorption capacity in 250–300 miles.
          (b) Wear patterns
          (c) Repaired vs. new footwear
       ii. Racing footwear should not be used in training because of lack of support and shock absorption.
       iii. In everyday footwear, look for patterns of wear and support characteristics.
    c. Systemic effects of overtraining
       i. Excessive fatigue and stiffness
       ii. "Staleness" and desire for rest
       iii. Deterioration of interest in training
B. **General treatment approach**
 1. **Classify degree of overuse** (Table 1).
    a. Early stages of overuse (Grades I and II)
       i. Evaluate training program for correctable problems.
       ii. Most athletes will not seek help at this stage.
    b. More advanced overuse (Grades III and IV)
       i. Pain limits competitive performance.
       ii. Training program is interrupted.
       iii. Rest and treatment are necessary.

TABLE 1. Staging of Overuse Syndromes*

Grade I	Post-activity soreness Duration of symptoms <2 weeks Generalized tenderness
Grade II	Pain during end of running and immediately after Duration of symptoms >2 weeks Localized pain, minimal inflammation
Grade III	Pain during early training Duration of symptoms >3 weeks Point tenderness, definite objective tissue inflammatory signs (erythema, edema, crepitus)
Grade IV	Pain with activities other than training, severity of which prohibits training or competition Grade II symptoms plus dysfunction of injured structure, muscle atrophy, tissue breakdown

* From Franz WB: Overuse syndromes in runners. In Mellion MB: Office Management of Sports Injuries and Athletic Problems. Philadelphia, Hanley & Belfus, 1988, with permission.

2. **Rest**
   a. The more severe the grade of overuse, the more rest is needed.
   b. Usually a decrease in weekly mileage is necessary.
   c. Training sessions should be divided into smaller increments, with rest between.
   d. Activities with less biomechanical strain can be substituted for running (e.g., swimming, bicycling).
3. **Cryotherapy and thermotherapy**
   a. **Ice** applied to inflamed body parts
      i. 20-minute applications or to tolerance, then rewarm and reapply as appropriate.
      ii. Ice is most useful in the acute phase of injury.
         (a) Decreases pain
         (b) Inhibits inflammation
      iii. Contraindicated with medical conditions that affect sensory nerve supply; e.g., diabetes, vascular disease, during use of local anesthetic.
   b. **Heat** is useful in later rehabilitation of injury.
      i. Increases tissue flexibility and elasticity
      ii. Allows athlete to stretch more comfortably
   c. **Compression and elevation** are used with cryotherapy.
      i. Decreases edema
      ii. Compression prevents accumulation of inflammatory products in tissue.
      iii. Elevation promotes venous and lymphatic flow.
4. **Pharmacologic treatment**
   a. NSAIDs and salicylates
      i. Useful both acutely and chronically
      ii. Pain relief initially and during longer term, indicating decrease in inflammation
   b. Injectable corticosteroids
      i. Indicated after more conservative measures fail
      ii. Often mixed with local anesthetic
      iii. Skin surgically prepared
      iv. Do not inject into tendons.
      v. Watch for systemic effect and infection.
5. **Orthotics for running**
   a. Consider for a specific biomechanical problem related to symptoms.
   b. Usually shoe inserts of plastic or rubber material
   c. Usual objective is to balance foot in neutral to inhibit pronation and supination.

    d. Initiate slowly, with multiple adjustments during break-in.
    e. Use in symptom-free athlete is contraindicated (may cause symptoms).
  6. **Shoes**
    a. Sports-specific shoes have enhanced performance.
    b. Running shoes should have good shock absorption, rigid heel control, good
       flexibility at midfoot break, provide good traction, and protect the feet.
       i. Wide heel with lift for shock absorption and support of Achilles tendon
       ii. Curve of sole conforms to foot shape, with greater curve for high arch or
           cavus foot.
       iii. Snug fit, allowing slight increase in volume during running
    c. Prescription of footwear is an important component of treatment program for
       overuse.
    d. Major problem is overworn shoes.
  7. **Promote appropriate warm-up and cool-down techniques.**
    a. Warm-up long enough to cause sweating and to feel mild exertion
       i. Enhances oxygen release from hemoglobin
       ii. Increases blood flow
       iii. Decreases blood viscosity
       iv. Enhances muscular contraction
       v. Increases speed of neuromuscular transmission (i.e., improved reaction
          time)
       vi. Increases tissue elasticity, with decreased viscosity of synovial fluid
       vii. Allows for better gains from subsequent stretching
    b. Nonballistic stretching
       i. Follows proper warm-up
       ii. Facilitates enhanced neuromuscular efficiency
       iii. Should be done gently, never past minimal discomfort to the point of pain
       iv. Careful attention to hamstring and gastrocnemius muscle group and to
           iliotibial band
    c. If running precedes stretching, warm-up should provide for flexibility.
       i. Alternate 220-yd jog with 20-yd walk for 0.5 mile.
    d. Cool-down
       i. Should be active vs passive
          (a) Facilitates removal of lactate from tissue
          (b) Heart rate and respiration decrease to preexercise levels.
          (c) Additional stretching can be done.

ACKNOWLEDGMENTS

Parts of this chapter were adapted extensively from the following sources: Part II from Costill
DL: Inside Running: Basics of Sports Physiology. Dubuque, IA, Brown and Benchmark, 1986,
pp 153–167; Part IV from Heiser TM: Track and field. In Mellion MB, Walsh WM, Shelton GL
(eds): The Team Physician's Handbook. Philadelphia, Hanley & Belfus, 1990, pp 585–598; and
Part V from Franz WB: Overuse syndromes in runners. In Mellion MB (ed): Office Management
of Sports Injuries and Athletic Problems. Philadelphia, Hanley & Belfus, 1988, pp 289–309.

REFERENCES

1. Costill DL: Inside Running: Basics of Sports Physiology. Dubuque, IA, Brown and Benchmark, 1986,
   pp 153–167.
2. Franz WB: Overuse syndromes in runners. In Mellion MB (ed): Office Management of Sports Injuries
   and Athletic Problems. Philadelphia, Hanley & Belfus, 1988, pp 289–309.
3. Heinonen J: Sports Illustrated Running for Women: A Complete Guide. New York, Time Inc., 1989.
4. Heiser TM: Track and field. In Mellion MB, Walsh WM, Shelton GL (eds): The Team Physician's
   Handbook. Philadelphia, Hanley & Belfus, 1990, pp 585–598.

Chapter 53: Bicycling

SUSAN R. HOPKINS, MD, PhD

The first bicycle race was 30 km and was held in France in 1869. The winning time was 3 hr 9 min, not surprising as the racing bicycle at that time weighed over 100 lbs! It was not until the 1932 World Championships that cycling was revolutionized by the introduction of derailleurs, which allowed the rider to change gears without dismounting from the bicycle. Since that time, amateur cycling has grown to include events ranging from the 1000-m matched sprint to the multiday, several hundred-kilometer stage race.

Although women's events are fully represented in off-road racing, female road and track cyclists have struggled for years to gain equal access to their sport. In 1984, the woman's road race was first included as an Olympic event, sprints were added in 1988, and the individual pursuit was added in 1992. The kilometer is still not recognized as an event for women either at the World Championships or Olympics, although the 500-m race was added for the 1993 World Championships. Team pursuit is similarly not represented in either competition, and the Olympics lack the points race and 500-m for women. Despite this, women's cycling has become extremely competitive, and North American racers are among the best in the world. Many elite female cyclists train up to 5 hours a day, and weekly mileages of 400–600 km is not uncommon. Very few scientific studies have been published relating to injuries in competitive cyclists of any gender, and none related specifically to women.

I. TYPES OF COMPETITION

A. **Cycling is a heterogeneous sport**, almost to the same extent as track and field events. In discussions with the athlete, the practitioner should seek information as to which type of cycling forms the bulk of time spend on her bike and at what level she competes.
   1. Cyclists are divided into categories depending on performance level. (Riders earn points by performance ranking in races to advance to the next level.)
   2. **Amateur road and track cyclists** are divided into:
      a. Elite: National Team or National Level cyclists
      b. Expert
      c. Sport
      d. Novice
      e. Beginner: Entry-level athletes
   3. **Women cyclists** in North America were originally categorized as male-equivalent riders (i.e., their performance was compared directly to men rather than to other women cyclists), but more states and provinces have changed their ranking systems so that the top-level women cyclists are given Category I designation.
   4. **Off-road cycling** designates four categories.
      a. Novice
      b. Sportswoman
      c. Expert
      d. Pro-Elite

B. **Road cycling** comprises the following events:
   1. **Road race:** A mass-start race often over open roads and may be a circuit race or point to point to point race. Typical distances for women are 50–120 km.
   2. **Criterium:** Mass-start race, often held in major cities where a block or two is entirely closed to traffic. Multiple short laps with high-speed corners, and distances up to 50 km.

3. **Time trial:** Individual races against the clock. Drafting (riding in another rider's slipstream or wake) is not allowed. A time trial may be of any distance and can be entirely uphill. Team time trial is two or more riders from the same team working together to race against the clock.

4. **Stage race:** Multiple races drawn from the previous described events. The winner is the rider who has the fastest combined time for all events. Tour de France is the best known example of this type of race.

C. **Track disciplines**

1. **1000-m sprint:** Pits one rider against another in a game of speed and strategy. Although the event is 1000 m long, only the last 200 m is timed. Times are not important; it is only necessary to defeat your opponent to advance to the next round.

2. **Kilometer (kilo):** A 1-km time trial

3. **500-m sprint:** A 500-m time trial. A world championship event for women new in 1993.

4. **Individual pursuit:** A 3-km time trial for women, 4-km for men, and 5-km for professional men. Two riders start on opposite ends of the track and try to catch each other, hence the name *pursuit*.

5. **Points race:** A longer race on the track, usually at least 10 km. Riders sprint for points at predetermined times during the race. The racer with the most points at the end of the race who has not been lapped by any other rider wins the race.

6. **Team pursuit:** A 4-km race that has two teams of 4 riders each working together to catch the opposing team.

D. **Off-road**

1. **Hill climb:** A time trial uphill

2. **Cross-country**: A mass-start race for mountain bikes over varied terrain

3. **Downhill:** A downhill time trial

4. **Trials:** A timed ride over an obstacle course. Penalties are assessed for crashing or touching the foot down during negotiation of the course.

5. **Dual slalom:** A downhill race through ski gates

II. **REVIEW OF LITERATURE**

A. **Overuse injuries:** Overuse injuries form the bulk of problems presenting to the primary-care sports medicine practitioner and are a significant cause of lost training time in elite athletes. Many good papers have described the nature of overuse injuries in these athletes, but few report injuries in competitive cyclists.

1. **Weiss**[10] surveyed nontraumatic injuries in participants in an 8-day, 500-mile cycle tour.
   a. These individuals typically rode <100 mi/week on a regular basis.
   b. The most common problem experienced:
      i. Buttock pain and saddle sores
      ii. Knee pain (35% of riders)
      iii. Neck and shoulder pain
      iv. Palmar numbness
   c. The types of problems experienced point to a lack of specific preparation for the cycle tour on part of the participants.

2. **Bohlmann**[1] reported on traumatic and overuse injuries in 100 competitive cyclists who responded to a questionnaire published in a popular bicycle paper.
   a. 20% reported pain and discomfort unrelated to trauma.
      i. Knee was the most frequent site of nontraumatic injury, accounting for 25% of nontraumatic problems.
   b. 77% reported injuries as a result of trauma.
   c. Survey population had a high percentage of less-experienced athletes and therefore problems that could be explained on the basis of bicycle fit and poor fitness.

      d. Survey solicited information regarding *any* pain and discomfort; in many cases, these problems may not have been severe enough to bring experienced athletes to seek advice from a physician.

  3. **Collins et al.**[4] reported survey information in 257 triathletes, 30 of whom were classified as elite.

      a. 12% of injured athletes listed cycling as the cause of their injury, illustrating the relatively low incidence of nontraumatic injuries in cycling compared to running.

      b. Training errors are cited much more commonly as cause of injuries to runners, being present in almost 60% of cases.

      c. Several explanations are possible for these differences in injury rates:

         i. In contrast to running, cycling is a weight-supported sport; the cyclist spends most time on the bike in a sitting position, and therefore less force is applied to the lower extremity.

        ii. The cycling motion is a very stereotypical movement, whereas the runner must constantly adjust stride length to account for changing terrain.

       iii. The cyclist has the option of modifying the stress applied by altering gear ratios.

       iv. The combination of changing terrain and the practice of drafting ensure that the effort required to propel the bicycle is not constant, and the cyclist may have the opportunity to "rest" periodically, even while engaged in competition.

B. **Traumatic injuries**

  1. **McLennan et al.**[7] prospectively studied the incidence of injuries in competitive road cyclists.

      a. Ranges from 0.57–1.2 injuries/100 hours of competition

      b. 75% of injuries involved less-experienced riders and 62% were in criterium racing.

      c. Most accidents occurred within 500 m of the start or finish.

      d. Most injured riders lost <1 week from training.

  2. **Survey information**[1] indicates that most abrasions and fractures involve the left side of the body.

      a. May reflect less experience with high-speed left-hand turns on the part of road cyclists.

      b. Most commonly cited causes of crashes were rider error or mechanical problems.

III. HELMETS AND PROTECTIVE EQUIPMENT

Helmets should always be worn for training and competition. Approved helmet use is mandatory for amateur competition in North America. More than 1000 people are killed in the U.S. each year while cycling, and 75% of deaths result from head injury. It is imperative to ask about helmet use routinely when treating or counseling cyclists.

A. **Modern helmets are extremely well-designed**, as light as 6 oz, and have excellent ventilation systems. Features of a well-designed helmet are:

  1. **Smooth stiff outer shell:** Resists penetration, protects liner, distributes impact. Helmets with soft Lycra covers are approved but are more fragile, and they should be upgraded to newer models with an outer shell.

  2. **Crushable styrofoam liner:** Absorbs shock.

  3. **Strong comfortable retention system**

  4. **Size-adjustment pads:** Removable washable pads that ensure a snug fit. These come in a variety of sizes to ensure a custom fit.

  5. **Snell approved:** Two main standards are in effect for certifying bicycle helmets: American National Standards Association (ANSI) and Snell Memorial Foundation.

  a. Snell standard is more stringent and represents maximal levels of protection in available helmets.
  b. ANSI should be considered the minimum acceptable standard.
  c. Helmets are tested by dropping them from different heights onto various surfaces, and the amount of force generated inside the helmet is recorded. Snell requires that helmets be dropped from a greater height, with the same recorded force, than does the ANSI test. A separate test covers strength of the retention system.
B. **Shirt:** A T-shirt covering the shoulders and worn under the cycling jersey will help prevent road rash over the upper body in the event of a crash, as the two layers of fabric will slide over each other and prevent some abrasion.
C. **Padded cycling gloves** prevent very painful palmar abrasions in the event of a fall on the outstretched hands. Abrasions, generally speaking, are minor injuries, but if located over most of the palmar surface may be sufficient to limit training and competition.

IV. COMMON CYCLING-RELATED COMPLAINTS

With some notable exceptions, such as road rash and saddle sores, cyclists do not get injuries that are different from those encountered in any primary-care sports medicine practice. In my clinical experience, I have seen only one cycling-related stress fracture, and that was in the wrist of a mountain biker. Therefore, the focus is not so much on the diagnosis and general treatment of the problem, but rather to emphasize areas where treatment is slightly different in cyclists and to give guidelines for return to full activity.

David Reid's recent book *Sports Injury Assessment and Rehabilitation*[9] is an excellent overall text and gives a more in-depth review of diagnosis and general treatment. **There does not seem to be a difference in the incidence of overuse injuries between male and female cyclists. Women bicycle riders seem to crash less and therefore may present less frequently with traumatic injuries.**

A. **Overuse injuries:** Cyclists have a clearly defined competitive season. Most racing starts between February and April, depending on regional weather, and finishes in the fall. Many athletes compete both days almost every weekend, in addition to local club training races once or twice a week in an area where cycling is very active. Some cyclists will take up to 5 weeks off their bike after the competitive season and participate in "active rest," where they pursue other athletic interests such as running, cross-country skiing, and weights. When endurance base training begins, cycling mileage may increase very rapidly from almost zero up to several hundred kilometers per week. Generally, cyclists develop overuse injuries when they make changes, either with equipment or training volume, and specific information should be sought about these factors:
  • What type of shoe and pedal system is the rider using?
  • How long has she had it?
  • How was the cleat adjusted?
  • Is it fixed or floating?
  • Have there been any changes to the saddle height or fore and aft position?
  • Has there been a recent crash which may have changed the frame alignment or bent the crank or pedal system?

  1. **Anterior knee pain**
    a. **Presentation:** The most common presenting complaint of cyclists of all ability levels. **Patellofemoral pain syndrome (PFPS)** is the most frequent problem (although patellar tendinitis is also common).
      i. Frequently related to changes in shoes and pedal systems or alteration in cleat alignment.
      ii. Characterized by anterior aching knee pain, often bilateral, exacerbated by climbing, going up and down stairs, and prolonged sitting. Slight swelling is not uncommon, but frank effusions would be unusual and should prompt investigation for other causes.

       iii. Plain radiographs are normal, and local tenderness underneath the patellar facets confirms the diagnosis.

  b. A tremendous amount of misinformation surrounds the problem of PFPS in the cycling community, and many athletes have been mistakenly informed that **chondromalacia** is present and accounting for their symptoms. Unless there is advanced changes on radiographs or arthroscopic confirmation of chondromalacia, this diagnosis should be avoided. It is very important to emphasize the benign nature of PFPS to the rider.

  c. **Treatment**

       i. First, ensure that the bicycle is set up appropriately with respect to **saddle height** and **fore and aft position** (Fig. 1). These adjustments are fairly standard and can be performed by most coaches or bicycle shops.[2]

       ii. In a rider with a **fixed cleat system**, cleat alignment adjustment using a Fit Kit®, available through many cycle shops and coaches, is sufficient to resolve most symptoms without further intervention.

         (a) Many athletes adjust their own shoes, but it has been my experience that an adjustment of only a few millimeters can often produce dramatic results.

         (b) If this is unsuccessful, a switch to a pedal system that allows some free rotation of the cleat may be beneficial.

         (c) Conversely, in an athlete who uses a rotating system, the switch to a fixed system with Fit Kit® adjustment may help.

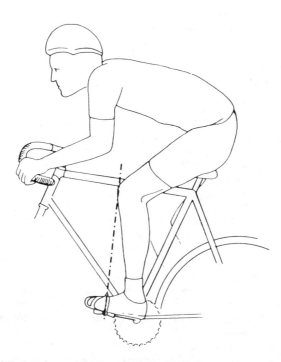

FIGURE 1. Saddle height and fore and aft position. Seat position relative to the pedals is determined by putting the pedals at the 3 and 9 o'clock positions with the ball of the foot firmly on the pedal. A plumb line dropped from the middle of the forward patella should fall on the pedal axle. (From Hill JW, Mellion MB: Bicycling injuries: Presentation, diagnosis, and treatment. In Mellion MB (ed): Office Management of Sports Injuries and Athletic Problems. Philadelphia, Hanley & Belfus, 1988, with permission.)

    iii. Simple measures such as **ice, ibuprofen,** and **analgesic creams** are also useful. Local physiotherapy can also be instituted if these are ineffective in controlling symptoms.

    iv. Individuals with foot pronation or very flexible feet may benefit from **semi-rigid foot orthotics.**

        (a) These should be made from a neutral suspension cast, with the subtalar joint in a neutral position and the midtarsal joint locked.

        (b) They should include forefoot posting, as cycling involves predominantly the forefoot and orthotics designed for running will not give adequate control.

        (c) Soft orthotics defeat the purpose of the rigid sole of a cycling shoe and should be avoided.

        (d) Fit Kit® adjustments should be repeated after an orthotic is obtained.

    v. **Strengthening exercises,** such as eccentric squatting exercises and leg press, should also be instituted.

  d. The vast majority of athletes will not have to stop riding but can **modify their training** by staying away from hills, using easy gears and emphasizing good technique. A good rule of thumb is to limit activity to a level where baseline symptoms are not increased the day following activity.

    i. Highly competitive road riders may spend as much as 25–30 hr/wk on their bike and cover as much as 500–600 km. Whereas runners consider 60 minutes to be a long distance, many cyclists will consider rides of <1 hour or 30 km to be very short, so adjust exercise prescription in accordance with previous volumes.

  e. Surgery should be considered a last resort and is rarely required.

  f. **Patellar tendinitis** presents very similarly to PFPS, but local tenderness will be in the region of the patellar tendon. Treatment is as for patellofemoral pain syndrome. Emphasize eccentric quadriceps rehabilitation.

2. **Posterior knee pain**

  a. **Presentation:** Posterior knee pain is the second most common overuse problem seen in elite cyclists in our clinic.

    i. The vast majority are biceps femoris insertional tendinitis.

    ii. Distinguished by local tenderness over the insertion of biceps femoris and pain on resisted hamstring flexion.

  b. **Treatment**

    i. Checking cleat position

    ii. Nonsteroidal antiinflammatory drugs (NSAIDs)

    iii. Ice

    iv. Physiotherapy consisting of strengthening and modalities

    v. Orthotics may help.

    vi. In athletes using rotating pedal systems, a switch to a fixed cleat may be helpful.

  c. **Treat this problem very aggressively,** as it tends to be refractory when well established. Be sure to rule out disk herniation in the athlete presenting with hamstring pain, even in the absence of back pain. Be especially vigilant if there is no local tenderness and pain on resisted hamstring contraction.

3. **Pelvic malalignment**

  a. **Presentation:** This entity consists of rotation through the sacroiliac joints, with one side of the pelvis rotated anteriorly and the other posteriorly.

    i. Usually the cyclist presents complaining of a leg-length discrepancy, saddle sores on one side, or low back or hip pain.

    ii. Rule out any underlying cause for back pain, such as disk herniation, seronegative arthropathy, etc. Frequently, there is a history of a recent crash.

        iii. On examination, the athlete will pronate more on the side of the anterior rotation, and the iliac crest on that side will appear higher when in the standing position. About 80% of pelvic malalignments have the left side rotated anteriorly.

        iv. Absolute leg lengths will be equal when measured from the anterior superior iliac spine, but when lying supine, the medial malleolus of the anteriorly rotated side will appear longer than the other side. When the athlete sits up, the leg length will become equal.

  b. **Treatment:** Manual therapy to restore normal alignment

  c. A cyclist with a pelvic malalignment will have an asymmetric cleat position, so consider pelvis malalignment in cases of refractory knee problems.

4. **Achilles tendinitis**

  a. **Presentation**

        i. Characterized by pain, swelling, and local tenderness in the Achilles region

        ii. May be more common in cyclists who do not use rigid-soled cycling shoes.

  b. **Treatment**

        i. Local physiotherapy

        ii. NSAIDs

        iii. A heel lift may help.

        iv. Cleat alignment is not usually required.

  c. Often presents with a long history and very well established. If advanced to the point that nodules have formed, **surgical tenolysis** may be required.

5. **Saddle sores**

  a. **Presentation:** Ranges from abrasions, small abscesses, to fibrous masses.

        i. Occurs more frequently in women than men.

  b. **Treatment**

        i. **A good saddle fit** is very important, and riders should be encouraged to keep trying until they find one that suits them. Many reputable bicycle shops will allow a customer to try different saddles until she finds one that is suitable.

          (a) Saddles specifically made for women do not seem to offer significant improvement over others and may actually cause chafing of the insides of the thighs because of the saddle's very wide rear profile.

          (b) **Sheepskin padding and gel-type saddles** are relatively ineffective and are disdained by competitive cyclists.

        ii. **A good pad inside the shorts** is crucial. The ultrasuede synthetic chamois is the most popular.

          (a) Shorts that have terrycloth or other cloth material as part of the chamois tend to get lumpy and rough with age and sometimes adhere to sensitive places, making removal extremely unpleasant.

          (b) Some women use a liner inside their cycling shorts, which takes the place of the chamois.

        iii. If the athlete complains of abrasions, particularly anteriorly over the clitoral area or anterior labia, trimming of long pubic hair and the use of a water-soluble cream (vitamin E-based, aloe vera, Noxema, etc.) will often help. Some riders prefer petroleum-based creams, as their lubricating effect lasts longer. Irritation tends to improve as the season goes on (as calluses develop).

        iv. Deep-seated boils and abscesses are treated as any other local skin infection and may require drainage, antibiotics, and time off the bike to heal.

        v. Occasionally, deep painful fibrous masses may develop which require surgical excision.

  c. If sores are unilateral, check leg length and pelvic alignment.

6. **Neuropathies in the hand**
   a. **Presentation**
      i. Usually seen following very long races, in cold weather, or with inadequate padding in protective gloves.
      ii. Compression of the ulnar nerve at or near the tunnel of Guyon is the most common site of nerve irritation (Fig. 2) and will produce pain and parathesia in the ulnar nerve distribution over the 4th and 5th fingers.
   b. **Treatment**
      i. Protection of the nerve using a doughnut pad made out of adhesive felt to reduce direct pressure over the hamate is usually all that is required to alleviate symptoms.
      ii. Local physiotherapy and NSAIDs may be used as adjuncts to reduce irritation.
      iii. Frequent changing of hand position during riding should be encouraged.
   c. Ask about saddle tilt, as a nose-down saddle will tend to displace the rider forward and put more pressure on the hands. This can be checked using an ordinary carpenter's level.

B. **Traumatic injuries:** Cycle racing is a high-risk sport and high-velocity crashes occur, although a surprising number of individuals walk away from crashes with little more than torn clothing and lost skin. Expect more crashes to come from criteriums on the road, mass-start races on the track, and downhill races off road. Road criteriums

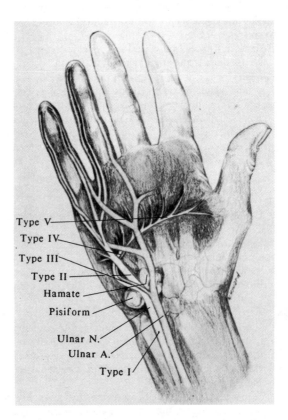

FIGURE 2. Anatomy of Guyon's canal showing the five potential areas of entrapment. (Modified from Wu I, et al: Ulnar neuropathy at the wrist: Case report and review of literature. Arch Phys Med Rehabil 66:787, 1985, with permission.)

tend to have more crashes than mass-start track events, but a rider who crashes on the track is more likely to have a serious injury.

The normal physiologic response to exercise masks considerable pain. I have twice seen riders get up and walk away from a crash concerned more about their bicycle than their bodies, only to have pelvic fractures on later radiographs. Remember to check for abdominal injuries that can occur from blunt trauma from handlebars or, in off-road riding, stumps or rocks. Athletes may not remember hitting their heads; if in doubt, check the helmet styrofoam liner for cracks and the surface of the helmet for abrasions indicating impact.

1. **Road rash**
   a. **Presentation**
      i. Classified from grade I to III, following the same classification as burns. Most that present for treatment will be grade I or II.
      ii. An easy diagnosis to make: Superficial skin abrasions.
      iii. In event coverage, it is the most common presenting complaint, particularly with criterium or mountain bike racing, but will not often present to the sports medicine practitioner in the office unless it is extensive or infected.
   b. **Treatment**
      i. Meticulous cleaning as soon as possible after the injury to remove embedded dirt and prevent tattooing. In the first few minutes following the injury, cleaning is surprisingly painless, but if repeated several hours later after local edema has started, analgesics or topical anesthetics may be needed. Many athletes will elect to complete their event before coming in for wound dressing.
      ii. For cleaning, simple soap and water is good enough, although some prefer hydrogen peroxide diluted with water, Hibitane and water, or other antibacterial solutions for skin cleansing. The spongy side of a surgical scrub brush is prepackaged, easy to carry, and works very well. Athletes can purchase their own prepackaged scrub brushes and keep them in their first aid kits, for situations where immediate medical attention is not available.
      iii. Following cleaning, a topical antibiotic such as bacitracin should be applied, the wound covered with Telfa, and the dressing secured with tape or stretchy tubular net. Petroleum or antibiotic gauze nets become adherent to road rash and should be avoided. Some physicians advise cyclists to leave the rash open to the air, but this causes drying, cracking, and bleeding of the wound as well as adherence of bed sheets and clothing.
      iv. The rider should be advised to clean the wound twice daily with soap and water or diluted hydrogen peroxide (in the shower is fine) and to redress using Telfa and a topical antibiotic.
      v. The wound will have a profuse exudate for 2–3 days, but the rider should return for follow-up if there are signs of infection. After about 5 days, when most of the local tenderness and exudate are gone, the wound may be left open to the air. A thin flexible scab will form, which will heal entirely within 10 days.
   c. Sunscreen will be required over the new scar to prevent burning, blistering, and possibly more scarring.
   d. A large or deep abrasion over a muscle could be indicative of an underlying muscle contusion, and the athlete should seek medical advice if she develops severe pain or neurovascular symptoms, indicating an underlying compartment syndrome.
2. **Clavicular fractures**
   a. **Presentation:** Clavicular fractures are among the most common injuries that will require the athlete to take time off their bicycle.

      i. Often the initial presentation is to the emergency department following a bicycle crash involving impact onto the shoulder.

      ii. Pain, deformity, and crepitus at the fracture site make the diagnosis apparent. Radiographs will confirm the diagnosis.

  b. **Treatment:** In a simple uncomplicated fracture, immobilization in a **clavicle strap** until the fracture is clinically united.

  c. The athlete should purchase two clavicle straps, so that one may be washed while the other is worn, particularly after she has returned to training.

  d. The athlete should be warned that the fracture will be painful during the first week and that she may want analgesics and to take time completely off training. Alternate training on a turbotrainer or stationary bike may be instituted to maintain fitness as soon as tolerated, provided the clavicle strap is worn.

  e. Road riding can be started at about 3 weeks postinjury, but with the advice to avoid hills (causes increased pain) or inclement conditions (risk of reinjury). The athlete is ready to return to competition when the fracture is clinically united, usually about 6 weeks postinjury.

3. **Acromioclavicular separations**

  a. **Presentation:** The acromioclavicular (AC) joint is most likely to be injured by a direct blow, such as a fall from a bicycle with direct impact. The diagnosis is usually straightforward with pain, swelling, tenderness, and possibly deformity at the AC joint.

  b. Acromioclavicular injury is graded into three stages. Higher degrees including compound injuries have been described.

      i. **Grade I:** Minor injury to the AC ligament and coracoclavicular (CC) ligament with little or no deformity. Radiographic stress views are normal.

      ii. **Grade II:** Injury to the AC ligament with little injury to the CC ligament, minimal displacement on radiographs.

      iii. **Grade III:** Complete disruption of both the AC and CC ligaments, with marked upward displacement of the distal clavicle, exacerbated on radiographic stress views.

  c. **Treatment**

      i. **Grade I:** Sling for comfort, ice, NSAIDs, and local physiotherapy. Training on the road can be resumed as tolerated; smooth flat surfaces are preferred. Racing can be resumed when the athlete has normal range of motion and a nontender AC joint, possibly as soon as 2 weeks.

      ii. **Grade II:** As above, but with training on the road usually at 3–4 weeks, avoiding climbing. Return to competition usually at 7–8 weeks within the above guidelines.

      iii. **Grade III:** Progression as for Grade II.

4. **Wrist fracture**

  a. **Presentation:** Scaphoid is the most commonly injured carpal bone, usually following a fall on an outstretched hand. Pain, local tenderness, and swelling will be present. Radiographs will usually show the fracture, although scaphoid injury may be occult initially.

  b. **Treatment:** Fiberglass cast

  c. Maintain a high index of suspicion.

  d. Bone scanning followed by CT scanning of a hot bone scan may be helpful in establishing an early diagnosis if plain radiographs are negative. The bone scan will take about 72 hours to become positive after bony injury.

  e. Casting will interfere significantly with racing and training. Training in a cast can be allowed provided there is no pain in the cast and adequate control of the bicycle and brake levels is possible. Racing in a cast is to be discouraged, especially in mass-start events because of difficulty in handling the brakes (many athletes will do it anyway).

V. MISCELLANEOUS CONSIDERATIONS
A. Yeast infections
1. Women cyclists may be more prone to perineal yeast because of the warm moist environment created by the chamois and the constant low-grade perineal irritation caused by riding.
2. Encourage meticulous hygiene. Riders should change shorts as soon as possible after riding. If a shower is not possible immediately after a race, perineal toilet can be performed using premoistened baby wipes or mild soap and water.
3. Prophylactic topical antifungals after long rides or races may help.
B. Breast support: The low impact nature of cycling enables many cyclists to use minimal breast support; many use a light cotton and Spandex tank similar to that used in aerobics wear or none at all. Athletic support bras of the jogging type are also popular.
C. Menstrual flow: The use of sanitary napkins is not compatible with cycling, as the bulk of the napkin renders this activity uncomfortable. Tampons are preferred by most women. Those who do not use tampons usually rely on the chamois to absorb flow.

VI. PREVENTION OF CYCLING INJURIES
Clearly the best way to treat an injury is not to have it in the first place.
A. Measure and record: The bicycle frame, saddle height, and fore/aft position should be measured and recorded in a safe place, such as the training diary.
B. Do not change a working system: A shoe and pedal system that is working satisfactorily should not be changed during the competitive season, but should be broken in when the rider is able to do slow steady rides. Ideally, the rider should have two pairs of shoes with identical set-up which are used equally, so that new shoes are not required in the event of breakage. For travel, shoes (and orthotics) should be kept in the carry-on luggage to prevent loss.
C. Maintain equipment: The bike should be kept in good mechanical order. Particular attention should be paid to brake adjustment and wear, derailleur adjustment, and tires. High performance racing tires are often glued onto the rim and must be very secure.
D. Wear protection: Gloves and helmets should be worn at all times, and sunscreen should be used on exposed skin.

REFERENCES
1. Bohlmann JT: Injuries in competitive cycling. Phys SportsMed 9(5):117–124, 1981.
2. Borysewicz E: Bicycle Road Racing: Complete Program for Training and Competition. Brattleboro, VT, Velo-News, 1985.
3. Burke ER: Safety standards for bicycle helmets. Phys SportsMed 16(1):148–153, 1988.
4. Collins K, Wagner M, Peterson K, Storey M: Overuse injuries in triathletes. Am J Sports Med 17(6):675–680, 1989.
5. Davis MW, Litman T, Crenshaw RW, Mueller JK: Bicycling injuries. Phys SportsMed 8(5):89–96, 1980.
6. Faria IE: Applied physiology of cycling. Sports Med 1:187–204, 1984.
7. McLennan JG, McLennan JC, Ungersma J: Accident prevention in competitive cycling. Am J Sports Med 16(3):266–268, 1988.
8. Mellon MB: Common cycling injuries: Prevention and management. Sports Med 11(1):53–70, 1991.
9. Reid DC: Sports Injury: Assessment and Rehabilitation. New York, Churchill Livingstone, 1992.
10. Weiss BD: Nontraumatic injuries in amateur long distance bicyclists. Am J Sports Med 13(3):187–192, 1985.

Chapter 54: Triathlon

KATHERINE KENAL, MD, MA

No one sport has gained such quick popularity with the athletic community as the triathlon. The most prestigious event, the Ironman Triathlon World Championship, had its beginning in 1978 when 15 participants entered the ocean in Hawaii. Three existing endurance events— Waikiki Rough-Water Swim (3.9 km), Around-Oahu Bike Race (180.2 km), and the Honolulu Marathon (42.2 km)—were combined to test the overall endurance of those athletes. Today, more than 1400 men and women compete in that race annually and 90–95% complete the events in the allotted time of 17 hours.

In 1979, the first female competitor, Lyn Lemaire, placed fifth overall, finishing just under 2 hours longer than the first-place male. As training, nutrition, race strategies, and equipment developed, women's times began to approach those of the men. The best female performance has been by Paula Newby-Fraser, who in 1988 finished just 30 minutes behind the fastest male at the Ironman.

Triathlons of shorter distance, of course, have the greatest popularity. As triathletes push harder to test the limits of performance, orthopedic and medical issues specific to the sport need to be addressed to ensure a healthy and safe pursuit. These athletes face not only the challenge of mastering the skills in swimming, biking, and running, but also the challenges which distance and environment present.

I. A GROWING SPORT

A. Participants
1. Over 1 million compete worldwide, the best as professionals.
2. In the U.S., 300,000 triathletes (23% female) compete in 1800 events/year.
3. Average age is 35 years.
4. **Training:** Athletes can average 15 hr/week in training for international-level events; 7 mi swimming, 200 mi cycling, 40 mi running.
5. **Championship events:**
   a. U.S. National Championship
   b. World Championship
   c. Masters World Games

B. Triathlon Federation/USA, located in Colorado Springs, is the national governing body:
1. Oversees >22,000 registered triathletes (17% females)
2. Organizes training and competition of the U.S. teams:
   a. U.S. Junior Team
   b. U.S. Elite National Team (men and women), compete in Pan Am Games

C. Four categories of races recognized by Triathlon Federation/USA
1. Sprint: 800-m swim, 13-mi bike (21-km), 5-km run
2. International: 1.5-km swim, 40-km bike, 10-km run
3. Long: 1.2-mi swim, 56-mi bike, 13.1-mi run
4. Ultra (ironman): 3.9-km swim, 180-km bike, 42-km run

II. ORTHOPEDIC INJURIES

Athletes first became attracted to the triathlon in part because of the belief that cross-training would allow them to minimize their injuries. Instead, the cross-training has allowed them to continue training in another sport, while their injured body part rests.

A. **Overuse injuries** are the most common diagnosis in triathletes seeking medical care.
  1. Running is the most cited cause of injury, followed by swimming, then cycling.
  2. Incidence has been reported as high as 91% during 1 year of training.
  3. 79% of athletes had injuries affecting more than one area.
  4. Incidence does not appear to be gender-related, but instead reflects training errors, biomechanic problems, extrinsic factors, and skeletal anatomy.
B. **Stress fractures:** Due to repeated microtrauma which overloads the body's normal ability to repair bone resorption (*see also* Chapter 42)
  1. Most occur in the tibial shaft at the junction of the middle and distal one third, and the distal one third; fibular shaft at the distal one third; and the metatarsals.
  2. Increased incidence in female triathletes: 25% of females are affected vs. 17% of males.
  3. **Risk factors**
     a. Menstrual dysfunction
     b. Disordered eating
     c. Training errors
     d. Extrinsic factors
  4. **Treatment:** Emphasize swimming, may include aqua-jogging.
C. **Patellofemoral stress syndrome:** Retropatellar pain due to patellar malalignment (tilt, rotation, lateral displacement) with increased Q-angles, weak vastus medialis obliquus function, imbalance of gluteal muscle strength, overpronation, hamstring/quadriceps inflexibility (*see also* Chapter 40).
D. **Other orthopedic problems**
  1. Iliotibial band syndrome
  2. Plantar fasciitis
  3. Shin splints
  4. Medial tibial stress syndrome
  5. Compartment syndrome
  6. Achilles tendinitis
  7. Swimmer's shoulder
  8. Traumatic injuries (cycling)
  9. Muscle cramps

III. **MEDICAL ISSUES**

Medical issues are similar to those of female athletes involved in the individual sports. They are dependent upon the distance undertaken and the environmental conditions during training and competition. The most common problems seen during competition are dehydration, electrolyte imbalance, and exhaustion. Rarely, deaths have been reported due to inherent cardiac problems during the swim and to bicycle–motor vehicle crashes. This underscores the need for appropriate preparticipation screening, adequate medical care coverage at the event, and traffic control.

A. **Dehydration**
  1. Cumulative effects of time, distance, heat, and inadequate hydration during race.
     a. Reduces endurance performance primarily by impairing cardiovascular function and thermoregulation.
     b. Acclimated athlete can lose 3.5 L sweat/hr with exercise in heat.
     c. Resulted in >50% of visits to the medical tent during the 1988 Hawaii Ironman.
  2. **Diagnosis:** Symptoms include:
     a. Dizziness
     b. Tachycardia
     c. Syncope
     d. Inability to urinate
     e. Hypotension

3. **Treatment**
   a. Blood should be drawn to measure electrolytes.
   b. Then give intravenous fluids.
      i. D5NS solution for races >4 hr
      ii. D51/2NS or NS for races <4 hr
4. May require **hospitalization** if triathlete has unrelenting muscle cramps or unable to tolerate oral fluids.
5. **Prevention:** Appropriate hydration during the race.
   a. Thirst is a poor warning sign of dehydration; average athlete must lose 2% of total body water before becoming thirsty.
   b. Regimented hydration should be followed:
      i. Water during events lasting <2 hr
      ii. Electrolyte/glucose replacement drink during events lasting >2 hr
      iii. Consider electrolyte/glucose replacement drink for international distance events >1.5 hr.
   c. Ideal electrolyte/glucose replacement drink:
      i. Glucose 6–10%; sodium 20–30 mEq/L; potassium 0–5 mEq/L
      ii. Serve cold.
      iii. Train using this drink for better tolerability during the race.
   d. Limitations in ability to consume or absorb fluid (maximum 1 L/hr) during exercise make **prehydration** and **early rehydration** of utmost importance.
B. **Hyponatremia** (sodium <130 mmol/L)
   1. Occurs in longer races (more common in Ironman than international distance) primarily as a result of voluntary intake of excessive water without replacement of electrolyte losses (via sweat).
      a. In response to prolonged exercise, heat stress, and dehydration, extrarenal factors controlling fluid retention predominate and prevent necessary excretion of excess hypotonic urine.
      b. Sodium values as low as 112 mmol/L have been reported after a triathlon.
   2. **Diagnosis**
      a. Delerium
      b. Personality changes
      c. Deteriorating states of consciousness
      d. Seizures
   3. **Treatment**
      a. D5NS solution intravenously
      b. Intravenous diazepam for seizures
      c. Hospitalization may be required
   4. **Prevention**
      a. Maintain balanced nutritional intake prior to event to ensure normal pre-race electrolyte balance.
      b. Maintain appropriate hydration with electrolyte/glucose replacement drink during races >2 hr.
C. **Thermoregulation:** Hypothermia and hyperthermia can occur during triathlons. Triathletes should acclimatize to the environmental conditions expected on race day (*see also* Chapter 43).
D. **Concussions:** Clinical syndrome characterized by immediate and transient impairment of neural function. May occur with traumatic injuries during cycling accident (*see also* Chapter 32: Neurologic Disorders).
   1. **Diagnosis**
      a. **Classification of concussion severity**
         i. Grade 1 (bell-ringer): No loss of consciousness, no post-traumatic amnesia, symptoms <10 min (see below)
         ii. Grade 2: No loss of consciousness, post-traumatic amnesia <30 min

       iii. Grade 3: Loss of consciousness <5 min, post-traumatic amnesia >30 min
       iv. Grade 4: Loss of consciousness >5 min, post-traumatic amnesia > 24 hr
    b. **Postconcussive symptoms** may include:
       i. Headache
       ii. Dizziness
       iii. Impaired orientation, cognition, or concentration
       iv. Memory deficit
       v. Any central nervous system dysfunction
  2. **Treatment**
    a. Remove athlete from competition and examine periodically to monitor neurologic and mental status.
    b. Return-to-competition decision depends on severity of injury (*see* Chapter 32).
    c. If the athlete is unconscious, precautions for cervical spine injury must be taken.
  3. **Prolonged unconsciousness**, persistent mental status alteration, worsening post-concussion symptoms, or abnormalities on neurologic examination require immediate neurosurgical consultation at trauma center.
  4. Consider differentiating between **head injury and heat illness**. A cycler may become hyperthermic, leading to dizziness and a fall from her bike. Obtain rectal temperature for confirmation.
E. **Other medical concerns**
  1. Amenorrhea
  2. Disordered eating
  3. Anemia
  4. Nutrition
  5. Overtraining
  6. Sports psychology
  7. Gastrointestinal (GI) dysfunction and GI bleeding

III. **SAFETY**

A. **Rules** have been implemented to reduce the rate of injuries during competition, including:
  1. "No-draft" rule during cycling (following another cyclist too closely), which has effectively reduced cycling entanglements
  2. Use of a helmet, which has reduced head injuries
  3. Allowing wet suits during the swim when water temperature is <78° F, reducing the incidence of hypothermia
B. **Pre-event information** is an important means of competitor education.
C. The International Triathlon Union has established **guidelines for medical coverage** during competition.[4]

REFERENCES

1. Collins K, Wagner M, Peterson K, Storey M: Overuse injuries in triathletes. Am J Sports Med 17:675–680, 1989.
2. Dolinar J: Triathlons—Not just for ironmen. Phys SportsMed 18(10):120–125, 1990.
3. Laird RH: Medical care at ultradistance triathlons. Med Sci Sports Exerc 21:S222–S225, 1989.
4. Medical care guidelines. In International Triathlon Union Manual. International Triathlon Union, North Vancouver, British Columbia, Canada, 1992, pp 54–58.
5. O'Toole ML, Douglas PS, Hiller WDB: Applied physiology of a triathlon. Sports Med 8:201–225, 1989.
6. O'Toole ML: Prevention and treatment of injuries to runners. Med Sci Sports Exerc 24:S360–S363, 1992.
7. Pierce PZ (Western Regional Medical Director, Tri Fed/USA): Personal communication.
8. Roberts WO: Managing concussions on the sidelines. Phys SportsMed 20(6):66–72, 1992.
9. Zambraski EJ: Renal regulation of fluid homeostasis and exercise. In Gisolfi CV, Lamb DR (eds): Perspectives in Exercise Science and Sports Medicine: Vol. 3. Fluid Homeostasis during Exercise. Chelsea, MI, Benchmark Press, 1990, pp 247–280.

Chapter 55: Aerobic Dance Exercise

ELIZABETH A. JOY, MD

Aerobic dance exercise is one of the most popular forms of exercise in the U.S. It is estimated that more than 30 million Americans participate in aerobic dance. A typical aerobic dance workout consists of a 10–15 minute warm-up, 30 minutes of aerobic-type exercise, 10–15 minutes of calisthenics, and a 5-minute cool-down. Numerous studies show that aerobic dance is an efficient, safe way to improve adult fitness.

I. HISTORY

A. Aerobic dance originated with Jackie Sorenson, wife of a navy pilot, who began teaching exercise classes at the U.S. Naval base in Puerto Rico in 1969.
B. By 1982, aerobic dance exercise was offered in 91.9% of all YMCAs in the U.S.
C. The rapid growth of aerobics has been attributed in part to the exercise video industry.
D. The original aerobic dance programs included activities such as running in place, jumping jacks, and hopping. This type of exercise was later referred to as **high-impact aerobics**. In an attempt to reduce the risk of injury, **low-impact aerobics** was developed, which encompass similar movements, but with one foot remaining in contact with the floor. Bench-step aerobics is the most recent innovation. This activity consists of choreographed movements stepping up and down on a platform.

II. PHYSIOLOGY

A. Two questions are often asked about aerobic dance:
1. Does it improve cardiorespiratory fitness?
2. Does it effectively promote weight loss?
B. **Cardiorespiratory fitness**
1. Multiple studies have shown **improvements in VO_2max** as a result of aerobic dance training. Most investigations evaluated participants who performed high-impact aerobic dance 3 days/week over a period of 8–10 weeks.
a. Improvements in maximal aerobic power ranged from 5–41% with a mean of 23%.
2. The **energy costs** of aerobic dance routines vary significantly depending on the type and intensity of exercise. A comparison of differing aerobic routines revealed that high-intensity high-impact aerobics required the greatest energy, followed by low-intensity high-impact aerobics, high-intensity low-impact aerobics, and low-intensity low-impact aerobics. Only the first 3 routines met American College of Sports Medicine (ACSM) standards for maintaining or improving cardiorespiratory fitness (i.e., VO_2max $> 50\%$ of maximum).
3. A recent study evaluated the cardiorespiratory response to **bench-step aerobics**, finding that oxygen requirement increased as the height of the bench increased and when propulsion movements were performed on and off the bench.
4. Studies evaluating the **metabolic cost of upper-extremity exercise** during aerobic dance have shown no significant increase in oxygen consumption with regard to either arm position or the use of 1–2 lb upper-body weights. However, increased work of the upper extremities does result in higher exercise heart rate. This heart rate response is attributed to an increase in sympathetic tone that results from exercise with the arms elevated.

5. Unlike running and biking, aerobic dance does not produce a linear increase in heart rate and oxygen consumption.
   a. Heart rates achieved during aerobic dance are 10% higher than those found during treadmill running at identical levels of oxygen consumption.
   b. For aerobic dance to exceed 50% of VO_2max, target heart rate must be 80% of the age-predicted maximum heart rate.
6. Due to the nonlinear relationship between heart rate and oxygen consumption, exercise intensity can be accurately monitored by using the Borg scale of perceived exertion.
7. Comparison studies of aerobic dance to walk-jog training programs have shown similar improvements in aerobic power. In an 8-week study during which subjects exercised 3 days/week, for 15–25 minutes aerobic activity, at an intensity of 60–80% of VO_2max, the running group experienced a 11% gain in peak oxygen uptake, and the aerobic dance group increased by 10%.

C. **Changes in body composition**
1. Exercise programs performed 3 days/week and expending at least 300 kcal/session meet ACSM guidelines for proper weight loss and fat reduction.
2. It is generally agreed that aerobic dance can meet these guidelines.
   a. Aerobic dance exercise expends approximately 8–10 kcal/minute.
   b. To burn 300 kcal, aerobic dance must be continuously performed for 30–40 minutes.
3. However, most investigations have not shown significant changes in either body fat or weight. These studies involved women of low to average fitness levels, performing aerobic dance routines 3 days/week, over an 8–12 week period. The short-term nature of these studies could explain why significant changes in body composition were not seen.
4. A descriptive study of **aerobic instructors** revealed that this group had a mean body fat of 17%.
   a. They used aerobic dance as their primary form of fitness and had been teaching on average 5.6 classes/week for 4 years.
   b. One could reason that aerobic dance performed in excess of 3 times/week over more than 12 weeks could result in favorable changes in body composition.
5. It is clear that more work is needed to determine a threshold volume of training to produce weight and fat loss.

D. **Serum lipids and lipoproteins**
1. One study investigated the effect of a 10-week aerobic training program on serum lipids and lipoproteins. No significant change was seen in triglycerides, total cholesterol, high-density lipoproteins, or low-density lipoproteins.

III. INJURIES ASSOCIATED WITH AEROBIC DANCE

A. **Injury studies** have evaluated both students and instructors participating in both high- and low-impact aerobic dance. There is currently no published data on the risk of injury in bench-step aerobics.
B. Despite differences in the definition of injury and the calculation of exposure, the results of injury studies show some consistency:
1. 75% of instructors report suffering an injury resulting from their aerobic dance activity, whereas students report 43%. This represents a nearly 2-fold difference in the number of injuries reported. However, when one looks at exposure data (injuries/100 hours of aerobic dancing), there is no significant difference in the rate of injury between students and instructors.
2. It is fairly evident that a linear relationship exists between risk of injury and time spent participating in aerobic dance. There seems to be a critical point of aerobic dancing beyond 3 times/week that places participants at greater risk of injury.

C. Most injuries suffered as a result of aerobic dance do not result in significant disability. In 75% of cases, musculoskeletal complaints resulted in **no alteration in activity.**

D. **Overuse** accounts for the vast majority of injuries, and 60–80% of injuries involve the lower extremity. Based on the type and location of injuries, it appears that they are caused by the aerobic or weight-bearing portion of the class.

E. **There are extrinsic and extrinsic factors which contribute to injury in aerobic dance.** Most overuse injuries are multifactorial. We know from running studies that the relative contribution each factor may contribute to injury is difficult to prove.

  1. **Intrinsic factors** are those beyond the immediate control of the participant. They include structural or biomechanical faults, age, sex, and previous injury.

    a. Structural and biomechanical faults such as scoliosis, leg-length discrepancy, femoral anteversion, ankle pronation, foot stability, poor flexibility, and muscle imbalance may contribute to injury.

    b. No correlation has been found between age and an increased rate of injury.

    c. Aerobic dance is an activity performed mostly by women. Studies involving men and women instructors have shown no correlation between gender and the incidence of injury.

    d. A history of previous injury predisposes participants to subsequent injury.

  2. **Extrinsic factors** which may contribute to injury include shoe wear, flooring, class type (high-impact vs low-impact vs bench-step), training errors (too much, too soon, too frequent), and the use of hand-held weights.

    a. It seems intuitively obvious that wearing appropriate footwear and exercising on a shock-absorbing floor surface would reduce the risk of injury. However, studies have not found that either shoe wear or flooring significantly impact one's risk of injury.

    b. **Low-impact** was designed to decrease the risk of injury during aerobic dance exercise. Few studies have compared injury rates between the two dance forms. Anecdotal reports abound that low-impact aerobics reduces the risk of injury. In a study of 375 individuals followed over 75–129 weeks, those engaging in high-impact aerobics suffered 38% of injuries reported, compared to only 24% of those participating in low-impact aerobics.

    c. There is currently no published literature examining the risk of injury with **bench-step aerobics.** Given the repetitive motion up and down off the bench, a considerable amount of stress is applied to the posterior lower leg. Considerable time should be spent stretching the lower leg prior to and after exercise.

    d. **Overuse** has been identified as the cause of 80% of all aerobic dance injuries. Attempts to relate training errors to injury in aerobic dance have not been successful. Participation in consecutive classes, concurrent involvement in other weight-bearing impact activities, and lack of experience or expertise in aerobic dance do not significantly increase one's risk of injury.

    e. Research has shown that the use of **hand-held weights** during aerobic dance does not significantly increase oxygen consumption. The risk of upper extremity injury associated with hand-weight use is considerably greater than that seen in conventional dance exercise classes. One study found a 15-fold increase in upper extremity injuries when hand-weights were used regularly.

    f. The **enthusiasm generated by instructors** and fellow participants has also been implicated as a potential cause of injury in aerobic dance. The thought being that less-fit and less-experienced participants are pushed or encouraged to exercise at levels beyond their capacity.

F. **Specific aerobic dance injuries**

  1. **Most injuries involve the lower extremity.** Survey studies of instructors and students reveal that the shin is the most frequently injured followed by the foot, ankle, knee, back, hip, and thigh.

2. **Muscle strain** was the most frequently diagnosed condition by physicians (25%), followed by tendinitis (21%), shin splints (18%), sprains (11%), and stress fractures (9%).

3. Anecdotal reports of injuries associated with bench-step aerobics have identified strain injuries of the gastrocnemius and Achilles tendinitis as two of the most common injuries.

G. **Evaluation of injury**

1. **A good history** will identify the problem in most cases.
   a. Overuse injuries are gradual in onset, whereas stress-related injuries result from an acute traumatic event.
   b. Identifying the activities which cause discomfort and when the discomfort occurs can help grade the severity of injury.
   c. Young women should be questioned in regard to menstrual history and dietary habits to rule out eating disorders and amenorrhea as possible contributors to injury.

2. **Physical examination** should begin with inspection and palpation of the injured area. Subsequent examination should focus on finding conditions which may be contributing to injury (e.g., muscle inflexibility, ligamentous laxity, postural and alignment abnormalities).

3. **Radiographs** should be ordered when indicated by the history and physical examination—specifically, if there is point tenderness on the bone.

4. **Laboratory studies** are not routinely indicated, and are performed only when deemed necessary.

H. **Treatment**

1. The vast majority of injuries suffered as a result of aerobic dance activities cause little or no disability. Thus, **treatment is generally conservative.**

2. Grading injury severity can help establish the extent of treatment and rehabilitation needed in overuse injuries.
   a. **Grade 1 injuries** are the most common. There is little to no pain, swelling or stiffness. Treatment would involve the use of RICE (rest, ice, compression, elevation). Activity may be continued as tolerated.
   b. **Grade 2 injuries** are moderate in nature. Pain occurs late in activity, or immediately afterward. Symptoms are present for 2–3 weeks. Examination reveals localized area of injury. Treatment consists of RICE, alteration in activity to avoid reinjury, and the use of nonsteroidal antiinflammatory drugs (NSAIDs). Prior exercise activity may be gradually resumed using pain as the guide.
   c. **Grade 3 injuries** are those in which the pain occurs early in activity. Symptoms have been present for 3–4 weeks' duration. Examination may reveal point tenderness, swelling, and warmth. Treatment involves a period of rest followed by the steps outlined for Grade 2 injuries.
   d. **Grade 4 injuries** may hurt at rest or during activities of daily living. Physical findings are similar to those described for Grade 3 injuries. Alteration in daily activities (e.g., casting, bracing) may be required to reduce discomfort and prevent further injury.

3. **When to return to activity**
   a. If it hurts at rest, do not exercise it.
   b. When it stops hurting at rest, you can exercise minimally, slowly.
   c. When you can exercise without pain, you can gradually increase the workload and intensity. If pain returns, cut back on intensity.
   d. In the meantime, maintain your cardiorespiratory fitness by doing an activity that does not aggravate the injury (e.g., swimming, cycling).

REFERENCES

1. American College of Sports Medicine: The recommended quantity and quality of exercise for developing and maintaining fitness in healthy adults [position statement]. Med Sci Sports Exerc 10:vii–x, 1978.
2. American College of Sports Medicine: Proper and improper weight loss programs [position statement]. Med Sci Sports Exerc 15:ix–xiii, 1983.
3. Belt CR: Injuries associated with aerobic dance. Am Fam Physician 41:1769–1772, 1990.
4. Berry MJ, Cline CC, Berry CB, et al: A comparison between two forms of aerobic dance and treadmill running. Med Sci Sports Exerc 24:946–951, 1992.
5. Blessing DL, Wilson GD, Puckett JR, et al: The physiologic effects of eight weeks of aerobic dance with and without hand-held weights. Am J Sports Med 15:508–510, 1987.
6. Francis PR, Poliner J, Bruno MJ, Francis LL: Effects of choreography, step height, fatigue and gender on the metabolic cost of step training [abstract]. Med Sci Sport Exerc 25(5):69, 1992.
7. Garber CE, McKinney JS, Carleton RA: Is aerobic dance an effective alternative to walk-jog exercise training? J Sports Med Phys Fitness 32:136–141, 1992.
8. Garrick JG, Gillien DM, Whiteside P: The epidemiology of aerobic dance injuries. Am J Sports Med 14:67–72, 1986.
9. Garrick JG, Requa RK: Aerobic dance: A review. Sports Med 6:169–179, 1988.
10. Janis LR: Aerobic dance survey: A study of high-impact versus low-impact injuries. J Am Pod Med 80:419–423, 1990.
11. Kravitz L, Dievert R: The safe way to step. Idea Today (April):47–50, 1991.
12. McCord P, Patterson P: The effect of low impact dance on aerobic capacity, submaximal heart rates and body composition of college-aged females. J Sports Med Phys Fitness 29:184–188, 1989.
13. Parker SB, Hurley BF, Hanlon DP, et al: Failure of target rate to accurately monitor intensity during aerobic dance. Med Sci Sports Exerc 21:230–234, 1989.
14. Reebok International: Step Reebok Training Manual, 2nd ed. Stoughton, MA, Reebok International, Ltd., 1991.
15. Rothenberger LA, Chang JI, Cable TA: Prevalence and types of injuries in aerobic dancers. Am J Sports Med 16:403–407, 1988.
16. Scharff-Olson M, Williford HN, Blessing DL, et al: The cardiovascular and metabolic effects of bench stepping exercise in females. Med Sci Sports Exerc 23:1311–1317, 1991.
17. Scharff-Olson M, Williford HN, Smith FH: The heart rate VO_2max relationship of aerobic dance: A comparison of target heart rate methods. J Sports Med Phys Fitness 32:372–377, 1992.
18. Williford HN, Blessing DL, Barksdale JM, et al: The effects of aerobic dance training on serum lipids, lipoproteins and cardiopulmonary function. J Sports Med Phys Fitness 28:151–157, 1988.
19. Williford HN, Blessing DL, Olson MS, et al: Is low impact aerobic dance an effective cardiovascular workout? Phys SportsMed 17(3):95–109, 1989.
20. Williford HN, Scharff-Olson M, Blessing DL: The physiological effects of aerobic dance: A review. Sports Med 8:335–345, 1989.

Chapter 56: Equestrian Events

MAUREEN A. FINNEGAN, MD

According to national organizations such as the American Horse Council, approximately 30 million Americans ride horseback on a regular basis—and 80 million will ride at least once in a 12-month period. Very little sports medicine literature is available on this activity, and what is available focuses on the acute and catastrophic events. While ailments of one-half of this athletic team (namely, the horse) have been addressed in fair detail, the rider has largely been ignored. In several studies, females sustained 50–75% of the injuries, particularly those under age 25. Unfortunately, all these studies were injury-based and none looked at the overall population of riders to see if there was a larger participation by women. The general impression, however, is that riders, especially under age 25, are predominantly girls. The medical and orthopedic issues in women equestrians can be divided into four categories: medical issues, overuse syndromes, degenerative problems, and acute trauma.

I. **MEDICAL ISSUES**
   A. **Asthma and allergies**
      1. Horses, as long-haired animals, are a significant source of allergens. Their food supply always includes some grasses, and their bedding in the stall may also include dried grasses.
      2. Athletes with **asthma or other allergies** may need assessment and possible prophylactic treatment by an allergist if they are serious about riding. Those riding, regardless of the level, should avoid antihistamines that sedate, as inattentiveness can lead to injury.
   B. **Skin problems**
      1. **Irritation:** Chapping along the inner thighs and medial aspect of the knees is common because of riding position as well as the tight, usually nylon, type of clothing. This usually clears with improved technique but can present difficulties during competition. Local skin care helps, padding does not.
      2. **Blisters:** Occur commonly in the hands, especially if the rider has not trained for a while. Gloves can help prevent these; treatment is otherwise local care and protection until the blisters heal.
      3. **Contact dermatitis:** Working with horses and the equipment such as tack involves using various solutions and chemicals. As well, a fair amount of riding is done outside and contact can also be made with various plant chemicals.
      4. **Intertrigo:** A combination of clothing, rider posture/position, and sweat make this a common problem. Addressing the clothing in the area involved (breasts, groin, or feet), changing hygiene schedule, and using local antifungals if needed clear most of these problems.
   C. **Infection**
      1. **Tetanus:** A common pathogen in stable and pasture soil. Scratches and small puncture wounds are common; therefore, it is recommended that anyone working or training in these areas have up-to-date tetanus vaccinations. Anyone treated for a penetrating injury to the skin should be prophylactically treated for tetanus.
      2. **Genitourinary infections:** The astride position and the clothing predispose the female rider to urinary tract infections. These respond well to standard treatment.
      3. **Fungal infections:** Several fungi are common residents in the soil of certain parts of the world. Riders in these areas can get systemic infection through either inhalation or inoculation through wounds. One should be aware of the native

pathogens as well as advising careful hygiene. The most common culprits are histoplasmosis, brucellosis, anthrax, and some forms of tuberculosis. The key is to suspect the possibility in your athletes and then treat appropriately after diagnosis.

4. **Encephalitis:** Equine encephalitis (Western, Eastern, and Venezuelan) is caused by a migratory bird virus that has both horse and rider as target hosts. Although the incidence appears to be geographic, there is also an association with stable conditions, which should adhere to local public health standards.

II. OVERUSE SYNDROMES

Unlike a good number of other sports, there has been little emphasis on conditioning and preseason personal training of the equestrian. Because of the nature of the sport, most overuse injuries are insidious and may not be attributed to the athletic activity unless the physician is aware that the patient rides and that these entities occur in riders.

A. **Adductor injuries**
  1. **Spasm:** Occurs with underconditioning or overtraining.
     a. Presents with pain, usually symmetric, on the inner aspect of both thighs. Pain is most frequently closer to the origin of the muscle than the insertion.
     b. Treatment consists of antiinflammatories and therapy with gentle stretching. During this time, training should be minimal if possible.
     c. Following resolution of the acute episode, the rider should maintain an adductor program of both stretching and strengthening.
  2. **Adductor contracture:** The astride position necessarily requires continued adductor contraction. This imbalance between agonist and antagonist muscles results in moderate adduction contractures.
     a. These are usually asymptomatic in their own right, but may play a role in both adductor spasms and in the low back problems that appear to be prevalent.
     b. Riders should be encouraged to specifically stretch this area.

B. **Ischial bursitis**
  1. **Symmetric buttock pain localized at the tip of the ischium** is the classic presentation. This represents friction irritation at this point of contact between the rider and the saddle. Although not entirely understood, it probably is the result of motion and is secondary to undertraining or improper equipment.
  2. Treatment with antiinflammatories and Sitz bath and correction of the causative factor help to solve the problem.

C. **Hamstring contractures**
  1. Except for Western riding and polo, most forms of equitation require a **flexed hip and knee, placing the hamstrings at shortened length.** On the other hand, the heel position, which is usually significant dorsiflexion, tends to keep the Achilles stretched out. Again, these are commonly asymptomatic, but are very likely contributing factors in the etiology of lumbar back pain. As with other athletes, riders should be encouraged to warm-up and cool-down with each training period.

D. **Patellofemoral syndrome**
  1. **Female riders are anatomically predisposed to patellofemoral syndrome** because the wide child-bearing pelvis and the "knees closer to the horse than the ankles" leg position automatically increase the Q-angle. This in turn increases the lateral forces on the patella causing it to track laterally in the groove. The vastus medialis is not worked while riding, although there is almost no literature in this area. This, coupled with a tight iliotibial band, will produce patellofemoral pain.
  2. **Treatment** consists of a therapy program which includes decreasing local pain with modalities such as ultrasound, selectively increasing vastus medialis mass and strength (which may be aided with electrical stimulation), and iliotibial band stretching.

E. **Upper-extremity overuse syndromes**
   1. **Shoulder pain:** Not common in most events, but seen where either repetitive motion (as in polo) or significant forces (as in rodeo) are placed across the shoulder. To date both of these events are very male-dominated, although women polo teams are becoming more prevalent.
      a. The four major pathologies are:
         i. Bicipital tendinitis
         ii. Acromioclavicular (AC) joint arthritis
         iii. Rotator cuff tendinitis
         iv. Impingement syndrome
      b. Each of these has fairly classic physical findings.
      c. The rotator cuff and impingement are more likely seen with the repetitive motions of polo, and the AC joint and bicipital tendon with the forces of rodeo.
      d. Treatment should include rest for the involved extremity, antiinflammatories, and a therapy program with both stretching and strengthening.
      e. Steroid injections are not recommended except in the AC joint because of the propensity for tendon rupture post injection.
   2. **Wrist pain:** Again, not common, and usually secondary to either improper technique or overtraining. Involves the flexor or extensor tendons.
      a. Treatment includes antiinflammatories and rest of the involved tendons. In a rider in the middle of competition, this may require a light splint to rest the tendons.

III. DEGENERATIVE SYNDROMES

A. **Low back pain:** Almost no literature is available on the occurrence of low back changes in the equestrian. However, there exists in the field suspicions that this is an entity. The question remains whether the incidence in riders is higher than a nonriding matched population.
   1. Several factors may put riders at risk:
      a. Although the amount varies with the type of equestrian event, **riders tend to load their lumbar spine significantly.** Neither the horse nor equipment provides any resistance to vibration. A number of lumbar spine studies done in populations that sit and sustain significant vibrations to their lower back (i.e., truck and tractor drivers) have shown that protection against vibration will decrease low back complaints.
      b. Abnormal pelvic motion and repetitive pelvic motion under load and with vibration may also contribute.
      c. Contractures of the hamstrings in particular will increase the nonmounted lumbar lordosis, which in turn loads the posterior facet joints causing symptomatic low back pain.
   2. This re-emphasizes the need for a good conditioning program for riders which includes lumbar spine maintenance.

IV. ACUTE TRAUMA

Epidemiologic studies have shown a lower incidence of injury in equestrian activities as compared to other sports. For instance, the incidence of injury per 1000 player exposures is 6.1 for football, 5.68 for track and field, and 4.5 for basketball, compared to **approximately 2.0 for equestrian events.** However, the forces involved in horse-rider activities include a four-legged animal weighing up to 2500 lbs and traveling at speeds up to 35 mph. The force of the horse's kick has been estimated to be more than 10 kilonewtons. In the adult on an appropriate-sized horse, the rider's head is 9 feet above ground, and the rider's center of gravity is well ahead of the horse's in most instances.

A. **Head injuries**
1. In all of the published studies on rider injuries, head injuries were the leading injury as well as the leading cause of death. Because the rider sits forward of the horse's center of gravity, the rider easily becomes a projectile.
2. Most of the available literature found that 20% or less of the studied population wore protective headgear. The quality of the available hard hats has been less than optimal, but they are definitely better than nothing. Recently there has been a push to design riding hats that fit ASTM (American Society for Testing Materials) standards. Recommended at present is a properly secured (i.e., chin strap) hard-shelled helmet with an expanded polystyrene insert. Work is continuing in this area.

B. **Spinal injuries**
1. **Cervical**: The neck is also at risk when the athlete is projected forward and downward. This has been less common than head injuries; probably because of the angle of projection. Medical teams covering an equestrian event should be prepared to evacuate a neck injury.
2. **Thoracolumbar junction injuries:** These tend to be the **commonest spine injuries seen with riders** and are somewhat unique to this sport.
   a. Again, the projectile thrown at the angle that most riders come off tends to land on the upper to mid-thoracic spine, creating a large flexion moment arm at the flexible thoracolumbar junction,
   b. A good number of these injuries have at least partial neurologic involvement, and they are all unstable with the potential for further paralysis.
   c. This requires a medical team that is prepared to handle and transport this type of injury.

C. **Upper-extremity fractures: These are the second most common injuries in riders,** especially when thrown. Most are straightforward; those that are compound need to be treated with thorough debridement and good antimicrobial therapy, as the flora of farmland, stables, and local waterways can be unique and nonresponsive to routine care.

D. **Chest and abdominal injuries:** Usually seen when the rider falls with the horse on top of her or when the rider is trampled. These need to be suspected and adequate resuscitation available prior to transport. Fractured ribs, especially in the younger riders, suggest a fair amount of force applied.

E. **Bites and kicks:** These injuries oddly enough occur when the athlete is neither training nor competing. They are, however, real and common problems around horses. Both produce localized injuries. Bites can often be associated with inoculation of organisms such as clostridia or anaerobes as well as gram-positive cocci. Care includes reduction of local swelling, local skin care, and appropriate antibiotics if needed.

F. **Lacerations:** Although not overwhelming in number, lacerations in the rider need special mention because of the unusual and potentially catastrophic microbes involved.
1. Tetanus status of all riders should be up-to-date and documented.
2. The treating physician should be aware of the local soil and water microbes.
3. When lacerations occur, the history needs to include where the incident took place.
4. Aggressive irrigation with sterile saline or Ringer's lactate should be followed by an antiseptic/antibiotic impregnated dressing.
5. The wound needs to be checked daily and referred immediately for surgical debridement if infection appears.
6. Wounds that appear to penetrate any depth, especially if they occurred in direct contact with soil or feces may need initial surgical debridement.

V. INJURY PREVENTION

A. **Apparel**
1. **Hat**: All riders should be required to wear protective headgear. To keep the hat on the rider, all headgear needs a chinstrap. Research needs to continue into improving the structural properties of equestrain headgear.

2. **Clothing:** Shirts and pants should be close fitting so they do not get caught on trees or equipment. Loose, flowing articles, such as scarves, should be avoided. Gloves will protect hands from both the weather and trauma.
3. **Boots:** Firm boots are more likely to protect the rider's foot from crush injuries than are rubber boots. However, the most important feature is the *heel*, which must have sufficient thickness that it can keep the foot from slipping through the stirrup, thus preventing the rider from being dragged if they fall off. Smooth soles are also recommended as they prevent the foot from becoming fixed to the stirrup.

B. **Equipment**
1. **Tack:** Fatigue failure of the rider's equipment is one of the most common causes of injury. This has been a particular problem in polo. Riders need to be trained not only to care for the tack but also to check it carefully for wear.
2. **Stirrups:** Breakaway stirrups have been available for a number of years and may be of some benefit in the younger or less-experienced rider. There is some controversy in the literature about the significance of their efficacy, but all agree that these stirrups have *no* efficacy if the breakout portion has been taped or wired closed.
3. **Protective devices:** To date, only polo players and racing jockeys wear any protective devices on a regular basis. Most polo players wear padding on their shins, knees, and knuckles. Jockeys have the option of wearing Kevlar spine protectors or flak jackets to protect their ribcages.

C. **Environment**
1. **Roads:** Hacking on country roadways is common practice; however, most car and truck drivers have no experience with horses and often tend to treat riders the same way they treat cyclists and motorcyclists. The horse is much more responsive to the crowding and noise of vehicles, and this is where a number of serious accidents occur. These rides are often a treat for young or inexperienced riders who frequently may be mounted above their skill level—this combination can be hazardous. One study found that 25% of the injuries seen occurred on roadways. Good roadway habits should be part of the learning process.
2. **Low branches:** Another favorite relaxing ride is to go out through the countryside, often through the brush. Too commonplace are the injuries incurred when an inattentive rider is knocked off by low limbs. Rider education as to the need for safety, even when not training, is essential.
3. **Alcohol and drugs:** As horses are not motorized vehicles, there has been little work done on drinking and riding. Because there is always a possibility that the horse, no matter how well trained, may misbehave, riding under the influence of anything should be strongly discouraged. At present, only jockeys appear to have addressed this. In some equestrian events, such as hunting, alcohol is part of the tradition and is felt by some to contribute significantly to the injury rate.

D. **Equestrian**
1. **Age/ability:** Young children should be age- and size-matched to their mount and closely supervised. The Chair of the U.S. Pony Club, in 1991, stated that in general children under the age of 6 should not ride independently. Reviews of injuries sustained while riding show that a number occur when the rider is mounted well beyond their skill level. As most animals do not willingly hurt themselves, these injuries are often because the rider has not the strength or agility to stay balanced on that particular mount. The enthusiasm of adolescent riders will frequently put them in these hazardous situations.
2. **Repeat injuries:** Several authors have noted a reinjury trend; those who were injured had had a previous injury—often a similar injury or a similar mechanism. The Pony Club noted that up to 27% were reinjuries, and these had occurred in the same manner as the initial injury. The racing world has recognized this as a problem and requires riders to keep an accurate log of their injuries. Physicians

treating riders should keep track of the injuries and determine that the rider has recovered sufficiently to return to training.

3. **Contraindications:** Because of the high incidence of head and neck injuries in this sport, it is recommended that athletes with previous severe injuries, sequelae from previous injury, or congenital deformities that put the head or neck at risk not participate further.

REFERENCES

1. Barone G, Rodgers B: Pediatric equestrian injuries: A 14-year review. J Trauma 29:245–247, 1989.
2. Bixby-Hammett D: Pediatric equestrian injuries. Pediatrics 89:1173–1176, 1992.
3. Bixby-Hammett D, Brooks W: Common injuries in horseback riding—A review. Sports Med 9:36–47, 1990.
4. Brooks W, Bixby-Hammett D: Prevention of neurologic injuries in equestrian sports. Phys SportsMed 16:84–95, 1988.
5. Firth J: Equestrian injuries. In Schneider R, Kennedy J, Plant M (eds): Sports Medicine: Mechanisms, Prevention, and Treatment. Baltimore, Williams & Wilkins, 1985.
6. Grossman J, Kulund D, Miller C, et al: Equestrian injuries: Results of a prospective study. JAMA 240:1881–1882, 1978.
7. Lloyd R: Riding and other equestrian issues: Considerable severity. Br J Sports Med 21:22–24, 1987.
8. McLatchie G: Equestrian injuries—A one year perspective study. Br J Sports Med 13:28–32, 1979.
9. Nelson D, Bixby-Hammett D: Equestrian injuries in children and young adults. Am J Dis Child 146:611–614, 1992.
10. Whitlock M, Whitlock J, Johnston R: Equestrian injuries: A comparison of professional and amateur injuries in Berkshire. Br J Sports Med 21:25–26, 1987.

Chapter 57: Tennis

CATHERINE M. FIESELER, MD

Tennis is a sport that requires skill, strength, speed, and endurance. Demands are placed on the upper and lower extremities and the trunk. Thus, total body fitness is necessary to compete, and the athlete is subject to a wide variety of injuries.

I. **GENERAL POINTS**
   A. Singles tennis meets the American College of Sports Medicine (ACSM) guidelines for intensity (heart rate) for cardiovascular fitness.
   B. A match consists of hundreds of short bursts of activity interspersed with intervals of submaximal effort and rest.
      1. Total match time may be several hours.

II. **EQUIPMENT**
   A. **Racquet**
      1. Weight: A heavier racquet is more stressful to the upper extremity.
      2. Proper grip size: The circumference of the handle should be equal to the measurement of the radial side of the ring finger, from the tip to the palmar crease.
      3. Size of the racquet head: Normal, midsized, and oversized.
      4. Strings: Natural gut, nylon, and synthetic.
         a. Gut is the choice for athletes recovering from upper-extremity overuse injuries.
         b. String tension should be decreased 3–5 lb when recovering from injuries.
   B. **Balls**
      1. Velocity may exceed 100 mph.
      2. Old, worn balls and wet balls require more energy to hit.
   C. **Shoes**: Ensure good fit, firm heel counter, and side stability. Insert orthotics as needed.
   D. **Courts:** Softer courts (clay, carpet, composition) are less stressful to the lower extremities.
      1. Clay: The ball bounces with a greater trajectory and is therefore easier to hit.
      2. Hard court: The ball bounces faster and lower to the ground and is therefore more stressful to hit.
      3. Grass: Stressful to the upper extremity due to irregular bounces and fast ball speed.

III. **INJURIES**
   Tennis is a sport consisting of multiple short bursts of activity and involving a multitude of movements—short sprints, rapid change of direction, overhead service, forehand and backhand volleys, and groundstrokes. For this reason, a wide variety of acute and chronic injuries may be seen.
   A. **Shoulder**
      1. When obtaining the history, it is important to inquire:
         a. Which stroke(s) and what part of the stroke is painful.
         b. Symptoms of dead arm, paresthesias, night pain, thoracic outlet syndrome, instability, mechanical clicking/popping.
         c. Symptoms consistent with cervical, cardiac, pulmonary, and neurologic causes of the problem.

2. **Tennis shoulder**: An adaptive postural change in the dominant shoulder of the tennis player (and other overhand athletes), characterized by a depression of the exercised shoulder; this is associated with an apparent scoliosis.
   a. Additional findings on examination may include:
      i. Apparent lengthening of the dominant arm
      ii. Asymmetry of the nipple line
      iii. Hypertrophy of the pectoralis major
      iv. Relative abduction of the dominant arm
      v. Widening of the distance between the spinous process and medial scapular border
   b. Tennis shoulder may cause cervical paraspinal muscle tenderness, decreased cervical motion, tender scapular support muscles (levator scapulae, trapezius, rhomboids), and constricted flexibility of pectoralis minor muscle.
3. **Rotator cuff inflammation** (rotator cuff tendinitis, impingement, subacromial bursitis)
   a. History of pain with service and overhead shots
   b. Examination findings:
      i. Positive impingement tests
      ii. Painful range of motion, especially above shoulder height
      iii. Rotator cuff and/or biceps weakness and pain
      iv. Lidocaine injection into subacromial space should relieve symptoms; if weakness persists, suspect rotator cuff tear.
   c. Treatment
      i. Relative rest, avoid aggravating strokes
      ii. Ice
      iii. Nonsteroidal antiinflammatory drugs (NSAIDs)
      iv. Rotator cuff stretching and strengthening program
      v. Corticosteroid injection into subacromial space
      vi. If not responding to conservative measures, use arthrogram or MRI to evaluate for rotator cuff or labral tear. Persistent symptoms may require surgical decompression of the subacromial space.
4. **Rotator cuff tear**
   a. History
      i. Usually older athletes
      ii. Complain of gradual loss of strength, night pain, persistent pain
   b. Examination findings:
      i. Weakness of rotator cuff and biceps; possible atrophy
      ii. Palpation of humeral head may reveal defect or point tenderness
      iii. Painful range of motion, especially abduction
      iv. Lidocaine injection into subacromial space will alleviate pain but not weakness.
      v. CT arthrogram will show leakage of dye.
   c. **Treatment**
      i. Ice
      ii. NSAIDs
      iii. Rotator cuff stretching and strengthening program
      iv. Surgical repair is often needed.
5. **Glenohumeral instability**
   a. Not a common cause of shoulder pain in tennis players
   b. Chronic instability symptoms are the most common presentation
   c. Long-term rotator cuff rehabilitation program is necessary.
   d. Often requires surgery for athlete to remain competitive.
B. **Elbow**
   1. **Lateral epicondylitis**

    a. 3–4 times more common than medial tennis elbow

    b. Thought to be due to small tears in the musculotendinous structures, especially at the insertion into bone. Healing is slow due to poor vascularity.

    c. History

        i. Repetitive rotary movements of the hand and wrist

        ii. Pain with backhand, shaking hands, turning doorknobs, lifting full cup of liquid

    d. Examination findings

        i. Pain localized over the lateral epicondyle

        ii. Increased pain with resisted wrist extension, forearm supination, and extension of the middle finger

    e. Treatment

        i. Correct underlying causes: Proper grip size, improve mechanics of strokes, larger racquet head, decrease string tension

        ii. Rest; avoid grasping in pronation; use supination when lifting.

        iii. NSAIDs

        iv. Ice

        v. Volar cock-up splint

        vi. Counterforce bracing (tennis elbow band)

        vii. Cross friction massage

        viii. Strengthening of wrist and hand musculature; stretching of forearm musculature

        ix. Corticosteroid injection

        x. Rarely needs surgery

2. **Compression of the radial nerve or its posterior interosseous branch as it courses through the supinator muscle**

    a. History

        i. Lateral elbow pain that radiates into the dorsal forearm.

        ii. Pain is often more diffuse than with lateral epicondylitis.

        iii. Pain is aggravated by supination-pronation activities.

    b. Examination findings

        i. Positive Tinel's sign 8 cm distal to the lateral epicondyle (tapping over the nerve reproduces symptoms).

        ii. Maximal tenderness is distal to the lateral epicondyle.

        iii. Weakness of wrist extensors (extensor carpi ulnaris, extensor carpi radialis)

        iv. Weakness of extension of the first three fingers at the metacarpophalangeal joint

        v. Entrapment of the posterior interosseous nerve may cause only pain and weakness of extension of the middle finger.

        vi. Electromyography (EMG) and nerve conduction velocity (NCV) studies are often negative.

    c. Treatment

        i. Relative rest; modify training

        ii. Conservative treatment as described for lateral epicondylitis

        iii. Often require surgical release

3. **Medial epicondylitis**

    a. Pathology is thought to be the same as in lateral epicondylitis.

    b. History

        i. Pain at medial aspect of elbow

        ii. More commonly seen in players with a top spin forehand and a hard serve

    c. Examination findings

        i. Pain over the medial epicondyle which increases with resisted wrist flexion or forearm pronation

        ii. Negative Tinel's sign at the cubital tunnel

d. Treatment: Same as in lateral epicondylitis except:
   i. Splint in neutral position
   ii. Counterforce brace (tennis elbow band) is applied over the flexor mass, not the extensor mass.

4. **Ulnar collateral ligament sprain**
   a. Injury is due to repetitive valgus stress on the elbow, which repeatedly loads the ulnar collateral ligament and results in microtears of this ligament.
   b. History: Insidious onset of medial elbow pain which is provoked by valgus stress activitites. Pain is relieved by rest.
   c. Examination findings
      i. Tender below the medial epicondyle over the humeroulnar joint
      ii. Increased pain with valgus stress to elbow at 20–30° of flexion
      iii. Radiographs may show spurring at ulna or ossification of the ulnar collateral ligament.
   d. Treatment
      i. Rest
      ii. NSAIDs
      iii. Ice
      iv. Strengthening and stretching of the wrist and hand musculature, especially the flexor-pronator group

5. **Ulnar nerve entrapment**
   a. Due to compression or subluxation of the nerve
   b. History
      i. Medial elbow pain which may radiate proximally or distally
      ii. Complaint of grip weakness
      iii. Complaint of numbness and dysesthesias on the ulnar one and a half digits
      iv. No complaints of neck pain or loss of motion
   c. Examination findings
      i. Positive Tinel's sign at the cubital tunnel
      ii. Forced elbow extension elicits pain.
      iii. Weakness of thumb–index finger pinch
      iv. Possible atrophy of the hypothenar eminence
      v. Normal neck examination
      vi. EMG/NCV positive 40–50% of the time
   d. Treatment
      i. Elbow pad
      ii. Rest; avoid aggravating motions
      iii. NSAIDs
      iv. Exercises to increase wrist and hand strength and flexibility
      v. Surgery

6. **Pronator teres syndrome**
   a. Compression of the median nerve at the elbow
   b. History
      i. Pain in the anterior proximal forearm which is insidious in onset
      ii. Parasthesias in the volar forearm and radial three and a half digits.
   c. Examination findings
      i. Pain increases with pronation and wrist flexion
      ii. Positive Tinel's sign over proximal forearm
      iii. Negative Tinel's sign and Phalen's test at the wrist (In Phalen's test, forced flexion of the wrist for 90 seconds reproduces symptoms.)
      iv. Tenderness over the pronator teres muscle
      v. Symptoms may increase with the following tests depending on the site of compression:

    (a) Resisted elbow flexion at 120-135° and forearm supination—lacertus
        fibrosus
    (b) Resisted forearm pronation and wrist flexion—pronator teres
    (c) Resisted flexion of the middle finger—arch of flexor digitorum super-
        ficialis
  vi. EMG/NCV may or may not be abnormal.
  d. Treatment
    i. Rest; modify activity, avoiding pronation
    ii. NSAIDs
    iii. Stretching of forearm musculature
    iv. Corticosteroid injection
    v. Surgery
7. **Posterior elbow pain** (uncommon)
  a. Overuse of the triceps caused by repetitive extension of the elbow
  b. History: Posterior elbow pain
  c. Examination findings
    i. Tenderness over triceps insertion
    ii. Increased pain with resisted extension of the elbow
  d. Treatment
    i. Rest
    ii. Ice
    iii. NSAIDs
    iv. Exercises to strengthen and stretch triceps
C. **Wrist and hand:** Tennis strokes require a stiff wrist, so wrist injuries are not very
   common. There are players (many beginners) who hit the ball (especially backhand)
   with a loose wrist, stressing the ligamentous structures of the wrist. Wrist motion does
   occur during service.
  1. **Fracture of the hook of the hamate**
    a. Not uncommon in tennis players
    b. The handle of the racquet lies over the volar area of the hook; a fracture may
       occur from a sudden impact when the handle is jammed into the hook.
    c. History
      i. Pain over the ulnar aspect of the wrist
      ii. Athlete may remember a specific stroke which caused the injury.
    d. Examination findings
      i. Tenderness over the hook of the hamate
      ii. May have associated tendinitis of the small finger flexor
      iii. Check the status of the ulnar nerve
      iv. Radiographs should include carpal tunnel and supination oblique views
      v. May need bone scan or CT to confirm suspicion
    e. Treatment
      i. If not displaced, cast with immobilization for 10–12 weeks, with frequent
        radiographic evaluation.
      ii. If displaced, surgical excision. (Due to the quicker recovery time, athletes with
        undisplaced fractures of the hook of the hamate may also opt for excision.)
  2. **Triangular fibrocartilage complex**
    a. The combination of impact and stresses due to twisting of the racquet can injure
      the triangular fibrocartilage complex, resulting in a tear.
    b. History: Pain in the area of the distal ulna
    c. Examination findings
      i. Tenderness over the ulnar styloid
      ii. May produce clicking with ulnar deviation and pronation
      iii. No gross wrist instability
      iv. Decreased grip strength

        v. Arthrography will demonstrate communication between the radial-carpal and distal radial-ulnar joint.
    d. Treatment
        i. Splint
        ii. NSAIDs
        iii. Corticosteroid injection
        iv. Surgery

3. **Extensor carpi ulnaris tenosynovitis**
    a. History: Pain over the dorsal ulnar aspect of the wrist
    b. Examination findings: Tenderness, swelling, and crepitus over the dorsal ulnar aspect of the wrist
    c. Treatment
        i. Splint
        ii. NSAIDs
        iii. Ice
        iv. Corticosteroid injection

4. **Extensor carpi ulnaris subluxation**
    a. Sudden supination, ulnar deviation, and volar flexion may result in rupture of the fibro-osseous tunnel of the extensor carpi ulnaris.
    b. History
        i. Pain over the dorsal ulnar aspect of the wrist
        ii. Complaint of clicking with movement of wrist
    c. Examination findings: As in extensor carpi ulnaris tenosynovitis
        i. Clicking with forearm rotation
        ii. Forced supination and palmar flexion will cause observable subluxation of the extensor carpi ulnaris.
    d. Treatment
        i. Acute: 6 weeks of immobilization in a long-arm cast with the wrist in supination and radial deviation
        ii. Chronic: surgery

5. **Flexor tenosynovitis (trigger finger)**
    a. Repetitive blunt trauma to the A1 pulley at the base of the finger due to direct compression by the handle of the racquet
    b. History: Painful locking of the finger in flexion
    c. Examination findings
        i. Locking
        ii. Palpable nodule over the A1 pulley
    d. Treatment
        i. Corticosteroid injection into the sheath but not the tendon of the flexor
        ii. Possible surgical release

D. **Trunk**
  1. **Thoracoabdominal injuries**
    a. Most commonly occur when the athlete reaches for an overhead shot or when serving. The spine is hyperextended when reaching overhead and the abdominal musculature undergoes forced contraction. The acute flexion that occurs when serving stresses the upper thoracic muscles.
    b. History: Will complain of chest or abdominal pain caused by certain motions
    c. Examination findings
        i. Have the athlete perform a Valsalva maneuver, *or* have the athlete reach overhead. If these maneuvers cause pain, the strain is *severe*. Palpate the painful areas.
        ii. Rectus abdominis: With the athlete supine, knees are bent and hands locked behind head. A partial sit-up is performed with the trunk 6–8 inches off the ground. The sit-up is then slowly completed. Then, have the

athlete perform a pushup and remain in the down position. If these maneuvers cause pain in the rectus abdominis, while the other maneuvers did not, the strain is *moderate* in severity.

    iii. Thoracic: With the athlete standing, the hands are held together with the elbows flexed in front of the body. Isometric pressure is applied until strain is felt in the thoracic region. Then, a pushup is performed against a wall with a small amount of pressure applied to the back. The elbows should be flexed and the hands spread widely apart. If these maneuvers cause thoracic pain while the others did not, the strain is *moderate* in severity.

  d. Treatment
    i. Rest; the greater the severity, the longer the period of rest required.
    ii. Ice
    iii. NSAIDs
    iv. Physical modalities
    v. As pain decreases, add gentle stretching, ground strokes, easy backhand, and forehand strokes.
    vi. Progress to more stretching, especially flexion and extension of the thoraco-lumbar spine, and then overhead reaching. Imitate service motion, first without and then with a racquet, gradually progressing to hitting a ball.
    vii. Rehabilitation exercises should work on overall strengthening and flexibility: e.g., sit-ups, pushups.

2. **Back**
  a. Upper back: See section on tennis shoulder.
  b. Lower back: The most common cause of low back pain in tennis players is strain of the lumbosacral muscles due to hyperextension of the spine. Herniated nucleus pulposus should also be in the differential diagnosis.
  c. History
    i. Pain in the lower back
    ii. Ask about radiation of pain, paresthesias, weakness, incontinence.
    iii. Does pain increase with Valsalva maneuver (i.e., sneezing, coughing, etc.)?
    iv. Is the pain worse when sitting or standing (with herniated nucleus pulposus, pain is worse when sitting)?
  d. Examination findings
    i. Decreased range of motion
    ii. Neurologic examination: If positive findings, consider herniated nucleus pulposus.
    iii. Straight leg raise tests
    iv. Check hamstring flexibility
  e. Treatment
    i. Rest
    ii. NSAIDs
    iii. Ice
    iv. Exercises to improve flexibility, especially hamstrings, and to strengthen abdominal musculature
    v. Instruction in back care (i.e., proper lifting techniques, etc.)

E. **Lower extremity**
  1. **Tennis leg:** Strain of the medial head of the gastrocnemius
    a. History
      i. Acute pain in the posterior calf following running or jumping. May state that it felt as if she was kicked in the calf.
      ii. Pain with pushing off
    b. Examination findings
      i. Tenderness at the juncture of the upper one-third and lower two-thirds of the medial head of the gastrocnemius

   ii. Check for palpable defect in the muscle
   iii. Swelling
   iv. Thompson test causes plantar-flexion of the ankle. (With the patient lying prone, the calf is squeezed. If the Achilles tendon is intact, plantar-flexion of the ankle occurs.)
   v. Foot is kept slightly plantar-flexed for comfort.
   c. Treatment
      i. Compression
      ii. Ice
      iii. Elevation
      iv. NSAIDs
      v. Crutches with progressive weight-bearing
      vi. 0.5 inch heel lift in the shoe
      vii. Stretching (dorsiflexion) and strengthening of gastrocnemius and soleus muscles

2. **Patellar and quadriceps tendinitis**
   a. History: Insidious onset of pain
   b. Examination findings
      i. Tenderness of superior or inferior pole of patella
      ii. Aggravated by quadriceps contraction and knee extension against resistance
      iii. Local swelling may be present
   c. Treatment
      i. Activity modification
      ii. Ice
      iii. NSAIDs
      iv. Neoprene sleeve
      v. Quadriceps strengthening and hamstring flexibility

3. **Achilles tendinitis**
   a. History
      i. Pain in Achilles tendon
      ii. Ask about an increase in training and change in shoes
   b. Examination findings
      i. Tendon is tender and thickened.
      ii. Pain with dorsiflexion
      iii. Palpate for defects in tendon
      iv. Thompson test causes plantar-flexion of the ankle.
   c. Treatment
      i. Modify training
      ii. Ice
      iii. NSAIDs
      iv. Heel lift
      v. Stretching
      vi. Correct anatomic problems (i.e., overpronation).
      vii. Occasionally needs surgical release of peritenon and debridement

4. **Achilles tendon rupture**
   a. History: Feels a pop and sensation of being struck in the heel
   b. Examination findings
      i. Weak plantar-flexion
      ii. Palpable defect in tendon (may be obscured by bleeding at site of rupture)
      iii. Thompson test does not cause plantar-flexion of the ankle.
   c. Treatment
      i. Surgery or cast immobilization (8–12 weeks)
      ii. Stretching and strengthening of lower leg muscles after either treatment.

5. **Lateral ankle sprain**
   a. More common on hard court because there is less foot slide.
   b. Usually grade 1 in severity
   c. History: Inversion of ankle resulting in pain and swelling
   d. Examination findings
      i. Localized tenderness
      ii. Check laxity: Anterior drawer and talar tilt tests (Pain may preclude this examination in the acute stage.)
      iii. Anterior drawer test: Stabilize the distal tibia and grasp the heel with your dominant hand; pull forward toward your body. Compare to the opposite ankle. Anterior talofibular ligament laxity causes significant excursion.
      iv. Talar tilt test: With the hand position as in anterior drawer test, an inversion stress is applied to the ankle and heel. Calcaneofibular ligament laxity causes increased excursion.
      v. Radiograph if there is any concern about a fracture (especially in patients with open growth plates).
   e. Treatment
      i. Ice
      ii. Compression
      iii. Elevation
      iv. NSAIDs
      v. Crutches with progressive weight-bearing as tolerated
      vi. Physical therapy: Early mobilization; range of motion; strengthening; proprioception
      vii. Grade 3 sprains require rigid support for 1–3 weeks.
6. **Plantar fasciitis**
   a. Constant starting, stopping, and changing directions stresses the feet.
   b. History: Pain in the bottom of the heel; it is especially painful on getting out of bed and diminishes after several steps.
   c. Examination findings
      i. Tenderness on palpation of the medial tubercle of the calcaneus
      ii. Pain with stretching of the plantar fascia
      iii. May have tight Achilles tendon, pes cavus, or pes planus
   d. Treatment
      i. Cross-training (non–weight-bearing)
      ii. Ice
      iii. NSAIDs
      iv. Heel cup
      v. Arch supports, arch taping, orthotics
      vi. Cross friction massage
      vii. Corticosteroid injection
      viii. Stretching of posterior calf muscles and plantar fascia; strengthening of foot flexors

IV. GENERAL PRINCIPLES OF PREVENTION AND REHABILITATION

A. To play tennis, total body strength and flexibility are required, especially for the dominant shoulder.
B. Upper extremity work should include the use of a racquet. A racquet attached to a Theraband may be used to simulate strokes against resistance.
C. Strength is especially important for the scapular retractors, rotator cuff, wrist extensors, and muscles involved in gripping.
D. Flexibility is especially important for the lower extremities, anterior area of the shoulder, shoulder flexors, and wrist extensors.

REFERENCES

1. Groppel JL, Roetert EP: Applied physiology of tennis. Sports Med 14:260–268, 1992.
2. Hawkins RJ, Hobeika PE: Impingement syndrome in the athletic shoulder. Clin Sports Med 2:391–405, 1983.
3. Harvey J, Glick J, Stanish W, Teitz C: Tennis elbow: What's the best treatment? Phys SportsMed 18(6):62–74, 1990.
4. Kamien M: A rational management of tennis elbow. Sports Med 9(3):173–191, 1990.
5. Lehman RC (ed): Racquet sports: Injury treatment and prevention. Clin Sports Med 7:229–370, 1988.
6. McCue FC, Meister K: Common sports hand injuries. Sports Med 15:281–289, 1993.
7. Nicholas JA, Hershman EB: The Upper Extremity in Sports Medicine. St. Louis, C.V. Mosby, 1990.

Chapter 58: Track and Field

CAROL L. OTIS, MD

The multiple events of a track and field meet require great commitment and many variations in training and performance from athletes, coaches, and sports medicine professionals. Track and field attracts large numbers of participants who have diverse backgrounds, abilities, training patterns, and injuries. The sports medicine professional needs to understand the different physiologic demands of training for each sport, the technical aspects of performance for each sport, sport-specific injury patterns, and fundamentals of covering a track and field meet.

Athletes in track and field may often be multi-sport athletes and train and compete year-round. Their potential for injuries is great. Surveys of injury patterns in high school sports in Washington state have shown that female cross-country and track athletes have the greatest injury rates, far exceeding rates in football, soccer, or gymnastics. Most injuries are overuse injuries that occur during training. Injuries during competition are much less common. Catastrophic injuries and fatalities are rare—e.g., massive head trauma from a fall while pole vaulting or from a thrown hammer or javelin. Acute muscle-tendon tears (e.g., hamstring injuries during sprinting) are dramatic events that occur during competition.

I. HISTORY

A. **Events of track and field are historically among the oldest events recorded in athletic competition:**
   1. An outgrowth of military training
   2. Male dominated
B. **Women's participation in track and field has been limited until recently.**
   1. Running events of >800 m were restricted to women until the 1970s out of concern that women were not physiologically capable of competing these distances.
   2. Women's marathon did not become part of the Olympic Games until 1984.
C. **Women have successfully trained and competed in almost all track and field events.**
   1. Pole vault, decathlon, 20-km and 50-km walk-race, triple jump, and hammer throw are *not* currently open for women in the Olympics.
   2. Women train in these events and participate in exhibitions of all these sports.
   3. Women's triple jump is included in collegiate, national, and world championship levels.

II. SPECIFIC EVENTS

A. **Throwing events**
   1. Involve the greatest risk of injury for spectators and others.
   2. Events include:
      a. Shot put
      b. Discus
      c. Javelin throw
      d. Hammer throw
   3. These sports involve careful attention to proper technique.
   4. **Training injuries:** Most injuries are overuse injuries sustained during training.
      a. Upper extremity
         i. Acromioclavicular joint: Sprains, separations, dislocations
         ii. Shoulder: Rotator cuff tendinitis, impingement, and tears; shoulder instability

455

       iii. Upper arm: Biceps tendinitis, tendon subluxation, ruptures, muscle strains
       iv. Elbow: Tendinitis, median nerve compression (pronator syndrome), medial epicondylitis
       v. Wrist and hand: Nerve compression, tendinitis, finger dislocations and sprains
   b. Back
       i. Imbalance of throwing side
       ii. Low back strain
   c. Lower extremity
       i. Hip and pelvis: apophysitis, bursitis
       ii. Leg muscles: Tears and strains of quadriceps, hamstrings, adductors, gastrocnemius
       iii. Knee: Ligament strains, bursitis, tendinitis
       iv. Ankle and foot: Sprains
5. **Competition concerns**
   a. Acute injuries to competitors are rare.
   b. Attention should be paid to maintaining proper hydration in athletes.
   c. Injuries possible to noncompetitors from thrown object (i.e., discus, javelin, hammer, or shot put).
   d. Hammer throw is usually conducted at a different site or earlier than other field events to avoid injuries to spectators.
B. **Jumping events**
  1. Injuries can occur equally in training and competition and include overuse injuries. Understanding what is involved in each event helps elucidate the types of injury possible.
  2. **Long jump**
   a. Four phases
       i. Approach
       ii. Takeoff
       iii. Aerial
       iv. Landing
  3. **High jump**
   a. Three styles
       i. Eastern scissors kick
       ii. Western roll, straddle roll
       iii. Fosbury flop
   b. Four phases
       i. Run-up
       ii. Planting
       iii. Aerial over bar
       iv. Landing
  4. **Triple jump**
  5. **Injuries:** Similar injuries occur in the different phases of each jump.
   a. Approach or run-up
       i. Muscle strains
       ii. Ligament sprains
       iii. Patellofemoral syndrome
       iv. Tendinitis (patellar and Achilles)
       v. Falls
   b. Planting and takeoff
       i. Knee injuries (including patellar tendinitis and patellofemoral syndrome)
       ii. Ankle injuries (including sprains and jumper's ankle)
       iii. Foot injuries (turf toe, plantar fasciitis)

     c. Landing: Involves impact and deceleration and related injuries as described above.

C. **Pole vault**
1. Technically difficult, requires speed, strength, timing, and balance.
2. Narrow margin of error. Catastrophic if injury occurs.
3. Equipment
    a. Fiberglass poles may snap at takeoff. Size and weight of the pole depend on the size and skill of the athlete.
    b. Vaulting boxes are constructed with angled walls to avoid contact with the pole.
    c. Foam landing mats should cover all sides of the vaulting box except pole entrance and should be 28–36 inches thick.
4. Four phases
    a. Run-up:. Runways range from 85–125 feet.
    b. Plant pole and takeoff: Complex motion, with the greatest risk for injury.
    c. Aerial over bar
    d. Landing
5. **Injuries**
    a. Injuries as seen in the approach phase in jumping events
    b. Most serious injuries occur from errors in landing or from pole breakage during takeoff and aerial phases.
    c. Falls can result in dislocations and fractures or, in the worst case, head and neck injury.

D. **Sprint events** (*see also* Chapter 52: Running)
1. Block starts. Spiked shoes used for racing.
2. Involves anaerobic activity.
3. Three phases of run
    a. Start
    b. Middle
    c. Finish
4. **Training injuries**
    a. Muscle balance (strains or tears of hamstrings and quadriceps)
    b. Toe running causes imbalance to gastrocnemius and toe flexors.

E. **Hurdles** (*see also* Chapter 52: Running)
1. Timing is critical in running (not jumping) over hurdle.
2. Flexibility important
3. Overuse injuries common to lower extremity and pelvis.
4. Contusions to the medial aspect of the trailing leg

F. **Endurance events** (1500 m and up) (*see also* Chapter 52: Running)
1. Aerobic training with distance, time, intensity, and surface are cofactors in injury.
    a. Running on pavement (concrete) is 3 times more likely to cause injury.
2. **Injuries are usually due to overuse:**
    a. Tendinitis
    b. Bursitis
    c. Stress fractures
3. Equipment
    a. Shoes lose shock absorption with wear after 200–300 miles.
    b. Spikes are used for racing.
4. Environmental factors are important.

III. ENVIRONMENTAL HAZARDS

A. Hypothermia
B. Hyperthermia
C. Event surface

IV. **SPECIAL CONCERNS FOR TRACK ATHLETES**
  A. Drug testing
     1. USA track and field: Random year-round testing
     2. National Collegiate Athletic Association (NCAA): At events
     3. International Amateur Athletic Federation (IAAF): At events
     4. U.S. Olympic Commission offers a Drug Information Hotline—800-233-0393.
  B. Vitamin B12 testing and other requests
  C. Psychology
  D. Sports massage
  E. Female athlete triad—amenorrhea, disordered eating, osteoporosis—is a concern for all female athletes but may be most prevalent in distance runners.
     1. Myth: Thinner is faster.
     2. Myth: Amenorrhea is a mark of training adequacy.
  F. Medical problems in athletes
     1. Asthma
        a. May present as exercise-induced asthma only
        b. Variable symptoms
        c. Multiple effective drug regimens available. Begin with pretraining inhalers.
        d. All medications should be cleared with the U.S. Olympic Commission Drug Information Hotline (800-233-0393).
     2. Gastrointestinal disturbance
        a. Reflux
        b. Gastritis: Look for use of nonsteroidal antiinflammatory drug as factor.
        c. Diarrhea: A common ailment
           i. Try diet modification
           ii. Use nonsedating antimotility agents, such as loperamide (imodium).
     3. Incontinence: Try Kegel exercises
     4. Screen for anemia
        a. Common in female runners
        b. Differential diagnosis should include pseudoanemia and iron deficiency.
     5. Hematuria
        a. May be due to bladder contusions (in male) or renal ischemia.
        b. If hematuria does not clear with stopping exercise for 1 or 2 days, do a full work-up.

RESOURCES

1. USA **Track and Field** (National governing body for track and field; formerly TAC, The Athletic Congress)
   One Hosier Dome, Suite 140
   Indianapolis, IN 46225
   (telephone: 317-261-0500)
   (fax: 317-261-0481)
2. *Track Techniques* (Official publication of USA Track and Field)
   Track and Field News, Inc.
   2570 El Camino Real, Suite 606
   Mountain View, CA 94040
3. *Track and Field News* (Monthly magazine, offering worldwide coverage of meets, results, etc.)
   2570 El Camino Real
   Suite 606
   Mountain View, CA 94040

Chapter 59: Softball

PATRICIA A. HEBERT, MD

Softball is one of the fastest growing recreational and competitive sporting activities enjoyed by women today. An estimated 10–15 million women participate annually in softball games, ranging from the organized collegiate level to the random pick-up game level. With such large numbers of participants, the possibility for injury is high, owing in part to the different skill levels and physical conditioning of participants playing in the same game. Moreover, even at the collegiate level, few women's softball teams have professional coaches, trainers, or team physicians at all games. With these facts in mind, it is no wonder that softball injuries account for more emergency department visits than any other sport. This chapter, focuses on the etiology of women's softball injuries and their prevention.

I. CLASSIFICATION OF INJURIES

Women's softball injuries can be categorized into four types including: sliding related injuries, collision-related injuries, fall-related injuries, and other injuries. Of these, sliding injuries account for the greatest number and often the more severe softball injuries.

A. Sliding-related injuries

1. **Mechanism**
   a. **"Head-first" sliding technique:** Ground contact is initiated by the hands, with deceleration occurring from ground contact with the chest and thighs. The outstretched hand then makes terminal impact with the base to complete deceleration.
      i. Injuries
         (a) Mostly hyperextension injuries to fingers and wrists as a result of terminal impact with the base
         (b) Digit and wrist sprains (treat with rest, ice, compression, elevation—RICE)
         (c) Navicular fractures. Covert fractures of the navicular must be considered with persistent wrist pain even if initial x-rays are negative. A repeat x-ray or bone scan in 7–10 days is indicated with continued wrist pain as severe arthritis is a likely consequence of an untreated navicular fracture.
   b. **"Foot-first" sliding technique:** The leading foot against the ground decelerates the runner, with terminal impact with the base resulting in complete deceleration.
      i. Injuries
         (a) Ankle sprains and fractures: These occur as the foot is forced into extreme plantarflexion upon impact with the base.
         (b) Knee injuries (medial and lateral collateral ligaments)
2. **Prevention of sliding injuries**
   a. Make sliding illegal: Players usually object.
   b. Low-profile bases: Reduces injuries caused by terminal impact with the base. However, often players overshoot the base and are thrown out when attempting to scramble back to base.
   c. Break-away bases (Roger's base, Fig. 1)
      i. Significantly decrease the number of sliding injuries
      ii. Mechanism

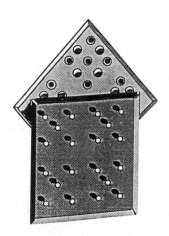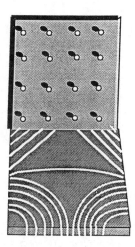

FIGURE 1.   The Roger's break-away base.

        (a) Base breaks away or releases with a pre-set amount of force, and this decreases injuries associated with terminal impact.

        (b) Youth, teen, adult, and professional models are available.

      iii. Cost: $400–$500

B. **Collision-related injuries**
  1. **Mechanism:** The player collides with a ball, fixed object, or another player.
  2. **Injuries:** Vary from minor injuries to long-bone fractures and head injuries.
  3. **Prevention**
    a. Batting helmets
    b. Proper coaching
    c. Discourage intentional blocking of the runner's path
    d. Pad fixed objects such as the backstop and outfield walls and fences.

C. **Fall-related injuries**
  1. Mechanism: Results from poorly groomed playing fields; litter, holes, etc.
  2. Injuries: Vary from minor injuries to serious fractures.
  3. Prevention: Careful examination of the entire playing field prior to the start of the game.

D. **Other injuries:** These consist of injuries sustained to the muscles and ligaments, *usually* as a result of limited flexibility or poor conditioning.
  1. **Overstretching of breast ligaments** can be prevented by a proper-fitting sports bra.
  2. **Muscle pulls:** Various body movements and maneuvers executed in softball include sprinting, hurdling, sliding, jumping, throwing, and side lunging.
    a. Injuries: Muscle pulls (hamstring, quadriceps, etc.)
    b. Prevention: Pregame stretching and warm-up period. Sport-specific tasks, i.e., throwing, sprinting, etc.
    c. A 5-minute unassisted preventative stretching program (Fig. 2).

II. SOFTBALL PITCHERS AND THE WINDMILL FAST-PITCH

Contrary to popular belief, underhand fast pitching does not protect the pitcher from arm- and shoulder-related injuries, but rather presents a new set of potential injuries to examine.

A. **Mechanics of the fast-pitch windmill delivery** (Fig. 3): Little is really known about the fast-pitch underhand delivery, as compared to the standard baseball pitch. The former, however, can be divided into four phases: early windup, windup, ball release, and follow-through.

The Shoulder Girdle Muscles

- Trapezius
- Levator scapulae
- Rhomboids

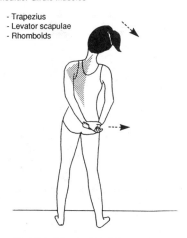

Stretching of the shoulder girdle musculature.

The Lateral Trunk Muscles

a. Quadratus lumborum
b. Tensor Fasciae Latae

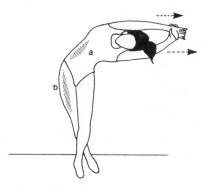

Stretching of the lateral trunk musculature.

The Medial Thigh Muscles

The Adductor group
- Adductor longus
- Adductor magnus
- Adductor brevis

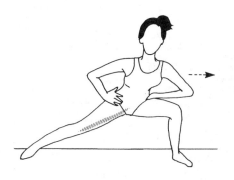

Stretching of the medial thigh musculature.

The Anterior Thigh Muscles

- Rectus Femoris
- Vastus medialis
- Vastus intermedius
- Vastus lateralis

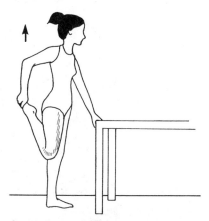

Stretching of the anterior thigh musculature - collectively known as the quadraceps.

FIGURE 2.   Preventive stretching program for pregame warm-up.

Calf Muscles

- Gastrocnemius
- Soleus

The Anterior Hip Muscles

- Iliacus
- Psoas

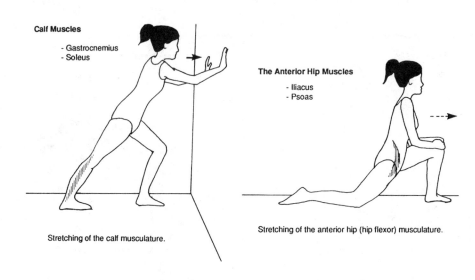

Stretching of the calf musculature.

Stretching of the anterior hip (hip flexor) musculature.

The Posterior Thigh Muscles

- Semitendinosis
- Semimembranosus
- Biceps femoris

a

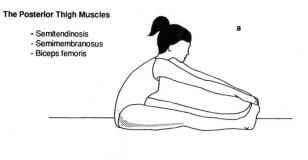

b

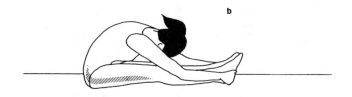

Stretching of the posterior thigh musculature - collectively known as the hamstrings.

a. partial stretch
b. maximal stretch

FIGURE 2. *(Cont.)*

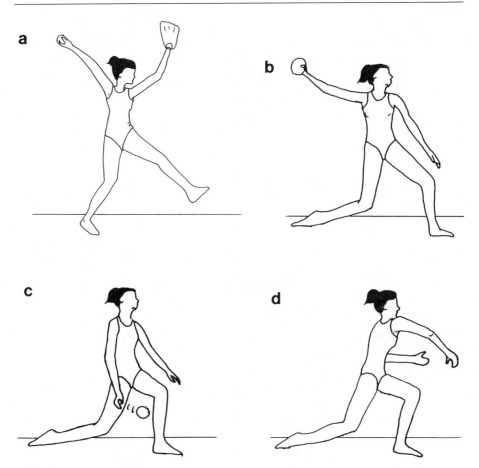

FIGURE 3. Four phases of the windmill pitch: a, early windup; b, windup; c, release; d, follow-through.

1. **Early windup** (Fig. 3A): Shoulder is maximally extended and internally rotated.
2. **Windup** (Fig. 3B): Elbow is slightly flexed and the forearm supinated.
3. **Ball release** (Fig. 3C): Wrist is dorsiflexed and forearm supinated.
4. **Follow-through** (Fig. 3D): Rapid arm deceleration. Forearm progresses from supination to maximal pronation.

B. **Injuries to pitchers**
   1. **Overuse injuries**
      a. Bicipital tendinitis
      b. Trapezius strain
      c. Rotator cuff injuries
      d. Fatigue/stress fractures of the ulna: Usually only found in elite pitchers. Results from tortional stress across the ulna during follow-through as the forearm goes from supination to maximal pronation. Bone scanning may be necessary to elucidate a hairline fracture of the ulna in a pitcher with persistant swelling or tenderness over the forearm or with painful pronation/supination.
   2. **Treatment**
      a. Limit innings pitched
      b. Proper coaching
      c. Rest, ice, nonsteroidal antiinflammatory drugs (NSAIDs)

III. SUMMARY

Inevitably, there will always be injuries in competitive sporting activities such as women's softball. However, prevention of a majority of injuries can be accomplished by proper coaching techniques, good flexibility and physical conditioning, limiting alcohol intake, the use of break-away bases and batting helmets, and careful inspection of the playing field prior to the start of each game.

REFERENCES

1. Duff JF: Youth Sports Injuries. New York, Macmillan, 1992, pp 233–235.
2. Eisenberg M, Allen WC: Injuries in a women's varsity athletic program. Phys SportsMed 6:112–120, 1978.
3. Gillette J: What kind of injuries occur in women's athletics? Schol Coach 1(2):51–52, 1976.
4. Janda DH, Wilde DE, Hensinger RN: Softball injuries: Aetiology and prevention. Sports Med 13(4):285–291, 1992.
5. Janda DH, Wojtys EM, Hankin FM, et al: A three phase analysis of the prevention of recreational softball injuries. Am J Sports Med 18:632–635, 1990.
6. Loosli AR, Requa RK, Garrich JG, et al: Injuries to pitchers in women's collegiate fast-pitch softball. Am J Sports Med 20:35–37, 1992.
7. Nadeau MT, Brown T: The prevention of softball injuries: The experience at Yokota. Milit Med 155:3–5, 1990.
8. Spring H, Illi U, Kunz HR, et al: Stretching and Strengthening Exercises. New York, Theime, 1991, pp 13–23.
9. Tanabe S, Nakahira J, Bando E, et al: Fatigue fracture of the ulna occurring in pitchers of fast-pitch softball. Am J Sports Med 19(3):317–321, 1991.
10. Whiteside PA: Men's and women's injuries in comparable sports. Phys SportsMed 8(3):130–140, 1980.

Chapter 60: Basketball

LISA STROUD KRIVICKAS, MD

Basketball is enjoyed by girls and women of all ages from grade school to the professional level. Most participants are age 10–22. Basketball is one of the few contact sports in which women participate. As a contact sport, injuries are incurred by contact with other players, the floor, walls, and bleachers. Data from the NCAA Women's Basketball Injury Surveillance System (1988–93) show that 51% of injuries involved contact, most frequently with another player. Female basketball players, especially those on highly competitive high school and college teams that train virtually year round, sustain a large number of overuse injuries, particularly to the lower extremities. In general, female basketball players sustain injuries to the same anatomic areas as their male counterparts; however, the percentage of sprains and strains is much higher. This chapter focuses on the most frequent medical and orthopedic problems of female basketball players and on those problems which are most easily prevented by proper training and rehabilitation—the overuse syndromes and recurrent injuries.

I. EPIDEMIOLOGY

- A. **Injury rate** (percent participants injured per season of play)
    1. **Youth programs:** Low, in one program 13.5% for girls aged 5–12 years, 6.2% for boys.[6]
        - a. Injury definition: Any problem requiring first aid or injury assessment.
        - b. Only 2.4% lost playing time because of injury.
        - c. Average playing time was 1.27 hr/week
    2. **High school:** 25% for girls vs 31% for boys in same schools[4]
        - a. Injury definition: Medical problem causing a participant to be withdrawn from a practice or competitive event.
        - b. Injury rate was 16% in competitions, 9% in practices.
    3. **College**
        - a. 2.5 injuries/1000 athlete exposures (20%) in study of 20 female college teams.[1]
        - b. NCAA surveillance data (1988–93) show 5.1 injuries/1000 athlete exposures
            - i. Third highest injury rate for a women's sport after gymnastics and soccer.
            - ii. Injury rate slightly higher for male basketball players (5.6 injuries/1000 exposures).
            - iii. NCAA injury definition: Medical problem resulting in restriction of activity for 1 or more days beyond the day of injury.
            - iv. Injury rate was 4.1% for practice, 8.8% for games.
    4. **Elite/professional**
        - a. 2.85 injuries/1000 hr of activity, 62% among elite Swedish players[2]
            - i. Injury definition: Problem resulting in absence from one game or practice.
        - b. 51.2 injuries/1000 exposures in American professional women's league[17]
            - i. 60% higher rate than for male professionals[19]
            - ii. Injury definition: Any trauma or illness evaluated by the trainer or physician; absence from practice or game not required.
        - c. Difference in definition of injury accounts for much higher injury rate in American study versus Swedish study.
    5. Roughly twice as many injuries per exposure in games as in practice sessions.
    6. In both games and practice, twice as many injuries occur in second half as in first half of session.

B. **Injury location**

	NCAA (1992–93 data)	Swedish elite players
Lower extremity	72%	96%
Ankle	26	56*
Knee	19	17
Foot	—	8
Achilles tendon	—	4
Upper extremity	13	—
Head and neck	8	—
Back and trunk	6	—

* 20% of Swedish players had recurrent ankle sprains.

C. **Injury type**

	Youth program	NCAA (1992–93 data)
Contusion	36%	8%
Sprain	28*	39
Strain	—	19
Epistaxis	13	—
Laceration	5	—
Tendinitis/tenosynovitis	—	5
Acute fracture	3 (finger)	3
Concussion	—	3
Joint dislocation	—	3
Stress fracture	—	2

* Strains and sprains combined.

D. **Injury severity**
  1. NCAA injury surveillance system (1988–93)
     a. 44% caused 1–2 days to be lost from play
     b. 22% caused >10 days to be lost
     c. No catastrophic or fatal injuries
     d. 7% required surgery
  2. Swedish elite players
     a. 20% severe (resulted in >4 weeks absence from training or games)
     b. 38% of knee and 12% of ankle injuries severe

II. **MEDICAL PROBLEMS**

There are no medical problems that are specific to female basketball players. Unlike female athletes in other sports where low body weight is advantageous, female basketball players do not have a higher prevalence of eating disorders or menstrual irregularities than found among the general population.

III. **SPECIFIC INJURIES**

A. **Head**
  1. **Concussion:** Traumatically induced alteration in mental status; does not require loss of consciousness.
     a. Multiple mild head injuries can cause cerebral hyperemia (brain swelling secondary to vascular engorgement).
     b. Assess mental status: orientation, attention, concentration, short-term memory. Have the player perform push-ups or sit-ups (Valsalva maneuver increases intracranial pressure) on the side-line to elicit symptoms.
     c. **Severity**—Colorado guidelines[10]
        i. Grade 1: Confusion, no amnesia. May return to play after the player is asymptomatic for 20 min.

      ii. Grade 2: No loss of consciousness, confusion and amnesia <24 hr. May play after asymptomatic for 1 week.

      iii. Grade 3 and Grade 4: Loss of consciousness. Requires hospital evaluation and head CT or MRI. No play for 1 month; return to play when asymptomatic for 2 weeks.

      iv. Terminate season if a recurrent Grade 3 or greater concussion occurs because of risk of second-impact syndrome.

    d. **Post-concussive syndrome:** Symptoms include recurrent headaches (migraine, tension, or cluster type) and dizziness, especially with exertion; irritability, fatigue, personality changes, memory and concentration deficits, decreased work performance and/or social functioning.

2. **Eye**

    a. Basketball is estimated to cause 7500 eye injuries/year in the U.S.

    b. Of 202 consecutive sports eye injuries seen by one ophthalmologist,[11] the highest percentage were caused by basketball (29%). Fourteen percent required hospitalization; 6% required surgery; 3.5% resulted in permanent visual loss (acuity <20/400 in 4 patients, <20/50 in others).

    c. **Injuries** include:

      i. Corneal abrasions and tears

      ii. Orbital contusions

      iii. Hyphema

      iv. Posterior segment hemorrhage

      v. Lens dislocation

    d. **Orbital blowout fractures:** Caused by anterior blow to orbit by nonpenetrating object (fist or ball).

      i. Orbital contents displaced posteriorly through medial wall or floor of orbit resulting in enopthalmos, diplopia, and subconjunctival hemorrhage.

      ii. Surgical referral necessary.

    e. **Optic nerve avulsion:** Caused by a finger-poke has been reported in a basketball player; little external damage present. Test acuity in each eye individually.

    f. **Commercial eye protectors:** Designed specifically for basketball, so that force of impact is redistributed to the anterior orbital bones. Polycarbonate lenses are 7 times stronger than any other lens material.

    g. Most eye injuries occur in children, who are least likely to wear protectors.

3. **Dental/oral**

    a. Injuries include tooth avulsion and fracture, alveolar bone fracture, tongue and lip lacerations.

    b. Nearly 100% of injuries preventable if all players wear mouthguards. Custom-fitted intraoral mouthguards constructed by dentists are made of clear plastic laminate and allow the player to speak and drink.

B. **Low back pain**

1. **Muscle strain**

    a. Most common cause of low back pain in adult female basketball players. Caused by a combination of jumping and rotation.

    b. May be acute or chronic. Pain or numbness will not radiate below buttock. Loss of lumbar range of motion due to muscle spasm.

2. **Herniated nucleus pulposus**

    a. Acute injury to L4–5 or L5–S1 discs most common, with compression of L5 and S1 nerve roots, respectively. Pain radiates below the ankle.

    b. On examination, look for extensor hallucis longus weakness (L5) or poor endurance with toe rise on affected leg (S1), dermatomal sensory loss, decreased medial hamstring (L5) or ankle (S1) reflex, positive straight-leg-raising test in 30–70° range.

3. **Facet syndrome**
   a. Low back pain radiates to the posterior buttock and thigh but not below the knee.
   b. Normal neurologic examination and negative straight-leg-raising test.
   c. Pain relieved by ambulation and worsened by hyperextension.
4. **Spondylolysis:** Fracture through pars interarticularis which may be acute or chronic.
   a. Most common in 10–15 year olds.
   b. Unilateral or bilateral pain which localizes to paraspinal muscles, exacerbated by hyperextension and rotation, especially with single-leg stance.
   c. When fracture is acute with positive bone scan, treat with rigid lumbosacral brace to promote fracture healing. Patient may come out of brace for flexibility and conditioning exercises and may play in brace as long as she remains pain-free.
5. **Spinal stenosis**
   a. Presents as intermittent low back pain with occasional radicular distribution.
   b. Pain relieved by lumbosacral flexion and sitting.
   c. Rare in young female athletes.
6. **Back rehabilitation program**
   a. **Pain-control phase**
      i. Limit activity producing pain.
      ii. If pain is severe, bedrest up to 48 hours.
      iii. Ice and nonsteroidal antiinflammatory drugs (NSAIDs).
   b. **Exercise training phase**
      i. Abdominal and pelvic-strengthening exercises.
      ii. Lumbar extension exercises if pain not aggravated.
      iii. Lower-extremity flexibility exercises emphasizing hamstrings. Also stretch quadriceps, iliopsoas, gastrocsoleus, hip internal and external rotators.
      iv. Improve body biomechanics.
      v. Stabilization training so that athlete can maintain neutral spine position that decreases radicular pain.

C. **Upper extremity**
   1. **Shoulder**
      a. **Rotator cuff:** Inflammation and/or impingement may occur as a result of repetitive shooting and overhead activities.
         i. Limit aggravating activities.
         ii. Stretch and strengthen rotator cuff in internal and external rotation.
      b. **Acromioclavicular joint separation:** Occurs traumatically from contact with other players or floor, often from a fall onto the point of the shoulder.
         i. Usually treated nonoperatively; a sling can be worn until pain subsides with grade I or II and for 6 weeks with a grade III.
         ii. Maintain shoulder strength, but avoid exercises that stress acromioclavicular joint (bench press, push-up) during period of healing.
   2. **Elbow**
      a. **Little leaguer's elbow:** Reported in young boys as a result of repetitive shooting and is likely also to occur in girls.
         i. Patients present with medial elbow pain, increased valgus carrying angle, and flexion contractures. Fragmentation of medial epicondyle, trochlea, and olecranon can occur. Most serious injury is osteochondritis dissecans of capitellum, radial head, or both.
         ii. Treatment is avoidance of shooting, arthroscopic removal of loose bodies, and exercises to stretch flexion contracture.
   3. **Wrist and hand:** Most injuries caused by fall on outstretched arm.
      a. **Colles' fracture**

      i. Posterior displacement of distal fragment of radius. May be intra- or extra-articular. May also involve the ulna.

      ii. Closed reduction and casting must achieve and maintain near-anatomic reduction.

  b. **Scaphoid fracture**

      i. Pain in anatomic snuffbox. Need high index of suspicion to make diagnosis.

      ii. If initial radiographs are negative, place in thumb spica cast and repeat radiograph in 10–14 days or obtain bone scan.

      iii. High risk of nonunion and/or avascular necrosis.

      iv. Nondisplaced fractures require long periods of immobilization (at least 8–12 weeks).

      v. Displaced fractures require reduction and internal fixation.

  c. **Wrist sprain**

      i. A rare diagnosis of exclusion.

      ii. Radiograph to rule out fracture; should include stress views. Multiple ligaments may be involved.

      iii. Minimum of 6 weeks' immobilization or surgical repair required for acute instability.

4. **Finger**

  a. Radiographs are the only way to differentiate a significant fracture requiring operative treatment from a minor sprain.

  b. **Proximal interphalangeal joint (PIP) dislocation**

      i. **Dorsal dislocation** most common. Due to hyperextension.

        (a) Perform closed reduction.

        (b) Protective splinting prevents further injury and may facilitate return to play. Splint in 15–30° flexion if volar plate tear suspected.

        (c) Need early range-of-motion exercises to prevent stiffness which can be a major problem.

      ii. **Volar dislocation:** Results from hyperflexion and can cause tear of central slip and **boutonnière deformity** with hyperflexion of PIP and extension of distal interphalangeal joint (DIP).

        (a) Palpate for tenderness over central slip insertion site on proximal middle phalanx.

        (b) Splint PIP in extension 6 weeks.

  c. **Flexor digitorum profundus avulsion** (jersey finger): Caused by catching finger on another player's uniform.

      i. Either tendon or tendon and bone is avulsed from insertion on distal phalanx.

      ii. Must test isolated DIP joint flexion to diagnose.

      iii. Requires operative repair to prevent loss of flexion.

  d. **Mallet finger:** Extensor tendon rupture or avulsion from distal phalanx resulting in loss of DIP extension. Injury mechanism is forced hyperflexion of joint.

      i. Immobilize DIP in extension 6 weeks; extension must be maintained at all times, even when splint is changed.

      ii. Dorsal splints are more functional than volar. Finger casts may also be used.

      iii. PIP should be actively exercised.

D. **Lower extremity**

1. **Quadriceps or hamstrings contusion**

  a. Aggressive icing: 20 minutes 4 times per day; contrast baths.

  b. Observe for development of compartment syndrome in the first 24 hours.

  c. Compress with elastic wrap; immobilize muscle in lengthened position for up to 48 hours if severe injury.

d. Regaining full range of motion important in preventing future injuries and in preventing myositis ossificans.

e. NSAIDs

f. Begin strengthening once full range of motion is regained.

2. **Knee**

   a. **Anterior cruciate ligament (ACL)**

      i. Higher **incidence** of injury in women's than men's basketball.

         (a) A survey showed 72% of referrals of female players were for knee problems, 25% for ACL tears (19/76 injuries), vs 2.6% for ACL tears (4/151 injuries) in male players.[5]

         (b) 1988 U.S. Olympic trials: 8 of 64 (12%) female players had undergone ACL reconstruction vs. 2 of 88 (2%) male players.

         (c) NCAA Injury Surveillance System 1989–90 data for basketball shows 50 ACL injuries in women vs. only 7 in men, an 8-fold higher injury rate in women.

      ii. **Mechanism**[5]

         (a) 58% landing from jump (centers)

         (b) 38% pivoting (guards)

         (c) 4% player knocked down

      iii. **Treatment**

         (a) Older, less-active individuals may function well with conservative management of an isolated ACL tear. Knee is most likely to give way during pivoting actions; this can cause meniscal injury.

         (b) Instability, timeframe for return to play, and player's future goals must be considered in deciding on nonoperative vs operative treatment.

         (c) Hamstring strengthening to restrain anterior tibial translation is the cornerstone of rehabilitation program.

      iv. **Bracing:** Controversial

         (a) Functional braces have not been shown to protect the knee from reinjury but may make athlete more cautious and decrease the frequency of giving-way episodes.

         (b) Anterior translation and external rotation of tibia are decreased only with subphysiologic loads.

         (c) Increased energy utilization with brace.

         (d) No effect on proprioception.

   b. **Collateral ligaments:** Nonoperative treatment for isolated medial (MCL) and lateral collateral ligament (LCL) injuries of all grades.

      i. Rehabilitation program should stress early protected mobilization (tend to lose extension with MCL tear), quadriceps and hamstring strengthening.

      ii. Rehabilitation brace to protect knee with MCL injury from valgus stress during period of healing. Functional braces have not been shown to reduce injury or reinjury incidence.

      iii. Often accompanied by other injuries. Triad of O'Donoghue includes MCL tear, ACL tear, medial meniscus injury. Patient usually requires ACL reconstruction for instability.

   c. **Meniscal tears**

      i. If suspected based on physical examination, use MRI to make specific diagnosis and delineate treatment plan.

      ii. Some peripheral, partial thickness, nondisplaced tears will heal spontaneously, and patients do well with functional rehabilitation program; on examination, these patients have tenderness for <1 cm along joint line.

      iii. Locking, loss of range of motion, and recurrent effusions are surgical indications.

   iv. Peripheral tears, especially in young athletes, can be repaired arthroscopically; otherwise, arthroscopic partial menisectomy relieves symptoms.

d. **Overuse syndromes:** Result from repetitive microtrauma.

   i. Overuse injuries are the most persistent and most preventable type of injury.

   ii. General etiologic factors include rapid increase in training volume, change in technique, change in footwear, lack of adequate flexibility, muscle weakness, and lower extremity malalignment.

   iii. Female basketball players are at high risk because they typically have very poor flexibility and do not incorporate stretching into their training program.

   iv. **Patellofemoral pain syndrome**

     (a) Symptoms: anterior knee pain, pain with prolonged sitting with knees flexed, pain with ascending or descending stairs, subjective feeling of swelling, giving-way secondary to pain-induced quadriceps inhibition.

     (b) Predisposing factors:

       (i) Biomechanical malalignment: increased femoral anteversion, increased Q-angle, foot pronation.

       (ii) Iliotibial band tightness: places stretch on lateral retinaculum; clinically see positive Ober test and weak hip abductors.

       (iii) Rectus femoris tightness: increases patellofemoral contact pressures.

       (iv) Hamstring tightness: increases demand on quadriceps resulting in increased patellofemoral contact pressures.

       (v) Gastrocsoleus tightness: encourages pronation.

       (vi) Quadriceps weakness, especially vastus medialis.

       (vii) Prior history of trauma or immobilization.

   v. **Jumper's knee:** Insertional tendinopathy with pathology at oseotendinous junction in skeletally mature athletes, apophysitis in skeletally immature athletes.

     (a) Location: 65% insertion of patellar ligament into inferior pole of patella, 25% quadriceps tendon insertion into superior pole of patella, 10% patellar ligament insertion into tibial tubercle.

     (b) Predisposing factors: Repetitive jumping, hard playing surface (concrete vs. wood), and thigh muscle tightness and weakness as with patellofemoral pain.

     (c) End-stage, untreated jumper's knee can result in patellar ligament or quadriceps tendon rupture.

   vi. **Traction apophysitis:** Occurs in skeletally immature athletes at sites of growth cartilage, or apophyses. Peak incidence is at time of growth spurt because strength and flexibility of muscles have not caught up to increase in bone length. In addition, the apophysis may be relatively weak. Same predisposing factors as for jumper's knee.

     (a) **Osgood-Schlatter disease:** Apophysitis at tibial tubercle. Pain can persist into adulthood if problem is neglected and free ossicles form. Treatment is surgical removal of ossicles.

     (b) **Sinding-Larsen-Johansson syndrome:** Traction on apophysis at inferior pole of patella.

     (c) **Quadriceps tendon avulsion:** Apophysitis at superior pole of patella.

   vii. **Iliotibial band friction syndrome:** Posterolateral knee pain produced as knee extends from 30–0°. Tight iliotibial band passes over lateral femoral condyle, irritating underlying bursa.

     (a) Treatment is iliotibial band stretching and gluteus medius strengthening. Ice and NSAIDs useful for underlying bursitis.

viii. **Rehabilitation program** for patellofemoral pain, jumper's knee, and traction apophysitis
   (a) Modify activity until symptoms improve.
   (b) NSAIDs
   (c) Ice
   (d) **Flexibility program**
      (i) Iliotibial band: Should have negative Ober test.
      (ii) Rectus femoris: Lie prone, pull heel to buttock.
      (iii) Hamstrings: should be able to straight leg raise past 90° and have popliteal angle of $<10°$.
      (iv) Gastrocsoleus: Should be able to dorsiflex ankle to 15° with foot slightly supinated. Test with knee extended and flexed.
   (e) **Quadriceps strengthening:** Some practitioners advocate using only open kinetic chain exercises, some only closed chain exercises, and some a combination. Excellent results have been obtained with both methods, although closed kinetic chain exercises better simulate physiologic activity.
      (i) Open kinetic chain exercises: Isometric quad sets, straight leg raises with ankle weights (work up to 3 sets of 10 with 20% of body weight), short arc knee extensions (0–30°).
      (ii) Closed kinetic chain exercises: Squats from 0–45° of knee flexion; static squatting at 30° of knee flexion with a ball held between the thighs to strengthen the vastus medialis.
   (f) **Gluteus medius strengthening:** Gluteus medius weakness allows overpull by tensor fascia lata causing tightening of iliotibial band. Perform straight leg raise from side-lying position keeping hips extended.
   (g) **Basketball-specific drills:** Jumping eccentrically loads extensor mechanism. Rehabilitation program must involve eccentric strengthening.
      (i) New isokinetic machines have eccentric modes.
      (ii) Jumping drills can initially be done in pool to decrease stress; advance to shallower water and then land.
   (h) **Shoe** with good arch support.
   (i) **Bracing and orthotics:** May help alleviate symptoms, but mainstay of treatment is improving flexibility and strength.
      (i) Orthotic for hyperpronators
      (ii) Chopat strap for jumper's knee
      (iii) Lateral buttress brace for patellofemoral pain
      (iv) Protective pad over tibial tubercle for Osgood-Schlatter disease
3. **Leg**
  a. **"Shin splints"** are posteromedial tibial pain (inner distal two-thirds of tibia) due to medial tibial stress syndrome, stress fracture, or exertional compartment syndrome.
  b. **Medial tibial stress syndrome** (MTSS)
    i. **Symptoms:** 3–6 cm tender area on posterior medial edge of distal third of tibia. Most patients have pain with ankle plantar flexion and inversion against resistance.
    ii. **Etiology:** No single hypothesis has been scientifically proven.
      (a) Inflammation of attachment of posterior tibial muscle to tibia; however, muscle origin does not correspond anatomically with location of pain.
      (b) Microtrauma at origin of medial half of soleus (the main dynamic and static controller of ankle plantar flexion); again, this does not correspond anatomically to location of pain.
      (c) Periostitis of distal third of tibia; corresponds with pain location.
    iii. **Hyperpronation** a predisposing factor.

      iv. **Diagnosis:** Clinical examination and bone scan demonstrating increased uptake along posterior tibial cortex for >30% of length.

      v. **Treatment:** Rest, NSAIDs, heel cord stretching, orthotics for hyperpronators, temporary use of heel lift while heel cord is still tight.

  c. **Stress fractures and stress reactions**

      i. Occur when normal bone is subjected to excessive stress or abnormal bone is subjected to normal stresses (the former is most likely in regularly menstruating female athletes).

      ii. Predisposing factors: Overtraining, poor footwear, temporary inactivity, inadequate calcium intake, menstrual irregularities, decreased bone density, muscle fatigue (muscles shield bone from stress).

      iii. **Diagnosis:** Examination shows more induration, warmth, erythema, and point tenderness than with MTSS. Bone scan shows more focal uptake than with MTSS. As few as 10% of stress fractures or stress reactions with positive bone scans are apparent on plain films.

      iv. **Treatment**

        (a) Pain-free weight-bearing; cast may be needed for 1–2 weeks if this is not possible. An exception is true fractures in the middle-third of the tibia, which require functional fracture brace or cast until callus formation is seen on plain film (approx. 6 weeks).

        (b) Strengthen tibialis anterior and gastrocsoleus to unload tibia.

        (c) May return to play when pain and all physical signs (warmth, erythema) are gone. Begin an every-other-day practice schedule with cross-training on alternate days.

        (d) Pneumatic brace may allow earlier return to activity by compressing the leg and unloading the tibia.

  d. **Exertional compartment syndrome**

      i. Players complain of paresthesias and weakness in addition to pain. Onset of pain occurs at a fixed interval after beginning exercise and worsens throughout the session.

      ii. Very rare in posterior compartments; much more common in anterior and lateral compartments.

      iii. Diagnosis made by measurement of compartmental pressure.

4. **Ankle sprains:** Single most common injury in women's basketball, with a high degree of chronicity.

  a. **Epidemiology:** Study of 84 male varsity basketball players[15]; comparable data are not available for women, but one would expect similarities.

      i. 70% had a history of ankle sprain

      ii. 80% of those with sprains had a history of multiple sprains.

      iii. 32% of sprains results in >2 weeks lost from play.

      iv. 50% of sprains resulted in residual symptoms; 15% felt residual symptoms compromised playing ability.

      v. Swedish study[2] showed 20% recurrence rate among elite female players.

  b. **Lateral sprains:** 85% of sprains. Medial ligaments are stronger than their lateral counterparts. Shape of talus and longer fibula protect against medial (eversion) injuries.

	ATF ligament tear	CF ligament tear	Anterior drawer test	Talar tilt test
Grade I	Partial	None	—	—
Grade II	Complete	Partial	+	—
Grade III	Complete	Complete	+	+

ATF = anterior talofibular ligament; CF = calcaneofibular ligament.

    c. **O'Donoghue Classification** of lateral sprains:

    d. **Recurrent lateral sprains:** causes include inadequate rehabilitation, peroneal weakness (may be due to L5 radiculopathy), chronic laxity, peroneal tendon subluxation (demonstrate with resisted inversion).

    e. **Associated hidden injuries** (can be ruled out by a very careful physical examination and anteroposterior, lateral, and mortise-view radiographs)

        i. **"High ankle sprain"** involves partial tear of tibiofibular ligament (syndesmosis); takes 2–3 times longer to heal. Pain when distal fibula is squeezed toward tibia (or with maximal dorsiflexion) is suggestive.

        ii. **Osteochondral talar dome fracture:** Present in 6.5% of ankle sprains.[14] Can cause nonunion, avascular necrosis, long-term disability; osteoarthritis develops in 20–50% of cases.

           (a) Signs and symptoms (none pathognomonic) include tenderness at anterolateral or anteromedial ankle corners, effusion, decreased range of motion, pain with inversion or eversion, crepitus.

           (b) Radiographs may be negative with acute lesion; subchondral sclerosis and cyst formation seen with chronic lesions. Bone scan and MRI helpful in acute situation.

        iii. Malleolar or epiphyseal fracture

        iv. Maisonneuve fracture: deltoid ligament sprain, syndesmosis injury, and high fibula fracture. Mechanism is external rotation of the talus.

        v. Cuboid subluxation

        vi. Distal fibula avulsion fracture

        vii. Fifth metatarsal fracture

    f. **Acute treatment**

        i. **Grade I:** Ice, compression (Unna boot, cryocompression boot, tape, Aircast), elevation; begin range of motion immediately, weight-bearing as tolerated. High-volt electrical stimulation begun immediately can decrease edema. Can usually return to play in a few days.

        ii. **Grade II:** Same plan as for Grade I, but needs 7–14 days before return to play. If Grade II sprain still significantly painful at 7–10 days, repeat radiographs to look for bony pathology not initially visible, and place ankle in brace (Aircast or other rigid support).

        iii. **Grade III:** Aircast or other rigid brace for 1–3 weeks, advance to weight-bearing as tolerated.

    g. **Rehabilitation**

        i. The key to preventing recurrent and chronic sprains.

        ii. Early mobilization allows more rapid return to play.[2a]

        iii. Range of motion should be equal to that of uninvolved ankle in inversion, eversion, dorsiflexion, and plantar flexion. Stretching of gastrocsoleus should be emphasized.

        iv. Strengthening

           (a) **Peroneal strengthening program:** The cornerstone of rehabilitation of lateral sprains.

              (i) Patient lies on table on side of unaffected ankle with injured ankle hanging over edge of table (the lateral malleolus is facing up).

              (ii) Ankle is plantarflexed, and weights are hung from the foot. Evert ankle to lift the weights.

              (iii) Begin by lifting 3 lbs 25 times; weight should be increased by 3 lbs/week until 15 lbs can be lifted 25 times.

           (b) Toe rises and walking, heel walking.

           (c) Theraband can be used to strengthen invertors, evertors, and ankle dorsiflexion.

      v. Proprioception and coordination training: multiplanar wobble board (BAPS board).

     vi. Functional skills: jumping drills, running in patterns—circles, figure of eight, boxes, cariocas (travel sideways, alternately crossing trailing foot in front and behind leading foot).

  h. **Return to play**

      i. Strength and muscle endurance must equal uninjured ankle.

     ii. Must be able to complete jumping drills and running in patterns without feeling unstable.

    iii. Lace-up style or other functional brace may be used initially; player should be weaned as soon as possible.

    iv. Taping may increase proprioception but not stabilization; high-top shoes may work similarly. The combination of a hightop shoe and tape or brace increases resistance to inversion.[13a]

5. **Foot:** Most injuries are of the overuse type.

  a. **Stress fractures**

     i. **Diagnosis**

       (a) Point tenderness on examination surrounded by an area of diffuse pain.

       (b) Radiographs positive at 3–4 weeks for metaphyseal fractures, 4–6 weeks for diaphyseal fractures.

       (c) Technetium bone scan will be positive but is nonspecific.

       (d) MRI highly sensitive and specific but can confuse stress fracture with neoplasm.

     ii. **Forefoot**

       (a) Second and third metatarsal neck and shaft are most common sites, especially in those with Morton's foot (second toe longer than great toe).

       (b) **Jone's fracture:** Occurs in proximal fifth metatarsal within 1.5 cm distal to the tuberosity. Area of poor blood supply, and nonunion is frequent. Treat with cast and non-weight-bearing 6–8 weeks, until radiographic union. Internal fixation may allow elite players to return to play more quickly.

       (c) Tibial sesamoid in flexor hallucis brevis tendon.

    iii. **Midfoot: Navicular fractures** cause foot cramping and point tenderness over the navicular. Treat with non-weight-bearing cast for 6 weeks, then weight-bearing cast or cast-brace for 6 weeks.

    iv. **Hindfoot:** talar dome, calcaneus. Treat with non-weight-bearing 4–6 week minimum. Operative internal fixation if no healing with nonsurgical treatment.

  b. **Plantar fasciitis**

     i. Pain along medial plantar fascia and medial calcaneus.

     ii. Predisposed by heel-cord tightness and pronation.

    iii. **Treatment:** Rest until pain-free to palpation; ice, NSAIDs, heel pad, arch support. Adhesive taping using Low Dye Technique,[17] which decreases pronation, stabilizes first metatarsal head, and serves as a guide to determine whether orthotics will be beneficial.

    iv. **Rehabilitation and prevention:** Stretching of heel cord and foot intrinsics and extrinsics, posterior tibialis strengthening to slow hyperpronation, orthotics to prevent pronation.

  c. **Achilles tendinitis**

     i. Point tenderness, thickening and/or crepitus over tendon. Palpable defect present with partial rupture.

     ii. Treatment: Heel lift, stretching, orthotic for pronated or cavus foot.

d. **Traction apophysitis**
   i. **Sever's disease:** Posterior heel pain due to rapid growth and increased tightness of gastrocsoleus. Accompanied by weak ankle dorsiflexion. May also have calf atrophy from pain, inhibiting gastrocsoleus.
     (a) Treatment: Stretch gastrocsoleus and tibialis posterior (ankle dorsiflexion with inverted foot), strengthen ankle dorsiflexors by heel walking and gastrocsoleus by toe rises. Heel cup often gives immediate relief. Shoes should have adequate heel cushioning.
   ii. **Islen's disease:** Apophysitis at peroneus brevis insertion at base of fifth metatarsal. May develop insidiously or begin after an inversion injury.
     (a) Tenderness to palpation over peroneus brevis insertion, pain with resisted eversion and extreme plantar flexion, pain with inversion in some cases. Aggravated by running, jumping, and cutting movements.
     (b) Radiograph may show enlarged apophysis, irregular and fragmented ossification pattern.
     (c) Treatment: Decrease load until pain-free and nontender. Aircast may be helpful in acute situations. Standard ankle rehabilitation program emphasizing peroneal stretching and strengthening.
e. **Blisters**
   i. Occur early in the season. Most common on posterior heel, ball of foot, and toes.
   ii. Prevention
     (a) Proper shoe fit and double socks to pad the shoe and decrease friction between the skin and shoe.
     (b) Talcum powder to decrease moisture.
     (c) Adhesive tape or moleskin over site of previous blister.
   iii. Management
     (a) Aspirate, do not de-roof, apply topical antibiotic such as polysporin, and cover with occlusive dressing such as duoderm, *or*
     (b) Open, apply adherent like Tuf-Skin, and cover with moleskin.

IV. CONDITIONING
A. A year-round conditioning program emphasizing aerobic, anaerobic, strength, and flexibility training improves performance and may decrease injuries.
B. NCAA data show twice as many injuries during early preseason as any other time.
C. **Program components**
  1. **Anaerobic power:** Major performance skills in basketball are anaerobic. Training involves alternate work (5–60 s) and rest bouts at 90–100% VO_2max.
  2. **Aerobic power:** Allows continuous play for 1.5–2.5 hours; increases the anaerobic threshold. Train with continuous activity at 80% VO_2max for 20–30 minutes. 50–100% of aerobic capacity gained by training can be lost in 3–6 months of deconditioning; 2 sessions/week required for maintenance.
  3. **Muscular strength, power, and endurance:** Crucial for jumping, controlling rebounds, maintaining position. Protect from some injuries. Can maintain strength with 1 session/week.
  4. **Flexibility:** Main function is joint protection and injury prevention. Lost rapidly without regular stretching.
D. **Training cycle**
  1. **Off-season:** Emphasize low-to-moderate intensity aerobic conditioning (60–80% VO_2max) and low-intensity, high-volume strength training. Flexibility should be maintained throughout the entire cycle.
  2. **Transition to preseason:** Begin anaerobic threshold training at 80% of VO_2max or above.

3. **Preseason:** Decrease volume but increase intensity of aerobic and strength training. Increase anaerobic training volume and intensity. Monitor players closely for signs of overtraining (fatigue, muscle soreness, sluggishness, loss of appetite and weight).
4. **In-season:** Maintenance of strength (1 session/week) and aerobic power (2 sessions/week); both may be accomplished by circuit training. Maintain peak anaerobic pwoer; may be achieved via specific skill drills.

ACKNOWLEDGMENTS

The author thanks Joseph Feinberg, MD, and Angela Smith, MD, for their review of this chapter and their helpful suggestions.

REFERENCES

1. Clarke KS, Buckley WE: Women's injuries in collegiate sports. Am J Sports Med 8(3):187–191, 1980.
2. Colliander E, Eriksson E, Herkel M, Skold P: Injuries in Swedish elite basketball. Orthopedics 9:225–227, 1986.
2a. Eiff MP, Smith AT, Smith GE: Early mobilization vs. immobilization in the treatment of lateral ankle sprains. Am J Sports Med 22:83–88, 1994.
3. Eisele SA, Sammarco GJ: Fatigue fractures of the foot and ankle in the athlete. J Bone Joint Surg 75A:290–298, 1993.
4. Garrick JG, Requa RK: Girls' sports injuries in high school athletics. JAMA 239:2245–2248, 1978.
5. Gray J, Taunton JE, McKenzie DC, et al: A survey of injuries to the anterior cruciate ligament of the knee in female basketball players. Int J Sports Med 6:314–316, 1985.
6. Gutgesell ME: Safety of a preadolescent basketball program. Am J Dis Child 145:1023–1025, 1991.
7. Herskowitz A, Selesnick H: Back injuries in basketball players. Clin Sports Med 12:293–306, 1993.
8. Ireland ML, Wall C: Epidemiology and comparison of knee injuries in elite male and female United States basketball athletes. Med Sci Sports Exerc 22:582, 1990.
9. Jones DC, James SL: Overuse injuries of the lower extremity: Shin splints, iliotibial band friction syndrome, and exertional compartment syndromes. Clin Sports Med 6:273–290, 1987.
10. Kelly JP, Nichols JS, Filley CM, et al: Concussion in sports—Guidelines for prevention of catastrophic outcome. JAMA 266:2867–2869, 1991.
11. Larrison WI, Hersh PS, Kunzweiler T, Shingleton BJ: Sports-related ocular trauma. Ophthalmology 97:1265–1269, 1990.
12. Micheli LJ: The traction apophysitises. Clin Sports Med 6:389–404, 1987.
13. Posner MA: Hand injuries. In Nicholas JA, Hershman EB: The Upper Extremity in Sports Medicine. St. Louis, Mosby, 1990, pp 495–594.
13a. Shapiro MS, Kabo JM, Mitchell PW, et al: Ankle sprain prophylaxis: An analysis of the stabilizing effects of braces and tape. Am J Sports Med 22:78–82, 1994.
14. Shea MP, Manoli A: Recognizing talar dome lesions. Phys SportsMed 21(3):109–121, 1993.
15. Smith RW, Reischl SF: Treatment of ankle sprains in young athletes. Am J Sports Med 14:465–471, 1986.
16. Stone WJ, Steingard PM: Year-round conditioning for basketball. Clin Sports Med 12:173–191, 1993.
17. Torg JS, Pavlov H, Torg E: Overuse injuries in sport: The foot. Clin Sports Med 6:291–320, 1987.
18. Torg JS, Vegso JJ, Torg E: The ankle. In Torg JS, et al (eds): Rehabilitation of Athletic Injuries. Chicago, Yearbook Medical Publishers, 1987, pp 26–68.
19. Zelisko JA, Noble HB, Porter M: A comparison of men's and women's professional basketball injuries. Am J Sports Med 10:297–299, 1982.

Chapter 61: Soccer

MARGOT PUTUKIAN, MD

Soccer is the world's most popular sport, and although it has only recently captured the attention of the U.S., it is the country's fastest growing team sport. Women's soccer has shown the most dramatic accomplishments, with the U.S. winning the World Championship in China in 1991. The reasons for its appeal are multifaceted—limited equipment, low incidence of injuries, absence of specific body-type selection, continuous action, etc. At the elite level, the physical demands are great. Soccer is a high-intensity, noncontinuous sport which demands both endurance and quick sprints, ball skills, and coordination and balance. It requires constant decision-making, individual skills, and team tactics which are as varied as the players themselves. Yet, all individuals young and old can participate and be physically challenged. Given the low injury rate and absence of body-type selection, soccer is an ideal sport for children and adolescents. This chapter introduces aspects of soccer as they relate to sports medicine. With a better understanding of the sport-specific concerns of soccer, recommendations for sport-specific training, prevention of injuries, and increased enjoyment are possible.

I. PARTICIPANTS

Soccer is truly the "world's game," with more than 70 million players worldwide.
  A. **United States**
    1. 15 million kids <18 years old kicked a soccer ball at least once over the past year.
    2. 1.9 million <19 years old participate in organized soccer.
    3. There are 150,000 registered men and women players >18 years old, and the number is increasing.
  B. **Women's soccer**
    1. Played by girls and women in 50 countries.
    2. In many countries, it is the most popular female sport.

II. THE GAME

  A. **Outdoor soccer** (10 field players, 1 goalkeeper)
    1. In general, the 10 field players are divided into defenders, midfielders, and forwards, as one moves from one's own goal forward. Goalkeeper is the only player allowed to use her hands. Winner of game is the one to score the most goals.
    2. Two 45-minute halves. Play is continuous unless the ball goes out of play, goes into the goal, or a foul occurs, whereby a kick is awarded to the other team.
    3. When the ball goes over the end line, it is kicked back into play by either the defending team (goal kick) or offensive team (corner kick). When the ball goes over the sideline, it is thrown back into play (throw in).
  B. **Indoor soccer** (5 field players, 1 goalkeeper)
    1. Usually played inside a hockey rink, with artificial surface and goals flush with the back wall. Ball goes out of play less often because of walls surrounding the field; it is kicked in if it goes outside the rink.
    2. Played primarily in the United States.
  C. **Characteristics of play**
    1. **Field players**
      a. Involved in series of short or longer sprints.
      b. Receiving the ball with various surfaces of the body (head, chest, legs).

      c. Striking the ball with the lower extremity in various positions.

      d. Jumping up to head the ball

      e. Throwing the ball with both hands overhead back into play.

  2. **Goalkeepers**

      a. Only players allowed to use their hands.

      b. Leap into the air or dive at players' feet to keep the ball out of the goal.

      c. Extensive contact with opponents.

      d. Stopping or catching a ball that can travel as fast as 90–100 mph.

      e. Punting the ball, or throwing it in a hurling or sidearm motion to a teammate.

  3. In a **typical 90-minute match**, each player will:

      a. Cover 10–12 km, with 5–10 km spent in short 7–25 m sprints.

      b. Jump 1–15 times, head the ball on average 5 times/game.

      c. Contact the ball 45–115 times, possessing it for only 40–200 seconds.

      d. Exhibit many skills (shooting, passing, receiving the ball out of the air) that require standing on one foot, and thus good balance and proprioception.

III. PHYSIOLOGIC ADAPTATIONS IN SOCCER PLAYERS

Most information is based on boys and men, with little information regarding the female soccer player. Physical characteristics of soccer players reflect the combination of aerobic and anaerobic demands, as well as the strength required in the legs, neck, and trunk.

  A. **VO$_2$max**

    1. In sixth-grade boys, VO$_2$max after 9 weeks of soccer is 50.22 mL/kg/min.

    2. In Canadian national under-16 and under-18 boys, VO$_2$max is 58.3 ml/kg/min.

    3. In adult men, VO$_2$max typically is 10–20% above average, 56–65 ml/kg//min

    4. During game, average oxygen consumption is close to 80% VO$_2$max, at both professional and recreational level.

  B. **Percent body fat** (men)

    1. U.S. professional male players: 7.1%

    2. Canadian national youths (under-16, under-18): 8.0%

    3. Canadian Olympic players: 9.8%

    4. 1982 Kuwaiti World Cup team: 8.9% (midfielders 6.2%, goalkeepers 13%, rest in between)

  C. **Anaerobic power**

    1. Lactate levels: 8–12.8 mmol/L. Higher levels with higher level play.

    2. Anaerobic speed test (AST—where time to exhaustion is measured on a treadmill at a fixed velocity of 3.58 m/s and 20% grade): Canadian national soccer players, 92.5 s; alpine skiers, 76.9 s; elite 800-m sprinter, 114.3 s.

  D. **Pulmonary function:** Similarly enhanced. Forced vital capacity, 4.8–5.81 L.

  E. **Cardiovascular function**

    1. Heart rate: Often reaches 132–204 beats/min.

    2. Systolic blood pressure: 160–200 mmHg.

    3. Can develop increased left ventricular end-diastolic volume (LVED), increased left ventricular wall thickness (LVWT), as well as other characteristics of **"athlete's heart."**

      a. Italian Olympic soccer athletes[22]: LVED, 54.9 mm (normal, 40–52); LVWT, 9.9 mm (normal, 8–12); and LV mass index, 105 g/m^2 (normal, <134).

      b. "Athlete's heart" (Table 1) can be confused with pathologic conditions such as hypertrophic cardiomyopathy if the physician is not familiar with electrocardiographic (ECG), radiographic, and echocardiographic changes that represent the physiologic adaptations to physical training.

  F. **Musculoskeletal system**

    1. Athletes utilize entire body during play, relying on trunk and lower extremities.

    2. Goalkeeper utilizes upper extremities for dives, catching ball, and releasing it.

TABLE 1.   Changes Seen in Athlete's Heart

ECG changes

Bradycardia and sinus pauses	Correlated to training level
First- and second-degree alpha block	Usually reverse with exercise
Incomplete right bundle branch block	One of most frequent changes
Left ventricular hypertrophy	Seen in 10–18% of athletes
Right ventricular hypertrophy	Seen in 18–69% of athletes
T negativity	Seen in up to 30% of athletes, reverses with exercise
ST peaks	Seen in 10–100% of athletes, regresses with inactivity, age-dependent

Radiographic changes

Increased cardiac silhouette	Not very sensitive
Increased pulmonary vasculature	Reflects increased pulmonary blood flow

Echocardiographic changes*

Increased left ventricular wall thickness
Increased left ventricular end-diastolic dimension
Increased ventricular septal thickness
Increased left ventricular mass and mass-index
Increased aortic root dimension
Increased left atrial dimension

* Although the ratio of septal to posterior wall thickness >1.3 has been used to differentiate hypertrophic cardiomyopathy from "normal," a more useful ratio is septal thickness to left ventricular end-systolic diameter (normal is <0.48).

3. Strength: Soccer players have increased measurements with isometric and isokinetic testing of both knee flexion and extension at various angular velocities. Vertical jump also higher than age-matched active controls.
4. Flexibility: One study revealed increased hip flexibility in Canadian soccer players compared to controls, but most other studies are to the contrary. Only 50% of senior-division soccer players had flexibility exercises in training programs.[6]

V. INCIDENCE OF INJURY

Data for injuries in soccer are difficult to compare because of differences in definitions of injury, age groups, and regular season as well as tournament play assessed. Little data are available in the U.S., particularly for girls and women and for indoor soccer.

A. **Injury definitions**
   1. Mild: <1 week lost from practice or play.
   2. Moderate: >1 week but <1 month lost from practice or play.
   3. Severe: >1 month lost from practice or play.
   4. Tables 2 and 3 summarize the incidence and type of injuries incurred.
B. **Female soccer injuries**
   1. Most studies including females are less strict in their injury definition, but allow comparison to the incidence of injuries in males.
   2. The incidence of injuries for girls is almost twice as high as for boys (Table 4).
   3. Some studies claim that the increased rate of injuries in female soccer is due to less skill or training, but there is no scientific documentation. Leg alignment differences and strength deficits or imbalances have also been offered as possible explanations. Finally, there may be differences in the biomechanics of jumping in women vs. men, with women more often landing with the knee in extension, increasing the likelihood of anterior cruciate injuries.
   4. In one study of elite women's teams followed over a year, 88% of injuries occurred in the lower extremity, with ankle sprains and knee ligament sprains most common.[9]

TABLE 2. Incidence of Injuries in Soccer

Study	Population	Incidence of Injury
Backous et al., 1988[2]	Soccer camp: 681 M/458 F, age 6–17 yrs	10.6/1000 hr in males 7.3/1000 hr in females
McCarroll et al., 1984[18]	14-month season: 253 teams, M + F, age 8–18 yrs	176 injuries (4.38%), with incidence increasing with age
Ekstrand, Gillquist, 1983[5]	1-year season: 180 male players, age 17–38 yrs	0.88 mild injuries/player 0.38 moderate injuries/player 0.16 major injuries/player (69% traumatic, 31% overuse)
Nielsen, Yde, 1989[20]	10-month season, Danish teams: 34 male division players (>18 yrs) 59 male lower-senior (>18 yrs) 30 youth (16–18 yrs)	 18.5/1000 in games; 2.3/1000 in practice 11.9/1000 in games; 5.6/1000 in practice 14.4/1000 in games; 3.6/1000 in practice
Engstrom et al., 1991[9]	2 elite Swedish teams: Female, age 21–35 yrs	24/1000 in games; 7.0/1000 in practice (49% minor, 36% moderate, 15% major)
Putukian et al., 1994[23a]	402 Men's Open 155 Women's Open 169 Over 30 min 101 Coed	1.45/1000 hrs* 1.96/1000 hrs 1.64/1000 hrs 1.80/1000 hrs

* Injury defined as time lost from play.

    a. Of the 12 severe injuries, 10 were trauma-induced and 7 involved knee ligaments or menisci.
    b. 72% of injuries were traumatic, 28% overuse injuries, 22% were re-injuries.
    c. Major knee ligament injuries in 17%, or 1 in 6 athletes.
    d. This study had very low numbers, making conclusions questionable, but it does raise concern and indicates that more research is badly needed.
  C. **Indoor soccer injuries:** Few data are available.
    1. Hoff and Martin[11] found 4.5 times more injuries in indoor soccer vs outdoor.
      a. Most injuries secondary to collision, with injury defined as any problem requiring medical attention as well as time lost from play.
    2. Albert found the incidence of injury higher in outdoor soccer than indoor—1.45 vs 0.8 injuries/player, respectively (did not assess injury/playing hour).
    3. Putukian et al.[23a] looked at the incidence of injury during a 3-day Indoor Tournament at Lake Placid, New York. There were only 38 injuries where time was lost from play for men, during a total of 7955 minutes of play. The kinds of injuries that occurred were very similar to those in outdoor soccer, with lower extremity injuries accounting for most (76.6%) injuries, and ankle sprains and knee sprains predominating the severe injuries. 65% of the injuries were mild, 44% were contact injuries, and in 46% of injuries a history of preexisting injury was given.

TABLE 3. Types of Injuries in Soccer (%)

	Lower Extremity	Contusion	Strain	Sprain	Fracture/ Dislocation	Tendinitis
Backous et al.[2]	70.8	35.2	27.8	19.4	2.0	—
McCarroll et al.[18]	80.2	11.4	6.8	20.5	12.0	9.0
Ekstrand, Gillquist[5]	88.0	20.0	18.0	29.0	6.0	23.0
Nielsen, Yde[20]	4.0	9.2	21.1	48.6	5.9	9.2
Engstrom et al.[9]	88.0	15.0	10.0	33.0	4.0	24.0
Putukian et al.[23a]	76.6	21.1	10.5	44.7	7.9	5.3

TABLE 4. Incidence of Injury (per 1000 playing hours) in Boys vs. Girls

	Boys	Girls
Engstrom et al., 1991[9]*	5	12
Nilsson and Roaas, 1978[19]	14	32
Maehlum et al., 1986	8.9	17.6
Schmidt-Olsen et al., 1985[29]	7.4	17.6
Sullivan et al., 1980[33]*	0.5	1.1

* Definition of injury = time lost from play. Other studies uses different definitions for injury.

D. **General observations**
  1. Progressive decrease in injury rate with age below 18 years.
  2. Most injuries are mild, 20% the number of injuries seen in American football.
  3. More injuries occur in games than practice.
  4. Most injuries occur in the lower extremity, usually contusions and ankle sprains.
  5. Knee and ankle sprains account for most severe injuries.
  6. Use of shin pads markedly decreases the incidence of lower leg injuries.
  7. Upper extremity injuries occur more commonly in goalkeepers.
  8. Fractures more likely in upper extremity, resulting from fall on outstretched hand or direct impact.
  9. Maxillofacial and dental injuries account for up to 5% of injuries, usually the result of contact and occurring more commonly in goalkeepers. Mouthguards can reduce severity.
  10. Traumatic injuries often associated with foul play, with the player fouling more likely to be injured.
  11. Abrasions, lacerations, blisters, calluses, and nail problems are common, yet do not often result in time lost from play.

E. **Head injuries**
  1. Account for only 4–10% of injuries.
  2. Repetitive heading may result in similar condition to "punch drunk" syndrome seen in boxers.
  3. **Mechanism** of head injury
      a. Direct contact with the ball when the player heads the ball.
      b. Direct contact when the ball is forcefully kicked and strikes the head.
      c. Direct head-to-head or head-to-goalpost contact.
      d. Goalkeepers rarely head the ball, but have risks for head contact with opponent's body as well as goalpost and ground.
  4. Ball weighs 14–16 oz (396–453 g), pressure of 15 lb/in (1 kg/cm²)
  5. When kicked, the ball averages a speed of 52 mph and, at 10 m, strikes with impact of 116 kpm.
  6. Improper technique increases the impact of the ball.
      a. Better heading leads to prolonged contact with ball, resulting in decreased force of impact to head. In animal studies, the head being freely mobile results in increased concussive force. If the head is in extreme flexion or extension, concussion is increased.
      b. Important to teach proper technique and strengthen neck musculature. Use smaller ball for youngsters in whom musculature is not yet developed and technique being refined.
  7. Despite proper technique, concern still remains on long-term consequences of heading.
      a. CT scanning revealed central cerebral atrophy in one-third of Norwegian professional players (329 games at national, 29 games at international level). Occurs more likely in those considered to be "typical headers." Degree of damage is less than in boxing, yet still raises concern.

TABLE 5.   Common Injuries in Soccer Players

Achilles tendon rupture	Common major injury
Achilles tendon strain	Often associated with hard-sole shoe
Adductor strain	Common with inside-of-foot kick, block tackle
Ankle sprain	Most common injury in soccer
Anterior cruciate ligament (ACL) injury	Planted foot, acceleration and change
Anterior tibialis strain	Often early in season, running
Head injuries	Symptoms often delayed, mechanisms multiple
Iliopsoas strain	Can present with groin/abdominal pain
Iliotibial band friction syndrome	Common with outside-of-foot kick; assess leg-length discrepancy, oversupination
Low back strain	Assess pelvis and leg alignment, muscle flexibility
Medial collateral ligament (MCL) injury	Valgus stress
Meniscal tear	Twisting mechanism, often associated with ACL or MCL injury
Posterior cruciate ligament injury	Blow to anterior tibia with foot planted
Quadriceps contusion	Direct blow to quadriceps
Quadriceps strain	Often secondary to kicking
Sartorius strain	Often secondary to kicking
Skin, nail lesions (blisters, subungual hematoma)	Proper shoes helpful, avoid nail removal if possible
Turf toe	Associated with hyperextension of great toe

      b. EEG changes were seen in soccer players with acute or protracted complaints secondary to heading, some persisting months to years.[33]

   8. Symptoms of head injury are often mild: headache, nausea, confusion, dizziness, neck pain, irritability, insomnia, hearing or visual disturbances, weakened memory.

   9. Use of protective headgear is controversial. Most feel it is impractical for field players, though reasonable for goalkeepers. However, most injuries occur in field players. It is more practical to emphasize proper technique and to pad goalposts.

F. **Specific injuries**

Certain injuries appear to occur more frequently in soccer players because of the nature of the game (Table 5).

   1. **Contusions**

      a. Several surfaces of the body used to control the ball as well as to strike it. Thus, if the ball is incorrectly controlled, strikes forcibly, or if a player is struck by an opponent, the result is a contusion.

      b. Thigh contusion common. Can lead to myositis ossificans if not properly diagnosed and treated.

   2. **Overuse injuries**: If a new skill utilizing an unusual body position is practiced over and over, an overuse injury can result. There are many soccer-specific skills, which account for most injuries in soccer. Predominantly the lower extremities are affected.

      a. **Outside-of-foot pass or shot:** Entails plantar flexion and inversion of the foot and internal rotation of the hip (Fig. 1). Can lead to overuse of peroneal tendons, anterior tibialis, and iliotibial tract. Leg-length discrepancies and oversupination may predispose individuals to this injury.

      b. **Inside-of-foot pass:** Entails external rotation of the leg to almost 90° and foot dorsiflexion. The ball is struck over the area between the medial malleolus and navicular (Fig. 2). Can lead to overuse injuries of adductors and sartorius.

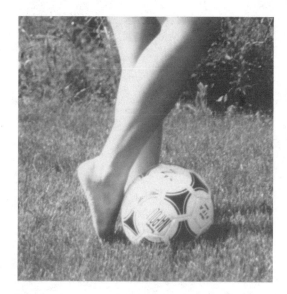

FIGURE 1. Outside-of-foot kick, showing plantarflexion and inversion of the foot as well as internal rotation of the hip. (Demonstrated bare-footed for clarity.)

c. **Block tackle:** Contact with inside-of-foot pass. Opposing players both strike the ball with the inside of the foot and weight over ball, in an attempt to win the ball. If done improperly with leg reaching out away from body, it can produce significant torque and valgus stress at the knee, leading to medial collateral and even anterior cruciate ligament injuries.

3. **Knee ligament injuries:** Screw-in cleats or other factors which increase the torque will increase the severity of these injuries.

a. **Anterior cruciate ligament injuries** are most feared and devastating. Mechanism in soccer is no different from other sports—acceleration and change in direction on planted foot.

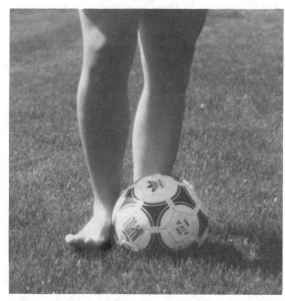

FIGURE 2. Inside-of-foot kick, showing external rotation of the hip, mild dorsiflexion, and ball contact between medial malleolus and navicular. Same technique also used in block tackle. (Demonstrated bare-footed for clarity.)

    b. **Medial collateral ligament injuries** result from valgus force.

    c. **Posterior cruciate injuries** result from a blow to the anterior tibia with planted foot.

    d. **Meniscal injuries** are common. Mechanism is often sudden twisting motions.

4. **Ankle/foot injuries:** Occur in soccer as they do in other sports which involve running, cutting, and sprinting.

    a. Achilles tendon injuries, quadricep and hamstring strains, anterior tibialis strains, stress syndromes, and ankle sprains.

    b. Ankle sprains are the most common injury in soccer. Mechanism and treatment are the same as for other sports.

G. **Heat injuries**

1. Soccer is often played in hot climates, and international tournament may not allow for acclimatization.

2. In the 1988 U.S.A. Cup Youth Soccer Tournaments, the number of heat-related injuries was decreased during the 6-day tournament by shortening playing periods, adding more water breaks, and adding more player substitutions.

3. Early signs of heat stress

    a. Nausea

    b. Irritability

    c. Headache

    d. Dizziness

    e. Confusion

    f. Cramping

    g. Fatigue

    h. Goosebumps

4. Predisposing factors

    a. Prepubertal age or age >50

    b. Dehydration

    c. Poor conditioning

    d. Previous history of heat injury

    e. Current or recent febrile illness

    f. Inadequate acclimatization.

5. Additionally, alcohol, diabetes, malnutrition, medications, and drugs can impair thermoregulatory function.

6. Maintain proper hydration prior to game, and allow for hydration every 15–20 minutes during activity.

H. **Cold injuries:** Soccer is also played in cold climates with risks of hypothermia.

1. Proper warm-up essential

2. Protective clothing

3. Adequate nutrition and hydration

VI. EVALUATING SOCCER INJURIES

A. **Intrinsic factors**

1. Leg alignment, leg-length discrepancy, foot alignment, and gait

2. Laxity, inherent or secondary to previous or preexisting injury

3. Age: Osgood-Schlatter disease, Sever's disease, and avulsion of growth plates are common in younger athletes.

4. Nutrition

5. Thermoregulation

6. Individual styles of play

7. Flexibility

8. Physical conditioning

9. Strength

B. **Extrinsic factors**
  1. **Proper equipment:** Proper footwear with good heel and arch support is essential.
     a. Many shoes are specific for indoor and outdoor soccer, including different grass surfaces (soft vs hard).
        i. Flat shoes are for indoor soccer and artificial turf.
        ii. Small multi-cleated shoes are used for artificial turf and hard natural grass surfaces.
        iii. Molded cleats are designed for soft natural grass surfaces.
        iv. Screw-in cleats are for very soft natural grass surfaces. Otherwise, these cleats tend to increase knee injuries.
     b. Heel confinement increases shock absorption at heel.
     c. Use of shin guards which cover malleoli significantly reduces number and severity of injuries.
  2. Playing surface
  3. Quality of supervision and referees
  4. Temperature, other weather conditions
  5. Movable goals: Between 1983 and 1991, 8 children died as a result of movable goals which fell on them. Goals should be anchored and children should not be allowed to hang from them or move them.
C. **Flexibility**
  1. Hamstring and groin strains can be reduced with implementation of 15-minute warm-up and stretching program before practices and games.
  2. In a prospective study of female collegiate athletes, flexibility and lower extremity strength imbalances of more than 15% were associated with a 2.6 times increase in the injury rate.[15]

VII. **INJURY PREVENTION**
  A. Ekstrand et al., in 1983, studied efficacy of injury prevention program.[6]
     1. Optimal shoes, shin guard required for practice and games
     2. Ankle taping for those with a history of ankle sprains or laxity on examination
     3. Exclusion of players with grave knee instability
     4. Structured warm-up followed by flexibility exercises prior to practice
     5. No shooting at the goal prior to warm-up
     6. Education of athletes regarding injuries and their association with foul play
     7. Close supervision and rehabilitation of injuries by physiotherapist and physician
  B. Implementation of the above program leads to a 75% reduction in injuries.

VIII. **NUTRITIONAL RECOMMENDATIONS**
  A. Recommendations geared toward mixture of aerobic and anaerobic demands that soccer entails.
     1. Muscle glycogen levels are invariably drained at the end of game. Leatt and Jacob showed increased muscle glycogen levels at post-game in soccer players if a glucose polymer was ingested before and during the match compared to placebo.
     2. Carbohydrate loading
     3. 300–500 ml of water 0–15 minutes before the game and 800–1600 ml/hr of a 6–8% carbohydrate solution with 10–20 mEq of sodium/L recommended during exercise.[10]
     4. Follow guidelines in the American College of Sports Medicine's position statement on fluid replacement, and those recently put forward by Sawka and Greenleaf.[28]

IX. **CONCLUSIONS**

Soccer is a sport which requires both aerobic and anaerobic work, individual ball control skills, coordination, balance, and team tactics. The demands it places on the cardiovascular and musculoskeletal systems can be immense, yet the injury rate is comparatively low.

TABLE 6. Guidelines for Successful Participation in Soccer

1. Preparticipation physical examination (PPPE): Focus on previous history of ankle sprains or knee injuries, and careful assessment for ligamentous laxity. Follow other guidelines for PPPE.*
2. Prophylactic taping or bracing for ankle laxity.
3. Further evaluation and strength testing for knee ligamentous laxity. Orthopedic consultation recommended.
4. Preseason cardiovascular training. Can be sport-specific with endurance and interval sprints incorporating ball skills (dribbling, juggling, feints and moves, passing partners).
5. Proper warm-up prior to all practices and games. Can be sport-specific with ball skills, gentle passing, dribbling.
6. Well-designed 15–20 minute flexibility program stressing adductors, hamstrings, quadriceps, gastrocsoleus complex, iliotibial tract, and trunk, upper extremity, and neck.
7. Flexibility program *after* warm-up or conclusion of practice.
8. Do not allow shooting at goal prior to warm-up or initiate practice with shooting drills.
9. Ensure adequate equipment including proper shoes and clothing suitable to weather conditions. Consider mouthguards.
10. Ensure use of protective shin guards.
11. Proper nutrition and hydration. Often, there is more success in advocating these if athletes know influences on performance.
12. Adequate strength of major muscle groups, primarily trunk, abdomen, and lower extremities.
13. Adequate strength of neck musculature for heading the ball.
14. Ensure proper technique for heading the ball.
15. Use a smaller ball for younger participants (sizes 3, 4)
16. Do not allow children to move goals.
17. Communication with parents and coaches prior to and throughout the season regarding methods to decrease injuries and treatment and rehabilitation of injuries when they occur.
18. Proper education of athletes regarding injuries and their prevention. Explain increased risk with fouling.
19. Proper supervision of practice sessions and games by trainer and physician when possible.

* See Putukian and McKeag.[23]

Nevertheless, soccer can be enjoyed by both young and old for its physical and mental challenges. It is important for physicians to be familiar with the physical demands that soccer entails and the types of soccer-specific skills that lead to common injuries. Preparticipation physical examination should closely assess the cardiovascular system (especially in older individuals), ligamentous laxity, and strength or flexibility deficits. Recommendations for securing safe and enjoyable participation in soccer are given in Table 6.

It is crucial to have adequate communication between health care providers and coach. If fortunate, one will have an athletic trainer, therapist, and physician working with and covering the team. Communication is necessary for injury prevention, proper rehabilitation, and safe return to competitive play.

REFERENCES

1. American College of Sports Medicine: Position statement: Prevention of thermal injuries during distance running. Phys SportsMed 12(70):43–51, 1984.
1a. Albert M: Descriptive three-year data study of outdoor and indoor professional soccer injuries. Athletic training 18:218–220, 1983.
2. Backous DD, Friedl KE, Smith NJ, et al: Soccer injuries and their relation to physical maturity. Am J Dis Child 142:839–842, 1988.
3. Berg KE, LaVoie JC, Latin RW: Physiological training effects of playing youth soccer. Med Sci Sports Exerc 17:656–660, 1985.
4. Ekblom B: Applied physiology of soccer. Sports Med 3:50–60, 1986.
5. Ekstrand J, Gillquist J: Soccer injuries and their mechanisms: A prospective study. Med Sci Sports Exerc 15:267–270, 1983.
6. Ekstrand J, Gillquist J, Liljedahl S: Prevention of soccer injuries. Am J Sports Med 11(3):116–120, 1983.
7. Elias SR, Roberts WO, Thorson DC: Team sports in hot weather: Guidelines for modifying youth soccer. Phys SportsMed 19(5):67–78, 1991.
8. Engstrom B, Forssblad M, Johansson C, et al: Does major knee injury definitely sideline an elite soccer player? Am J Sports Med 18:101–105, 1990.

9. Engstrom B, Johansson C, Tornkvist H: Soccer injuries among elite female players. Am J Sports Med 19:372–375, 1991.

10. Gisolfi CV, Duchman SM: Guidelines for optimal replacement beverages for different athletic events. Med Sci Sports Exerc 24:679–687, 1992.

11. Hoff GL, Martin TA: Outdoor and indoor soccer: Injuries among youth players. Am J Sports Med 14:231–233, 1986.

12. Huston TP, Puffer JC, Rodney WM: The athletic heart syndrome. N Engl J Med 313:24–32, 1985.

13. Jorgensen U, Ekstrand J: Significance of heel pad confinement for the shock absorption at heel strike. Int J Sports Med 9:468–473, 1988.

14. Keller CS, Noyes FR, Buncher CR: The medical aspects of soccer injury epidemiology. Am J Sports Med 15:230–237, 1987.

15. Knapik JJ, Bauman CL, Jones BH, et al: Preseason strength and flexibility imbalances associated with athletic injuries in female collegiate athletes. Am J Sports Med 19:76–81, 1991.

16. Leatt PB, Jacobs I: Effect of glucose polymer ingestion on glycogen depletion during a soccer match. Can J Sports Sci 14(2):112–116, 1989.

17. Leatt P, Shepard RJ, Plyley MJ: Specific muscular development in under-18 soccer players. J Sport Sci 5:165–175, 1987.

17a. Maehlum S, Dahl E, Daljerd OA: Frequency of injuries in a youth soccer tournament. Phys SportsMed 144(7):73–79, 1986.

18. McCarroll JR, Meaney C, Sieber JM: Profile of youth soccer injuries. Phys SportsMed 12(2):114–117, 1984.

19. Nilsson S, Roaas A: Soccer injuries in adolescents. Am J Sports Med 6:358–361, 1978.

20. Nielsen AB, Yde J: Epidemiology and traumatology of injuries in soccer. Am J Sports Med 17:803–807, 1989.

21. Oberg BE, Moller MHL, Ekstrand J et al: Exercises for knee flexors and extensors in uninjured soccer players: Effects of two different programs. Int J Sports Med 6:151–154, 1985.

22. Pellicia A, Maron BJ, Spataro A, et al: The upper limit of physiologic cardiac hypertrophy in highly trained elite athletes. N Engl J Med 324:295–301, 1991.

23. Putukian M, McKeag DB: The preparticipation physical examination. In Buschbacher R, Braddon EL (eds): Sports Medicine and Rehabilitation: A Sport-Specific Approach. Philadelphia, Hanley & Belfus, 1994.

23a. Putukian M, Knowles W, Severe S: Injuries in Indoor Soccer: The Lake Placid Dawn to Dark Indoor Tournament, 1993. Submitted for publication, 1994.

24. Ramadan J, Byrd R: Physical characteristics of elite soccer players. J Sports Med 27:424–428, 1987.

25. Raven PB, Gettman LR, Pollock ML, et al: A physiological evaluation of professional soccer players. Br J Sports Med 10:209–216, 1976.

26. Rhodes EC, Mosher RE, McKenzie DC, et al: Physiological profiles of the Canadian Olympic soccer team. Can J Appl Sports Sci 11:31–36, 1986.

27. Robertson JW: Preventing heat injury in sports. Phys SportsMed 19(5):31–35, 1991.

28. Sawka MN, Greenleaf JE: Current concepts concerning thirst, dehydration, and fluid replacement. Med Sci Sports Exerc 24:643–687, 1992.

29. Schmidt-Olsen S, Bunemann LKH, Lade V, et al: Soccer injuries of youth. Br J Sports Med 19:161–164, 1985.

30. Smodlaka VN: Cardiovascular aspects of soccer. Phys SportsMed 6(7):66–70, 1978.

31. Smodlaka VN: Medical aspects of heading the ball in soccer. Phys SportsMed 12(2):127–131, 1984.

32. Sortland O, Tysvaer AT: Brain damage in former association football players. Neuroradiology 31:44–48, 1989.

33. Sullivan JA, Gross RH, Grana WA, et al: Evaluation of injuries in youth soccer. Am J Sports Med 8:325–327, 1980.

34. Tysvaer A, Storli O: Association football injuries to the brain: A preliminary report. Br J Sports Med 15:163–166, 1981.

35. U.S. Youth Soccer Association: Peter Ehlers, Personal communication, 17 May 1993.

36. Winter D, Snell PG, Stray-Gunderson J: Effects of 100% oxygen on performance of professional soccer players. JAMA 262:227–229, 1989.

37. Zeppilli P: The athlete's heart: Differentiation of training effects from organic heart disease. Pract Cardiol 14(8):61–84, 1988.

Chapter 62: Volleyball

CRAIG J. DAVIDSON, MD
DENISE J. HARTY, ATC

Volleyball, first called *mintonette,* was invented in the U.S. in 1885 by YMCA physical director William G. Morgan, who used the inside of a basketball for a ball. The game was initially created as a recreational activity for businessmen, designed to be "not too strenuous." Original rules allowed for an unlimited number of players on each side, continuous "air dribbling" up to 4 ft from the net, and an unlimited number of hits on each side of the court.

Today, volleyball is one of the most popular games in the world. The International Volleyball Federation represents more than 150 million players in 170 countries.[5] International competition is relatively new, first introduced in the 1955 PanAmerican Games in Mexico City. Volleyball made its debut as an Olympic sport in Tokyo in 1964. In 1975, volleyball became the first professional team sport to have men and women competing on the same team. In 1981, the National Collegiate Athletic Association (NCAA) held its first volleyball championship for women. It was not until the early 1980s that the U.S. Olympic Volleyball Team's success in "medal play" fueled increased media attention and boosted interest in volleyball in both athletes and spectators across the country.

Since 1895, the game has seen a number of changes. Volleyball has slowly evolved into the game of "power volleyball," a physically demanding game requiring quick movement, frequent direction changes, strength, coordination, stamina, and mental toughness. Today, it is very much a "contact sport." Injuries may occur when a player comes into contact with the ball, another player, or the floor, especially with the increasingly aggressive play.

I. BACKGROUND AND RATE OF INJURY

A. **Increased participation has led to a greater number of injuries.**
  1. 1.97 injuries/100 hours of play in one study of tournament injuries[14]
  2. Injury rates higher in the preseason
  3. No evidence for gender difference in rate of injury in one study looking at NCAA intercollegiate sports
  4. High-level players average approximately 150 one-meter jumps per match with ball velocities in upwards of 80 mph.

B. **Injury risk factors**
  1. Technique and training errors
  2. Playing surface: Significant differences occur with impact on parquet, composite, or concrete surface.
  3. Strong jumping element in volleyball; hence players are prone to injury since one can easily land off balance, misstep, or fall.
  4. Shock absorbing shoes (or lack of)
  5. Level of physical conditioning

C. **Common injuries**
  1. Overuse injuries more common than acute injuries
  2. Front-row positions and attempts to block or spike the ball account for most injuries
  3. Ankle, knee, hand, shoulder, and low back most frequently injured (Fig. 1).

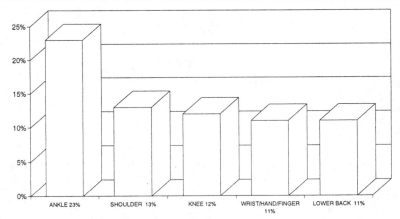

FIGURE 1. Anatomical distribution of injuries in women's volleyball. (Data from the NCAA Injury Surveillance System 1992–93.)

II. UPPER EXTREMITY INJURIES

A. Finger

1. **Background**
   a. 41% of all volleyball-related injuries for all age groups involve the wrist, hand, or finger.
   b. Sprains and strains are the most common, followed by fractures and contusions.
   c. In one study of long-term sequelae of volleyball-related hand injuries,[1] a high percentage of patients cited stiff and/or crooked fingers, limited range of motion, and tenderness as complaints.
   d. Most injuries occur near the net when a player performs a block or stop.
   e. Fingers, especially the thumb and little finger, are vulnerable, as they are usually spread fully apart to provide maximum area for blocking (Fig. 2).
   f. Impact of the ball with the finger usually results in a hyperextension-related injury.

2. **Gamekeeper's thumb**
   a. **Mechanism**
      i. Trauma to the ulnar collateral ligament
      ii. Involves forced abduction of the thumb; may occur with thumb exposed, such as with a block, or may occur with a fall on an outstretched hand with the thumb caught in abduction.
   b. **Examination**
      i. Pain and localized swelling along the ulnar aspect and base of the thumb
      ii. If significant laxity is seen on ulnar collateral ligament testing, obtain radiographs.
   c. **Radiographs**
      i. Will occasionally show a small avulsion fracture at the base of the proximal phalanx.
      ii. Avoid stress radiographs in the presence of an avulsion fracture due to the risk of extending the severity of the injury.
      iii. If no avulsion fracture is present, may proceed with stress radiographs. May need to image both thumbs for comparison.
      iv. If stress views show >20–30° of radial deviation compared to the uninjured side, then a complete tear of the ligament is likely.
      v. If stress views show <20–30° of radial deviation and there is no endpoint on physical examination, then proceed with conservative treatment.

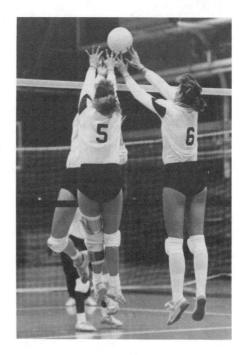

FIGURE 2. Finger injuries are common in volleyball due to the fingers being fully spread for contact with the ball. (From Fandel D, Mellion MB: Volleyball. In Mellion MB, Walsh WM, Shelton GL (eds): The Team Physician's Handbook. Philadelphia, Hanley & Belfus, 1990, pp 510–518; with permission.)

    d. **Treatment**
       i. Surgical treatment is necessary for completely torn ligament.
      ii. Thumb spica cast for 4–6 weeks for avulsion fracture
     iii. May consider thumb spica splint or cast for injuries with equivocal endpoints and/or negative radial deviation on stress testing.
3. **Ulnar collateral ligament sprain of the thumb**
    a. **Mechanism:** Same presentation and mechanism as for gamekeeper's thumb.
    b. **Examination:** No laxity of the ulnar collateral ligament is seen on physical examination.
    c. **Radiographs** are negative.
    d. **Treatment**
       i. Rest
      ii. Ice
     iii. Nonsteroidal antiinflammatory durgs (NSAIDs)
     iv. Range of motion exercises
      v. Protective taping, "check rein"
     vi. Return to competition using pain threshold as a guide
4. **Finger sprains and strains—"jammed finger"**
    a. **Mechanism**
       i. Usually involves hyperextension
      ii. Most commonly involve proximal interphalangeal (PIP) joint
     iii. More frequent on radial side of finger
     iv. Common; most are uncomplicated
    b. **Examination:** Localized tenderness, edema, and/or ecchymoses of PIP joint or collateral ligaments.
    c. Obtain radiographic films to rule out fracture.
    d. Treatment: Ice, buddy taping
5. **Volar plate injury**
    a. **Mechanism**
       i. Forced hyperextension injury of the PIP joint

ii. Edema and tenderness of the PIP joint (palmar aspect)
b. **Examination:** May see hyperextension of the PIP joint compared to the uninjured side (may need to perform this test utilizing a digital block for pain control before stressing the joint).
c. **Radiographs** often show an associated avulsed fragment of bone at base of middle phalanx.
d. **Treatment**
   i. Splint PIP in 20–30° of flexion for 3 weeks, followed by protective splinting (buddy taping) for an additional 3 weeks.
   ii. Unrecognized distal volar plate disruption may result in a swan neck deformity.
   iii. Volar plate injury with subsequent flexion deformity may result in the pseudo-boutonnière deformity.

6. **Mallet finger**
   a. **Mechanism**
      i. The term *mallet finger* implies disruption of the extensor mechanism of the dorsum of the distal interphalangeal (DIP) joint.
      ii. Seen frequently when the ball hits the tip of the exended finger, forcing the DIP joint into hyperflexion. Subsequently, the extensor mechanism is either torn or thinned.
   b. **Examination**
      i. Diffuse tenderness of DIP with palpation
      ii. Inability to actively extend the DIP joint
      iii. Swelling and ecchymoses at the DIP joint
   c. **Radiographs**
      i. May show the DIP joint in flexion
      ii. Often the terminal extensor tendon avulses a bony fragment from the base of the distal phalanx.
      iii. May be negative if tendon injury is via complete disruption through the body of the tendon.
   d. **Treatment**
      i. Ice
      ii. NSAIDs
      iii. Splint DIP in extension for 6 weeks. Prefabricated plastic splints (stack splint) are available. Avoid hyperextension.
      iv. DIP must be in extension for *entire* 6 weeks. If the joint is allowed to flex, some of the healing time will have been lost, thereby increasing the risk of failure.
      v. Following the initial splinting period, the splint should be worn an additional 2–4 weeks at night and with athletic activities.

B. **Wrist**
   1. **Wrist sprain**
      a. **Mechanism**
         i. Nonspecific term. Should be a diagnosis of exclusion.
         ii. May be due to single trauma, such as fall on outstretched hand or secondary to repetitive stress of ball handling (i.e., setting).
      b. **Examination**
         i. Few distinct clinical signs
         ii. Subjective pain with active or passive range of motion
         iii. Occasionally diffuse tenderness; otherwise little or no tenderness with palpation
      c. **Radiographs:** Usually negative. Must exclude fracture or dislocation.
      d. **Treatment**
         i. Rest

ii. Ice

iii. NSAIDs

iv. Wrist splint. Usually see total resolution after 1–2 weeks of immobilization with a splint.

2. **Scaphoid fracture**

a. **Mechanism**

i. Often overlooked and complaint is dismissed as minor

ii. Usually secondary to fall on a hyperextended hand

iii. Increased risk of avascular necrosis and nonunion secondary to a tenuous blood supply

b. **Examination**

i. Reveals tenderness and swelling over the dorsoradial aspect of the wrist

ii. Point tenderness over the anatomic snuffbox

c. **Radiographs**

i. Scaphoid series (6-view series: posteroanterior, lateral, right, left oblique, posteroanterior of wrist in radial and ulnar deviation) may confirm fracture.

ii. Maintain high clinical index of suspicion, even if radiographs are negative. May consider bone scan 24 hours or more from injury to confirm or rule out fracture.

d. **Treatment**

i. If no fracture, then immobilize in a splint and repeat films in 2 weeks.

ii. Nondisplaced fractures

(a) Thumb spica cast for 2–3 months

(b) Rate of healing varies depending on fracture location. Orthopaedic consultation is advised.

iii. Displaced fractures

(a) Displaced or unstable if anteroposterior or oblique views show >1 mm of offset.

(b) Surgical referral for open reduction and internal fixation.

3. **Pisiform fatigue fracture**

a. **Mechanism**

i. Pisiform located along ulnar aspect of wrist

ii. Repetitive impact and trauma over pisiform may contribute to stress, resulting in fatigue fracture.

iii. Usually no specific trauma recalled by athlete

b. **Examination**

i. Point tenderness over pisiform

ii. May or may not have accompanying swelling

c. **Radiographs**

i. Routine anteroposterior and lateral views of wrist usually normal, because it is difficult to detect fracture secondary to superposed carpal bones.

ii. Carpal tunnel view (axial) and hyperextension view of wrist may reveal fracture.

d. **Treatment**

i. Immobilization in cast for 4–6 weeks

ii. Arthritic pain at the pisotriquetral joint from fracture or repetitive trauma may be treated with surgical excision of the pisiform.

C. **Shoulder**

1. **Background**

a. The shoulder is one of the most anatomically and biomechanically complex joints in the body.

b. Shoulder is vulnerable to injury in volleyball due to the explosive hitting motion and repetitive overhead activity utilized in serving and spiking (Fig. 3).

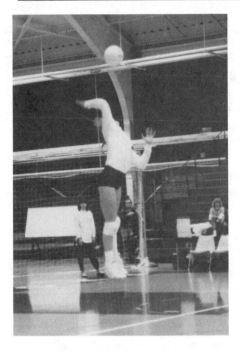

FIGURE 3. Repetitive overhead hitting, blocking, and serving can cause impingement and overuse syndromes. (From Fandel D, Mellion MB: Volleyball. In Mellion MB, Walsh WM, Shelton GL (eds): The Team Physician's Handbook. Philadelphia, Hanley & Belfus, 1990, pp 510–518; with permission.)

  c. Yohoe found shoulder involvement in 44% of volleyball players.[9]
  d. Injury may be secondary to chronic repetitive microtrauma, acute injury, or a combination of both.
 2. **Rotator cuff tendinitis, Impingement syndrome**
  a. **Mechanism**
   i. Inflammation of rotator cuff tendons (most commonly supraspinatus) from friction against coracoacromial ligament secondary to overuse
   ii. Trauma secondary to forced abduction, as with a dive for a ball
   iii. Rotator cuff musculature often overlooked in strength and conditioning programs. Result is a relative muscular imbalance of the shoulder, predisposing to injury or inflammation.
  b. **History**
   i. Recent change in activity or intensity of training, especially with overhead activities
   ii. Pain and/or weakness with overhead activities
   iii. May complain of a dull ache in middle deltoid region
   iv. History varies from minimal pain with activity, with no deficits in strength or range of motion, to marked tendinitis, with significant pain and decreased range of motion.
  c. **Examination**
   i. May have tenderness over rotator cuff musculature
   ii. Painful arc between 80–120° of abduction
   iii. Weakness, most commonly supraspinatus
   iv. Pain with impingement maneuver—90° forward flexion and internal rotation of shoulder
   v. Scapular instability. See increased lateral excursion of scapula with forward flexion of arm compared to opposite scapula.
  d. **Radiographs**
   i. Usually normal
   ii. May see subacromial spurring

       iii. With significant weakness of rotator cuff musculature, may see superior migration of humeral head in relation to glenoid labrum.

  e. **Treatment**

      i. Discontinue painful activities

      ii. Ice

      iii. NSAIDs

      iv. Range of motion exercises

      v. Rotator cuff strengthening and scapular stabilizing exercises

      vi. Consider corticosteroid injection if conservative therapy fails (*complete rest, ice, NSAIDs, strengthening, local modalities*).

3. **Acromioclavicular (AC) joint sprain or separation**

  a. **Mechanism**

      i. Trauma to AC ligament from fall on outstretched arm (force transmitted to AC joint)

      ii. Blow to lateral shoulder, as with a fall on the lateral aspect of shoulder (i.e., with a dive for a ball)

  b. **Examination**

      i. May have visible deformity and edema or ecchymosis over AC joint

      ii. Tenderness at AC joint with palpation

      iii. May have crepitance with shoulder range of motion

      iv. Pain with crossover maneuver (touch uninjured shoulder with hand of injured extremity)

  c. **Radiographs**

      i. Grade I AC sprain: Normal radiographs

      ii. Grade II AC sprain: Slight elevation of distal clavicle compared to noninjured side

      iii. Grade III AC sprain: >1.3 cm between clavicle and coracoid process

  d. **Treatment**

      i. Rest

      ii. Ice

      iii. NSAIDs

      iv. Range of motion exercises

      v. Grade I and II: Consider brief course of arm sling or shoulder immobilizer for symptom control

      vi. Grade III: Consider use of figure-of-8 sling or immobilize as above.

      vii. Return to activity when pain-free with full range of motion and full strength

4. **Suprascapular neuropathy**

  a. **Definition/background**

      i. Weakness and atrophy of the infraspinatus muscle

      ii. Relatively rare; however, is unique to volleyball and other sports with shoulder "overuse" syndromes

      iii. 13% of volleyball players competing in the 1985 European championships were found to have asymptomatic isolated paralysis of the infraspinatus muscle on the dominant side.

  b. **Mechanism**

      i. Exact mechanism unknown; lesion of the suprascapular nerve at the spinoglenoid notch has been postulated.

      ii. Compression by the supraspinatus muscle, ganglia, and hypertrophied spinoglenoid ligament have all been implicated.[11]

  c. **History**

      i. Usually seen in those individuals who regularly play and train

      ii. No history of shoulder trauma or pain. May develop posterior shoulder discomfort late in course (atrophy already present). Pain is poorly localized.

       iii. Usually no complaint of loss of function
       iv. May notice pain and/or weakness with serving or spiking
       v. May be alerted to atrophy by friends, relatives, or team members

  d. **Examination**
       i. Visible atrophy of infraspinatus muscle
       ii. Nontender with palpation
       iii. Upper extremity weakness with abduction and external rotation

  e. **Treatment**
       i. Address rotator cuff weakness; otherwise no treatment necessary.

III. TRUNK/TORSO INJURIES

A. Back

1. **Background**
   a. Low-back injuries are common, accounting for 10% of all injuries in the NCAA Women's Volleyball Injury Surveillance System for the 1992–93 season.
   b. Lumbar spine is prone to injury in volleyball due to the repeated trauma from jumping/landing and forced hyperextension in hitting, blocking, and setting.
   c. Underhand passing and "ready position" put hips into flexion, stressing the lumbosacral spine.

2. **Lumbar strain/sprain**
   a. **Mechanism**
      i. Repeated trauma or acute event from jumping/landing, twisting, or forced hyperextension of lumbar spine
      ii. Sprain/strain of spinal facet joints and/or soft tissues
      iii. Weak abdominal musculature and/or tight hamstrings may predispose low back to injury.
   b. **Examination**
      i. May have limited range of motion secondary to pain
      ii. May detect paraspinal and/or midthoracic muscle tenderness and/or spasm with palpation
      iii. Loss of lumbar lordosis with severe muscle spasm
      iv. Normal lower extremity strength, reflexes, and sensation
      v. Check hip range of motion and hamstring flexibility. Check for radicular symptoms with straight leg raise test on left and right.
   c. **Radiographs** are normal. Usually unnecessary to obtain lumbar spine series unless history of pain with hyperextension activities (to rule out spondylolysis) or bony tenderness on examination.
   d. **Treatment**
      i. Rest
      ii. Ice (including ice massage)
      iii. NSAIDs. May consider narcotic analgesics or sedating muscle relaxants at night if patient is having difficulty sleeping due to pain.
      iv. Range of motion exercises. May utilize heat to lumbar region *before* stretching, *followed* by ice.
      v. Local modalities as needed or available for pain control
      vi. Hamstring flexibility, abdominal strengthening, particularly lower abdominals
      vii. Return to activity using pain threshold as a guide

3. **Spondylolysis**
   a. **Mechanism**
      i. Fracture of pars interarticularis
      ii. Increased risk in volleyball with repetitive lumbar extension
      iii. Most common at L5
      iv. Spina bifida occulta may predispose to an increased risk of spondylolysis

b. **History**
   i. Pain with activities involving hyperextension (i.e., serving, hitting)
   ii. May complain of "midline" ache at lumbosacral junction
   iii. Suspect in any adolescent with "low-back pain," especially if it has not responded to conservative therapy (rest, ice, NSAIDs).
   iv. Some hereditary component

c. **Examination**
   i. Pain with one leg hyperextension test (ipsilateral side)
   ii. Hamstring spasm common.

d. **Radiographs**
   i. Lumbar series, *including oblique views.* Oblique views may show pars defect ("scotty dog") and/or reactive sclerosis of opposite pars.
   ii. Consider bone scan if radiographs are inconclusive (SPECT scan more sensitive).

e. **Treatment**
   i. Same as noted above for lumbar strain, **plus**
   ii. Boston brace, a plastic custom-made, anterior-opening brace that fits around torso. Brace prevents hyperextension and thus promotes healing through splinting of the pars.
      (a) Brace worn for 18 out of 24 hours of the day, including all athletic activities and with sleep
      (b) 3 months in brace usually adequate for healing
   iii. May return to activity in the brace when pain-free

B. **Other trunk/torso injuries**
   1. **Hip pointer** (contusion): Caused by fall onto iliac crest or direct contact with another player.
   2. **Greater trochanter bursitis:** Secondary to recurrent trauma to the hip sustained by floor contact with diving maneuvers.

IV. LOWER EXTREMITY INJURIES

A. **Knee**
   1. **Background**
      a. Knee is vulnerable to injury in volleyball due to frequent jumping, subjecting the extensor mechanism to high stress. Increased risk of injury subsequent to landing "off balance" on one foot.
      b. The most common reason for anterior knee pain in volleyball players is the "jumper's knee" syndrome.
      c. The majority of traumatic injuries of the knee are sustained during a jump, most occurring during offensive play (smashes) vs defensive play (blocking). Traumatic injuries frequently involve the anterior cruciate ligament.
      d. Several studies have suggested that serious knee ligament injuries may be more common in women volleyball players than in men.[5]
      e. Isolated meniscal injuries of the knee occur predominantly during defensive play, when players are required to perform rapid twisting movements. When this is done with the knee in 90° of flexion or more, the meniscus is subject to compression and torsion stress and subsequent injury.

   2. **Patellofemoral syndrome**
      a. **Mechanism**
         i. Overuse injury, more common in females than males, especially in preadolescent and adolescent athletes
         ii. Weak vastus medialis obliquus (VMO) contributes to "poor tracking" as this portion of the quadriceps muscle is responsible for proper tracking of the patella. A weak VMO results in a relative muscular imbalance, with

increased lateral force, resulting in abnormal patellofemoral tracking and
retropatellar irritation/inflammation.

   iii. Wider pelvis in the female athlete may increase the Q-angle $>15°$ and
predispose to abnormal patellofemoral tracking.

   iv. Tight lateral structures (lateral retinaculum, iliotibial band) may also
contribute to abnormal patellofemoral tracking.

  b. **History**

    i. Complaint of retro- or peripatellar knee pain

    ii. Activity related

   iii. May have history of intermittent effusion

   iv. Pain may be worse after prolonged sitting, such as in a car or movie
(positive "car" and "theater" sign)

  c. **Examination**

    i. May have positive "patella femoral grind test"—i.e., pain with pushing
patella distally and having the athlete contract the quadriceps as examiner
applies direct pressure to the kneecap.

    ii. May have effusion

   iii. May have decreased tone of VMO

   iv. May have decreased medial excursion (tight lateral retinaculum)

  d. **Treatment**

    i. Relative rest—substitute pain-free activity

    ii. Ice, especially after activity

   iii. NSAIDs

   iv. VMO strengthening

    v. Hamstring and iliotibial band stretches as appropriate

   vi. Neoprene sleeve with patellar stabilizer may be beneficial in some patients.

3. **Patellar tendinitis—"jumper's knee"**

  a. **Mechanism**

    i. Usually results from excessive jumping. Results in inflammation of
patellar tendon, usually at insertion of inferior pole of the patella (Fig. 4).

    ii. The number and variety of jumps, often to the limits of a player's strength
during games and practice sessions, predispose the knee extensor apparatus
to significant mechanical stress.

   iii. Pathologic changes most often at insertion sites (bone–tendon junction),
the weakest point of the knee extensor mechanism.

   iv. Injury characterized by inflammatory and degenerative changes of distal
quadriceps tendon and patellar tendon (tendinitis) as well as at their site
of insertion (apicitis).

    v. Hard playing surface (such as concrete) contributes significantly to
increased injury rate. Incidence of jumper's knee in athletes training or
competing on concrete was 37.5% vs 4.7% in those playing or training on
wood (parquet) surface.[3]

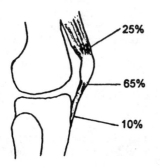

FIGURE 4. Location of pain in jumper's knee.

    b. **History**

        i. Gradual onset of anterior knee pain, exacerbated by running, jumping, or descending stairs. More severe cases may have pain with walking.

        ii. Sharp pain of variable intensity

    c. **Examination**

        i. Pain at the insertion either of the quadriceps tendon, upper or lower pole of the patella, or over the tibial tuberosity

        ii. Localized swelling in severe/chronic cases

        iii. VMO atrophy

        iv. May see weakness of ankle dorsiflexors

        v. Check for hamstring, quadriceps tightness

    d. **Radiographs**

        i. May see elongation of inferior pole of patella in chronic cases

        ii. MRI may be useful in diagnosing chronic patellar tendinitis by defining patellar thickening. MRI may also be useful for demonstrating focal areas of involvement and chronic tears.

    e. **Treatment**

        i. Relative rest (decrease painful activities)

        ii. Ice

        iii. NSAIDs

        iv. VMO strengthening

        v. Quadriceps/hamstrings flexibility and stengthening exercises

        vi. Local modalities, such as ultrasound, cross-frictional massage

B. **Anterior shin pain**

  1. **Background**

    a. Anterior shin pain may be secondary to a number of conditions, including periostitis, stress fractures, compartment syndromes, tendinitis, contusions, and others.

    b. The term *shin splints* is used frequently to describe anterior shin pain between the knee and ankle. However, shin splints is a relatively nonspecific term and should not be used as a diagnosis.

    c. Overuse, inadequate flexibility, and poor conditioning, may contribute to injury.

    d. Common early in the season

  2. **Posterior tibialis tendinitis**

    a. **Mechanism**

        i. Recurrent impact from jumping/overuse

        ii. Excessive pronation, rigid pes cavus foot, and improper footwear may contribute to stress on posterior tibial tendon.

        iii. Relative imbalance between anterior and posterior shin musculature

    b. **History**

        i. Often history of poor conditioning prior to increase in activity

        ii. Begins with pain at beginning of activity or practice, lessens after warm-up, then returns after practice

        iii. May have constant pain as condition worsens

    c. **Examination**

        i. Tenderness along the course of the posterior tibial muscle tendon (distal one-third early in course, proximal involvement with prolonged course or increased inflammation).

        ii. May see localized swelling

        iii. Pain or weakness with resisted inversion/plantar flexion

    d. Obtain **radiographs** to rule out stress fracture or periostitis. Otherwise films normal.

    e. **Treatment**

        i. Rest. Avoid painful activities

       ii. Non-weight-bearing on crutches if walking with a significant limp
      iii. Ice massage
      iv. NSAIDs
      v. Anterior shin strengthening
      vi. Stretching of gastrocsoleus complex
      vii. Orthotics to correct hyperpronation or consider orthotics if fails to improve with conservative therapy.

  3. **Other anterior shin disorders**
    a. **Periostitis**
      i. Presentation and treatment similar to posterior tibial tendinitis
      ii. Localized tenderness along medial or lateral, anterior tibia
    b. **Stress fractures** of the tibia and fibula
      i. Localized bony tenderness on examination
      ii. Radiographs may not be positive for up to 2 weeks after onset of symptoms
    c. **Compartment syndrome**
      i. Broad group of "syndromes," may be either acute or chronic
      ii. Pain with exercise secondary to intrinsic swelling, followed by compression of muscular and vascular structures
      iii. Treatment varies from conservative to surgical intervention, depending on severity.

C. Ankle
  1. **Background**
    a. Most common injury seen in volleyball.
    b. Accounted for 23% of all injuries in the NCAA Women's Volleyball Injury Surveillance Survey for the 1992–93 season.
    c. Ankle sprains or strains common, occurring with body rotation over a planted foot.

  2. **Ankle sprain**
    a. **Mechanism**
      i. Primarily inversion with plantar flexion
      ii. May have inversion mechanism with dorsiflexion while blocking or hitting at net and landing on opponent's foot (Fig. 5).
    b. **History**
      i. Often "roll-over" history (inversion type injury) with immediate onset of pain and swelling.
      ii. Check for recurrent history of ankle sprains. Underlying weakness.
      iii. May have heard a "pop" with grade II or grade III sprains.
    c. **Examination**
      i. Mild to severe swelling depending on severity and grade
      ii. Positive "anterior drawer test," with grade II and grade III sprains
      iii. Pain with palpation over ligamentous damage
      iv. Ecchymosis
      v. Decreased range of motion
    d. **Radiographs** usually normal. Fracture unlikely in absence of significant swelling or ecchymosis.
    e. **Treatment**
      i. Rest: Crutches until the patient can walk without a significant limp.
      ii. Ice
      iii. Compression with elastic wrap
      iv. Elevation helpful first 48 hours until swelling stabilized
      v. Protection with Aircast initially
      vi. Range of motion exercises
      vii. Strengthening of ankle musculature (inversion, plantar and dorsiflexion) and proprioceptive training.

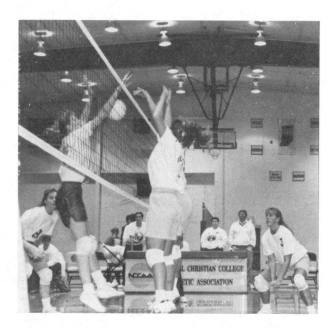

FIGURE 5. Net players are at increased risk of ankle sprains. (Photograph courtesy of C. Davidson.)

D. **Foot injuries**
1. **Stress fractures**
   a. **Mechanism**
      i. Foot subjected to recurrent trauma with repetitive jumping of volleyball
      ii. Playing surface and shoes play an important role in mechanism of injury.
      iii. High rigid arch and/or excessive pronation may contribute to increased stress over metatarsals and increase risk of stress fracture with overuse.
   b. **History**
      i. May start with dull ache, commonly over metatarsal region
      ii. Often gradual onset
      iii. Overtraining errors
      iv. Increased pain with activity, improved with rest
   c. **Examination**
      i. Usually pinpoint pain with palpation
      ii. Localized swelling and/or ecchymosis
   d. **Radiographs**
      i. May be normal initially
      ii. Bone scan may be necessary to detect early stress fracture.
   e. **Treatment**
      i. Discontinue painful activity until pain-free.
      ii. Crutches until the patient can walk without a limp.
      iii. Ice
      iv. Orthotics for correction of biomechanics as needed
      v. Sorbothane shoe inserts upon return to play
2. **Sesamoiditis**
   a. **Mechanism**
      i. Repetitive jumping
      ii. Landing on dorsiflexed first metatarsophalangeal (MTP) joint (recurrent trauma with overuse)

b. **Examination**
    i. Pain with palpation over sesamoids under first metatarsal head
    ii. Mild swelling/erythema
    iii. Pain with dorsiflexion of great toe
c. **Radiographs**
    i. Important to rule out fracture
    ii. Bipartite sesamoid common, may appear similar to fracture
    iii. Bone scan may be useful to determine fracture.
d. **Treatment**
    i. Avoid painful activity
    ii. Ice
    iii. NSAIDs
    iv. Sorbothane shoe inserts or metatarsal pad upon return to activity. May consider corticosteroid injection if fails conservative therapy. Surgical excision rarely needed.

V. CONCLUSION

Volleyball has changed a great deal since its origin in 1895. Over the last decade, it has evolved from a "recreational activity" to a highly skilled, fiercely competitive sport. Increased popularity and emphasis on an aggressive style of play have led to a greater number of injuries. An increased awareness of injury trends and mechanisms in the game of volleyball are the first steps toward injury prevention.

ACKNOWLEDGMENTS: Conclusions in this paper drawn from or recommendations based on data provided by the National Collegiate Athletic Association are those of the authors based on analyses or evaluations of the authors and do not represent the views of the officers, staff, or membership of the NCAA.

REFERENCES

1. Bhairo NH, Nijsten MWN, ten Duis HJ: Hand injuries in volleyball. Int J Sports Med 13:351–354, 1992.
2. Bodne D, Quinn SF, Murray WT, et al: Magnetic resonance images of chronic patellar tendinitis. Skel Radiol 17:24–28, 1988.
3. Ferretti A: Epidemiology of jumper's knee. Sports Med 3:289–295, 1986.
4. Ferritti A, Cerullo G, Russo G: Suprascapular neuropathy in volleyball players. J Bone Joint Surg 69A(2):260–263, 1987.
5. Ferretti A, Papandrea P, Conteduca F: Knee injuries in volleyball. Sports Med 10(2):132–138, 1990.
6. Ha KI, Hahn SH, Chung M, et al: A clinical study of stress fractures in sports activities. Orthopedics (Oct):1089–1095, 1991.
7. Israili A, Engel J, Ganel A: Possible fatigue fracture of the pisiform bone in volleyball players. Int J Sports Med 3:56–57, 1982.
8. Kujala UM, Aalto T, Osterman K, et al: The effect of volleyball playing on the knee extensor mechanism. Am J Sports Med 17:624–631, 1990.
9. McKeag DB, Hough DO: Primary Care Sports Medicine. Dubuque, IA, Brown and Benchmark, 1993.
10. Mellion MB, Walsh JM, Shelton G (eds): The Team Physician's Handbook. Philadelphia, Hanley & Belfus, 1990.
11. Montagna P, Colonna S: Suprascapular neuropathy restricted to the infraspinatus muscle in volleyball players. Acta Neurol Scand 87:248–250, 1993.
12. Scates AE: Winning Volleyball, 3rd ed. Newton, MA, Allyn and Bacon, 1972, pp 3–10.
13. Schafle MD: Common injuries in volleyball. Sports Med 16(2):126–129, 1993.
14. Schafle MD, Requa RK, Patton WL: Injuries in the 1987 National Amateur Volleyball Tournament. Am J Sports Med 18:624–631, 1990.
15. Strickland JW, Rettig AC: Hand Injuries in Athletes. Philadelphia, W.B. Saunders, 1992.
16. Viera BL, Ferguson BJ: Volleyball—Steps to Success. Champaign, IL, Leisure Press, 1989, pp 1–6.
17. Watkins J, Green BN: Volleyball injuries: A survey of Scotish national league male players. Br J Sports Med 26(2):135–137, 1992.

Chapter 63: Considerations for Women in the Wilderness

ROSEMARY AGOSTINI, MD

Women, as well as men, have been seeking out and continue to seek out wilderness to explore and enjoy. The purpose of this chapter is to educate and dispel myths about women's abilities to cope, survive, and enjoy wilderness environments.

I. HISTORY

A. Colorado congresswoman **Pat Schroeder**, in a speech in Seattle, has reminded us that women have been left out of historical accounts of settlement and exploration.
   1. When celebrating **Christopher Columbus'** discovery of America, we need to remember that **Queen Isabella** of Spain footed the bill.
   2. When our forefathers came to America, our foremothers accompanied them. They did not come later on a cruise ship having their hair and nails done!
   3. **Lewis and Clark** might still be wandering around the Pacific Northwest if it were not for a certain Indian woman, **Sacajawea**.
B. In 1808, **Marie Paradis**, of Chamonix, became the first woman to reach the summit of Mont Blanc, the highest point in Europe. She owned a tea shop at the bottom and was interested in increasing her business.
C. **Lucy Walker** explored the high Alps in 1858–64 and was known as the first really dedicated woman climber. Her climbing career spanned 20 years at a time that was not the easiest for mountaineers in general and women in particular.
D. **Fanny Bullock Workman** and her husband traveled and explored the Himalayas between 1889 and 1915 and wrote six books about their adventures.
E. **Alexander David Neal** made a series of journeys across the high Tibetan plateaus from 1911 to 1944 which have been characterized as the most remarkable ever made by any explorer in Tibet, man or woman. At age 55 years, she disguised herself as a Tibetan beggar woman and walked 2000 miles to the forbidden city of Llasa.
F. On May 16, 1975, in the International Women's Year, **Junko Tabei**, a 36-year-old Japanese woman in an all-women's expedition, was the first woman to reach the summit of Mount Everest.
G. **Wanda Rutkiewicz**, one of the most accomplished woman mountaineers of the present era (1961–1992), became the first European woman to ascend Mount Everest and then K2 without oxygen.
H. On September 29, 1988, **Stacey Allison** became the first American woman and the world's seventh woman to scale Mount Everest.
I. In 1928, **Amelia Earhart** was the first woman to cross the Atlantic by air.
J. In 1978, **Dr. Sally Ride** was the first American woman astronaut to venture into outer space.

II. PHYSIOLOGY

Men are larger sized and have more muscle mass, less subcutaneous fat, and higher hematocrits. When strength is measured relative to lean body mass, men and women are more similar. However, the ability to reach a summit, cross Antartica, or survive in the wilderness depends on many more factors than absolute strength.
A. **Adaptation to heat and cold**
   1. In studies in which men and women of similar fitness levels were compared, **few**

differences in thermal regulation between the genders were observed, except that men perspire more than women in humid environments.

2. **Women allow their skin temperatures to fall to lower levels than men when exposed to cold environments.** Because the average woman has more subcutaneous body fat, the greater tissue insulation allows women to maintain their core temperatures during cold exposure.

B. **Women and altitude**
   1. Women have the same experiences at altitudes as men.
   2. **Women can suffer from acute mountain sickness, high-altitude pulmonary edema (HAPE), and high-altitude cerebral edema (HACE).**
   3. Another life-threatening problem of high altitude combined with dehydration, increased hematocrit, and sometimes immobilization (snowstorms, injuries, etc.) is **deep-vein thrombosis** and subsequent pulmonary embolus.
      a. Women taking **birth control pills** or **hormone replacement therapy** need to consider the potential increased risk of deep-vein thrombosis.
      b. The benefits of birth control pills (not getting pregnant, decreased bleeding) vs the potential increased risk of deep-vein thrombosis should be discussed with any woman planning an extended high-altitude expedition.

III. HYGIENE AND SANITATION

A. **Water**
   1. Do not drink untreated surface water, despite its pure appearance. *Giardia lamblia* is a common contaminant from human and animal feces and can cause severe diarrhea.
   2. Boil, filter, or chemically treat all drinking and cooking water. Boil water for at least 1 minute at a full rolling boil.
   3. Avoid using soaps or detergents for personal, clothes, or dish washing in streams or lakes, as these soaps pollute. Carry water at least 100 ft from shore for washing.

B. **Toileting**
   1. For a pit toilet, dig a hole away from camp and at least 200 ft from any stream or lake. The hole should be at least 6 inches deep and should be covered when finished. Bring back any toilet paper to camp for burning. Leaves, of course, make excellent toilet paper, but avoid poison ivy!

C. **Personal hygiene:** Genitourinary infections can easily ruin a trip and women should be educated about the importance of vaginal cleanliness.
   1. **Vaginal infections:** Keep the vaginal area clean. Avoid tight pants, opting for loose-fitting cotton or wool ones. Change underwear regularly.
   2. **Urinary infections:** Unusual frequency and slight burning on urination are warning signs of infection. Drink fluids liberally and urinate frequently. Consider pyridium for symptoms and antibiotics for infection (*see* Medical Kit later).
   3. **Cleanliness:** Frequent bathing on the trail is usually unavailable and unnecessary.

D. **Menstruation:** Women have broken all kinds of records in every stage of menstruation.
   1. When hiking or camping, pack out **pads and tampons**. Mothballs in the trashbag will help control odors.
   2. Mild exercise is usually good for **cramps**. Bring medications (nonsteroidal antiinflammatory drugs, NSAIDs) if you need them. A hot water bottle or hot rocks wrapped in clothing help ease cramps.
   3. Tampons can be used for nosebleeds. Sanitary pads are great bandages for wounds.
   4. **Bears *do not* selectively munch on menstruating females.**
      a. The myth stems from an incident on August 13, 1967, when two women were killed by grizzly bears in separate parts of Glacier National Park. A *New York Times* reporter asked an unidentified member of the park staff (probably a maintenance man) what he thought was the reason for the bear attacks; he responded, "Oh, they must have been having their periods." The next day, it was in the headlines of the *Times*.

    b. Bear attacks occur when a bear with a history of **habituation** (repeated exposure to people so that the bear no longer readily flees from them) and **food conditioning** (history of feeding on people's food or garbage), plus a certain **predisposing personality** on the bear, encounters a person in a vulnerable situation where the bear perceives the possible "food" gain to be worth the risk of attacking a person.

    c. Other animals, likewise, do not seek out menstruating females.

IV. MEDICAL KIT

A. **Include medications for** (*see also* Chapter 36. Infections):

  1. **Vaginal infections**

    a. Candida: Antifungal vaginal creams can be bought over-the-counter (e.g., Monistat, miconazole)

    b. Herpes: Acyclovir (Zovirax), 400 mg 3 times daily for 5 days

    c. Sexually transmitted diseases

       i. Prevention: Abstinence, condoms

      ii. Gonorrhea: Cefixime (Suprax), 400 mg in 1 dose

     iii. Chlamydia: Azithromycin (Zithromax), 1 g in 1 dose 1 hr before or 2 hrs after a meal

  2. **Vaginal bleeding:** If unable to evaluate, temporary measures include:

    a. High-dose NSAIDs

    b. Birth control pills (Lo/Oval)

  3. **Dysmenorrhea:** NSAIDs

  4. **Urinary tract infections:**

    a. Increase fluids

    b. Pyridium, 200 mg 3 times daily for 3 days, for symptoms

    c. Antibiotics

       i. Trimethoprim/sulfamethoxazole, double-strength tablets (Bactrim DS, Septra DS), one tablet orally twice daily for 3 days

      ii. Ciprofloxacin (Cipro), 500 mg orally twice daily for 3 days

V. PREGNANCY

A. **Several issues need to be discussed with a pregnant woman who plans to go to wilderness:**

  1. Remoteness of the planned trek

  2. How important is the pregnancy?

  3. Health effects on the mother from altitude sickness, exhaustion, traveler's diarrhea, etc. can also adversely affect the developing fetus.

  4. The pregnant woman needs to think about her responsibility to herself, the fetus, and other members of the expedition.

B. **Other issues of concern for the pregnant woman should be discussed with her physician:**

1. Immunization	5. Medications	9. Physiologic and anatomic
2. Physical activity	6. Malaria	changes of pregnancy
3. Altitude	7. Flying	10. Obstetrical risk factors
4. Traveler's diarrhea	8. Maternal health	

VI. TRAIL SAFETY

Often, getting to the park is more dangerous than being in the park or on the trail, but crime can happen anywhere and it is best to be aware of its possibility. Common sense and a willingness to listen to intuitive feelings often afford the best protection.

A. **Pay attention to danger signals and situations.**

  1. **If a person or situation makes you uneasy or gives you bad feelings, pay attention to it.** Either leave the area or trail, end the conversation, or move on. Most important is to act quickly and remove yourself from the threatening area. If necessary, do not hesitate to ask a stranger to leave or seek the help of a park ranger or security.

2. **Avoid alcohol or drugs and people using these on the trail.** As in urban areas, alcohol and drugs are involved in a large percentage of crimes committed in park lands.

3. **Avoid high trash or littered areas,** as these are often gathering areas for locals, who may harass hikers or campers. Avoid confrontations both on and off the trail with hikers or locals.

4. **Realize that not everyone you meet on the trail is your friend.** Be especially wary of overly inquisitive strangers who seem too curious about the number in your party or your plans. Avoid single males.

5. **Avoid hiking alone.** In addition to assaults, accidents and illness can strike the lone hiker.

6. **Be careful in parking your car.** Break-ins and vandalism to cars are much more common than crimes against persons in parks. Avoid parking your car in unattended or remote areas.

B. **Personal protection on the trail**

1. **Sound alarms:** Alarms are lightweight and portable; these can be heard up to ¼–½ mile and offer good protection when in proximity to other people.

2. **Dogs:** Although many parks restrict or forbid dogs within their boundaries (where they pose a threat to wildlife), dogs, even on leashes, offer women excellent protection against attacks and harassment. Even dogs that are not vicious will bark and deter troublemakers.

3. **Guns and knives:** Despite giving a great sense of security, guns are of dubious value for protection. The user must be trained in *how* as well as *when* to use a gun, and accidental shootings remain a major risk. Knives assume close combat, where a woman likely will be overmatched by a larger and stronger male attacker.

4. **Sprays:** Mace or pepper sprays are easily portable but require a "direct hit" in the attacker's face to be an effective deterrent. "Deter" capsules, which release a powerful pungent odor when ruptured, are a good alternative.

VII. EQUIPMENT

Many manufacturers are realizing that there is a woman's market and are attempting to design equipment that fits women.

VIII. PSYCHOLOGY

A. Women may **not** be taken as **seriously** when they are injured or ill.

B. Women may **not** listen to their **intuitive** self when injured or ill and try to keep going when that can lead to being at more risk of severe and life-threatening consequences.

C. **What does a woman want?** In response to Freud's question, Drs. Ann Bernstein and Gloria Warner do not think it is presumptuous to suggest the answer is a simple one: "Women want to be considered separate, autonomous individuals with their own set of characteristics, determined biologically and stemming from their early infantile relationships. They do not want these characteristics to be pejoratively labeled or considered to be merely a compensation for their damaged anatomy, not less good, nor less desirable, nor less important—merely different."

REFERENCES

1. Barry M, Bia F: Pregnancy and travel. JAMA 261:728–731, 1989.
2. Blanton B: Trail safety. Women's Outdoor Journal (Jan/Feb):8–12, 1991.
3. Hackett P, et al: High altitude medicine. In Auerbach P, Geehr E (eds): Management of Wilderness and Environmental Emergencies. St. Louis, Mosby, 1989, pp 1–35.
4. Haymes E: Environmental factors as they affect women. In Hale R (ed): Caring for the Exercising Woman (Current Topics in Obstetrics and Gynecology). New York, Elsevier, 1991.
5. Heinonen J: Dogged defense. Runner's World (July):1986.
6. Hutch R: Pregnancy and altitude: Physical activity at high altitude. In Mittelmark RA (ed): Exercise in Pregnancy. Baltimore, Williams & Wilkins, 1991, pp 247–260.
7. Neilly S: Female hygiene in the backwoods. Women's Outdoor Journal (May/Jun):1990.

INDEX

Page numbers in **boldface** type indicate complete chapters.